FOOD, EATING AND NUTRITION:
a multidisciplinary approach

Sabina Saccomanno - Licia Coceani Paskay (eds.)

FOOD, EATING AND NUTRITION: a multidisciplinary approach

edi·ermes

AOMT
ACADEMY of OROFACIAL MYOFUNCTIONAL THERAPY

edra
PUBLISHING

FOOD, EATING AND NUTRITION: a multidisciplinary approach
Sabina Saccomanno, Licia Coceani Paskay (eds.)

ISBN: 978-1-962679-09-1

eISBN 978-1-962679-00-8

Knowledge and best practice in this field are constantly changing: As new research and experience broaden our knowledge, changes in practice, treatment, and drug therapy may become necessary or appropriate. Readers are advised to check the most current information provided (i) or procedures featured or (ii) by the manufacturer of each product to be administered, to verify the recommended dose or formula, the method and duration of administration, and contraindications.
It is the responsibility of the practitioners, relying on their own experience and knowledge of the patient, to make diagnoses, to determine dosages and the best treatment for each individual patient, and to take all appropriate safety precautions.
To the fullest extent of the law, neither the Publisher nor the Editors assume any liability for any injury and/or damage to persons or property arising out of or related to any use of the material contained in this book.
This publication contains the author's opinions and is intended to provide precise and accurate information.
The processing of the texts, even if taken care of with scrupulous attention, cannot entail specific responsibilities for the author and / or the publisher for any errors or inaccuracies.
The Publisher has made every effort to obtain and cite the exact sources of the illustrations. If in some cases the Publisher has not been able to find the right holders, it is available to remedy any inadvertent omissions or errors in the references cited. All registered trademarks mentioned belong to their legitimate owners.

Book Publishing Manager: Costanza Smeraldi
Paper, Printing and Binding Manager: Paolo Ficicchia
Proofreading: Sandra Calarota
Layout: Edi.Ermes srl
Cover: Laura Barzacca

The procedures described and recommended in this book are the result of the research and the work of a group of competent physicians, dentists and orthodontists, speech-language pathologists, in compliance with the current trends in the scientific world. Needless to say, the information provided, including diagnoses and therapeutic interventions, should not be considered as being valid in absolute terms, but should be appropriately evaluated by the individual professional and adapted to the real clinical conditions of the patient. Therefore, the Authors and the Publisher disclaim any responsibility for any problematic situation to be directly or indirectly referred to the procedures described, to the possible presence of any mistake or to any misunderstandings of the text by the reader.

edra
PUBLISHING
Edra Publishing US LLC
3309 Northlake Boulevard, Suite 203
Palm Beach Gardens, FL, 33403
EIN: 844113980
info@edrapublishing.com
www.edrapublishing.com

Printed in Italy by LegoDigit S.r.l., Lavis (TN), May 2024

Foreword – Siloes and Foxholes

Silo: *A structure, system, process, or department that operates in isolation from others.*
Foxhole: *A hastily constructed dugout which can serve as both shelter and fortress.*

After air and water, food is the third most important human necessity. Food is the currency that pays for everything else. For most of human life on this planet, there has been an *underabundance* of food, and therefore an oversize desire to accumulate it. For centuries, undernutrition killed millions, and wars were fought over access to food. But in the second half of the 20th century, due to changes in food production, processing, procurement, and unfortunately propaganda, the tables turned, and now in many regions food is *overabundant*, with the chronic diseases of overnutrition occupying most of the headlines. The difference is that with undernutrition, it was God's fault or a political fault. Now, with overnutrition, it's always the *victim's* fault. Smaller target. And not having God to contend with provides cover. Much easier to climb into the foxhole and start firing.

One of the reasons that this attack mentality is so prevalent today is that the various disciplines that are touched by food have remained siloed – that is, there has been little attempt at horizontal integration of the science, the sociology, and the politics of food. One group doesn't know what the others are doing, and there are enormous abysses in combining our knowledge. Scientists work in the ivory tower, dietitians work in the hospital or clinic, nutritionists work in social media, public health experts work in the journals, advocates work in the barrios and schools, and politicians work on TV talk shows. Attempts at cross-fertilization and applying the science and culture to rational policy have come up short time and again. And when you don't have an answer, it's easy to descend from the silo, crawl into a foxhole, and lob grenades at everyone else.

Also, within each of these siloes, there is little vertical integration of information as well. One example – the science can be divided up into three disciplines. *Food science* is what happens to food between the ground and the mouth. *Nutrition* is what happens to food between the mouth and the cell. *Metabolic health* is what happens to food inside the cell. Alterations in food quantity can affect nutrition, but alterations in food quality affect metabolic health. Each informs the other, but they are not the same. Even scientists don't know this. Another example – the sociology can be divided up into *agriculture*, which explains why certain people farm, ranch, or fish a certain way; *food culture*, which explains why certain people eat a certain way; and *social disparities*, which explains why certain people get sick a certain way. None of these people are talking to each other, yet they are all interdependent. And the third example – the politics can be divided up into *economics*, which is how much money is spent on food; *healthcare*, which is how much money is spent on disease; and *marketing*, which is how much money is wasted on both.

These siloes are opaque and impenetrable, and the foxholes are easily dug and then abandoned as needed. It's also a long way down from the top of a silo to the bottom of a foxhole, you can't even yell at each other and expect the other to hear you. No wonder our food system and our healthcare system are in such disarray. The only way to solve this problem is to, metaphorically, topple the siloes and fill in the foxholes. A daunting task, to be sure.

This is the challenge that Sabina Saccomanno and Licia Coceani Paskay have embraced. This textbook, *Food, Eating and Nutrition: A Multidisciplinary Approach*, attempts to broach the chasms between the science of food, the sociology of food, and the politics of food. That's why there are 38 chapters. They have called upon the world's leading experts to lend their expertise for this comprehensive yet approachable treatise. Even though it's a textbook, it's written for any and all food stakeholders, and it's written in a clean and cogent style that will translate across international borders. For clinicians, there are sections on the roles various foods play in the pathogenesis of disease; not just *what* they eat, but also *how* they eat. For sociologists, there are sections on food across the lifespan, and specific cultural differences in the food supply. For politicians, there are sections on gender, the future of food, and the marketing and disinformation of food and the food industry.

No one person, one discipline, one society, or one industry can solve our current food debacle. The only way to solve it is bringing the multiple stakeholders to the same table, imbue them with a common knowledge base, and attempting to forge a common belief system and narrative. But that means they have to speak the same language, both figuratively and literally. Can anyone dismantle the siloes and fill in the foxholes to level the playing field? Saccomanno and Paskay insert themselves into this noble cause, hoping that one discipline will rub off on the others; thus a *multidisciplinary* approach. If the food protagonists want to find a way forward, at least this book will point them in the right direction.

September 4, 2022

Robert H. Lustig, MD, MSL

Prefaces

"Proper nutrition is the medicine of the future", said Nobel laureate Linus Carl Pauling, speaking of nutrition.

Is it possible to deny that today (the future cited by Pauling) the most popular topic is food? Just turn on the TV and each channel offers us its flagship cooking program, the newscasts often have in-depth features on gastronomy, even the most popular hashtags on Instagram are #foodporn #foodblogger #foodlover and are strictly accompanied by the usual photo. I don't deny it myself. I love to relax cooking and trying new recipes. Food is a pleasure for me. And if all that is "social" it must be followed and must be a model that influences. We often notice the claim that everything you cook must be healthy often being low in calories or "low carb". You invite followers to eliminate some substances so that you can be fit and healthy. But I wonder, as a doctor, is it really true?

We all know that certain foods can certainly influence certain pathologies (a celiac cannot eat gluten, as a diabetic will have to limit the use of sugar), but these are broad ideas and we need experts to tell us more.

This book aims to address the topic in its entirety, focusing on the individual as a complex being and interconnected unity, following it from birth to old age, recognizing its biological differences (sex) and possible pathologies. We will analyze eating from the newborn to the elderly and how we can prevent some problems and treat others with the help of food while not forgetting the social and cultural aspect of the food that must be taken into consideration. Each chapter will be addressed by an expert who, in addition to presenting the various topics in a scientific manner, will challenge myths and legends that often hover around the topic "eating".

Beyond my personal passions, as a doctor and an orthodontist, I care a lot about the influence of food on the craniofacial complex and its development. When we talk about food and the mouth, the first link that comes to mind is sugar and food but in reality the question is more complex.

Sugar does not simply cause tooth decay, it is the increasingly refined foods, the modality and frequency of eating them that can cause, associated with a bad oral hygiene, a carious pathology in permanent teeth, and even on "baby teeth".

In addition to the sugar composition, we must think of the consistency of foods and the fact that sticky, sugary foods more easily remain adhered to teeth and therefore can do more damage.

With regard to this, the question becomes complex. Yes, sticky foods can adhere more easily to dental enamel, but think of the muscular effort that is made in chewing soft foods. It is almost nothing. We carry this physiological disruption into a growing child and if muscles do not work properly they cannot "guide" bone growth properly and therefore disrupt the eruption of baby teeth first and permanent teeth later on.

Our journey within the food topic will therefore address all these aspects, with a specific focus on the mouth, where it all begins. We will even venture into the future of humans eating while traveling to other planets. Have you ever wondered what astronauts eat? Are foods in space like those on the Earth? How hard is it to eat without gravity? We will also answer these questions and more.

Sabina Saccomanno

As a speech-language pathologist who specializes in chewing and swallowing disorders I have bemoaned for many years the lack of some "centralized" information about the impact of food choices on people of all ages, the mechanics of eating and their implications on nutrition, therefore their well-being and health. I had so many questions without finding easy or even available answers. Similarly, Dr. Sabina Saccomanno, as an orthodontist, was aware since the beginning of her career of the impact of chewing, swallowing and eating in general on the overall growth and development of the craniofacial complex. She knew that ignoring this reality was not boding well for the outcome and stability of any orthodontic treatment.

This is what motivated Sabina and myself to compile this book with chapters written by international experts in the various medical and dental arena. The information contained in some chapters seem to contradict what is stated in other chapters, but that's just the reality of science, of clinical practice and of life in general: there is a lot of "wiggle room" between various treatments and practices. It's not up to Sabina nor myself to say who's right or not. That's up to the readers to decide. That is up to science to come up with a consensus.

We take food for granted but we shouldn't. Currently, food production, delivery and consumption are so much different that it was at any other times in human history, and, as such, the impact of industrialized food is also unprecedented, as it's explained in Section 1.

The types of food and the mechanics of eating it have had a direct impact on our lives since day one and continues until our last day and several chapters written in Section 2 pinpoint these issues but also possible solutions.

Obviously eating begins in the mouth and although modern medicine managed to bypass the mouth with enteral feeding, the implications of bypassing the complex oral neurosensory system are many, and many oral conditions affect eating and nutrition, as is illustrated in Section 3.

Food directly affects our health and there is no part of our body nor function that is not affected by what we eat. The impact of food and nutrition on the kidney, the heart, the nervous system or the immune system are just some examples of the many chapters in Section 4 that address the multifaceted, prismatic nature of the connections between food and health.

Because food and eating are constantly evolving, Section 5 looks at the future and at new frontiers such as the future colonization of space and microgravity which will bring its own features and challenges to nutrition. As a medical community we can assist future denizens of space to optimize their ability to eat in unprecedented and literally "alien" conditions for the human body. Similarly, in the future mankind may be spending even more time underwater and currently scuba diving worker spend many hours in long shifts underwater. Therefore, what scuba divers eat is addressed as well, as food choices can be a life-or-death issue for anyone spending time underwater.

Eating is not just a physiological need upon which our very existence relies, but it's also a social and cultural construct. We sit and share meals with family, friends, colleagues, strangers and ever rivals, to signal love, appreciation, trust, collaboration and peace. Therefore, it is appropriate to include a few chapters in Section 6 devoted to these world differences in types of foods and religious rituals that have one thing in common: food and eating.

Clearly, it's impossible to write an absolutely complete book on the subject, and we realized that there is so much more that can be said about the subjects of food, eating and nutrition. But maybe that's material for a second book. For now, go ahead and savor every chapter. I know I did, and I could not wait to share all that I learned with you through this wonderful book.

Licia Coceani Paskay

Acknowledgements

This book "Food, Eating and Nutrition: A Multidisciplinary Approach", born from the fact that I strongly believe in a multidisciplinary approach, has involved several specialists in such a convivial field as food. I thank my friend Licia C. Paskay who has worked with me for years on this ambitious project; I thank my dad who - even though he's gone - was my biggest fan; I thank my mother and my sister who have always accompanied me with their loving support. I thank all the co-authors who collaborated with wonderful chapters and who had the patience to wait for their publication. I thank all those who, while often hindering me in my professional career, stimulated my creativity and pushed me to do more and more by not making me see a victory as the point of arrival but defeat as a departure.

Sabina Saccomanno

This book would have never seen the light of day without the constant loving support from my husband Steve to whom I'm profoundly grateful. He lovingly took care of our daily life so I could spend hundreds of hours on this project, plus doing the editing, discussing some of the topics and overall being the wonderful person he has always been. I'm also grateful to my sisters Germana, Donatella Giulia and Nicoletta for their constant encouragement. They are my cheer leaders who always give me happiness and love.

I'm grateful to Sabina for giving me the chance to join her in this endeavor. She is a great professional and a great friend, and this book is just one of the many projects for which we joined forces. Thank you, Sabina.

Licia Coceani Paskay

Our gratitude goes to all the various authors of this book, for their passion, expertise and patience in providing their corresponding chapters.

Our gratitude and a heartfelt *thank you* go to: Nicole Archambault, MS, CCC-SLP; Joan Ryan, MS, CCC-SLP; Hila Robbins, DMD, DDS; Samantha Weaver, MS, SLP; and especially Steve Paskay, BA for overall editing; Rabbi Dr. Joseph Schames, for additional editing of the section on Jewish food and traditions; to Ms. Hena Mohiuddin, for additional editing of the section on Islamic food and traditions; and to Mahadev Parameswaran, PhD, for additional editing of the section on food and traditions in Hinduism.

AOMT
ACADEMY *of* OROFACIAL MYOFUNCTIONAL THERAPY

The Academy of Orofacial Myofunctional Therapy (AOMT, www.AOMTinfo.org) is an institute based in California, USA that is the global leader in the emerging field of orofacial myofunctional therapy. Having worked with leading universities, hospital systems, and governments around the world, the AOMT is most publicly known for training healthcare professionals worldwide, the facilitation of research, dissemination of scientific information for public health, and consulting for health systems and models. Our mission is to offer the best foundation for health professionals to learn this critical therapy and bring its benefits to those who need it. The AOMT and its global faculty is proud to support the formation and dissemination of this textbook.

Editors

Sabina Saccomanno, DDS
Department of Life, Health and Environmental Sciences,
University of L'Aquila, L'Aquila, Italy

Licia Coceani Paskay, MS, CCC-SLP
Speech-Language Pathologist, Private Practice
Los Angeles, USA

Contributors

Emiliano Angeloni, MD
Sant'Andrea University Hospital, Rome, Italy
Chapter 23

Diane Bahr, MS, CCC-SLP, CIMI
Specializing in Feeding, Motor Speech, & Mouth Development/Function
Ages and Stages, LLC, Resources for Feeding, Motor Speech, & Mouth Function,
Las Vegas, USA
Chapter 6

Davide Bellini, MD
Department of Radiological Sciences, Oncology and Pathology, Sapienza University of Rome; I.C.O.T. Hospital, Latina, Italy
Chapter 33

Luigi Bennardo, MD
Università Magna Graecia, Catanzaro, Italy
Chapter 25

Mauro Bernabei, MD
Department of Dental Clinic, Università Cattolica del Sacro Cuore, Rome, Italy
Chapter 32

Ersilia Biondi, MD
Fondazione Policlinico Universitario A. Gemelli IRCCS,
Università Cattolica del Sacro Cuore, Rome, Italy
Chapter 35

Francesco Bove, MD, PhD
I.N.I. Italian Neurotraumatology Institute, Grottaferrata, Rome, Italy
Chapter 22

Gabriele Bove, MD
I.N.I. Italian Neurotraumatology Institute, Grottaferrata, Rome, Italy
Chapter 22

Lucia Bovicelli, DDS
Private Practice
Chapter 13

Kevin Boyd, DDS, MSc
Dentistry for Families and Children, Chicago, USA
Chapter 1

Cinzia Myriam Calabrese, MD
Private Practice, Rome, Italy
Chapter 3

Giorgio Calabrese, MD, PhD
Grand Officer of the Italian Republic
Lecturer in Human Nutrition and Dietetics
Medical Offices in Asti, Turin, Milan and Rome, Italy
Chapter 3

Marlei Braude Canterji, SLT
Speech Therapist at the Study Group on Obesity and Metabolic Surgery
Porto Alegre, Brazil
Chapter 31

Damiano Caruso, MD, PhD
Department of Medical Surgical Sciences and Translational Medicine,
Sapienza University of Rome; Sant'Andrea University Hospital, Rome, Italy
Chapter 33

Roberto Cauda, MD
Professor of Infectious Diseases
Chairman of the Department of Healthcare Surveillance and Bioethics
Section of Infectious Diseases
Università Cattolica del Sacro Cuore, Rome, Italy
Chapter 4

Annafranca Cavaliere, MD
Università Cattolica del Sacro Cuore, Rome, Italy
Chapter 5

FEDERICA COSTANTINI
Private Practice
Chapter 24

ANTONIO D'ADDONA, DDS
Professor, Department of Head and Neck and Sensory Organs, Division of Oral Surgery and Implantology, Fondazione Policlinico Universitario A. Gemelli IRCCS,
Università Cattolica del Sacro Cuore, Rome, Italy
Chapter 12

ANA MARIA BETTONI RODRIGUES DA SILVA, DDS, MD, PhD
Department of Restorative Dentistry, School of Dentistry of Ribeirão Preto, São Paulo University, Ribeirão Preto, São Paulo, Brazil
Chapter 17

MARCO ANTÔNIO MOREIRA RODRIGUES DA SILVA, DDS, MD, PhD
Department of Restorative Dentistry, School of Dentistry of Ribeirão Preto, São Paulo University, Ribeirão Preto, São Paulo, Brazil
Chapter 17

PAOLO DE ANGELIS, DDS
Department of Head and Neck and Sensory Organs, Division of Oral Surgery
and Implantology, Fondazione Policlinico Universitario A. Gemelli IRCCS,
Università Cattolica del Sacro Cuore, Rome, Italy
Chapters 12 and 16

RITA DE ANGELIS, MD
Medical Surgeon, Specialist in Pediatrics, Specialist in Puericulture, Pediatrician ASL Rome 2, Scientific Committee FIMP, Rome, Italy
Chapter 9

CARLO DE COLLIBUS, MD
INPS General Medical Legal Coordination, Rome, Italy
Chapter 30

FRANCESCA DE LEVA, MD
University Policlinico Foundation A. Gemelli, Università Cattolica del Sacro Cuore, Rome, Italy
Chapter 24

PAOLA DEL GIACOMO, MD
Infectious Diseases Unit,
Fondazione Policlinico Universitario A. Gemelli IRCCS, Rome, Italy
Chapter 4

MAURO DI LEO, MD
University Policlinico Foundation A. Gemelli, Università Cattolica del Sacro Cuore, Rome, Italy
Chapter 24

SIMONETTA DI PAOLA
Educator specialized in the Montessori Method
Former director of the early childhood education facility at the Conferenza Episcopale Italiana (CEI), Rome. Italy
Chapter 10

ANNA DI TULLIO, SLT
Speech Therapist in Private Practice
Chapters 30 and 38

MARIA CRISTINA FABBRI, MD
Fondazione Policlinico Universitario A. Gemelli IRCCS,
Università Cattolica del Sacro Cuore, Rome, Italy
Chapter 34

ALESSIO FILIPPONE, MD, PhD
Center for Integrative Oncology
Fondazione Policlinico Universitario A. Gemelli IRCCS, Rome, Italy
Chapter 29

SIMONE AUGUSTA FINARD, SLT
Speech Therapist at the Physiatrics and Rehabilitation Service of Hospital de Clínicas de Porto Alegre, Brazil
Chapter 31

SILVIA GIANCASPRO, DDS
Department of Life, Health and Environmental Science, University of L'Aquila, L'Aquila, Italy
Chapter 37

CARMEN GRAVINA, MD
Fondazione Policlinico Universitario A. Gemelli IRCCS,
Università Cattolica del Sacro Cuore, Rome, Italy
Chapter 28

DONATELLA GUARINO, MD
Center for Integrative Oncology
Fondazione Policlinico Universitario A. Gemelli IRCCS, Rome, Italy
Chapter 29

SOFIA GUIDI, MD
Università Cattolica del Sacro Cuore, Rome, Italy
Chapter 5

Maria Concetta La Milia, MD
Università Cattolica del Sacro Cuore,
Rome, Italy
Chapter 5

Daniele Laganà, DDS
Full Professor, Dental School, University of L'Aquila, L'Aquila, Italy
Chapter 36

Andrea Laghi, MD
Department of Medical Surgical Sciences and Translational Medicine,
Sapienza University of Rome;
Sant'Andrea University Hospital,
Rome, Italy
Chapter 33

Antonio Lanzone, MD
Head of Complex Operational Unit Obstetrics and Obstetric Diseases 2, Università Cattolica del Sacro Cuore,
Rome, Italy
Chapter 5

Alfredo Laudani, MD
Unit of Nephrology and Dialysis, University of Messina, Italy
Chapter 21

Wes Leffingwell, DDS Retired
Leucadia, CA, USA
Chapter 19

Robert H. Lustig, MD, MSL
Professor emeritus of Pediatrics, Division of Endocrinology, University of California, San Francisco (UCSF), USA
Foreword

Rebecca Jewel Manenti, DDS
Department of Life, Health and Environmental Science, University of L'Aquila,
L'Aquila, Italy
Chapter 37

Paolo Francesco Manicone, DDS
Professor, Department of Head and Neck and Sensory Organs,
Division of Oral Surgery and Implantology,
Fondazione Policlinico Universitario A. Gemelli IRCCS,
Università Cattolica del Sacro Cuore,
Rome, Italy
Chapter 16

Giuseppe Marzo, MD
Director of Post Graduate School of Orthodontics
Department of Life, Health and Environmental Science, University of L'Aquila,
L'Aquila, Italy
Chapters 13 and 37

Giovanni Melina, MD
Sant'Andrea University Hospital, Rome, Italy
Chapter 23

Giacinto A.D. Miggiano, MD
Director of Human Nutrition Research Center - Catholic University, Rome, Italy
Director of Clinical Nutrition - Fondazione Policlinico Universitario A. Gemelli IRCCS,
Rome, Italy
Chapter 2

Joy L. Moeller, RDH, OMT
Academy of Orofacial Myofunctional Therapy (AOMT), California, USA
Chapter 18

Steven Paul Nisticò, MD
Università Magna Graecia, Catanzaro, Italy
Chapter 25

Hernán Felipe Palomino V., Research Assistant
University of Chile; Faculty of Medicine, Human Genetics Program, Institute of Biomedical Sciences (ICBM), Santiago, Chile
Chapter 8

Nicola Panvini, MD
Department of Radiological Sciences,
Oncology and Pathology, Sapienza University of Rome; I.C.O.T. Hospital, Latina, Italy
Chapter 33

Licia Coceani Paskay, MS, CCC-SLP
Speech-Language Pathologist, Private Practice
Los Angeles, USA
Chapters 13, 14, 15, 20, 36, 37 and 38

Silvia Perossini, MD
Università Cattolica del Sacro Cuore,
Rome, Italy
Chapter 5

Dario Pitocco, MD
UOSA Director of Diabetology University Policlinico Foundation A. Gemelli, Università Cattolica del Sacro Cuore, Rome, Italy
Chapter 24

Valentina Prete, MD, PhD
Policlinico A. Gemelli, Rome, Italy
Chapter 11

Daniela Prosperi, MD
Nuclear Medicine Unit, Sant'Andrea University Hospital, Rome, Italy
Chapters 23 and 33

Vincenzo Quinzi, DDS
Department of Life, Health and Environmental Science, University of L'Aquila, L'Aquila, Italy
Chapters 13 and 37

Gill Rapley, PhD
Canterbury Christ Church University, Canterbury, Kent, UK
Chapter 7

Luca Revelli, MD
Professor, Fondazione Policlinico Universitario A. Gemelli IRCCS,
Università Cattolica del Sacro Cuore,
Rome, Italy
Chapters 28, 34 and 35

Cristina Rossi, MD, PhD
Center for Integrative Oncology
Fondazione Policlinico Universitario A. Gemelli IRCCS, Rome, Italy
Chapter 29

Maria Maddalena Rossi, MSc
Center for Integrative Oncology
Fondazione Policlinico Universitario A. Gemelli IRCCS, Rome, Italy
Chapter 29

Gabriele Rumi, MD
Area Gastroenterologia ed Oncologia Medica
UOC di Allergologia
Fondazione Policlinico Universitario A. Gemelli IRCCS,
Università Cattolica del Sacro Cuore,
Rome, Italy
Chapter 27

Sabina Saccomanno, DDS
Department of Life, Health and Environmental Sciences, University of L'Aquila, L'Aquila, Italy
Chapters 13, 15, 30, 36, 37 and 38

Angelo Santoliquido, MD
Professor, Fondazione Policlinico Universitario A. Gemelli IRCCS,
Università Cattolica del Sacro Cuore,
Rome, Italy
Chapter 28

Domenico Santoro, MD
Full Professor, University of Messina, Italy
Director Postgraduate School of Nephrology
Director Unit of Nephrology and Dialysis, AOU G. Martino, Messina, Italy
Chapter 21

Stefano Saran, DDS
Department of Human Sciences, Innovation and Territory, School of Dentistry, Postgraduate of Orthodontics, University of Insubria,
Varese, Italy
Chapter 13

Giovanni Scambia, MD
Head of Complex Operational Unit Cancer Gynaecology, Università Cattolica del Sacro Cuore,
Rome, Italy
Chapter 5

Rossella Siligato, MD
Unit of Nephrology and Dialysis,
University of Messina, Italy
Chapter 21

Martina Silvestri, MD
Università Magna Graecia,
Catanzaro, Italy
Chapter 25

Federica Tamburi, MD
Università Cattolica del Sacro Cuore,
Rome, Italy
Chapter 25

AnnaClara Tamburrelli, MD
Sapienza University of Rome, Clinica Oculistica Ospedale Umberto I, Rome, Italy
Chapter 26

Ciro Tamburrelli, MD
Professor, Oftalmico Hospital of Rome,
Rome, Italy
Chapter 26

Linda Tartaglione, MD
UOSA Director of Diabetology University Policlinico Foundation A. Gemelli, Università Cattolica del Sacro Cuore,
Rome, Italy
Chapter 24

Emanuela Traini, MD
Fondazione Policlinico Universitario A. Gemelli IRCCS,
Università Cattolica del Sacro Cuore,
Rome, Italy
Chapter 35

Antonio Valassina, MD
Fondazione Policlinico Universitario A. Gemelli IRCCS,
Università Cattolica del Sacro Cuore, Rome, Italy
Chapter 34

Laís Valencise Magri, DDS, MD, PhD
Department of Restorative Dentistry, School of Dentistry of Ribeirão Preto, São Paulo University, Ribeirão Preto, São Paulo, Brazil
Chapter 17

Annalisa Vidiri, MD
Complex Operational Unit Obstetrics and Obstetric Diseases, Università Cattolica del Sacro Cuore, Rome, Italy
Chapter 5

Pía Villanueva B., MD, SLP
Professor, University of Chile; Faculty of Medicine, Speech, Language & Hearing Science Department, Santiago,
Chile
Chapter 8

Marina Angela Visco, PhD
Faculty of Psychology, eCampus University, Novedrate,
Como, Italy
Chapter 32

Table of contents

SECTION 1

Food: everything we think we know

1 Varieties of nutrient acquisition strategies over the course of human evolution: an epigenetic perspective

Kevin Boyd

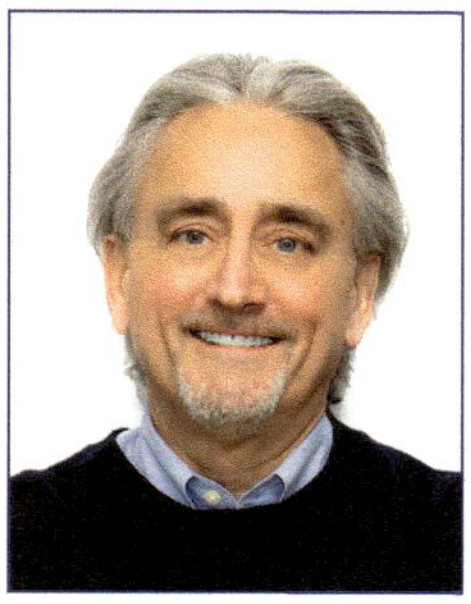

1.1 Universal common ancestry

According to Forterre et al., "...one of the most important outcomes of modern biology has been the demonstration of the unity of life. All living beings are in fact descendants of a unique ancestor commonly referred to as Luca (the Last universal common ancestor)" [1]. In fact, *Luca* is not at all a *recent* concept; in his 1859 publication of Origin of Species [2], Charles Darwin wrote, "Probably all of the organic beings which have ever lived on this earth have descended from one primordial form, into which life was first breathed". In addition, many pre-/non-*industrialized* cultures (e.g., Native Americans, San Bushman, Celtic Druids, etc.) believe(d) *all of life* is interrelated. Over the course of *Homo sapiens sapiens* (i.e., anatomically modern humans, AMH), the component of the AMH craniofacial complex (i.e., the tissues associated with the head, face, teeth and jaws), dedicated to internal food processing (i.e., chewing, grinding, tearing, etc.), is often referred to as the *masticatory apparatus* (MA). The mammalian MA is comprised of several different biological tissues that collectively function, under coordination from the circulatory and central nervous systems, primarily to acquire, taste, lubricate and biomechanically process food, ingest water and also perform communication skills necessary for speech and facial expression; furthermore, the mammalian MA can also function as a secondary (to the nose) airway portal. As our *pre-modern* human ancestors evolved away from their most recent common ancestor with modern chimpanzees (*Pan troglodytes* and *Pan paniscus*) some 5-7 million years ago [3], the MA had been indispensable to their survival and *evolutionary fitness* (i.e., ability to survive childhood and produce offspring). The genomic sequence (genes/suites of genes) required for producing the modern human MA phenotype over the past 300,000 (+/–) years is therefore not likely to have undergone appreciable macrogenetic alteration (nucleotide rearrangement, mutation, etc.); and accordingly, our genome has certainly remained intact over the past few hundreds of years after *mechanical* and *cultural industrialization* had first begun to appear in England, North America and Europe. Interestingly, coinciding with first appearances of industrialization are two phenomena: first, women begin to enter the workforce in ever-increasing numbers; and human malocclusion (HM, the narrowing of the jaw and facial bones

Kevin Boyd, DDS, MSc
Dentistry for Families and Children, Chicago, USA

Email: kbo569@googlemail.com

– dentofacial complex – with their associated crowding and misalignment of teeth) begins to appear more frequently than any other time in human history.

1.2 The tetrapod tongue

In 2014 this author delivered a keynote lecture, "Impact of tongue-tie over a lifetime: an anthropological perspective" at the IATP World Summit in Montreal [4]. Therein, evidence had been presented in support of anthropologists and archaeologists who have claimed for decades that *the tongue*, as a biologically distinct component of at least two survival mechanisms, specifically, the intimately interconnected masticatory and speech apparatuses, if not also a third, the respiratory apparatus, had been non-existent in fish until some 3.75 million (+/–) years ago [5] when certain early *lobe-finned* fish became capable of changing their *food acquisition strategy* in order to survive upon the land (after having *crawled* out of shallow ponds) to acquire food, water and air with the aid of their newly evolved togues having originated from their Hyomandibular, Basihyal and Ceratohyal cartilages. Once established in pre-amphibian fish progenitors, the tongue, as an integral component of the aforementioned survival apparatuses, gene nucleotide sequences responsible for the coding of this vital biological structure, have remained within the genomes of *all* succeeding amphibian, reptile and mammalian tetrapods.

1.3 Nutrient acquisition

When this author was pursuing a Master of Science degree in Human Nutrition at Michigan State University in the early 1980's, didactic and clinical academic experiences were mainly focused upon how individual macronutrient energy and structural substrates (e.g., proteins, carbohydrates and lipids), water (i.e., a hydration substrate) and ambient air/oxygen (i.e., respiratory substrates) and micronutrients (e.g., vitamins, minerals, phytochemicals, other trace elements) were consumed, digested, absorbed into the hepatic portal system, delivered to systemic tissues and metabolized by individual cells to support growth, development, repair and maintenance of homeostatic equilibrium; but not much at all was offered regarding how the nutrients were acquired from environmental sources. Largely because Biological Anthropology and Evolutionary Biology are not, as of now anyway, considered as being similarly useful to healthcare professionals' (HCPs) educations as are other life science subjects such as Biology, Chemistry, Biochemistry and Microbiology, etc., most HCPs will struggle at best to evaluate modern diseases from an evolutionary perspective [6].

Nowadays, *foraging* for (mostly overly processed) foods merely involves visiting supermarkets, having groceries delivered, seasonal visits to local Farmer's Markets, ordering from within/without restaurants, occasional hunting and/or fishing trips, and/or growing/raising your own crop or animal food sources [7]. Before the advent of agriculture, some 10,000-15,000 years ago, first within the Fertile Crescent in the Middle East region near Iraq, and then gradually radiating outwards over thousands of years spreading to the rest of the world [8]. Another pre-agricultural nutrient acquisition strategy that persists in many extant *traditionally*-living cultures, and to a lesser extent some modern industrialized cultures, is what is often called *subsistence fishing* with various marine resources [9].

1.4 Epigenetics and the recent appearance of human malocclusion and cultural industrialization

Within the widely used textbook *Contemporary Orthodontics* [10], coauthor William Profit posed the question: "Is it possible that a child's masticatory (chewing) effort plays a major role in determining dental arch (jaw) dimensions?", and then provides a response to his own query: "That seems unlikely". Profit's conclusion seems at odds with many anthropologists' observations; Corruccini [11] has hypothesized: "An epidemiologic transition to high prevalence of such diseases as diabetes and coronary heart disease accompanies the process of modernization/industrialization. I suggest that an equally clearly defined epidemiologic transition characterizes misaligned and discrepant dental occlusal relations in Western societies, and others undergoing urbanization, and that the rapidity of the transition is proportional to the rapid expansion of urbanization. This phenomenon rather throws the weight of suspicion toward environmental, not genetic, etiologic factors".

As previously mentioned, HM – narrowed jaws and facial bones and crowded teeth – is a condition that was nearly non-existent only a few hundred years ago. Larsen [12] reports, "...a shift to agriculture or more intensified agriculture was accompanied by an increase in dental crowding and malocclusion."; Gilbert [13] states, "...jaw anomalies (malocclusions wherein the teeth cannot fit properly in the jaw) are relatively new to European populations. Well-preserved skeletons from the 15th and 16th centuries show almost no malocclusion in the population."; and Lieberman [14] reports in his recent book, Evolution of the Human Head, "...there is much circumstantial evidence that jaws and faces do not grow to the same size that they used to...".

1.5 Ancestral versus modern strategies of nutrient acquisition in infancy and early childhood

The etiology of malocclusion is best understood within the educational framework of Nesse and Williams' *Mismatch* hypothesis for explaining modern human disease vulnerability [15]; amongst anthropologists (and many other *anthropologically-informed* dental and medical health professionals), *mismatch* (between a Pleio-Pleistocene-adapted MA and a *modern* overly-processed food supply) is one of the leading explanations for why worldwide prevalence of malocclusion have recently spiked, and most rapidly in *Western*-exposed cultures. As I alluded to earlier, their also seems to be a possible association between when women began to enter into the emerging industrial workforce in the mid-18th thru late19th-Centuries and ever-increasing numbers of individuals with malocclusion. One hypothesis being considered for this speculated inter-relationship is changed nursing and weaning strategies. Specifically, over the 2.4 million years of the genus *Homo*, if a child had not been fed according to an *ancestral* pattern of nutrient acquisition (i.e., nursing, weaning and post-weaning) during the first years of life, she/he could not have survived childhood as there were no nursing/weaning substitutes (infant formula, commercially-made baby foods, artificial feeding nipples, etc.) available until around the mid-18th thru late19th-Centuries. Pressures exerted by the *on-demand* suckling of breast milk, usually into the 3rd year of life, and mastication/chewing of fresh and minimally processed wild foods, provided for optimal development of the craniofacial respiratory complex (CFRC, Fig. 1.1) and thus had been conducive to maximization of *evolutionary fitness*.

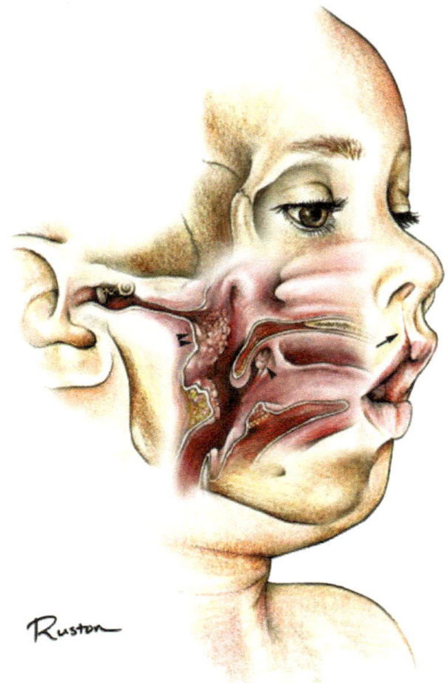

Fig. 1.1 The craniofacial respiratory complex.

REFERENCES

1. Forterre P, Herve P. The last universal common ancestor (LUCA), simple or complex? Biol Bull 1999; 196(3): 373-5; discussion 375-7.
2. Darwin C. On the Origin of Species by Means of Natural Selection, or the Preservation of Favoured Races in the Struggle for Life. John Murray, London, 1859.
3. Kumar S, Filipski A, Swarna V, Walker A, Hedges SB. Placing confidence limits on the molecular age of the human-chimpanzee divergence. Proc Natl Acad Sci USA 2005; 102(52): 18842-7.
4. Boyd K. Impact of tongue-tie over a lifetime: an anthropological perspective. Presentation at the IATP 2nd World Summit. Montreal, Quebec, 2014.
5. Shubin NH, Daeschler EB, Jenkins FA Jr. Pelvic Girdle and Fin of Tiktaalik Roseae. Proc Natl Acad Sci USA 2014; 111(3): 893-9.
6. Stearns SC, Nesse RM, Govindaraju DR, Ellison PT. Evolution in health and medicine Sackler colloquium: Evolutionary perspectives on health and medicine. Proc Natl Acad Sci USA 2010; 107 Suppl 1(Suppl 1): 1691-5.
7. Paglia L. The sweet danger of added sugars. Eur J Paediatr Dent 2019; 20(2): 89.
8. Fertile Crescent. Edited by History.com Editors, History.com, A&E Television Networks, Dec 20, 2017. www.history.com/topics/pre-history/fertile-crescent.
9. Busilacchi S, Russ GR, Williams AJ, Sutton SG, Begg GA. The role of subsistence fishing in the hybrid economy of an indigenous community. Mar Policy 2013; 37: 183-91. https://doi.org/10.1016/j.marpol.2012.04.017
10. Proffit W, Fields H, Larson B, Sarver *D*. Contemporary Orthodontics. 6th Edition. Philadelphia, Elsevier, 2019.
11. Corruccini RS. An epidemiologic transition in dental occlusion in world populations. Am J Orthod 1984; 86(5): 419-26.
12. Larsen CS. Biological Changes in Human Populations with Agriculture. Annu Rev Anthropol 1995; 24: 185-213. https://www.jstor.org/stable/2155935
13. Scott F. Gilbert. (2003). "The Reactive Genome". Origina-

tion Of Organismal Form: Beyond The Gene In Developmental And Evolutionary Biology. 87-101. https://works.swarthmore.edu/fac-biology/431
14. Lieberman D. The Evolution of the Human Head. Belknap Press of Harvard University Press, pp. 276-7, 2011.
15. Nesse RM, Williams GC. Why We Get Sick: the New Science of Darwinian Medicine. New York: Vintage Books, 1996.

2 Food, health and well-being

Giacinto A.D. Miggiano

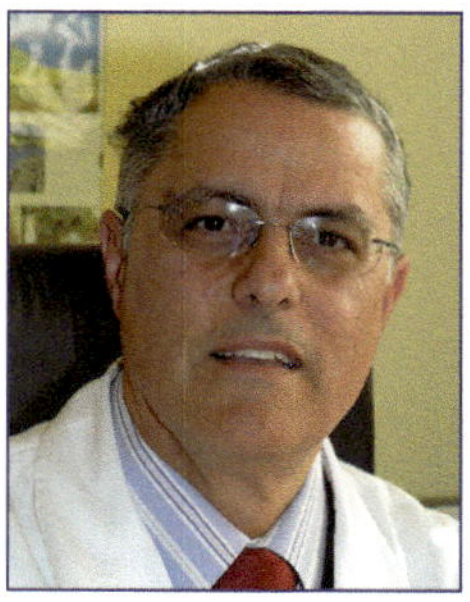

2.1 Introduction

The concept of well-being, in existence since the 1950s, indicates that a human being must be considered as a whole, both physically and mentally. The "feel good" has become a way of life indicated as a method to prevent the development of diseases, according to the old motto for which "it is better to prevent than to cure". This philosophy concerns various aspects of human life and primarily is based on a correct lifestyle, which combines healthy eating behavior and regular physical activity, while also covering psychological aspects and social implications (such as the relationship with the others). Today, the World Health Organization defines health not only as the absence of illness but rather as a "state of complete physical, mental and social well-being", that is, to feel good and feel fit with oneself and with others.

2.2 Eating to feel good in a healthy lifestyle

People, like all living beings, derive from food the substances necessary for living and living well. The daily preoccupation of eating for survival has led, since the beginning, to an incessant search for food, since it has been shown that a well-nourished organism has the possibility to live longer, to resist diseases better, to procreate more easily thus prolonging the species. Eating is therefore essential. Today, fortunately, in the civilized world, a strict need to search for food does not exist (at least for most people); however, a proper way of eating is essential to keep healthy and perform normal daily activities. We do not just try to "survive", as our ancestors did, but we tend to thrive, satisfying our desires and satisfying even non-material needs. Food thus acquires the values of a personal symbolism (of pleasure) and of social relationship with fellow members of one's community.

The pursuit of well-being pushes the person to perform actions in daily living useful for that purpose: nutrition and physical-sporting activity, in this sense, constitute a very close union and are mutually interconnected. In fact, while on the one hand with proper nutrition the body has everything necessary for physical activity, on the other hand it allows to achieve and maintain a healthy body

Giacinto A.D. Miggiano, MD
Director of Human Nutrition Research Center - Catholic University, Rome, Italy
Director of Clinical Nutrition - Fondazione Policlinico Universitario A. Gemelli IRCCS, Rome, Italy

Email: gmiggiano@libero.it

composition, which is a prerequisite for the well-being of the body and mind.

Proper nutrition rests on three main cornerstones: 1) use of safe food (from the hygienic and toxicological point of view); 2) diet (i.e., lifestyle), adequate in nutrients and possibly enriched with functional compounds; 3) correct eating behavior. Only if these three cornerstones are respected, nutrition contributes to health and well-being. In the absence of one or more of these factors, there is the risk of losing the state of health and of slipping more or less quickly towards an illness [1]. Leaving aside the first point (food safety), the relationship between food and eating, nutritional adequacy and eating behavior of individuals is outlined below.

2.3 Nutrition or eating?

"Nutrition" and "eating" are not synonymous, as Food Science studies have shown there is a complex relationship between food and the individual. One could say that "animals feed themselves, men eat" or in other words "eating is not just eating". Hunger, appetite, sense of satiety at the end of the meal and sense of satiety between meals are different and important concepts in the regulation of food intake.

2.3.1 State of nutrition (or organ of nutrition?)

With nutrition, the substances that are necessary and indispensable (nutrients) are supplied to the organism in order to maintain health, to grow and to avoid the decay of the organism. Even if there is not a well-defined anatomical organ, such as the heart or muscles, quickly identifiable, it may be helpful to think of an "organ of nutrition", (it would be better to talk about "nutrition apparatus"), which does not have physically distinct anatomical dimensions. However, it must be regularly maintained and safeguarded, as all the organs can get sick (causing illness) putting health and life at risk.

The organ of nutrition consists of nutrients and works for the presence of these. The 45 essential compounds must be introduced with food, as our body does not have the ability to build them in various ways. The foundation of these studies on essential compounds is the "Budget Principle", which applies to each of these 45 compounds: in a nutshell the daily intake of nutrients with the diet must correspond to the body outputs (obligatory). If this principle is respected, then the balance will be achieved, otherwise in the absence of this simple rapport the Budget may move away from the equilibrium point, going towards growth (positive balance) or towards a decrease (negative balance), with both situations compromising health and therefore life too.

Since the 45 nutrients appear in the body in different quantities (operationally we speak of macro- and micronutrients), it follows that changes in the balance of the former will have more or less gross repercussions on the structure of the organs, while for the latter (micronutrients/microconstituents, such as vitamins and microminerals), more sensitive methods are needed to detect scarcity or need. These methodologies obviously do not exclude more sophisticated techniques, in which the input (eating) is correlated with the output (excretion) (considered the "gold standard"). However, in practice these techniques are supplanted by others that are based on a different assumption: if the body's content is balanced, it is the outflows (excretion) that determine the inflows of food and nutrients. The constant level (within established limits) of these nutrients therefore bears witness to a balanced budget condition.

For the chemical composition (in nutrients) there are specific tables elaborated by prestigious institutions, easily available on electronic form or in hard copy, which are updated periodically. The differences in the composition (or bromatological) values, which depend on various factors including the composition and origin of food, are never such as to affect the biological variability. Also, for this reason the variety of foods is a key principle in food choices.

2.4 Eating behavior and nutrition

There are many ways to eat and yet eating behavior has repercussions on how much is then consumed. We must eat calmly, so as to taste the food and feel the feeling of satiety (eating quickly does not allow, in fact, to control how much you eat). This becomes more difficult today at a time when everything is fast, from the place of work to the various activities of life. Eating while standing, walking and talking, causes the loss of the socializing and convivial dimension of a meal consumed at home with one's family.

On the other hand, care must also be taken not to load the food with values and symbolisms that go beyond the fact that it must nourish us. If it is normal – precisely because of the symbolic meaning of food – to eat a little more on special occasions, one must not fall into the habit of gratifying oneself, however, always with food. Eating (a little) more what we like is also a means of overcoming a momentary state of discomfort; but if you exaggerate with this consolatory behavior, serious health damage can result. In these cases, it is necessary to recognize the causes of the discomfort, understanding that one enters a vicious circle and, above all, not pouring on the food a meaning that it must not have.

Eating disorders are many and more or less known, such as anorexia [2], bulimia [3], uncontrolled nutrition, orthorexia (being obsessed with the quality and genuineness of food), vigorexia (being obsessed with physical and athletic appearance and therefore with the type of food admitted) and psychogenic obesity [4, 5].

2.5 Eating disorders

Various conditions increase the risk of a compromised nutritional state, as the daily introduction of food increases or more often decreases: the loss of the nutrient balance is accompanied by an alteration of the metabolic state of the individual (malnutrition). It should be emphasized that extreme variations appear visually, as alterations in the body composition and profile/image of the person make it clear to everyone the danger of this condition and the need for nutritional restoration. However, it should be remembered that some alterations, linked to mineral and vitamin imbalance, are still important even if more subtle and less easy to recognize as these situations can severely impact the well-being condition of those affected.

Caloric malnutrition (or more often protein-calories malnutrition) is a condition that not only affects the categories of subjects with psychiatric disorders, but it is the consequence of a reduced introduction of energy (calories) and/or proteins necessary to compensate for daily losses [6]. Faced with this situation, the body responds initially with an adaptation by reducing, for example, the activity of basic metabolic processes, as indicated by a lower level of thyroid hormones, or by improving the efficiency of intestinal absorption of some nutrients, and lastly by resorting to use the body's reserves. This condition of total, partial or variously modified fasting gradually reduces body weight which begins to become visually evident. The image of an individual with anorexia is similar to the sadly famous pictures of prisoners in concentration camps, reduced to skeletal appearance due to severe malnutrition. Alongside the obvious deficiencies, which affect the body image, other nutrients may be lacking partially or totally creating individualized situations, diagnosable with sophisticated biochemical techniques that document the deficiency of many, if not all, of the 45 nutrients.

Caloric malnutrition, due to reduced proteins (a clinical situation known as Kwashiorkor) or especially due to a reduction in protein-calories (a clinical situation known as Marasmus), compromises the person's health, affecting multiple organs and especially the cardiovascular system, whose failure is the ultimate cause of death. To prevent this extreme condition in the most serious cases, the 45 nutrients are administered directly intravenously, or through the Parenteral (Forced) Nutrition procedures.

The hidden malnutrition, on the other hand, represents a reduced supply of one or more micronutrients (minerals and/or vitamins) that apparently are not accompanied by a decreased intake of proteins and above all of energy (the subject can also appear normal or even overweight). These deficiency diseases, even if they do not reach such degrees as to lead to death, nevertheless compromise the functionality of all the organs and consequently contribute to the insufficiency of these organs. Even in such situations, it is obviously necessary to remedy the problem by replacing the missing nutrient, either by correcting the diet or by boosting it with supplements [7].

Malnutrition due to excess is the consequence of a food behavior that is characterized by an excess of food intake, of a different type and according to different methods that are not reported here but which are easy to perceive (haphazardly eating, bingeing, etc.). In this case we are faced with people who actually "eat more than they should".

Even in the presence of food surplus, the body initially puts in place defense mechanisms both reducing, where possible, the absorption of nutrients in excess and above all, but not always, increasing the outputs. This shows how the body has, within certain limits, the ability to maintain internal homeostasis by acting on the inputs and outputs in different ways depending on the individual nutrients. For example, for iron there is the possibility of increasing the percentage absorbed, but without being able to affect the increase in elimination. Therefore, the control of the iron balance occurs at the level of intestinal absorption. On the other hand, for others like sodium, its control occurs only at excretory level (kidney), with nothing on the absorption quota (sodium is almost completely absorbed). Even an excess of individual nutrients can be risky for health and for life.

In food behavior disorders, nutritional deficiency pictures accompany certain situations, such as anorexia nervosa, athletic anorexia, vigorexia, orthorexia, dieting, etc., while nutritional accumulation diseases (energy, fats, etc.) can be found in cases of bulimia nervosa, uncontrolled eating and psychogenic obesity [8].

2.6 Treatment: which therapy?

The therapy for malnutrition is obviously multidisciplinary and multidimensional (diet, physical activity, drugs and cognitive-behavioral therapy) [9]. In these cases, it is necessary to treat the person with malnutrition and not only malnutrition by itself! Neglecting the psychological aspects and focusing attention only on the physical-biological problems risks intervening only on the symptoms and ignoring the causes. Therefore, the first concern is to not underestimate the problem, thinking of being able to solve it without the intervention of an expert, or worse, not to recognize it at all. The identification of malnutrition by defect or excess is the first step, which immediately follows the identification of a true path of re-nutrition that is presented as a food re-education aimed at correcting the most harmful aspects.

Times, methodologies and counseling, of course, are not standardizable, as therapy should be individualized. An optimal approach avoids being too hasty in imposing the correct feeding, but rather looks to establish since the beginning a few and simple rules that can produce, in the end, a satisfactory result on both the physical and the behavioral level. By proceeding step by step, it is possible, on the one hand, to avoid rapid changes in body composition, which the patients may live as compromising their body images, and, on the other hand, it is possible to avoid pursuing impossible objectives, both theoretical and ideal.

REFERENCES

1. Stråvik M, Barman M, Hesselmar B, Sandin A, Wold AE, Sandberg AS. Maternal Intake of Cow's Milk during Lactation Is Associated with Lower Prevalence of Food Allergy in Offspring. Nutrients 2020; 12(12): 3680.
2. Schaumberg K, Anderson D. Dietary restraint and weight loss as risk factors for eating pathology. Eat Behav 2016; 23: 97-103.
3. Ágh T, Kovács G, Pawaskar M, Supina D, Inotai A, Vokó Z. Epidemiology, health-related quality of life and economic burden of binge eating disorder: a systematic literature review. Eat Weight Disord 2015; 20(1): 1-12.
4. Molinari E. (2020). La clinica dei disturbi del comportamento alimentare: l'intervento psicologico. Istituto Lombardo - Accademia Di Scienze E Lettere - Incontri Di Studio. https://doi.org/10.4081/incontri.2020.632
5. Petroni M. (2020). L'intervento nutrizionale nei disturbi del comportamento alimentare. Istituto Lombardo - Accademia Di Scienze E Lettere - Incontri Di Studio. https://doi.org/10.4081/incontri.2020.633
6. Stice E. Interactive and Mediational Etiologic Models of Eating Disorder Onset: Evidence from Prospective Studies. Annu Rev Clin Psychol 2016; 12: 359-81.
7. Cooper SL, Pelly FE, Lowe JB. Construct and criterion-related validation of nutrient profiling models: a systematic review of the literature. Appetite 2016; 100: 26-40.
8. Toulany A, Wong M, Katzman DK, Akseer N, Steinegger C, Hancock-Howard RL, Coyte PC. Cost analysis of inpatient treatment of anorexia nervosa in adolescents: hospital and caregiver perspectives. CMAJ Open 2015; 3(2): E192-7.
9. Fairburn CG. Cognitive Behavior Therapy and Eating Disorders. New York: Guilford Press, 2008.

3 Misinformation about food

Giorgio Calabrese and Cinzia Myriam Calabrese

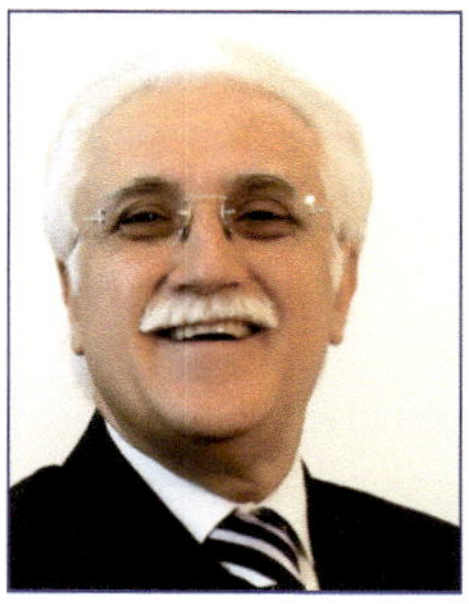

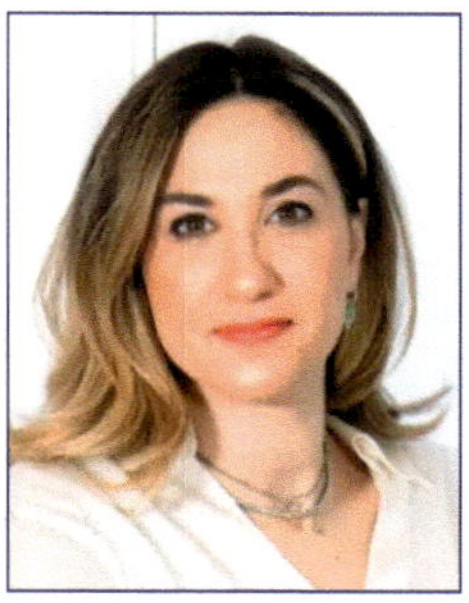

3.1 Introduction

"Fake news" about food, or rather flawed indications that lead to the lowest point of food information are more and more common. Fakes, lies or falsehoods, have now taken the place of food myths and legends. The media and social networks then act as a sounding board and give voice to what should not even be taken into consideration. Thus, news without any scientific validity is debated in newspapers and TV, so much so that the Italian National Institute of Health, in the food sector, had to propose the new section "False myths and hoaxes" which tried to dispel some incorrect opinions on nutrition that are the result of "hearsay" or opinion.

Unfortunately, many of these myths are so ingrained in our society that they are difficult to eradicate. A series of short food fakes are now in the public domain and science is struggling to bring back on the right tracks the truth established by research carried out by us medical scientist, nutritionists, who are at the service of science. Here are some fakes: pineapple burns fat, milk is bad for adults and gluten is everyone's enemy, banana is by far the richest food in potassium, and so on. Dr. Internet and Dr. Google act as immense amplifiers, alternating old made-up information with new hoaxes. The use of the internet cannot be criminalized in its entirety. It is a new working tool, and it can certainly be useful, but not all news sites are reliable or unbiased. Information is good if the truth is not omitted or distorted due to economic or social or political interests or partisan beliefs. It is better to rely on official sites such as those of the Ministry of Health, the Italian National Institute of Health, the Italian Research Center for Food and Nutrition or the equivalent entities in other countries.

In case of doubts or health problems, do not hesitate to contact directly your doctor or a medical specialist in Food Science by specifying your ailments and indicating foods that are difficult to digest. Certainly, the recommendations will be specific and tailored to the individual, and therefore more reliable than generic information sometimes not exactly objective if not outright suspect. The

Giorgio Calabrese, MD, Ph.D
Grand Officer of the Italian Republic
Lecturer in Human Nutrition and Dietetics
Medical Offices in Asti, Turin, Milan and Rome, Italy

Email: giorgiocalabrese@gcalabrese.it

Cinzia Myriam Calabrese, MD
Private Practice, Rome, Italy

Email: cinzia.calabrese@gmail.com

food we bring to our table can be a source of benefits but also of pitfalls. It happens that sometimes the culinary tradition was unable to guess the true characteristics of food, thus generating "false myths". So, it is better not to cling to one's own beliefs, perhaps erroneous, and not to overly rely on popular "legends". To ensure a healthy and balanced diet, it is important to be well aware of what you eat and not to be dazzled by clichés: with a little critical sense and the right information, you can make the right choices for proper nutrition.

3.2 Eating Kamut® makes you lose weight!

Kamut® is a brand or a trademark and is not the scientific name of a plant species. This duly registered American trademark refers to a specific variety of wheat called khorasan (*triticum turanicum*). Everyone can grow, sell and buy this khorasan wheat, but only the company that owns the brand can market it under the name Kamut®. In Italy there are already various companies that sell products made with this grain, which are easily recognizable because the name khorasan appears on the label. The other myth to dispel is that of its origin: khorasan is not native to ancient Egypt, but it is considered ancient because it did not undergo the genetic selection carried out in the mid-20th century to improve productivity. In addition, it is characterized by its high protein content but, like all wheat, it contains gluten and is therefore not a good food for people with celiac disease. It is not uncommon that in many stores Kamut® is promoted just to celiacs, which is a nonsense.

3.3 The fake on the water – our blue gold

3.3.1 Tap water

Tap water causes kidney stones. There is still a widespread fear that the calcium salts and magnesium present in the water may favor the development of kidney stones, but there is no scientific evidence that can confirm this correlation. The formation of stones depends mainly on the individual and family predisposition, on the eating habits and on the daily amount of liquids taken. Generally, drinking tap water is considered unsafe, but this is also a false belief. Tap water (drinking water) and natural mineral water are no different from a safety point of view. In fact, in the case of both natural mineral waters and drinking water or water treated after the delivery point (for example, in "water kiosks" or public water fountains), tests and controls ensure the absence of risks for consumers, which are guaranteed in all cases. The only difference between regular drinking water and natural mineral waters comes from their "nature". In fact, drinking water is a universal human right to be always guaranteed through the availability of good quality water for all, in the places of life and work, in a necessary quantity and at affordable costs for all human use, not just for drinking [1]. For this reason, the origin of water intended for human consumption can be different: for instance, in Italy 85% of water comes from underground sources but also from rivers or reservoirs or from mixtures of different sources. The chemical (hardness, acidity or alkalinity, i.e., pH, presence of mineral salts) and organoleptic characteristics (smell and taste) of the water can sometimes change over time, but the safety standards are in any case guaranteed by the rigorous controls carried out under the approval of the Ministry of Health, the water managers and the Local Health Authorities responsible for the water along its entire path, from the source to the tap. Natural mineral waters, on the other hand, represent consumer goods freely placed on the market and purchased by consumers' choice. Mineral water must meet quality standards which, in addition to guaranteeing the safety of use from a health point of view, ensure that the quality and characteristics of the bottled water are the same as the various original waters, which come from officially authorized sources. It is often said that *it is preferable not to drink water with meals.* It is not so. A right amount of liquid improves the digestibility of ingested foods and promotes an overall good digestion.

3.3.2 Drink only when you are thirst?

It is said: *You only need to drink when you are thirsty*, but this is a falsehood. If this were the case, our elderly people who do not feel the sense of thirst, would face significant damage from dehydration, if they did not induce themselves to drink the amount of water appropriate to their age and build. Drinking water is a fundamental action to be healthy and fit because water represents about 60-65% of the body mass for an adult individual. Its quantity is greater in the newborn (approximately 77%) and tends to decrease with age (in the elderly it decreases to 50%). Drinking water brings important mineral elements that the body cannot produce, such as, among others, calcium and magnesium. Water is a necessary element for the proper maintenance of vital functions and plays essential physiological roles [2]. Thanks to water the body maintains its constant temperature regardless of the outside temperature (this can prevent severe effects during heat waves). It allows essential processes to happen, such as digestion and blood circulation along with the transport of nutrients and the elimination of "waste" through the urine. Water also lubricates muscles and joints, it keeps the skin supple, and does much more. Its presence in the body must be kept constant and that is why it is possible to remain without drinking it for only a short time. When water begins to lack, the thirst mechanism intervenes which, however, is not always felt (especially in children and the elderly) and which is activated when a phase of stress and dehydration has already begun in the body. For example, in the case of physical and sporting activities or intellectual commitment, the lack of a sufficient quantity of water also significantly penalizes performance. For all these reasons, it is necessary to drink even if we do not feel the sense of thirst [3].

3.3.3 "Cluster-breaking" pretreated water

The need to pretreat and improve water leads to the application of bottle covers with a "cluster-breaking" function in order to separate the aggregates of molecules considered harmful. Yes, of course, water can contain groups of molecules (clusters), which form and disintegrate very quickly but do not create any obstacles to the absorption of this important element by our body. These groups of molecules would be held together by chemical bonds and, due to their excessive size, would not allow water to adequately penetrate the cells of our body. According to this belief, *it would be necessary to use special devices to break up water clusters,* breaking them down into smaller groups (5 or 6 molecules), considered more suitable for spreading in the organism. It is known that water molecules in a liquid state can be held together by chemical bonds. However, these are rather weak and very dynamic bonds, so much so that groups of water molecules are formed and destroyed continuously, in a process that is defined as "dynamic equilibrium". It is therefore unthinkable that the presence of such unstable groups of water molecules has any effect on the ability of water to penetrate into the cells of our body. In conclusion, there is no need to pretreat the water with cluster-breaking devices. This fake is induced by the belief that water coming both from domestic supplies and from bottles, once ingested, it would have difficulty penetrating into the cells of our body [2, 3].

3.3.4 Water without chemical substances

Another fake concerning water claims that *drinking water to be defined as "good" should be free of any chemical substance*. Leading this false news is the term "chemical" which in everyday life is opposed to the so-called "natural". As for water, many chemicals contained in it are beneficial to health. Water free of minerals, dissolved gases and even microorganisms is distilled water, which is not drinking water. It is used in the medical field to prepare, for example, the physiological solution to be used for eye drops and injectable products. Even at home, distilled water is useful to generate vapor in irons. Eliminating all the substances present in drinking water, in fact, would cause the reduction of nutritional elements essential for health and naturally present, such as boron, selenium, fluorine, chromium or copper, along with numerous other minerals such as calcium, magnesium, iodine or potassium. The legislation on water aims to ensure that water meant for human consumption is healthy and clean and aims to prevent chemicals, potentially harmful to health, from reaching dangerous levels [4-6].

3.3.5 A diet of water?

There is no water diet. There is a false belief that by drinking a lot of water without eating you can lose weight [2]. The organism would suffer for sure. Drinking too much water, as well as drinking too little, is harmful to one's health because, among other effects, it can determine the dilution of electrolytes in the blood, especially sodium and potassium with their essential function of balancing liquids between internal and external compartments. To maintain a good state of health, the human body needs the right amount of water in order to replenish water losses, thus ensuring optimal conditions for most of the physiological processes. Signs of excessive water intake are headache, nausea and vomiting, increased blood pressure, confusion, sleepiness, difficulty breathing and fatigue. The Scientific Panel on Dietetic Products, Nutrition and Allergies of the European Food Safety Authority (EFSA) [1] has recently redefined the dietary reference values of several nutrients, including water, recommending the amount a person needs to take to stay healthy, depending on age and gender. The reference values [7], which consider the water taken as a whole, both through direct consumption and through food and beverages of all kinds, in conditions of moderate environmental temperatures and average levels of physical activity, are defined as follows:

- In infants up to six months of life: 100 milliliters per kilogram of weight per day (mL/kg/day)
- In children:
  - between 6 months and one year of age: 800-1000 milliliters per day (mL/day)
  - between 1 and 3 years of age: 1100-1300 mL/day
  - between 4 and 8 years of age: 1600 mL/day
  - ages 9-13: 2100 mL/day (just above half a gallon) for boys and 1900 mL/day for girls
- In adolescents, adults and the elderly:
  - for females 2 liters per day (L/day) or half a gallon
  - for males 2.5 L/day.

These values are indicative; in hot climates and during intense physical activities, or other situations that induce dehydration, the levels of water to be drunk can vary significantly (it can also be considered more than double the quantities indicated). This also occurs in conditions of stress and gastrointestinal disorders that lead to vomiting and diarrhea, such as infant's diarrhea.

3.3.6 Safe water with pretreating equipment?

Another fake information regarding water concerns the need for water treatment devices. The manufacturers of such equipment indicate that these are necessary to render normal tap water "safe". While in Italy these are not at all necessary, as every municipality must guarantee the healthiness of the water in its water supply, in many different countries and local communities these may be indeed necessary. In general, the water distributed in Italy is of an adequate quality for human consumption and does not require other treatments to make it drinkable or to avoid health risks [6]. It may happen that specific accidental circumstances make the water unsuitable for drinking, making some restrictions necessary. When that happens, the water source operator and the authorities are required to promptly restore the quality of water and, in the period necessary to do so, to supply the consumers concerned, through alternative supplies (e.g., tankers), with adequate quantities of water suitable for human consumption. The water treatment devices authorized and legislated have the sole purpose of making the taste and smell of tap water more pleasant or to make it fresh and sparkling, to satisfy the tastes of consumers. It is also useful to read the documentation accompanying each device.

3.3.7 Water in pitchers at the restaurant

In most restaurants, it is not unusual to find pitchers of filtered water instead of bottled water. The legislation, especially in Italy, on the supply of natural mineral water in a public establishment provides that the same must take place with a hermetically sealed bottle and with the label showing all the legal indications [6]. In no case should any ambiguity be generated in the consumer about the water administered. In the event that drinking water is supplied in jugs or pitchers and undergoes treatments before getting on the table, it ought to clearly show on the container the words "treated drinking water or treated and sparkling drinking water", if carbon dioxide has been added to the water [8]. Natural mineral water is usually subject to strict regulations not only with respect to its origin, recognition and control but also on the information associated with its administration, to protect the health and information rights of consumers.

3.3.8 Our grandparents' water

Another fake about water concerns the belief that water was once better, in other words, that our grandparents drank better water. This is not the case. On the contrary, once upon a time, proximity to sewer networks that were not always perfectly sealed caused contamination and disease. In Italy we can certainly say that today's water is good. We know much of what can make water "unsafe" for health and, through constant technical and scientific improvement, we know how to keep the various dangers or harmful events under control, for example, by preventing the presence of bacteria and viruses or toxic substances [9]. Unfortunately, these same "dangers" continue to kill around two million people (especially children) every year in the rest of the world, even if progress in prevention is ongoing [10].

In Italy, in order to ensure the sustainability of the UN Millennium Goal number 6: *Access to safe drinking water and adequate sanitation*, the collaboration between environmental and health interventions has increased, in an effort to consider the possible environmental and climatic impact on water resources, with potentially significant effects on everybody's health [11].

3.4 Fruit

Fruit is experiencing a moment of confusion, if not contradiction, and is primarily the subject of fake news. A first fake is that eating fruit at the end of a meal is like eating poison. It would carry a load of sugars into our digestive system that ferment and ruin digestion. But our body is trained to digest fruit very well after a meal because it has been doing this for centuries. Indeed, that minimum of any fermentation helps digestion (which is then the reason given by those who drink sparkling water with meals: because they digest better...). The same people who discard the traditional placement of fruit consumption, however, do not disdain dessert at the end of a meal. But are sweets less sugary than fruit? Of course not, moreover they certainly are loaded with fats, which fruit does not have, except in rare cases such as with avocado.

Another ancient myth is that eating citrus fruits in the evening is bad. If the person is healthy, there is no scientific evidence that indicates the right time of day to eat them or factors that interfere with digestion. It is different for those with gastroesophageal reflux disease (GERD): in this case, it is not recommended to ingest acidic fruits such as citrus fruits, but also equally acidic foods such as chocolate, tomatoes, mint or coffee.

Another story tells of fruit that does not contain sugar but fructose and therefore can be eaten in quantity even by people with diabetes. Fructose is a sugar that, together with glucose, forms sucrose, which is the common table sugar. Diabetics should not deprive themselves of fruit, which is indeed an indispensable food for our body, due to the fact that together we ingest vitamins, mineral salts and excellent fiber. For diabetics in particular, however, it is necessary to exclude or strongly limit some types such as figs and grapes, taking care not to take it together with other foods with a high glycemic index. The discussion on quantity also applies to those who are healthy: fruit is rich in simple sugars that can raise blood sugar quickly.

3.5 Iron

It is widely believed that the excellent spinach, rich in fiber and mineral salts, is a useful food for people with anemia problems because they contain high amounts of iron. The problem is that this iron, actually present, cannot be used by the body because together with it there are other substances that prevent its absorption. For example, foods rich in iron and useful for anemics are liver, offal, bitter cocoa, lentils, dried fruit and seafood. But the question of absorption should not be underestimated: iron is better assimilated by the body when it is combined with vitamin C and, in general, with acidifying foods.

3.6 Meat

The "super-spreader" equivalent in current times. Attacks on this food ignore scientific truths. The "popular feeling" replaces, in fact, scientific research. It has been established that eating meat twice a week not only does not cause damage to health, but it also helps children to grow, adults to resist and the elderly to live better and longer. Those who prefer to avoid for religious reasons or personal choices will certainly do without it, but they cannot demonize the product if consumed in the right quantity, much less deny its quality for human health. Animal proteins are important for mankind but also for our pets. In fact, we need to stock up on ready-to-eat cans of both meat and fish for our pets who need to consume them for their well-being. Those who prefer different animal proteins, such as vegetarians, can consume eggs, milk and derivatives. The extreme view of red meat is misleading and underplays the qualities of this important food. *There is no scientific evidence that unprocessed red meat, taken in the right quantities and as part of a varied diet, is a certain carcinogen. For some categories, such as children and pregnant women, it is a very important food to provide the necessary nutrients such as iron and vitamin B12.*

Red meat is a much-discussed food. The debate on its real risks and benefits is increasingly heated, supported by scientific studies that associate its consumption with a "probable" increase in the risk of developing certain cancers and other diseases. In 2015, the IARC (International Agency for Research on Cancer) – Agency of the World Health Organization that deals with evaluating and classifying the evidence of carcinogenicity of substances – defined red meat as *probably* carcinogenic (Group 2A) and *processed* meat as a carcinogen (Group 1) especially with respect to the emerging of colorectal cancer, but also of other types of cancer (for example, affecting pancreas, breast, stomach and prostate). Regarding prostate cancer, the data collected is still insufficient. All the studies considered were conducted only on the adult population, however there are no studies that show the total absence or drastic decrease of the tumors listed above in vegetarian subjects [12-16].

Basically, we can distinguish meat as processed or "not processed". Whole and distinct anatomical parts are understood to be unprocessed, such as: muscle sections of beef, veal, pork, lamb, mutton and goat. In some countries unprocessed meat includes large chunks of llama, moose, horse, camel, buffalo or yak. By processed meats we mean meats subjected to salting, maturing, fermentation, smoking or other processes such as the addition of preservatives (nitrites and nitrates) to improve their flavor or conservation (cured meats, sausages, canned meat, etc.).

In most cases it is red beef or pork that is more likely to be processed, but it can also be poultry or other types of meat. However, it is not clear whether the increased risk is related to the meat itself (heme-iron), to the salting process or to the additives used to preserve it such as nitrites and nitrates. It should be noted that epidemiological studies offer scientific correlation data that cannot be interpreted as evidence of a cause-and-effect relationship. This means that we can speak of an increased risk, and therefore an increase in the probability of the disease appearing, when consuming red or processed meat, but it cannot be said that the disease will certainly appear as a consequence of their consumption. It should be noted that the increased risk of cancer depends on the quantity and frequency of consumption of these foods [17, 18].

In general, the consumption of red or processed meat should not exceed the limits recommended by the guidelines for healthy eating. The adult population should not eat more than twice a week a portion, equal to 50 grams, of processed meat and no more than three times a portion, equal to 100-150 grams, of red meat, for a maximum of 350-500 grams per week.

The consumption of red meat, however, must always be defined on the basis of individual health conditions and the need for iron and vitamin B12, of which red meat is a valuable "supplier". In particular, the need for these indispensable nutrients, difficult to find and assimilate from foods of plant origin (in which vitamin B12 is absent), increases in pregnant women and children.

3.7 Fats must be completely eliminated from diets

It is a common belief that fats are bad for you. This theory, partial in itself and therefore incomplete, finds a fertile substratum in the various pathologies present in a large segment of the population. It is more correct to say that *excessive* fat is bad. Fats are essential nutrients for our body and eliminating them from the diet can put your health at risk. The important thing is not to abuse them (they can represent 25-30% of the daily calories intake) and select the ones with the best qualities, such as extra virgin olive oil.

Fats are often denigrated because they are very caloric (1 g of fat = 9 kcal) and for this reason they are accused of promoting weight gain and cardiovascular problems. Fats make foods tasty and reducing or eliminating fats make the food too bland, so they are usually replaced with sugar, hence the "fattening" problem. Instead, they are essential for the body to function properly, provided you know how to dose and choose them. It is extremely important not to overdo it, especially with those of animal origin.

Fats can belong to different families; depending on their chemical formula, there are *saturated fatty acids*, called "bad fats", which have the drawback of increasing the synthesis of cholesterol and promoting cardiovascular problems, especially in the case of hereditary predisposition. Then there are *unsaturated fatty acids*, called "good fats," divided into *monounsaturated* and *polyunsaturated* ones. Among the latter we find the famous essential fatty acids, that is, those that our body cannot produce, but which are essential for its functioning. Clearly, fats provide a significant caloric contribution, that is, useful energy for our body, but to make the difference, in addition to the quantity and the type of fat, diet and lifestyle such as a sedentary lifestyle, bad habits or overeating must be included into the equation. The fats in our body have multiple functions, so they should never be missing from the diet: 1) they form the membrane of our cells, guaranteeing fluidity; 2) allow nerve impulses in the brain to travel all over the body; 3) they protect the internal organs, covered by a thin layer of fat, which forms a sort of insulating sheath against external trauma; 4) they help us to keep the skin young, as it is covered with a thin lipid layer, which allows it to defend itself from external attacks, guaranteeing elasticity and brightness, softness and hydration; 5) thanks to fats it is possible to absorb the "fat-soluble" vitamins which need, in fact, a vehicle of fat to be absorbed; therefore a diet that is too low in fat could create problems with vitamin malabsorption.

3.8 Milk causes cancer!

It starts with a bizarre idea that is raging on the internet according to which milk would be harmful because it is a food intended for growth that only humans, among animals, eat for life. In fact, milk is a primordial food, it has been part of the human diet for thousands of years, indeed it has always been used by humans, from any mammal it comes from: cow, goat, sheep, camelids. The nomadic peoples of the desert have always consumed camel and dromedary milk. This atavistic consumption has allowed humans to modify their genome, allowing even in adulthood the production of the enzyme responsible for breaking down lactose, that is, milk sugar. In the Bible, to indicate the characteristics of the Promised Land, it is said that it is a land where milk and honey flow. Milk and cheeses have accompanied the subsistence of many peasant and non-peasant peoples. In

Italy, when red or white meats were a rarity in the post-war period, good milk guaranteed good nutrients for children and adults. The Italian breakfast, appreciated and imitated all over the world, always includes cappuccino, i.e., frothed milk and coffee, at home, in hotels and coffee shops.

3.8.1 Those who are intolerant to lactose should not eat cheese

The prolonged maturation of many cheeses leads to a radical decrease if not almost the disappearance of lactose. Furthermore, even lactose intolerant people are generally able to tolerate doses up to about 125 milliliters of milk per day without problems and discomfort. All this based on data from the European Free Trade Association (EFTA).

3.8.2 Food without lactose is healthier

Lactose-free foods, such as gluten-free foods and "free" foods in general, are considered to be "better". This is a tendency in total contrast with how products were once advertised emphasizing the richness of their contents, for example, milk with more vitamins, more calcium, etc. Consuming lactose-free foods by people who are not actually intolerant, costs more and does not add value to one's nutrition; on the contrary, the word "without" means taking something away. In the long run, the lactase enzyme, that is normally produced to break down and digest lactose, gradually decreases until it disappears. In this last case it is really no longer possible to digest the milk [19].

Those intolerant to lactose, due to reduced or absent ability to digest it in case of ingestion, register a state of fermentation in the intestine and gas formation that leads to bloating and abdominal pain. This is one of the most common food intolerances and can come in two types: primary and secondary. In most cases primary intolerance is caused by a generally hereditary enzyme disorder. A secondary intolerance may only be temporary due to gastrointestinal tract infections, or lesions, or very rapid and sudden changes in the usual diet [20]. The food industry has recently increased the offer of products specifically designed for the needs of individuals with allergies and intolerances. It is now very easy to find milk derivatives on the market, manipulated in such a way as to reduce the presence of lactose. These foods represent a precious resource for people affected by the most severe forms of lactose intolerance. However, the habit of consuming lactose-free foods is also spreading among those who do not suffer from these disorders, in the mistaken belief that they eat healthier and feel "lighter". In the absence of a proven (diagnosed) lactose intolerance, it is advisable to consume milk and its derivatives in order not to deprive yourself of the nutrients contained in them. Eliminating dairy products and cheeses from the diet, in the absence of reasons ascertained by the doctor, in fact, risks depriving the body of essential nutrients, such as calcium and vitamin D, without any scientifically proven advantage [21, 22].

3.9 Cane sugar is not fattening

Many believe that cane sugar is healthier than white sugar and contains fewer calories, so much so that it is more suitable for those on a diet. In reality, cane sugar has the same nutritional and caloric characteristics as refined white sugar.

3.10 Breadsticks and rusks to replace bread

These substitutes for bread very often are "fake" allies of staying in shape, because they are dry and less rich in water, but they involve a higher calorie intake than traditional bread. They also do not satisfy like a nice bite of bread and one is inclined to eat more than one should. It is therefore better to indulge in a small wholemeal sandwich, rather than throwing yourself on breadsticks to keep the calories under control. On the other hand, rusks are often considered synonymous with dietetic food, but on balance compared to bread, they contain on average 100-150 kcal more per hundred grams, due to the higher lipid content necessary for optimal roasting.

3.11 The "enemy": gluten

The boom in the gluten-free market, which is associated with many other "free" foods, has led to the demonization of gluten, which we know should only be avoided by celiacs and by those who have demonstrated a gluten sensitivity (about 2% of Italian population). All the others who, without clinical indication, choose to completely remove gluten from the diet, are wrong! In fact, on the nutritional level they renounce to good vegetable proteins, exposing themselves to the onset of other symptoms and diseases of the intestine, such as dysbiosis, that is, alterations of the intestinal flora, with impoverishment of the microbiome which is one of our best allies for health.

3.12 Is white flour a poison?

Some say that it would hurt, because of its high glycemic index, it is deprived of nutrients and even bleached. At least in Italy, bleaching flour is prohibited and no one, of course, eats it raw or feeds almost exclusively on flour. It must be taken alternately or together with other foods, which integrate its nutritional value and make meals balanced. At the same time, there is a campaign to sanctify good wholemeal flour, which has pluses but also some contraindications, especially for children, because there are substances in the bran (the grain kernel) that can hinder the absorption of minerals such as calcium and iron. Excessive use of wholemeal flours may have some contraindications even for adults.

In "dressed" cereals (wheat, barley, rice, etc.), which require dehusking to obtain a refined product, the external part is the one that is in contact with all the pesticides and fertilizers in the field, and whatever product that does not decay is deposited right on the husk. Therefore, wholemeal products should preferably be organic, that is, with a low use of chemical treating agents.

3.13 Pineapple burns fat

This is also a rumor. The pineapple has alleged fat-burning properties, thanks to the presence of an enzyme, bromelain, which, however, is contained in the core of the pineapple, the same that is eliminated with special tools, so almost no one eats it. In any case, even when ingested, its action is to promote the digestion of proteins and not the neutralization of calories and fats.

3.14 Bananas are the richest food in potassium

This myth is to be attributed first to Björn Borg, a famed tennis player who, during a final, continued to eat bananas, between one set and another, winning. Then, tennis player Michael Chang, who became famous for defeating Ivan Lendl in the memorable final of Roland Garros 1989, introduced the habit of eating bananas during breaks between sets. Bananas are certainly rich in potassium and also have the advantage of being easy to consume, but at the top of the list of foods richer in potassium raw spinach appears first, followed by rocket and raw sprouts. Bananas are placed in ninth place, far away from the "medal zone". Among fresh fruit, kiwis firmly hold the leadership.

3.15 Some fake news that have been identified and clarified by the Italian National Institute of Health

3.15.1 In case of diarrhea, eat "bland"

In the case of acute gastroenteritis, it is advisable to follow some indications that cannot be reduced to a generic one: eat "white" (usually white rice). Surely the first rule is hydration. Diarrheal discharges cause loss of a lot of fluids and, more likely, sick people don't really want to eat but rather drink and, depending on the season, one can drink cold or hot. In the case of diarrhea of infectious origin, especially in children, immediate treatment has always been based on prolonged fasting or *bland* diets, meaning light and easy digestible foods to avoid burdening the digestive system, while ensuring the minimum nutrients. The diet thus administered involves the elimination of milk (which paradoxically is white!), of foods rich in fiber, in order not to increase intestinal motility too much, and the reduction of foods with high energy values such as sweets. The Italian Society of Pediatrics (SIP) [23] states that restrictive diets have not proved useful. In the case of acute gastroenteritis, the normal rules of healthy eating can be followed, and nutrition can resume as soon as the appetite improves. It is very important to ensure good rehydration with proper fluid intake, as intestinal infections can more easily cause dehydration in children (especially in infants). Meals should be small and frequent with a progressive increase in caloric intake. It is good to avoid foods with high sugar content which can make diarrhea worse, but these should always be limited, even in the absence of gastrointestinal problems!

3.15.2 Coffee harms the liver

Not true. On the contrary, several scientific studies show that a moderate consumption of coffee can even have beneficial and protective effects.

A healthy liver is essential for the well-being of our body: it helps cleanse the blood by eliminating the harmful substances produced by our body; secretes bile, which is used to break down the fat contained in food, promoting its absorption; stores glucose so that it can be used when we need energy quickly. It is often thought that there is a negative correlation between coffee and the onset of liver cirrhosis, the fearful chronic inflammation of the liver, which is difficult to treat, and which can lead to cancer. In recent years, many studies have tried to understand the relationship between coffee consumption and liver health.

In the past, drinking coffee was considered a bad habit, like drinking alcohol or smoking. In 1991, the World Health Organization, on the basis of research and scientific knowledge of the time, included coffee in the list of substances defined as "possibly carcinogenic to humans". In 2016, the IARC determined that there is insufficient evidence to define coffee as a "possibly carcinogenic" substance to humans [24]. The negative relationship between coffee consumption and the onset of liver damage has not been confirmed. On the contrary, coffee is said to be an excellent protector against liver cirrhosis [25]. In addition, scientific evidence has accumulated over time demonstrating that not only coffee is not harmful (except in subjects with some pathologies) but that, if consumed in moderate doses of 2-3 cups a day, it can represent a good source of antioxidants. But be careful not to think that a few cups of coffee are enough to reduce the risk of liver damage. To keep our liver healthy, it is very important to reduce the consumption of alcohol, cigarette smoking and to follow a balanced and varied diet along with regular exercise. Furthermore, primary liver tumors are largely avoidable both with the hepatitis B virus vaccine and by eradicating the hepatitis C virus. Finally, it is essential to take medications only after consulting your doctor and, in any case, never abuse them [26].

3.15.3 Is a refreezing defrosted product harmful?

Not if the defrosted product has undergone cooking. It is therefore possible to defrost, cook and refreeze a product. In case of defrosted product due to lack of electricity, or due to inattention, refreezing the product itself without cooking it is risky.

The defrosted product, without the protection of the cold as a conservation practice, risks becoming contaminated with bacteria or viruses that were originally present in the raw food. Freezing food at –18 °C stops microbial development but does not kill bacteria or viruses. With defrosting, the bacteria present can regain their vitality and, if time and temperature conditions allow, they can multiply exponentially enough to reach quantities that are harmful to health. With cooking, most of the microorganisms that may be present are inactivated. Defrosted and cooked food is, so to speak, a *new food* capable of being frozen again. The correct way to defrost does not concern food safety but it is important to maintain the organoleptic conditions of the product, depending on the size of the food. Defrosting can be skipped altogether with food that goes directly from the freezer to the stove top or oven. The faster it is cooked, the less nutrients are lost in the process.

3.15.4 Is heating or cooking food in the microwave oven dangerous? False!

Cooking in the microwave oven does not alter the food and does not cause cancer [27]. Microwave ovens heat food thanks to the action of radiofrequency radiation, radio waves with wavelengths ranging from 1 mm to 30 cm (about 12 cm), with a low amount of energy. This is the mechanism of action of the microwave: the microwaves are absorbed by the molecules of water and fat which, thanks to the energy received, are able to vibrate: the molecular friction caused by rubbing generates heat and the heat in turn cooks the food. It is clear from all this that food does not absorb radioactivity because cooking is not based on a radioactive action that cooks the food but the application of principles of physics. In a microwave oven, the heating rate depends on the power of the oven and the water content, density and quantity of food to be heated. Microwave energy does not penetrate well into thicker parts of the food, resulting in uneven cooking. Food cooked in a microwave oven is safe and has the same nutritional value as food cooked in a traditional oven. The main difference between these two cooking methods is certainly the cooking speed. Microwaves penetrate deeper into the food thus reducing cooking time.

3.15.5 Vitamin supplements are not always healthy

Vitamins or vital amines are essential substances for life, therefore essential for our body, which does not know how to produce them by itself and therefore must be taken with food. If the introduction is insufficient then there is a deficiency called "vitamin deficiency" [28]. Thanks to this important role, vitamins generally enjoy the reputation of substances that "can only do good", and the consumption of vitamin supplements is spreading more and more. For this reason, excessive consumption of vitamin supplements is now considered normal and harmless. But this can lead to even serious diseases, called hypervitaminosis. Humanity has been plagued for a long time by diseases caused by avitaminosis, without knowing what caused them [29]. Starting in the late 1700s, vitamins were progressively identified precisely by observing that the introduction of some foods and substances eliminated diseases whose cause was not previously understood. For example, in 1753 the English navy doctor James Lind was the first to understand that scurvy, a very serious disease that at the time decimated the crews of ships engaged in long commercial or exploratory voyages, was cured by giving the sailors lemon or lime juice. However, it was only in 1932 that the "anti-scurvy" substance was isolated and chemically identified, receiving the names of ascorbic acid or vitamin C. In 1937 it was discovered that pellagra was caused by the deficiency of a substance now known as vitamin B3. Pellagra is a very serious disease that for a long time have afflicted poor populations of Northern Italy, whose diet was based exclusively on polenta (maize-meal or corn-meal) because there was no wheat flour. Wheat, in fact, unlike corn, contains good quantities of vitamin B3.

While vitamin deficiencies still afflict the poor regions of the world today, in the West they have now practically disappeared, except for the rare cases in which a disease can prevent their absorption, or if a particularly unbalanced diet is followed, or in cases of need increased, as happens in pregnancy. The consumption of vitamin supplements is therefore superfluous in healthy individuals who eat a varied diet. Not everyone knows, however, that excessive consumption of vitamins can lead to diseases, called hypervitaminosis, which can sometimes have very serious consequences [30]. The most frequent hypervitaminosis occurs by taking in excess the fat-soluble vitamins A, D, E or K. While some vitamins, such as C and B, are soluble in water, if in excess they are rapidly eliminated in the urine, vitamins A, D, E and K, which are not water soluble due to their chemical nature, are stored in the liver and body fat, and are eliminated very slowly. The symptoms linked to hypervitaminosis are variable and substantially depend on which vitamin accumulates. In case of hypervitaminosis A there is headache, vomiting and lethargy, with premature ossification or malformations, in the child and fetus, respectively. In excess of vitamin D there is an increase in calcium levels in the blood, with thirst, abdominal pain and fatigue, up to more severe cases of alterations in the state of wakefulness. Hypervitaminosis E is not toxic but can lead to intestinal disorders. Excess of vitamin K is rarer but can cause hot flashes, thrombosis and anemia. Taking excessive doses of these vitamins through food is extremely difficult if not impossible: most of the reported cases of hypervitaminosis are due to excessive consumption of supplements. It is therefore good to always keep in mind that vitamin supplements must not be taken indiscriminately and without a real need, and that it is advisable to always inform our doctor of all the supplements we take or have our children take [31, 32].

3.15.6 Cinnamon to treat diabetes

It is a full-blown fake from which people should distance themselves. No food can replace a drug and that is true for cinnamon as well. Adding cinnamon powder to the foods we consume can make them more palatable, but there is no scientifically valid evidence that this habit helps fight diabetes [33].

Cinnamon, a spice made from the bark of the homonymous plant, is considered by some to have beneficial properties, presumably by virtue of some antioxidants of which it is particularly rich. The use of this spice as a food supplement has very ancient origins in Chinese and traditional medicine. Even today it is sometimes recommended to use it in case of gastrointestinal problems, against bacterial infections.

Indeed, studies have been conducted to ascertain a possible action of cinnamon on blood glucose levels [34, 35] but, contrary to what seemed to indicate the preliminary studies of a few years ago, recent studies, carried out on a greater number of people, have provided conflicting results regarding the effect of cinnamon intake on blood glucose levels (blood sugar) [36]. In addition, there is no indication of specific doses and duration of administration of it so that cinnamon intake is effective. At the moment, therefore, there is no solid scientific basis to support the systematic use of cinnamon-based preparations to treat diabetes [37, 38]. This disease, therefore, must be treated with established therapies, according to the indications of the attending physician.

REFERENCES

1. European Food Safety Authority (EFSA). Scientific Opinion on the substantiation of health claims related to water and maintenance of normal physical and cognitive function (ID 1102,1209,1294,1331), maintenance of normal thermoregulation (ID 1208) and "basic requirement of all living things" (ID 1207) pursuant to Article 13(1) of Regulation (EC) No 1924/2006. EFSA Journal 2011; 9(4): 2075.
2. Italian Ministry of Health. Water and diet.
3. Italian National Research Institute for Food and Nutrition (INRAN). Drink plenty of water every day. Guidelines for a healthy Italian food habits, 2003.
4. World Health Organization (WHO). Guidelines for drink-

ing-water quality, 4th edition, incorporating the 1st addendum. 2017.
5. Italian Ministry of Health. The checks on the waters.
6. Italian Ministry of Health. The quality of the water distributed in Europe and Italy.
7. Italian National Research Institute on Food and Nutrition (INRAN). Drink plenty of water every day. Guidelines for healthy Italian food habits, 2003. Scientific Opinion on Dietary reference values for water. EFSA Journal 2010; 8(3): 1459.
8. Legislative Decree 23 June 2003, n. 181. Implementation of Directive 2000/13 / EC concerning the labeling and presentation of food products, as well as the relative advertising (OJ no. 167 of 21 July 2003).
9. Italian Ministry of Health. Water contamination and potential risks.
10. World Health Organization (WHO). Drinking water. 2006.
11. World Health Organization (WHO). Nutrients in drinking water. 2005.
12. IARC Monographs. Evaluation of consumption of red meat and processed meat, Volume 114.
13. Bouvard V, Loomis D, Guyton KZ, Grosse Y, El Ghissassi F, Benbrahim-Tallaa L, Guha N, Mattock H, Straif K; International Agency for Research on Cancer Monograph Working Group. Carcinogenicity of consumption of red and processed meat. Lancet Oncol 2015; 16(16): 1599-600.
14. Norat T, Scoccianti C, Boutron-Ruault M-C, Anderson A, Berrino F, Cecchini M, Espina C, Key T, Leitzmann M, Powers H, Wiseman M, Romieu I. European Code against Cancer 4th Edition: Diet and cancer. Cancer Epidemiol 2015; 39 Suppl 1: S56-66.
15. Diallo A, Deschasaux M, Latino-Martel P, Hercberg S, Galan P, Fassier P, Allès B, Guéraud F, Pierre FH, Touvier M. Red and processed meat intake and cancer risk: Results from the prospective NutriNet-Santé cohort study. Int J Cancer 2018; 142(2): 230-7.
16. World Cancer Research Found and America Institute for Cancer Research – CUP (Continuous Update Project) Diet, nutrition, physical activity and colorectal cancer, 2017
17. Farvid MS, Stern MC, Norat T, Sasazuki S, Vineis P, Weijenberg MP, Wolk A, Wu K, Stewart BW, Cho E. Consumption of red and processed meat and breast cancer incidence: A systematic review and meta-analysis of prospective studies. Int J Cancer 2018; 143(11): 2787-99.
18. Crippa A, Larsson SC, Discacciati A, Wolk A, Orsini N. Red and processed meat consumption and risk of bladder cancer: a dose-response meta-analysis of epidemiological studies. Eur J Nutr 2018; 57(2): 689-701.
19. Deng Y, Misselwitz B, Dai N, Fox M. Lactose Intolerance in Adults: Biological Mechanism and Dietary Management. Nutrients 2015; 7(9): 8020-35.
20. Wilt TJ, Shaukat A, Shamliyan T, Taylor BC, MacDonald R, Tacklind J, Rutks I, Schwarzenberg SJ, Kane RL, Levitt M. Lactose intolerance and health. Evid Rep Technol Assess (Full Rep) 2010; (192):1-410.
21. Kanis JA, Johansson H, Oden A, De Laet C, Johnell O, Eisman JA, Mc Closkey E, Mellstrom D, Pols H, Reeve J, Silman A. A meta-analysis of milk intake and fracture risk: low utility for case finding. Osteoporos Int 2005; 16(7): 799-804.
22. Lomer MC, Parkes GC, Sanderson JD. Review article: lactose intolerance in clinical practice--myths and realities. Aliment Pharmacol Ther 2008; 27(2): 93-103.
23. Italian Society of Pediatrics (SIP). Illness of the month: acute gastroenteritis.
24. Loomis D, Guyton KZ, Grosse Y, Lauby-Secretan B, El Ghissassi F, Bouvard V, Benbrahim-Tallaa L, Guha N, Mattock H, Straif K; International Agency for Research on Cancer Monograph Working Group. Carcinogenicity of drinking coffee, mate, and very hot beverages. Lancet Oncol 2016; 17(7): 877-8.
25. Bravi F, Bosetti C, Tavani A, Bagnardi V, Gallus S, Negri E, Franceschi S, La Vecchia C. Coffee drinking and hepatocellular carcinoma risk: a meta-analysis. Hepatology 2007; 46(2): 430-5.
26. Larsson SC, Wolk A. Coffee consumption and risk of liver cancer: a meta-analysis. Gastroenterology 2007; 132 (5): 1740-5.
27. World Health Organization (WHO). Electromagnetic fields & public health: microwave ovens. 2007.
28. EpiCentro (ISS). Vitamines. www.epicentro.iss.it
29. The James Lind Library. www.jameslindlibrary.org
30. Svirbely JL, Szent-Györgyi A. The chemical nature of vitamin C. Biochem J 1932; 26(3): 865-70.
31. Elvehjem CA, Madden RJ, Strong FM, Wooley DW. The isolation and identification of the anti-black tongue factor. 1937. J Biol Chem 2002;277(34): e22.
32. Manson JE, Bassuk SS. Vitamin and Mineral Supplements: What Clinicians Need to Know. JAMA 2018; 319(9): 859-60.
33. Khan A, Safdar M, Ali Khan MM, Khattak KN, Anderson RA. Cinnamon improves glucose and lipids of people with type 2 diabetes. Diabetes Care 2003; 26(12): 3215-8.
34. Baker WL, Gutierrez-Williams G, White CM, Kluger J, Coleman CI. Effect of cinnamon on glucose control and lipid parameters. Diabetes Care 2008; 31(1): 41-3.
35. Davis PA, Yokoyama W. Cinnamon intake lowers fasting blood glucose: meta-analysis. J Med Food 2011; 14(9): 884-9.
36. Allen RW, Schwartzman E, Baker WL, Coleman CI, Phung OJ. Cinnamon use in type 2 diabetes: an updated systematic review and meta-analysis. Ann Fam Med 2013; 11(5): 452-9.
37. Ranasinghe P, Jayawardana R, Galappaththy P, Constantine GR, de Vas GN, Katulanda P. Efficacy and safety of "true" cinnamon (Cinnamomum zeylanicum) as a pharmaceutical agent in diabetes: a systematic review and meta-analysis. Diabet Med 2012; 29(12): 1480-92.
38. Talaei B, Amouzegar A, Sahranavard S, Hedayati M, Mirmiran P, Azizi F. Effects of Cinnamon Consumption on Glycemic Indicators, Advanced Glycation End Products, and Antioxidant Status in Type 2 Diabetic Patients. Nutrients 2017; 9(9): 991.

4 Food safety

Paola Del Giacomo and Roberto Cauda

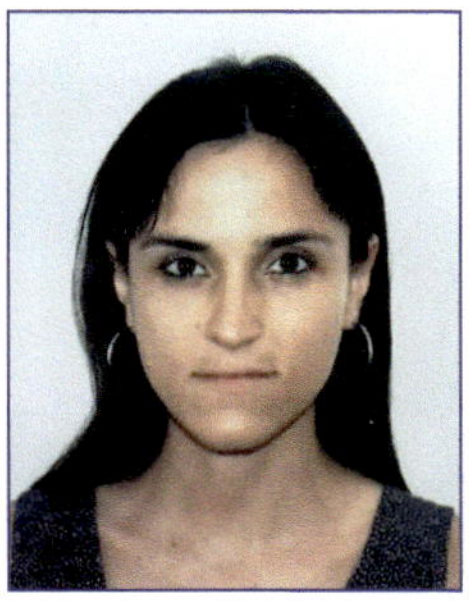

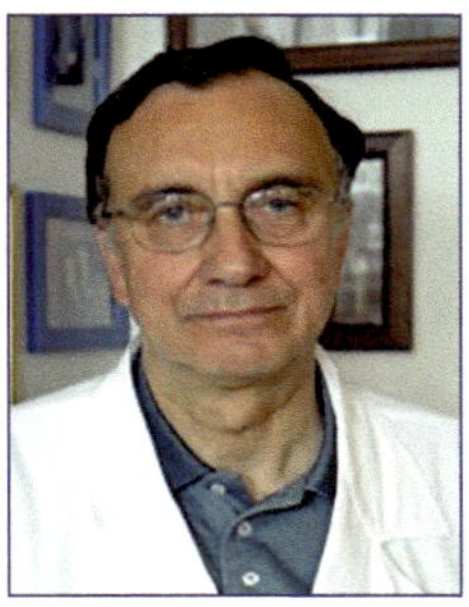

4.1 Introduction

Currently each year, an estimated 600 million people worldwide (almost 1 in 10) get sick eating contaminated food and approximately 420,000 die, with a much higher loss in terms of healthy life years or Disability-Adjusted Life Years (DALYs). Children under 5 years of age are among the most affected by this problem [1]. Access to safe food is a key factor to sustaining life and promoting good health. Improving food safety is also crucial in achieving Sustainable Development Goals. Furthermore, the right to food is protected in Article 25 of the Universal Declaration of Human Rights [2].

The Second International Conference on Nutrition, held in Rome in November 2014, reiterated the importance of food safety in achieving better human nutrition. Sharp geographic, economic and sociocultural inequalities persist between developed and developing countries and between urban and rural settings. Socioeconomic status of the population in poorer economies is one of the major determinants for the availability of safe food to the vulnerable population [3].

In this context, most Foodborne Diseases (FBDs) develop as a result of consuming fresh, perishable foods sold in informal markets and with poor hygiene control, which is a risk for human health. Despite the strong trend of the intensification of agricultural production, so far agro-industrial production and modern retail have not demonstrated clear advantages in food safety and disease control [4].

In developing countries, lack of food and water hygiene has been linked not only to the transmission of a variety of infectious diseases, but also to the low growth outcomes in children and to the slow social and economic development of these countries, because of their huge impact on human capital and productivity [5]. However, in developed countries, despite higher standards of living, large-scale production and the preparation and distribution of food could represent a higher risk for epidemics caused by pathogens of gastrointestinal origin [6].

Globalization of the food supply chain can lead to the introduction of infectious pathogens into new geographical areas. Travelers, refugees and immigrants

Paola Del Giacomo, MD
Infectious Diseases Unit,
Fondazione Policlinico Universitario Agostino Gemelli IRCCS, Rome, Italy

Email: paola.delgiacomo@policlinicogemelli.it

Roberto Cauda, MD
Professor of Infectious Diseases
Chairman of the Department of Healthcare Surveillance and Bioethics
Section of Infectious Diseases
Università Cattolica del Sacro Cuore, Rome, Italy

Email: roberto.cauda@unicatt.it

as well may be exposed to unfamiliar risks in new environments. In many countries, as people increasingly consume food prepared outside the home, growing numbers are potentially exposed to the hazards of poor hygiene in commercial foodservice settings [7].

4.2 Definitions

Food security has been defined at the World Food Summit of 1996 as: "When all people at all times have access to sufficient, safe, nutritious food to maintain a healthy and active life". Food safety or food hygiene refers to the conditions and practices that preserve the quality of food to prevent contamination and foodborne illnesses throughout the entire food supply chain, from primary production to consumption. In developed countries, despite well-detailed guidelines for proper food preparation and handling [8, 9], there are many opportunities for food contamination along the food chain: during production, processing, distribution or preparation.

The five key principles of food hygiene, according to World Health Organization, are so defined:

- **keep clean**: washing hands, sanitizing surfaces and protecting kitchen areas from pathogens spread by insects, pests and other animals;
- **separate raw and cooked foods to prevent contamination of cooked foods.** Food mixing is also particularly hazardous, because a pathogen present in a single one of the components may contaminate the whole batch. For example, unpasteurized fruit juices, hamburgers or omelets can contain fruit, meat or eggs, respectively, deriving from hundreds of harvests or animals which may contain pathogens;
- **cook foods** (especially meat, poultry, eggs and seafood) **for the appropriate length of time and at the appropriate temperature to kill pathogens.** It must be mentioned that heating food to an internal temperature above 160 °F (or 78 °C), for even a few seconds, is sufficient to kill almost all parasites, viruses or bacteria. *Clostridium* bacteria that produce spores are only killed at temperatures above boiling (that is why canned foods must be cooked to a high temperature under pressure as part of the canning process). Boiling temperatures are not sufficient to inactivate the staphylococcal enterotoxin and *Bacillus cereus* toxin cereulide. For fresh produce that is consumed raw, there are few options for reducing pathogens after harvest, and thus food safety management should begin at the farm long before harvest begins;
- **keep food at the safe temperatures** as most microorganism can multiply between 41 °F and 140 °F (or 5 °C and 60 °C). Many bacterial microbes need to multiply to a large number in the food to cause disease but, as an example, given optimal conditions of warmth and moisture as well as of a supply of nutrients, one bacterium that reproduces by dividing itself every half hour is able to produce 17 million progeny in 12 hours. As a result, lightly contaminated food left out overnight can be highly infectious by the next day. If the food is refrigerated promptly, the bacteria will not multiply because refrigerating temperatures generally preserve bacteria in a non-replicating state. Unfortunately, some pathogenic bacteria, such as *Listeria monocytogenes* and *Yersinia enterocolitica*, are able to grow at refrigeration temperatures. Keeping cooked food piping hot before serving is another rule of food hygiene. However, it is important to mention that in several countries refrigeration of foods is either logistically absent or unaffordable, making the safe and correct storage of food impossible and increasing the risk of foodborne infectious diseases;
- **use safe water and raw materials.** Water itself can become the main source of contamination. Raw foods of animal origin (e.g., raw meat and poultry, raw eggs, unpasteurized milk and raw shellfish) are the most likely to be contaminated. Washing and peeling can reduce the risks. High salt, sugar or acid concentration levels naturally prevent bacterial growth; thus, salted meats, jams and pickled vegetables are traditionally preserved foods [8].

Although the contamination of food products with pathogens can occur along any link of the food chain, it must be underlined that the scope and size of produce-associated outbreaks tend to decrease the closer the point of contamination is to the time of consumption [10].

4.3 Foodborne diseases: epidemiological and clinical aspects

Researchers have identified more than 250 FBDs and their spectrum is constantly changing. Unfortunately, precise estimates of the burden of FBDs are complicated. Major limitations include different definitions of acute diarrheal illness used in studies, data gaps and the uncertainty around the proportion of diseases that are foodborne: the reported outbreaks of food-associated illness for which a specific source was identified are a small fraction of all foodborne illnesses (0.05%) [11].

Moreover, a consequence of the current rapid rate

of food globalization is that a single food product may contain ingredients from many different parts of the world. Such diversity makes tracing the exact source of contamination even more challenging and despite the number of resources available for investigation of FBD outbreaks, few are directed at developing countries.

One of the new challenges in the matter of FBDs is indeed the development of new diagnostic techniques. Culture-independent diagnostic tests (CIDTs) can be included in the diagnostic armamentarium recently introduced into the field of FBDs. Fast and easy to use, CIDTs detect some illnesses that would otherwise be missed (i.e., *Cyclospora*, *Yersinia*, *Vibrio*, and non-O157 Shiga toxin-producing *Escherichia coli* – STEC). These tests do not need a laboratory to be performed. According to the Center for Disease Control (CDC), the overall number of the most frequent foodborne infections diagnosed by CIDTs increased 96% in 2017 when compared to the average diagnosed during 2014-2016. Compared to the culture-based methods, CIDTs do not identify the serotype (the specific kind of microorganism based on its surface structure) that cause infections [12, 13].

Norovirus is the leading cause of foodborne illness causing 125 million cases worldwide, while *Campylobacter spp.* causes 96 million cases of foodborne illnesses. Of all foodborne diseases, diarrheal and invasive infections due to non-typhoidal *Salmonella enterica* infections resulted in the highest burden, causing 4.07 million DALYs. Regionally, DALYs per population are highest in the African region followed by the South East Asian region [14].

Norovirus infection causes an acute gastrointestinal illness, usually with more vomiting than diarrhea, that generally resolves within three days. Norovirus, unlike many foodborne pathogens, does not have an animal reservoir but spreads from one infected person to another, often through contaminated food, water or environmental surfaces. Epidemic outbreaks can happen when infected people working in restaurant kitchens spread the virus through their hands while preparing sandwiches or salads.

Campylobacter spp. are bacterial pathogens that live in the intestines of healthy birds, commonly found on raw poultry meat. Eating undercooked chicken, or other food that has been contaminated with juices dripping from raw chicken, is the most frequent source of infection. It causes fever, diarrhea and abdominal pain. Guillain-Barré syndrome can complicate the infection.

Among others, *Salmonella spp.*, *S. enteritidis* and *S. typhimurium* are of major concern. Salmonellosis typically includes fever, diarrhea and abdominal cramps and, in persons with poor underlying health or a weakened immune system, it can be responsible for life-threatening bloodstream infections.

Norovirus, *Clostridium botulinum*, *Salmonella* and verocytotoxin-producing *Escherichia coli* (VTEC) are more frequently documented in industrialized rather than in developing countries. Enterotoxigenic *Escherichia coli* (ETEC), enteropathogenic *Escherichia coli* (EPEC), *Shigella*, *Vibrio cholerae* and parasites are the main scourges in developing countries. Epidemics are generally due to *Shigella dysenteriae* serotype 1 and *Vibrio cholerae*.

A bacterial pathogen is often identified with bloody diarrhea. *Shigella* is the most common one to be isolate (49%), followed by *Campylobacter* (20%), *Salmonella* (19%) and *E. coli* O157:H7 (8%). The latter is involved in the development of hemolytic-uremic syndrome [15].

Other clinically relevant foodborne infections, with various clinical presentations, can be caused by bacteria which produce toxins such as *Clostridium perfringens*, a spore-forming gram-positive bacterium that can contaminate beef or poultry, especially large roasts and gravy, along with dried or precooked foods. It is an anaerobe, i.e., can survive in conditions with very low oxygen levels or in the absence of oxygen, and is responsible for diseases characterized by intense abdominal cramps and diarrhea. The type C strains of *C. perfringens* produce a beta toxin, which can cause hemorrhagic necrosis of the jejunum, called enteritis necroticans or pigbel, that usually occurs in resource-limited countries (particularly Papua New Guinea) following pork consumption. *Staphylococcus aureus* can grow in some foods and produce a toxin that causes intense vomiting within a few hours after ingestion of contaminated products.

Foodborne botulism caused by *Clostridium botulinum* is due to the ingestion of food (usually home-canned foods such as fruits, vegetables and fish) already contaminated by botulinum toxin, which is responsible for a severe paralytic syndrome [16].

Viruses that are known foodborne threats include enteroviruses, adenovirus, hepatitis E virus, tick-borne encephalitis virus and astroviruses, among others. Viruses emerging as foodborne pathogens are a result of modern agricultural practices which can concentrate livestock and bring them in contact with wild animals. Examples of such emerged viruses are influenza, the Nipah virus and coronaviruses, such as Severe Acute Respiratory Syndrome (SARS) coronavirus (SARS-CoV), Middle East Respiratory Syndrome (MERS) coronavirus (MERS-CoV) and the most recent SARS-CoV-2. While there is currently no evidence that food is a likely source or route of transmission of SARS-CoV-2, it should be noted that, at the beginning of the outbreak, about two-thirds of the initial cases of pneumonia due to SARS-CoV-2 presented an epidemiological link to the live animal and seafood market in Jianghan District, Wuhan, Hubei Province, China. It is still controversial whether the market was the origin or just a key link in the epidemic [17].

The role of bats, bush meat, rodents, pigs, cattle and poultry as reservoirs from which infectious pathogenic viruses emerge must be taken into account [18].

In the case of Ebola virus, the importance of the foodborne route of transmission to humans has been already highlighted, with the virus being transmitted through the increased hunting of "bushmeat" wildlife [19]. Among parasites, the most common foodborne diseases in the United States are due to protozoa *Cryptosporidium spp.*, *Giardia intestinalis*, *Cyclospora cayetanensis* and *Toxoplasma gondii*; roundworms such as *Trichinella spp.* and *Anisakis spp.*; and tapeworms such as *Diphyllobothrium spp.* and *Taenia spp.* [20].

4.4 Antibiotic resistance

About one in five resistant infections are caused by foodborne pathogens [21]. Although some people are at greater risk than others, no one is immune to the risk of antibiotic-resistant infections. Many of these infectious diseases result in severe illness and death and require the use of new antibiotic compounds, with increased recovery time and medical expenses.

Many antimicrobials used in breeding and agriculture are identical, or closely related, to antimicrobials used in medicine. Antimicrobials are used in food-producing animals to treat and control bacterial infections both in the presence of disease and for disease prevention. During the mid-1950s, it was discovered that small, subtherapeutic quantities of antibiotics, delivered to animals in feed, could enhance the feed-to-weight ratio for poultry, swine and beef cattle. This use, intended to increase the rate of weight gain or to improve feed efficiency, contributed to the emergence of antibiotic-resistant bacteria in food-producing animals. The misuse of antibiotics can lead to selection and dissemination of antimicrobial-resistant bacteria in food-producing animals, which can then be transmitted to humans through food and other transmission routes [22, 23]. According to data published by the Food and Drug Administration (FDA), in 2011 there were more kilograms of antibiotics sold in the United States for food-producing animals than for humans [24].

There is concern that the use of antibiotics in any setting can select for resistance in other bacteria that do not themselves cause disease but can transfer those resistant genes to bacteria that do. Historically, this transmission of genetic material and the emergence of antibiotic resistance have occurred faster from aquatic bacteria to humans than from terrestrial animal bacteria to humans [25]. In many parts of the world, fish farming is integrated with sewage of industrial wastewater or with land agriculture, as manure and other agricultural residues are commonly employed in fish feed [26].

Fish overcrowding, unhygienic measures and other manipulations in this intensive, industrial-scale production act as stressors to the fish and promote an increased use of antibiotic prophylaxis, particularly in the shrimp and carnivorous fish (such as salmon) related industries. Moreover, even though the use of growth promoting antibiotics in aquaculture has been stopped in North America and Western Europe, therapeutic treatment of fish generally occurs through the introduction of antibiotics in fish food. This results in exposure of the entire body of water to the drugs exerting selective pressure on the sediment and water microflora at distant sites, exposing wild fish and shellfish to antimicrobials.

Preventing resistant enteric infections requires a multifaceted approach. The World Health Organization (WHO) continues to highlight the urgency to fight antibiotic resistance through a holistic, intersectoral and multifaceted approach that includes the abolition of the unnecessary use of antibiotics, including those used in food production.

Guidelines on use of medically important antimicrobials in food-producing animals has been extensively delineated by the WHO, with the last edition in 2017. Recommendation number 3 of the new guidelines underlines that antibiotics should not be used as a preventive tool in the absence of disease in animals. The use of antimicrobials for disease prevention may be justified only when a veterinary professional evaluates that the hazard of the spread of a particular infectious disease is too high, if such a judgement is made on the basis of recent culture and sensitivity testing results [27, 28].

4.5 Mycotoxins

Certain types of molds naturally produce toxic compounds called mycotoxins capable of growing on numerous foodstuffs such as cereals, nuts, dried fruits and spices, penetrating deep into food not just on the surface. Toxigenic fungi and mycotoxins entered human food supplies about the time when mankind first began to cultivate crops and to store them from one season to the next.

Hundreds of different mycotoxins have been

identified so far, but about a dozen have been shown to occur in food and to exert severe effects on human health. Exposure to mycotoxins can happen either directly by eating infected food or indirectly from animals fed with contaminated feed. This problem affects both developed and developing countries [29].

The effects of some foodborne mycotoxins are acute with symptoms of severe illness appearing quickly after consumption of contaminated food products. Other mycotoxins have been linked to long-term effects on health, including cancers and immune deficiency.

For example, large doses of aflatoxins can lead to acute poisoning (aflatoxicosis) and can be life threatening, usually causing liver damage of different severity. Aflatoxins have also been shown to be genotoxic, meaning they can damage DNA and cause cancer in animal species as well as in humans. Aflatoxins are produced by certain molds (*Aspergillus flavus* and *Aspergillus parasiticus*) which grow in soil, decaying vegetation, hay and grains, oilseeds, spices (chili peppers, black pepper, coriander, turmeric and ginger), tree nuts or in the milk of animals that are fed with contaminated feed.

Patulin is a mycotoxin produced by a variety of molds, particularly *Aspergillus*, *Penicillium* and *Byssochlamys*. Major human dietary sources of patulin are apples and apple juice made from contaminated fruit. The acute symptoms in animals include liver, spleen and kidney damage and toxicity to the immune system. Gastrointestinal symptoms have been reported in humans. Patulin is considered to be genotoxic; however, a carcinogenic potential has not been demonstrated in humans so far.

Ochratoxin A is produced by several species of *Aspergillus* and *Penicillium* and is a common food-contaminating mycotoxin. Contamination of food commodities, such as cereals and cereal products, coffee beans, dry vine fruits, wine and grape juice, spices and licorice, occurs worldwide. The most sensitive and notable effect in animals is kidney damage and kidney cancer, but the toxin may also have effects on fetal development and on the immune system. The association between ochratoxin A exposure and kidney disease in humans is unclear; however, effects on kidney have been demonstrated.

Fusarium fungi are common to the soil and produce a range of different toxins, on a variety of different cereal crops. Different fusarium toxins are associated with certain types of cereal. Trichothecenes can be acutely toxic to humans, causing rapid irritation to the skin or intestinal mucosa and lead to diarrhea. Reported chronic effects in animals include the suppression of the immune system. Zearalenone (ZEN) has been shown to have hormonal, estrogenic effects and can cause infertility at high intake levels, particularly in pigs. Fumonisins have been related to esophageal cancer in humans, and to liver and kidney toxicity in animals.

These are some rules to minimize the health hazards related to mycotoxins:

- buy grains and nuts as fresh as possible;
- inspect whole grains (especially corn, sorghum, wheat, rice), dried figs and nuts for evidence of mold and discard any that look moldy, discolored or shriveled;
- avoid damaging grains before and during drying and storage, as damaged grain is more susceptible to invasion of molds;
- make sure that foods prone to mold contamination are stored properly (free of insects, dry and not too warm) and for short periods of time [30-32].

4.6 Conclusion

Despite significant advances in food science and technology as well as in consumer knowledge of safe food preparation, FBDs continue to have harmful consequences in both developed and developing countries. It is an open question whether future food safety concerns will shift priorities given the imperatives to supply sufficient food [9].

Governments should make food safety a public health priority, establishing and implementing effective policies and regulatory frameworks ensuring that food producers and suppliers, along the whole food chain, operate responsibly and supply safe food to consumers.

In addition to these measures, a crucial element for ensuring a correct food security policy is the education of the consumers about safe food handling and storage which should reflect the different cultural and geosocial realities on the ground, such as unreliable electricity for refrigeration, distance to and from markets, climate.

REFERENCES

1. https://www.who.int/news-room/fact-sheets/detail/food-safety
2. http://www.un.org/en/universal-declaration-human-rights/index.html
3. Akhtar S, Sarker MR, Hossain A. Microbiological food safety: a dilemma of developing societies. Crit Rev Microbiol 2014; 40(4): 348-59.
4. Grace D. Food Safety in Low and Middle Income Coun-

tries. Int J Environ Res Public Health 2015; 12(9): 10490-507.
5. Del Giacomo P, Trecarichi EM, Cocconcelli PS, Cauda R. Safety of water and food: a key factor for development. In: Bertoni G. (ed.). World Food Production: Facing Growing Needs and Limited Resources. Milan: Vita e Pensiero; 2015: 27-53.
6. Scallan E. Activities, achievements, and lessons learned during the first 10 years of the Foodborne Diseases Active Surveillance Network: 1996-2005. Clin Infect Dis 2007; 44(5): 718-25.
7. https://www.who.int/foodsafety/publications/foodborne_disease/contents_intro.pdf
8. https://www.who.int/foodsafety/publications/consumer/en/5keys_en.pdf?ua=1
9. Kang HJ, Lee MW, Hwang IK, Kim JW. Development of Safe Food Handling Guidelines for Korean Consumers. J Food Prot 2015; 78(8): 1541-6.
10. Byrd-Bredbenner C, Cohn MN, Farber JM, Harris LJ, Roberts T, Salin V, Singh M, Jaferi A, Sperber WH. Food safety considerations for innovative nutrition solutions. Ann N Y Acad Sci 2015;1347: 29-44.
11. Painter JA, Hoekstra RM, Ayers T, Tauxe RV, Braden CR, Angulo FJ, Griffin PM. Attribution of foodborne illnesses, hospitalizations, and deaths to food commodities by using outbreak data, United States, 1998-2008. Emerg Infect Dis 2013; 19(3): 407-15.
12. Marder EP, Cieslak PR, Cronquist AB, Dunn J, Lathrop S, Rabatsky-Ehr T, Ryan P, Smith K, Tobin-D'Angelo M, Vugia DJ, Zansky S, Holt KG, Wolpert BJ, Lynch M, Tauxe R, Geissler AL. Incidence and Trends of Infections with Pathogens Transmitted Commonly Through Food and the Effect of Increasing Use of Culture-Independent Diagnostic Tests on Surveillance - Foodborne Diseases Active Surveillance Network, 10 U.S. Sites, 2013-2016. MMWR Morb Mortal Wkly Rep 2017; 66(15): 397-403.
13. https://www.cdc.gov/foodnet/reports/prelim-data-intro-2017.html
14. Kirk MD, Pires SM, Black RE, Caipo M, Crump JA, Devleesschauwer B, Döpfer D, Fazil A, Fischer-Walker CL, Hald T, Hall AJ, Keddy KH, Lake RJ, Lanata CF, Torgerson PR, Havelaar AH, Angulo FJ. World Health Organization Estimates of the Global and Regional Disease Burden of 22 Foodborne Bacterial, Protozoal, and Viral Diseases, 2010: A Data Synthesis. PLoS Med 2015; 12(12):e1001921.
15. Talan D, Moran GJ, Newdow M, Ong S, Mower WR, Nakase JY, Pinner RW, Slutsker L, EMERGEncy ID NET Study Group. Etiology of bloody diarrhea among patients presenting to United States emergency departments: prevalence of Escherichia coli O157:H7 and other enteropathogens. Clin Infect Dis 2001; 32(4): 573-80.
16. Sobel J, Tucker N, Sulka A, McLaughlin J, Maslanka S. Foodborne botulism in the United States, 1990-2000. Emerg Infect Dis 2004; 10(9): 1606-11.
17. https://www.efsa.europa.eu/en/news/coronavirus-no-evidence-food-source-or-transmission-route
18. Kingsley DH. Emerging Foodborne and Agriculture-Related Viruses. Microbiol Spectr 2016; 4(4).
19. Tsuda Y, Caposio P, Parkins CJ, Botto S, Messaoudi I, Cicin-Sain L, Feldmann H, Jarvis MA. A replicating cytomegalovirus-based vaccine encoding a single Ebola virus nucleoprotein CTL epitope confers protection against Ebola virus. PLoS Negl Trop Dis 2011; 5(8):e1275.
20. https://www.cdc.gov/foodsafety/symptoms.html
21. https://www.cdc.gov/drugresistance/threat-report-2013/pdf/ar-threats-2013-508.pdf
22. Stokstad ELR, Jukes TH. Further observations on the "Animal Protein Factor". Proc Soc Exp Biol Med 1950; 73(3): 523-28.
23. van den Bogaard AE, Stobberingh EE. Antibiotic usage in animals: impact on bacterial resistance and public health. Drugs 1999; 58(4): 589-607.
24. https://www.fda.gov/downloads/forindustry/userfees/animaldruguserfeeactadufa/ucm338170.pdf
25. Marshall BM, Levy SB. Food Animals and Antimicrobials: Impacts on Human Health. Clin Microbiol Rev 2011; 24(4): 718-33.
26. Petersen A, Andersen JS, Kaewmak T, Somsiri T, Dalsgaard A. Impact of integrated fish farming on antimicrobial resistance in a pond environment. Appl Environ Microbiol 2002; 68(12): 6036-42.
27. http://apps.who.int/iris/bitstream/handle/10665/258970/9789241550130-ng.pdf;jsessionid=F1ED6A7B1B6CCCC8BA1867B8A8985E11?sequence=1
28. Hoelzer K, Wong N, Thomas J, Talkington K, Jungman E, Coukell A. Antimicrobial drug use in food-producing animals and associated human health risks: what, and how strong, is the evidence? BMC Vet Res 2017; 13(1): 211.
29. Wagacha JM, Muthomi JW. Mycotoxin problem in Africa: current status, implications to food safety and health and possible management strategies. Int J Food Microbiol 2008; 124(1): 1-12.
30. https://www.who.int/news-room/fact-sheets/detail/mycotoxins
31. Pitt JI, Miller JD. A Concise History of Mycotoxin Research. J Agric Food Chem 2017; 65(33): 7021-33.
32. Bryden WL. Mycotoxins in the food chain: human health implications. Asia Pac J Clin Nutr 2007; 16 Suppl 1: 95-101.

SECTION 2 Food, eating and nutrition from day one

5 Role of nutrition in pregnant women

Annafranca Cavaliere, Silvia Perossini, Maria Concetta La Milia, Annalisa Vidiri, Sofia Guidi, Antonio Lanzone and Giovanni Scambia

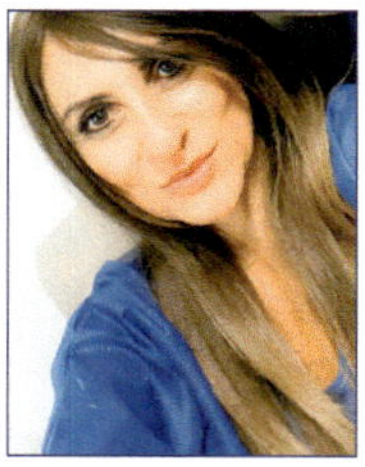

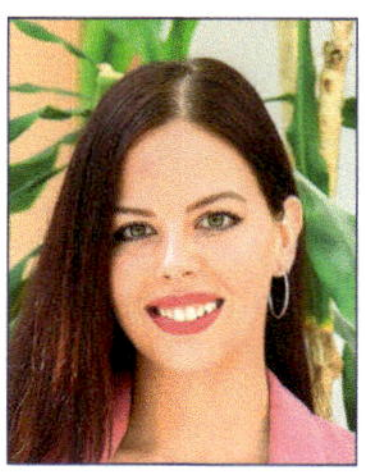

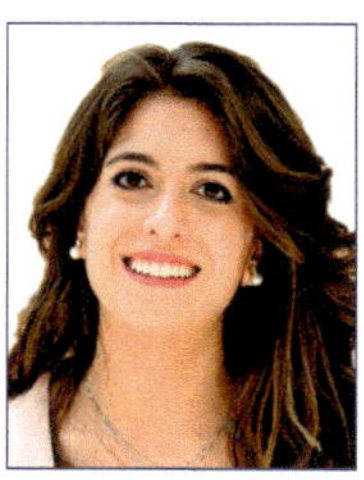

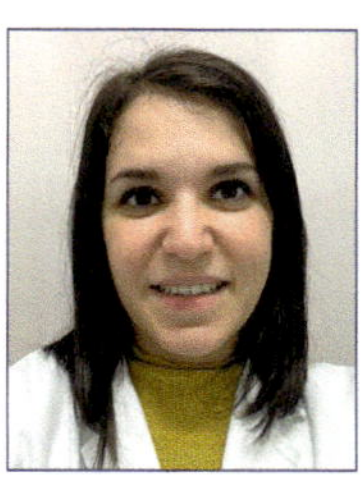

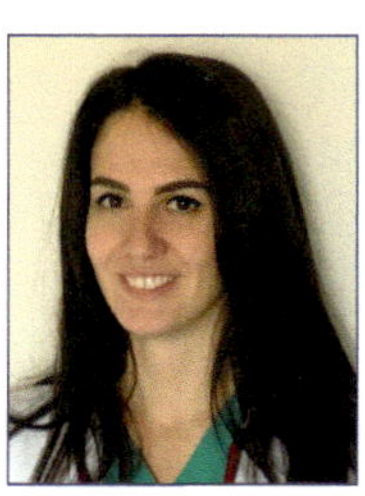

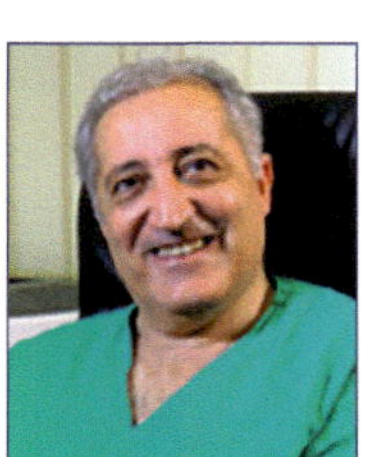

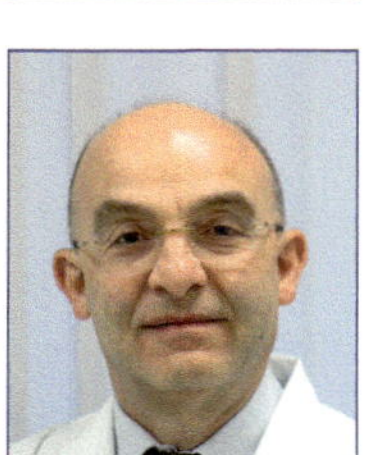

5.1 Introduction

Maternal metabolism, especially of glucose and lipids, undergoes substantial changes during pregnancy. Early gestation is characterized by an anabolic state with increased maternal fat storage and a small increase in insulin sensitivity, aimed at meeting maternal and fetal-placental nutrient demand of late gestation and lactation. Late pregnancy, instead, resembles a catabolic state, showing decreased insulin sensitivity with increased insulin resistance, resulting in increased maternal glucose and fatty acid concentrations, allowing for a greater substrate availability for fetal growth [1].

5.1.1 Glucose metabolism

Pregnancy is a "diabetogenic state" and the adaptations in glucose metabolism promote the development of the fetus while maintaining adequate maternal nutrition [2]. Basal and postprandial glucose metabolism gradually changes over the course of gestation, according to fetal-maternal needs. In non-pregnant physiological conditions, the liver produces glucose through gluconeogenesis at approximately the rate of its usage. During pregnancy, fasting glucose progressively decreases with advancing gestation due to factors such as increased plasma volume and consequent dilutive effect, increased utilization by both the fetal-

Annafranca Cavaliere, MD
Università Cattolica del Sacro Cuore, Rome, Italy

Silvia Perossini, MD
Università Cattolica del Sacro Cuore, Rome, Italy

Email: silvia.perossini@gmail.com

Maria Concetta La Milia, MD
Università Cattolica del Sacro Cuore, Rome, Italy

Annalisa Vidiri, MD
Università Cattolica del Sacro Cuore, Rome, Italy

Sofia Guidi, MD
Università Cattolica del Sacro Cuore, Rome, Italy

Antonio Lanzone, MD
Università Cattolica del Sacro Cuore, Rome, Italy

Giovanni Scambia, MD
Università Cattolica del Sacro Cuore, Rome, Italy

placental unit and the mother herself and/or inadequate production with respect to circulating glucose concentration [1].

In pregnant women with normal glucose tolerance, there are decreased fasting glucose levels and increased hepatic production of glucose, with a concomitant increase in fasting insulin. Hepatic glucose production is supposed to be suppressed by insulin. However, despite the increase in fasting insulin, hepatic glucose production is increased due to a reduction in hepatic insulin sensitivity, exacerbated by obesity, which impairs the inhibition of hepatic glucose production [1]. Studies have shown that lean pregnant women with normal glucose tolerance have a 10% reduction in insulin sensitivity during early pregnancy, reaching 30% in later phases [3]. In contrast, there is a 15% increase in insulin sensitivity in obese women in early pregnancy as compared with pre-gravid estimates, because of baseline insulin resistance [4].

Maternal insulin resistance begins in the second trimester and peaks in the third trimester. The physiologic factors responsible for the decrease in insulin sensitivity or increased resistance during pregnancy are related to the metabolic effects of several diabetogenic hormones (human placental lactogen or hPL, prolactin, progesterone, human chorionic gonadotrophin or HCG, estradiol, cortisol) and cytokines (tumor necrosis factor-alpha or TNF-α) that are elevated in the maternal circulation during gestation due to their secretion by the fetal-placental unit [5, 6].

The effect of the placental hormones on insulin sensitivity is made evident postpartum when there is a sudden decrease in insulin resistance [7].

In order to compensate for the insulin resistance state during physiological pregnancy, insulin-secreting pancreatic beta-cells undergo hyperplasia and hypertrophy, augmenting insulin secretion. If a woman's endocrine pancreatic function is impaired, and she is unable to overcome the insulin resistance associated with pregnancy, then gestational diabetes develops [2].

5.1.2 Lipid metabolism

Alterations in glucose metabolism are considered the primary metabolic adaptation of pregnancy; however, significant alterations occur in lipid metabolism as well. These changes accommodate the needs of the developing fetus, increasing triglyceride levels for the mother's energy needs, while sparing glucose for the fetus, and increasing LDL (low-density lipoprotein) cholesterol for placental steroidogenesis [2].

Modifications at the level of the liver and adipose tissue determine variations in the concentration of triglycerides, fatty acids, cholesterol and phospholipids, characterized by an initial decrease over the first eight weeks of gestation followed by an increase [8, 9]. The mechanisms responsible for these variations are mainly an increased synthesis of VLDL (very low-density lipoproteins) by the liver and decreased lipoprotein lipase activity, attributable to the action exerted by estrogens on the liver itself and low lipase activity due to insulin resistance [10]. All these factors lead to a decreased catabolism of adipose tissue [2].

During pregnancy, adipose tissue is increased in terms of both preperitoneal and subcutaneous fat and is primarily centrally distributed (mid-thorax to mid-thigh area) [1]. Moreover, the ratio between preperitoneal and subcutaneous fat is increased, suggesting intra-abdominal fat increase in pregnancy. Subcutaneous fat stores are an important source of calories for both the mother and the fetus during pregnancy and lactation. Instead, the increased visceral fat may relate to the reduced insulin sensitivity typical of late gestation [11, 12].

The understanding of the role of adipocytes has extensively evolved over time. Adipose tissue not only stores calories but is a metabolically active tissue playing a key role in a person's metabolism by producing cytokines and inflammatory mediators that can increase (TNF-α) or decrease (adiponectin) insulin resistance [1].

5.1.3 Protein metabolism

Pregnant women require an increased protein intake during pregnancy. Amino acids are actively transported across the placenta to fulfill the needs of the developing fetus. However, the transport of amino acids from endogenous deposits is reduced over the first trimester of gestation, indicating a reduction in proteolysis, and increasing again later in pregnancy [2].

The reduction of maternal proteolysis in the first trimester seems functional for future maternal and fetal needs. At the beginning of gestation, in fact, an increase in the lean (protein) mass occurs in the mother in relation to fetal mass. Therefore, adaptive responses of nitrogen compounds turnover and maternal body composition seem to precede the demands of the fetus [13].

During pregnancy, changes are observed in circulating amino acids levels, both during fasting and in the postprandial period, reflecting adaptation mechanisms, such as an increase in body fluids and therefore a reduction in volume distribution of amino acids [14].

The reduction of proteolysis in the first trimester may also reflect a condition of relative caloric deprivation due to the development of the fetus, which is accompanied by insulin resistance and an increase in free fatty acids that can, in turn, inhibit proteolysis [15, 16]. Maternal proteolysis returns to normal values in the third trimester, because of greater demand for amino acids by the fetus [17].

Finally, over the course of a normal pregnancy, there is an increase in concentrations of other proteins such as the alkaline phosphatase of placental origin (especially in the third trimester), transferrin and globulin-like glycoproteins. There is also an increase in acute phase proteins (such as alpha-1-antitrypsin, transferrin, ceruloplasmin) and some coagulation proteins such as fibrinogen, fibrinopeptide A and fragments of prothrombin, responsible for the hypercoagulative state of pregnancy [18].

5.1.4 Salivation, nausea, vomiting and periodontal diseases

During pregnancy, women can experience excessive salivation (sialorrhea), nausea and vomiting (hyperemesis gravidarum). Hyperemesis gravidarum is one of the most common disorders affecting the quality of life of pregnant women. Symptoms occur mainly during the first trimester with a peak between 9 and 16 weeks of gestation and resolve by the 22nd week, although in a minority of women it can last through the entire pregnancy [19]. Vomiting is usually accompanied by a sense of nausea, which can be exacerbated in cases of excessive salivation [20]. Sialorrhea can be related to hormonal changes occurring during pregnancy; progesterone and estrogens produced by the placenta may have a vasodilatory effect on the major arteries with an increased local blood flow. Saliva is altered both in quantity and composition and pH. Physiologically, it contains enzymes, immunoglobulins, cytokines, antimicrobial components and buffering agents that contribute to maintain the integrity of oral tissue. Gingival inflammation is heightened by vascular and gingival changes caused by typical hormonal variations which occur during pregnancy, affecting the immune response to bacterial plaque [21]. Pregnancy predisposes to an increased inflammation of gums, gingival bleeding, periodontal pocket inflammation and dental caries [22]. Pregnant women's susceptibility to dental caries and gingivitis is affected by change in their diet, frequent snacking due to food craving and oral health negligence and it is higher compared to their non-pregnant counterparts [23].

Moreover, it was found that women with periodontal diseases and active infections are at major risk of adverse pregnancy outcomes, such as preterm birth, preeclampsia, gestational diabetes, fetal loss and Low Birth Weight (LBW) babies [24]. Periodontitis may lead to inflammation, thus triggering the common pathway of preterm delivery including increased uterine contractility, cervical ripening and decidua/membrane activation [25]. This is probably due to an alteration of oral flora and a diffusion of bacteria into the bloodstream with the release of endotoxins and inflammatory cytokines, which can target the fetus [26]. Dental health of both mother and baby may be influenced by her diet during pregnancy [27]. It is important to educate pregnant women about dental and oral hygiene and health professionals should provide this information during preconception, prenatal and postpartum care [28, 29].

Moreover, oral cavity alterations can be worsened by gastroesophageal reflux. Its increased prevalence during pregnancy is attributable to a reduction of gastroesophageal sphincter tone, prolonged gastric emptying times and an increase in intra-abdominal pressure caused by an enlargement of the uterus.

5.2 Body mass index and weight gain

Body Mass Index (BMI) provides an estimate of body fat in males and females of any age. The World Health Organization (WHO) developed a classification that uses this statistical index to define a subject as underweight, normal weight, overweight or obese (Box 5.1).

In recent years, a global obesity epidemic has been recorded, resulting in an increasing number of

5.1 Classification and Body Mass Index (BMI) number*

- Severely underweight: BMI < 16.5 kg/m^2
- Underweight: BMI < 18.5 kg/m^2
- Normal weight: BMI ≥ 18.5 to 24.9 kg/m^2
- Overweight: BMI ≥ 25 to 29.9 kg/m^2
- Obesity: BMI ≥ 30 kg/m^2
  - class I: BMI 30 to 34.9 kg/m^2
  - class II: BMI 35 to 39.9 kg/m^2
  - class III: BMI ≥ 40 kg/m^2 (also referred to as severe, extreme or massive obesity)
- Asian and South Asian population
  - Overweight: BMI between 23 and 24.9 kg/m^2
  - Obesity: BMI > 25 kg/m^2

* Adapted from [53].

Table 5.1 Recommendations for gestational weight gain during pregnancy*

Recommendation	*Pre-pregnancy weight*			
	Underweight	*Normal weight*	*Overweight*	*Obese*
Body Mass Index (kg/m^2)	< 18.5	18.5-24.9	25-29.9	≥ 30
Total weight gain range (kg)	12.5-18	11.5-16	7-11.5	5-9

* Adapted from [31].

Table 5.2 Weight gain distribution among gestation trimesters*

Preconception BMI (kg/m^2)	*Total weight gain (kg)*	*Weight gain in the 2nd and 3rd trimester of gestation (kg/week) Mean (interval)*
Underweight (< 18.5)	12.5-18	0.51 (0.44-0.58)
Normal weight (18.5-24.9)	11.5-16	0.42 (0.35-0.50)
Overweight (25.0-29.9)	7-11.5	0.28 (0.23-0.33)
Obesity (≥ 30)	5-9	0.22 (0.17-0.27)

* Adapted from [31].

overweight and obese women of childbearing age, leading to an important increase of baseline BMI of women entering pregnancy and subsequent gestational weight gain [30].

An association between either excessive or insufficient gestational weight gain and adverse pregnancy outcomes has been observed. The most common maternal and fetal complications related to an altered weight gain are Small for Gestational Age (SGA), Large for Gestational Age (LGA), macrosomia, cesarean delivery, Gestational Diabetes Mellitus (GDM), preeclampsia, postpartum weight retention and offspring obesity.

Specific recommendations regarding the ideal weight gain during pregnancy have been provided by the Institute of Medicine (IOM). The WHO categories of maternal body mass index have been included in the 2009 updated IOM guidelines, which recommend less gestational weight gain for obese women (Table 5.1) [31].

As mentioned before, gestational weight gain greater than or less than what is recommended in the 2009 IOM guidelines is associated with a higher risk of adverse maternal and infant outcomes. For this reason, the achievement of ideal preconception BMI and the prevention of excess gestational weight gain became a WHO priority. Research implementations are required to integrate into routine health care the identification of women who are seeking pregnancy, in order to promote healthy lifestyle strategies before and during gestation [32].

Appropriate nutrition and balanced energetic intake should lead to a total gestational weight gain which is in accordance with what is recommended for each different BMI category. Weight gain should occur gradually throughout the pregnancy. During the first trimester, weight increase is determined by the hematic volume expansion and the growth of the uterus. During the second trimester it is defined by the increased adipose mass and mammary tissue, while in the third trimester, weight gain is due to the augmented placenta volume and fetal growth.

Having said that, weight gain should be minimal during the first trimester of gestation, while in the other trimesters maternal weight should increase gradually depending on the preconception BMI (Table 5.2).

In light of the data present in the literature, it is evident that lifestyle counseling should be delivered to all pregnant women, in order to intervene during pregnancy and prevent both maternal and infant short-term and long-term health risks.

5.3 Caloric intake

According to the WHO, correct and balanced maternal nutrition is fundamental for fetal growth, birth weight, infant morbidity, as well as for the woman's health, productivity and caring capacity. Proper maternal nutrition is therefore an important prerequisite for a successful pregnancy, achieved through an adequate caloric intake and an increase in body weight. For each expectant mother, it is important to establish daily energy needs, which will then be broken down into the different nutrients.

According to the 2015-2020 Dietary Guidelines for Americans (DGA), pregnant women have to consume a variety of foods to maintain energy and nutrient requirements and to gain recommended amounts of weight [33].

According to the Dietary Reference Intakes (DRIs) and the IOM, caloric necessities are no higher than the estimated energy requirement for non-pregnant women until the second trimester. In fact, in the first trimester, caloric intake does not need to be increased, unless the woman is underweight. Starting from the second trimester, the increase in maternal tissues and fetal growth determine a progressive increase in energy requirements: a normal weight pregnant woman in her second trimester of pregnancy needs to increase her caloric intake by 350 kcal/day, up to 460 kcal/day in the third trimester [34]. The increase in energy requirement varies according to maternal preconception BMI and lifestyle, resulting in a very wide energy requirement, ranging from 1800 to 2400 kcal/day.

5.4 Underweight and overweight during pregnancy

Women of childbearing age should obtain a normal body mass index before pregnancy. In fact, it has been demonstrated that both maternal overweight and underweight are factors which negatively influence the course of the pregnancy, increasing the risk of adverse outcomes. Either preconception maternal obesity or excessive weight gain during pregnancy have been related to an increased risk of metabolic and non-metabolic disease in the offspring [35]. Overweight is particularly associated with an increased risk of stillbirth, large for gestational age, macrosomia, or in some cases LBW and a greater risk to be admitted to the neonatal intensive care unit. This condition is common in developed societies, while maternal underweight is a condition more common in developing countries. Underweight in pregnancy is a critical condition associated with a high risk of morbidity for both the mother and her fetus. Studies available in the literature on this topic are limited by small sample size. However, it has been reported that this condition exposes the offspring to an increased risk of chronic diseases development. The main leading mechanism, to develop chronic diseases during the offspring's adulthood, is represented by the discrepancy which exists between a poor nutritional in utero environment and a normal postnatal food supply, related to a subsequent rapid growth catch-up [35]. Literature data reported an association between being pre-pregnancy underweight and an increased risk of preterm birth, small for gestational age and LBW [36]. In addition, placental abruption risk is moderately increased among women who are underweight prior to or in early pregnancy [37]. In order to counteract these conditions, lifestyle interventions before and during pregnancy are advisable.

5.5 Dietary styles

During pregnancy, it is recommended to follow a balanced diet that includes a daily intake of the main food groups [34, 38]. In particular, it is important to improve the intake of certain macronutrients, such as:

- *Proteins*: they should provide about 20% of the daily energy intake. An important part of this intake should derive from foods with high biological value proteins, such as meat, milk and eggs. During pregnancy, protein requirements increase progressively of 1 g/day in the first trimester, 9 g/day in the second and up to 29 g/day in the third.
- *Lipids*: the energy deriving from them should be 20-35% of the total daily energy requirements [34]. Saturated fats should not exceed 10% of the total, with a cholesterol intake lower than 300 mg/day. Since during pregnancy it is important to maintain an adequate intake of fatty acids, the remaining percentage should be covered by omega-3 and omega-6 polyunsaturated fatty acids and monounsaturated fatty acids. Of particular interest is DHA (docosahexaenoic acid, an omega-3) due to its role in the development of the fetal retina and nerve structures [39]. A recommended intake in pregnancy has not been strictly identified; however, a reference range indicates a 100-200 mg/day intake [34].
- *Carbohydrates*: their contribution should account for 45-60% of daily energy requirements. During pregnancy, carbohydrate intake should not be less than 175 g/day to ensure adequate levels for both the mother and the fetus [40]. When choosing foods, it is useful to prefer whole grains, so that fiber intake also can be augmented. Consumption of sugary and sweet drinks, on the other hand, should be limited [34].
- *Fibers*: the diet should include a fiber intake of about 30 g/day, mainly water-soluble. Therefore, the consumption of foods naturally rich in dietary fiber, such as whole grains, legumes, fruits and vegetables should be recommended.

- *Vitamins*: if a pregnant woman follows a balanced diet, all vitamin requirements should be guaranteed, requiring no special recommendations of supplementation, with the exception of folic acid (see paragraph on Dietary supplements).
- *Minerals*: as for vitamins, proper nutrition with foods derived from all food groups allows for an optimal coverage of nutritional needs during pregnancy. The only exceptions are calcium, iron and iodine.
  - *Calcium* requirements remains unchanged with respect to the preconception period. However, an insufficient dietary supply of calcium is quite common and pregnant women are advised to consume calcium-rich foods on a daily basis. For women who do not drink milk or consume any dairy product, it is recommended to use calcium-fortified foods or calcium supplements. Adequate calcium intake is essential to reduce the risk of preeclampsia, especially in women at risk for gestational hypertension [41].
  - *Iron* intake during pregnancy should significantly increase, especially after the first trimester of gestation, due to increased fetal demand, making iron supplementation often necessary (see paragraph on Dietary supplements).
  - The recommended *iodine* intake during pregnancy is 220-250 μg/day [34, 42]. However, iodine intake through diet is often insufficient, and iodine enriched foods, such as salt and potatoes, are recommended. One gram of this type of salt contains 20-30 μg of iodine, and its daily use allows to reach optimal levels of iodine.

It is also very important to drink at least 2 liters of water during the day, increasing the quantity in case of profuse sweating. In this respect, the Mediterranean diet represents the best dietary style.

Other types of diets, such as vegetarian and vegan, have been studied in relation to pregnancy, and it has been documented that these women can develop zinc, vitamin B12, DHA and iron deficiencies. These deficiencies can negatively affect the course of pregnancy, increasing the risk of preeclampsia and miscarriage, and fetal-neonatal outcome by increasing the risk of neural tube defects, other neurodevelopmental deficits and fetal-neonatal hypothyroidism. Therefore, if a pregnant woman is vegan or vegetarian, it is extremely important that her diet is supplemented and followed up with an expert throughout gestation and lactation.

5.6 Microbiome and microbiota during pregnancy

The term microbiota, defined for the first time by Lederberg and McCray, describes the collection of microbial communities living in a defined environment/human body [43]. It has an important role on host physiology and disease risk, in particular the microbiota of the gastrointestinal (GI) tract.

With the term microbiome we refer to the entire habitat, including microorganisms with their genomes and the surrounding environmental conditions.

Evidence suggest that microbiota is critical to both maternal and fetal health. Maternal microbiome influences the risk of pregnancy outcomes and have critical impacts upon the health of the infant, in terms of preterm birth, cardiometabolic complications of pregnancy such as preeclampsia, gestational diabetes, gestational hypertension and gestational weight gain [44].

Composition of maternal microbiome is shaped by different factors, including the maternal diet, pre-pregnancy weight and gestational weight gain, and hygiene practices [45].

The existence of a clear association between altered nutritional intake and pregnancy outcome is supported by scientific evidence. In fact, it has been demonstrated that food intake is an important factor that influences and shapes the composition and configuration of the maternal gut microbiota. There is increasing evidence that maternal microbiota can make use of dietary components, pharmaceuticals and toxins, which are subsequently passed on to the developing fetus.

Both altered BMI and dysregulated nutritional intake are factors which have a negative influence on the composition of microbiota and microbiome [46, 47].

These findings highlight the importance of diet during pregnancy. All pregnant women should maintain an adequate BMI throughout gestation, adopting an appropriate and balanced diet that includes a daily intake of the main food groups. Promotion of a healthy diet, attainment of a healthy weight status and weight gain during pregnancy, and oral hygiene should be suggested by practitioners, in order to reduce the risks for both the mother and the infant [44].

5.7 Dietary supplements

All pregnant women need appropriate nutritional supplementation. Iron supplementation is essential for iron deficiency anemia during gestation [33]. The WHO recommends a supplementation between

30 and 60 mg per day of elemental iron. Folic acid supplementation should be started in the preconception period, about one month before pregnancy, and continued until the 12th week of gestation, in case of normal pregnancy [38]. Folic acid supplementation of 400 µg/day is important to avoid neural tube defects, such as spina bifida and anencephaly [48]. Adequate levels of vitamin D (600 IU/day) are important as well. Vitamin D supplements are not required by all women but should be prescribed to those at risk of hypovitaminosis D, such as women from Southeast Asia, Africa, the Caribbean Islands, or the Middle East, women with few opportunities for sun exposure and/or those who do not have an adequate intake of dietary vitamin D [38]. However, NICE (National Institute for Health and Care Excellence) guidelines suggest a supplementation of 10 µg/day of vitamin D for all pregnant women and during lactation. In addition, choline (450 mg/day) and iodine (220 mg/day) are needed for normal fetal growth and brain development [33]. During pregnancy and lactation, adequate calcium intake is considered to be 1000 mg/day. Women with calcium intake of less than 500 mg/day need additional amounts to achieve adequate maternal and fetal bone requirements [49].

5.8 Anemia during pregnancy

During pregnancy, iron demand increases according to the different trimesters of gestation.

- 1st trimester → 2 mg/day
- 2nd trimester → 4-5 mg/day
- 3rd trimester → 6 mg/day

The increased iron demand is related to both maternal red blood cells expansion and fetal placenta development. The definition of anemia varies according to the trimester of pregnancy (Table 5.3).

The WHO defines severe anemia in all persons as a Hb of 7 g/dL and any severe anemia as a Hb of 4 g/dL. During pregnancy iron deficiency anemia is the most common (75%). In the USA it represents the 3-9% of cases during the first trimester and 16-55% of cases during the third trimester of gestation. Anemia prevalence is increased by malabsorption, nutrition deficit and two or more pregnancies too close to one another. There are different risks factors leading to iron deficiency, among these [50]:

- a diet poor in iron content (found in clams, beef, turkey, cereals, beans, lentils);
- a diet poor in food which increase iron absorption (orange juice, grapefruit juice, strawberries, broccoli, peppers);

Table 5.3 Anemia defining hemoglobin or hematocrit levels during pregnancy*

Women	*Hemoglobin (Hb) or hematocrit (Hct) level*
Non-pregnant	< 12 g/dL
1st trimester	< 11 g/dL or Hct < 33
2nd trimester	< 10.5 g/dL or Htc < 32
3rd trimester	< 11 g/dL or Htc < 33
Postpartum	< 10 g/dL

* Adapted from [54].

- a diet rich in food that reduces iron absorption (found in soy, spinach, coffee, tea);
- gastrointestinal diseases that affect iron absorption; menorrhagia (heavy menstrual bleeding).

During pregnancy, anemia treatment includes oral iron administration and/or lactoferrin supplementation. Oral administration is the preferred treatment strategy, while intravenous iron administration, which is a rapid and effective treatment, can be considered only in selected severe cases due to the high risks related to the procedure.

5.9 Myths and false beliefs: dos and don'ts

Pregnant women often hold wrong concepts about nutrition during pregnancy. Whether derived from either false beliefs transmitted by their family or myths belonging to the popular tradition, the problem seems to be the lack of published data on this topic [51].

An unexpectedly high percentage of women reported at least one false belief in terms of nutrition during pregnancy. This appears to be inversely associated with educational level: nonetheless, these results suggest that the usual sources of information about dietary regimens during pregnancy are not adequate to overcome misinformation and myths transmitted by popular practices and traditions [52].

The most common misconceptions about what to eat or drink in pregnancy, or when to do it, appear to be that a glass of red wine a day is beneficial for blood circulation, that food portions should be doubled ("eating for two"), that herbal tea inhibits fluid retention and that sugar supplements such as juices and candies are needed in case of dizziness or weakness.

DOS:

- Well cooked meat
- At least three servings of proteins per day (meat

or legumes)
- Six or more servings of whole grains per day
- Five or more servings of fruits and vegetables per day
- Two or three servings a week of cooked fish (such as haddock, bass, crab, anchovies, lobster, scallops, clams, squid, trout, salmon, etc.)
- Three or more servings of dairy products per day (pasteurized milk, mozzarella, parmesan, cottage cheese, ricotta, spreadable cheese).

DON'TS:
- Alcohol (no amount of alcohol has been deemed safe)
- Excessive caffeine (max 300 mg/day, 2 espresso coffees)
- Uncooked processed meat, smoked meat, raw meat, carpaccio, salami, sausages
- Raw fish and seafood
- High-mercury fish such as tuna (max 340 g/week), swordfish, shark and other predator fish
- Unpasteurized dairy such as raw milk derivatives (Brie, Camembert, Feta, Gorgonzola and blue cheese)
- Liver and derivatives (due to high content of vitamin A, which has toxic effects on the central nervous system, liver, bone and skin if its levels are too high)
- Uncooked eggs
- Unpasteurized fruit juices
- Herbal teas made of plant extracts.

REFERENCES

1. Lain KY, Catalano PM. Metabolic changes in pregnancy. Clin Obstet Gynecol 2007; 50(4): 938-48.
2. Soma-Pillay P, Nelson-Piercy C, Tolppanen H, Mebazaa A. Physiological changes in pregnancy. Cardiovasc J Afr 2016; 27(2): 89-94.
3. Catalano PM, Tzybir ED, Wolfe RR, Calles J, Roman NM, Amini SB, Sims EA. Carbohydrate metabolism during pregnancy in control subjects and women with gestational diabetes. Am J Physiol 1993; 264 (1 Pt 1): E60-7.
4. Catalano PM, Huston L, Amini SB, Kalhan SC. Longitudinal changes in glucose metabolism during pregnancy in obese women with normal glucose tolerance and gestational diabetes mellitus. Am J Obstet Gynecol 1999; 180(4): 903-16.
5. Di Cianni G, Miccoli R, Volpe L, Lencioni C, Del Prato S. Intermediate metabolism in normal pregnancy and in gestational diabetes. Diab Metab Res Rev 2003; 19(4): 259-70.
6. Ryan EA, Enns L. Role of gestational hormones in the induction of insulin resistance. J Clin Endocrinol Metab 1988; 67(2): 341-7.
7. Mazaki-Tovi S, Kanety H, Pariente C, Hemi R, Yissachar E, Schiff E, Cohen O, Sivan E. Insulin sensitivity in late gestational and early postpartum period: the role of circulating maternal adipokines. Gynecol Endocrinol 2011; 27(9): 725-31.
8. Di Cianni G, Miccoli R, Volpe L, Lencioni C, Ghio A, Giovannitti MG, Cuccuru I, Pellegrini G, Chatzianagnostou K, Boldrini A, Del Prato S. Maternal triglyceride levels and newborn weight in pregnant women with normal glucose tolerance. Diabet Med 2005; 22(1): 21-5.
9. Herrera E, Ortega-Senovilla H. Disturbances in lipid metabolism in diabetic pregnancy – Are these the cause of the problem? Best Pract Res Clin Endocrinol Metab 2010; 24(4): 515-25.
10. Alvarez JJ, Montelongo A, Iglesias A, Lasunción MA, Herrera E. Longitudinal study on lipoprotein profile, high density lipoprotein subclass, and postheparin lipases during gestation in women. J Lipid Res 1996; 37(2): 299-308.
11. Ehrenberg HM, Huston-Presley L, Catalano PM. The influence of obesity and gestational diabetes mellitus on accretion and the distribution of adipose tissue in pregnancy. Am J Obstet Gynecol 2003; 189(4): 944-8.
12. Sattar N, Greer IA, Pirwani I, Gibson J, Wallace AM. Leptin levels in pregnancy: marker for fat accumulation and mobilization? Acta Obstet Gynecol Scand 1998; 77(3): 278-83.
13. Kalhan SC, Devapatla S. Pregnancy, insulin resistance and nitrogen accretion. Curr Opin Clin Nutr Metab Care 1999; 2(5):359-63.
14. Kalhan SC. Protein metabolism in pregnancy. Am J Clin Nutr 2000; 71(5 Suppl): 1249S-55S.
15. Dasarathy J, Gruca LL, Bennett C, Parimi PS, Duenas C, Marczewski S, Fierro JL, Kalhan SC. Methionine metabolism in human pregnancy. Am J Clin Nutr 2010; 91(2):357-65.
16. Tessari P, Nissen SL, Miles JM, Haymond MW. Inverse relationship of leucine flux and oxidation to free fatty acid availability in vivo. J Clin Invest 1986; 77(2): 575-81.
17. Kalhan SC. Protein metabolism in pregnancy. In: Cowett RM (ed.). Principles of Perinatal-Neonatal Metabolism. 2nd ed. New York, NY: Springer-Verlag; 1998: 207-20.
18. Brenner B. Haemostatic changes in pregnancy. Thromb Res 2004; 114(5-6): 409-14.
19. Bustos M, Venkataramanan R, Caritis S. Nausea and vomiting of pregnancy – What's new? Auton Neurosci 2017; 202: 62-72.
20. Lew KM, Younis RT, Lazar RH. The current management of sialorrhea. Ear Nose Throat J 1991; 70(2): 99-105.
21. Morelli EL, Broadbent JM, Leichter JW, Thomson WM. Pregnancy, parity and periodontal disease. Aust Dent J 2018 May 16. doi: 10.1111/adj.12623. Online ahead of print.
22. Naveen S, Asha ML, Shubha G, Atul Anand Bajoria, Anju Anu Jose. Salivary Flow Rate, pH and Buffering Capacity in Pregnant and Non Pregnant Women - A Comparative Study. JMED Research 2014; Vol. 2014 (2014), Article ID 506946, DOI: 10.5171/2014.506946.
23. Martínez-Beneyto Y, Vera-Delgado MV, Pérez L, Maurandi A. Self-reported oral health and hygiene habits, dental decay, and periodontal condition among pregnant European women. Int J Gynaecol Obstet 2011; 114(1): 18-22.

24. Gajendra S, Kumar JV. Oral health and pregnancy: a review. N Y State Dent J 2004; 70(1): 40-4.
25. Wagle M, D'Antonio F, Reierth E, Basnet P, Trovik TA, Orsini G, Manzoli L, Acharya G. Dental caries and preterm birth: a systematic review and meta-analysis. BMJ Open 2018; 8(3): e018556. doi: 10.1136/bmjopen-2017-018556.
26. Paglia L. Caring for baby's teeth starts before birth. Eur J Paediatr Dent 2017; 18(1): 5. doi: 10.23804/ejpd.2017.18.01.01.
27. Saini R, Saini S, Saini SR. Periodontitis: A risk for delivery of premature labor and low-birth-weight infants. J Nat Sci Biol Med 2010; 1(1): 40-2.
28. Rabinerson D, Krispin E, Gabbay-Benziv R. Dental care during pregnancy. Harefuah 2018; 157(5): 330-4. [Article in Hebrew]
29. Hashim R, Akbar M. Gynecologists' knowledge and attitudes regarding oral health and periodontal disease leading to adverse pregnancy outcomes. J Int Soc Prev Community Dent 2014; 4 (Suppl 3): S166-72.
30. Diemert A, Lezius S, Pagenkemper M, Hansen G, Drozdowska A, Hecher K, Arck P, Zyriax BC. Maternal nutrition, inadequate gestational weight gain and birth weight: results from a prospective birth cohort. BMC Pregnancy Childbirth 2016; 16: 224.
31. Institute of Medicine IOM (US) and National Research Council (US) Committee to Reexamine IOM Pregnancy Weight Guidelines. Weight gain during pregnancy: reexamining the guidelines. Rasmussen KM and Yaktine AL (eds.). Washington (DC): National Academy Press (US): 2009.
32. Goldstein RF, Abell SK, Ranasinha S, Misso M, Boyle JA, Black MH, Li N, Hu G, Corrado F, Rode L, Kim YJ, Haugen M, Song WO, Kim MH, Bogaerts A, Devlieger R, Chung JH, Teede HJ. Association of Gestational Weight Gain with Maternal and Infant Outcomes: A Systematic Review and Meta-analysis. JAMA 2017; 317(21): 2207-25.
33. Sebastiani G, Herranz Barbero A, Borrás-Novell C, Alsina Casanova M, Aldecoa-Bilbao V, Andreu-Fernández V, Pascual Tutusaus M, Ferrero Martínez S, Gómez Roig MD, García-Algar O. The Effects of Vegetarian and Vegan Diet during Pregnancy on the Health of Mothers and Offspring. Nutrients 2019; 11(3): 557
34. SINU: Società Italiana di Nutrizione Umana (https://sinu.it), Livelli di Assunzione di Riferimento di Nutrienti ed Energia per la popolazione italiana (LARN)
35. Bellver J, Mariani G. Impact of parental over- and underweight on the health of offspring. Fertil Steril 2019; 111(6): 1054-64.
36. Liu P, Xu L, Wang Y, Zhang Y, Du Y, Sun Y, Wang Z. Association between perinatal outcomes and maternal prepregnancy body mass index. Obes Rev 2016; 17(11): 1091-1102.
37. Adane AA, Shepherd CCJ, Lim FJ, White SW, Farrant BM, Bailey HD. The impact of pre-pregnancy body mass index and gestational weight gain on placental abruption risk: a systematic review and meta-analysis. Arch Gynecol Obstet 2019; 300(5): 1201-10.
38. Ministero della Salute, ISS, CeVEAS. Linee guida sulla Gravidanza Fisiologica. Aggiornamento 2011 http://www.salute.gov.it/imgs/C_17_pubblicazioni_1436_allegato.pdf
39. Morse NL. Benefits of docosahexaenoic acid, folic acid, vitamin D and iodine on foetal and infant brain development and function following maternal supplementation during pregnancy and lactation. Nutrients 2012; 4(7): 799-840.
40. Institute of Medicine (IOM). Food and Nutrition Board: Dietary Reference Intakes for Energy, Carbohydrates, Fiber, Fat, Fatty Acids, Cholesterol, Protein and Amino Acids (Macronutrients). Washington (DC): National Academies Press; J Am Diet Assoc 2003; 103(5): 563.
41. McGuire S. WHO Guideline: Vitamin A supplementation in pregnant women. Geneva: WHO, 2011; WHO Guideline: Vitamin A supplementation in postpartum women. Geneva: WHO, 2011. Adv Nutr 2012; 3(2): 215-6.
42. WHO Guideline: Calcium supplementation in pregnant women. Geneva: WHO, 2013.
43. Lederberg J, McCray AT. 'Ome sweet 'omics – A Genealogical Treasury of Words. Scientist. 2001; 15(7): 8.
44. Dunlop AL, Mulle JG, Ferranti EP, Edwards S, Dunn AB, Corwin EJ. Maternal Microbiome and Pregnancy Outcomes That Impact Infant Health: A Review. Adv Neonatal Care 2015; 15(6): 377-85.
45. Gregory KE. Microbiome aspects of perinatal and neonatal health. J Perinat Neonatal Nurs 2011; 25(2): 158-62; quiz 163-4.
46. Wu WK, Panyod S, Ho C-T, Kuo C-H, Wu M-S, Sheen L-Y. Dietary allicin reduces transformation of L-carnitine to TMAO through impact on gut microbiota. J Funct Foods 2015; 15: 408-17.
47. Dominianni C, Sinha R, Goedert JJ, Pei Z, Yang L, Hayes RB, Ahn J. Sex, body mass index, and dietary fiber intake influence the human gut microbiome. PLoS One 2015; 10(4): e0124599.
48. Centers for Disease Control and Prevention. Folic Acid: Recommendations. http://www.cdc.gov/ncbddd/folicacid/recommendations.html
49. Hacker AN, Fung EB, King JC. Role of calcium during pregnancy: maternal and fetal needs. Nutr Rev 2012; 70(7): 397-409.
50. Horowitz KM, Ingardia CJ, Borgida AF. Anemia in pregnancy. Clin Lab Med 2013; 33(2): 281-91.
51. Vieira Martins Mde F, Remoaldo PCA. Myths and beliefs during pregnancy in the northwest region of Portugal and the implications for women's health. Recherche en Soins Infirmiers 2007; 90: 75-85. [Article in French]
52. Guggino A, Barbero S, Ponzo V, Viora E, Durazzo M, Bo S. Myths about nutrition in pregnancy. J Obstet Gynaecol 2016; 36(7): 964-5.
53. Weir CB, Jan A. BMI Classification Percentile And Cut Off Points. 2021 Jun 29. In: StatPearls [Internet]. Treasure Island (FL): StatPearls Publishing; 2022 Jan.
54. Khoigani MG, Goli S, Hasanzadeh A. The relationship of hemoglobin and hematocrit in the first and second half of pregnancy with pregnancy outcome. Iran J Nurs Midwifery Res 2012; 17(2 Suppl 1): S165-70.

6 Feeding/mouth development from conception to age 2 years

Diane Bahr

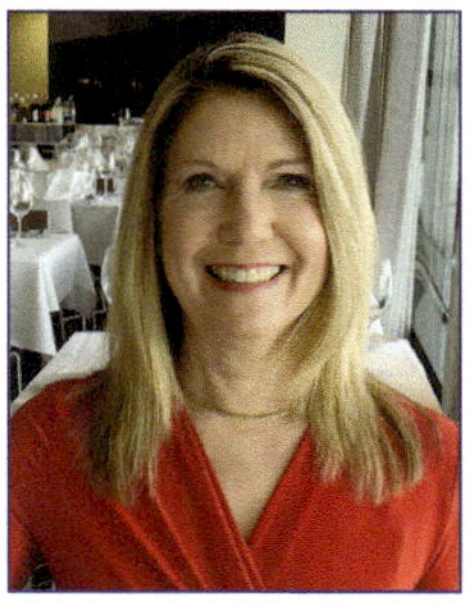

6.1 Introduction

The majority of feeding development occurs in the first two-years of life if a child is given the opportunity for this development. One problem in many of today's societies is children are not taught appropriate feeding skills with appropriate tools and food textures in a timely manner based on their cultures. This is a particular concern in Westernized civilizations where baby food products often do not reflect appropriate developmental information. In this chapter, we will examine good mouth and feeding development from conception to age 2.

6.2 Cranial, facial and oral development and function in utero

The precursors for feeding development begin early in utero. Information from many resources was used to attain the developmental sequence discussed in this part of the chapter [1-9]. It's essential to note different sources reflect slightly different timing of processes. However, an attempt was made by the author to provide the reader with a sense of when this development occurs and how it impacts feeding function. So, let's start at the beginning. We will cover the embryonic period (conception to week 8 of gestation) and the fetal period (week 9 to birth).

Around the 4th week of gestation, the face and oral cavity begin to emerge. During the 4th to 5th week, the mandible, lower lip and chin are formed and fused. The nasal and oral cavities become distinct areas around the 6th week of gestation. The upper lip and primary (front) palate is formed around the 7th week. Tongue muscles evolve, and the tongue lowers from the nasal area to the oral cavity around 7 to 8 weeks. The tongue's descent seems at least partially related to mandibular growth. At this time, the inside of the oral cavity has sensory receptors for touch, pressure, temperature, pain, etc. Approximately 50% of jaw and tongue growth occurs before birth [10].

Tethered oral tissues (tongue, lip and/or buccal ties) reportedly occur in utero between 2 and 8 weeks of gestation. Much is known about tongue tie while less is known about lip and buccal tie. However, lip and buccal tie seem to impact feeding and other aspects of mouth function. Ankyloglossia is a congenital condi-

Diane Bahr, MS, CCC-SLP, CIMI
Specializing in Feeding, Motor Speech, & Mouth Development/Function
Ages and Stages, LLC, Resources for Feeding, Motor Speech, & Mouth Function, Las Vegas, USA

Website: www.agesandstages.net. Email: dibahr@cox.net

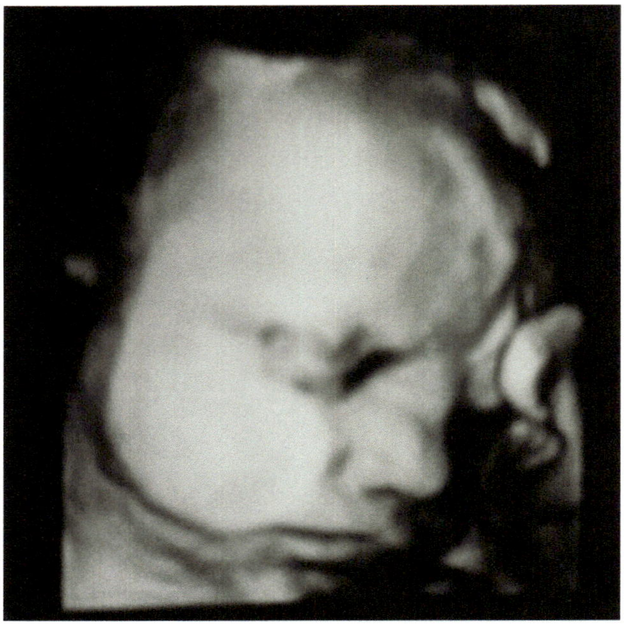

Fig. 6.1 Baby in utero with hand to face (Photo with parent permission).

tion limiting tongue mobility secondary to an atypical lingual frenum (the tissue connecting the bottom of the tongue to the floor of the mouth). Tongue tie may impact mandibular (lower jaw) as well as maxillary (upper jaw) growth. Three to 12% of newborns are believed to have this problem often resulting in breastfeeding difficulties. If left untreated, tongue tie may also result in food placement and collection issues, inhibition of the normal oral phase swallow, oral hygiene concerns and speech problems [11-28].

The palatal shelves rise to form the hard palate and the floor of the nasal cavity in the 8th or 9th week. The cartilaginous facial structure is seen around the 9th week. During the 10th to 12th week, the soft palate tissue fuses. Bone begins replacing cartilage to form the early cranial base and vault, mandible and maxilla around the 12th week. Taste buds mature by 13 to 18 weeks of gestation [6].

Cleft lip and/or palate occur between 6 and 12 weeks of gestation. There is a higher incidence in males than females with differing incidences among ethnic groups. Clefts are caused by both genetic and environmental factors, and the malformations vary significantly. They impact mouth, airway, overall cranio-facial and dental development; as well as velopharyngeal function, breathing, feeding, eating, drinking, swallowing, speaking, voicing, hearing and social interaction [5, 29-37].

Between 12 and 20 weeks of gestation, sucking, swallowing and overall oral functioning become organized as these processes are needed at birth. By 20 weeks of gestation, the brain has a "full complement of neurons" [38]. Around 16 weeks, the specific timing of sucking and swallowing develops along with the esophageal reflex, and the fetus swallows approximately 7 mL of amniotic fluid per day. The fetus sucks and swallows increasing amounts of amniotic fluid until birth (such as 500 mL of amniotic fluid per day) [2].

Many oral sensory-motor reflexes are activated in utero. The gag response appears between 26 and 27 weeks of gestation. Reflexive suckling and volitional sucking appear between 27 and 28 weeks. The rooting, phasic bite and transverse tongue responses appear around 28 weeks. The anterior tongue reflex is seen between 38 and 40 weeks, and this reflex is believed to be part of the suckling response. The cough occurs at 40 weeks when the baby is born full-term [39-42].

Lip contact with body parts such as the hand and foot results in mouth opening and tongue protrusion. Between 17 and 20 weeks of gestation, there is hand to face movement (Fig. 6.1). Between 28 and 31 weeks, finger sucking can be seen. Between 34 and 35 weeks, in utero hand to mouth movements are coordinated [43].

Sucking or buccal fat pads develop toward the end of gestation when the baby is full-term and other fat is developing on the baby's body. These crucial structures provide lateral oral support and stability during feeding. They assist in attaining adequate intraoral pressure in the mouth for sucking and keep the mouth from collapsing during feeding. If a baby is born with thin or missing sucking pads, the baby may compensate by humping and bunching the tongue to attain enough intraoral pressure for feeding. Babies born prematurely do not have sucking pads, and many close-to-term babies (37 to 39 weeks of gestation) have thin or missing sucking pads. Compensatory feeding strategies such as the Dancer Hand Position or carefully applied cheek support can be used in these cases to provide lateral oral assistance during feeding. Fully developed sucking pads are particularly important for breastfeeding [39, 44-51].

6.3 The full-term (40-week) baby's structures and functions for feeding

The newborn baby's mouth and throat structures are close together (e.g., when not crying, feeding, vocalizing or using a pacifier). There is little room or open space within the newborn's oral cavity at rest (Fig. 6.2). The tongue fills the mouth and rests against the palate (roof of the mouth) which helps maintain the wide "U" palatal shape [10, 57]. The newborn's larynx is high in the neck area, so it doesn't have far to move during the pharyngeal phase of the swallow. The baby's palate is relatively flat at birth resulting in a fairly straight horizontal lip line. While the nasal passages are initially small, the nasal turbinates quickly decrease in size after birth creating an open nasal airway if there is no inflammation [2, 58, 59].

Nose breathing (Fig. 6.3) is essential for nasal, orofacial, sinus and thoracic-ventilatory development [2]. Nitric oxide production in the body is a by-product of nose breathing and serves important purposes. It's produced in the paranasal sinuses to help maintain healthy sinuses through antimicrobial activity and to assist oxygenation of the body through vasodilation in pulmonary capillaries [60-62]. A newborn should be a nose breather with a resting respiratory rate of approximately 30 to 40 breaths per minute [63-65].

Additionally, the full-term baby should be born with a full set of sucking (buccal fat) pads. They are balls of fat in the newborn's cheeks and provide lateral (side) stability during feeding. The broad palate and cupped tongue provide upper and lower stability during feeding. A newborn's gums also reportedly enlarge to assist with the latch [66]. This is likely due to increased blood supply to the area. All of these structures help the baby attain adequate intraoral pressure for sucking, particularly during breastfeeding.

When a baby has a full set of buccal fat pads, one can barely place a finger between the newborn's cheek and gum areas. Babies born prematurely do not have sucking pads and will not develop them. Some babies born close-to-term (37 to 39 weeks of gestation) or even full-term (40 weeks of gestation) have been observed to have thin or missing buccal fat pads. A number of practitioners question whether this may be an epigenetic change related to the use of bottle-feeding over several generations as a baby can usually bottle-feed without adequate sucking pads.

The newborn baby's Eustachian tubes are relatively horizontal from the back of the nasopharynx to the middle ear space. A baby can breastfeed in any position that works for the mother and baby because there seem to be balanced pressures throughout the system during breastfeeding. However, when bottle-feeding, it's important to keep the infant's ear above the mouth, so liquid doesn't enter the Eustachian tubes causing middle ear problems. This is explained in the next paragraph of the chapter.

Most full-term newborn babies are ready to feed and naturally protected from swallowing difficulties based on their anatomy and physiology described above. They are also born with full-body, oral and hand-mouth reflexes. The oral reflexes and the hand-mouth reflexes specifically assist with feeding [46, 50-56, 66-72].

Readiness to feed is based on the baby's functional suck, swallow and breathe maturity and coordination [73-77]. Newborns have both nutritive sucking (approximately 1 per second) and non-nutritive suckling (around 2 per second). Nutritive sucking allows the baby to feed, and non-nutritive suckling can help the baby to calm [77-79].

When a newborn's lips or cheeks receive touch, the baby's mouth searches for the touch. This is the

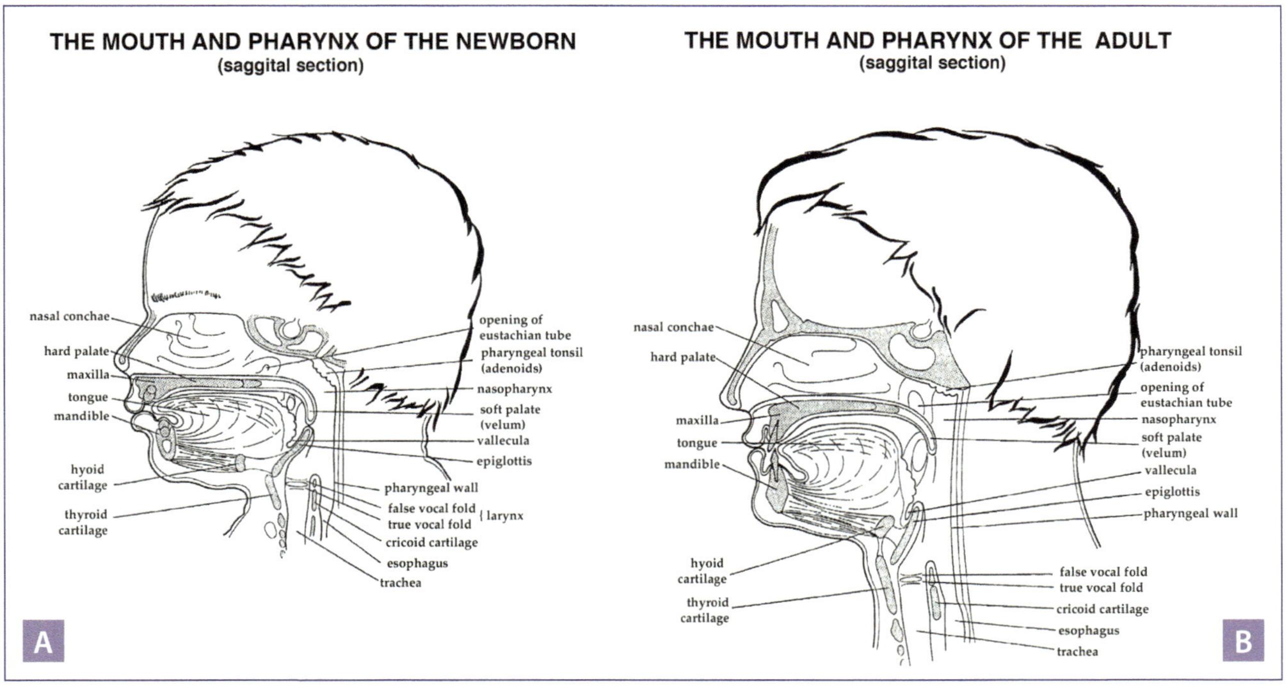

Fig. 6.2 Newborn versus adult mouth and throat (Drawings by Betsy True for Suzanne Evans Morris who granted permission). Newborn (**A**). Adult (**B**).

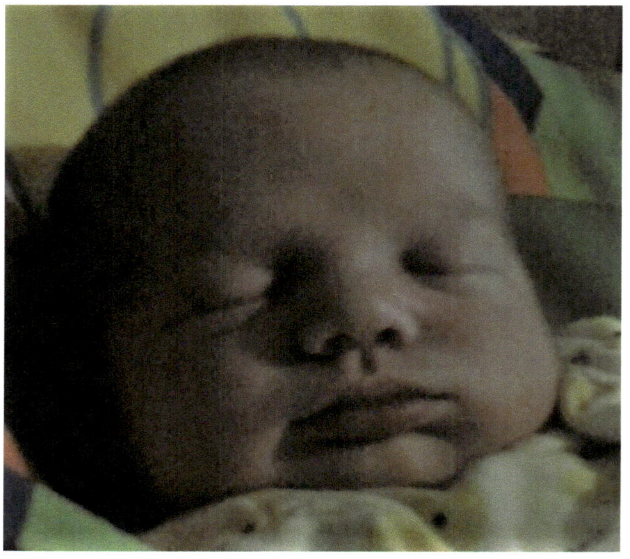

Fig. 6.3 Nice broad eye area, straight lip line and nasal breathing in full-term newborn (Photo with parent permission).

rooting reflex which seems to help the baby find the breast, finger or bottle (if paced baby-led bottle feeding is used). The rooting response also appears to lead to nutritive sucking or non-nutritive suckling. A baby gains control over the rooting reflex around 1 month of age, and the response seems to be integrated by the brain between 3 and 6 months as the baby prepares for food introduction.

The non-nutritive suckling reflex (2 per second) is stimulated when something enters the newborn's mouth. The baby begins to gain control of this response around 2 to 3 months of age. It seems to be integrated by the brain between 6 and 12 months of age as the baby learns to eat appropriate foods and drink properly from cups and straws.

The anterior tongue reflex (likely part of the suckling response) occurs when the newborn's tongue or lips receive touch. For breastfeeding, this response allows the baby's tongue to grasp the breast and draw it into the mouth. It may also serve a protective function by pushing items out of a baby's mouth when the infant is not ready for them. The anterior tongue reflex seems to fade around 3 to 4 months of age when the baby is ready to mouth safe and appropriate mouth toys. It seems to be integrated by the brain between 12 and 18 months as the toddler eats safe foods of increasing texture.

The swallowing reflex is triggered as amniotic fluid (before birth), saliva, liquid and eventually food move toward the baby's throat. A baby gains control of this reflex around 18 months, and it's an important reflex to maintain throughout life. Proper function of the back and base of tongue is crucial for good swallowing.

A newborn's phasic bite response occurs when the baby receives firm but gentle pressure on the gum surfaces. The baby opens and closes the jaw in a rhythmic munching pattern (approximately 1 per second). This reflex exercises the jaw elevator (muscles that raise the jaw) and depressor muscles (those that lower the jaw). A baby begins to gain control over this reflex between 5 and 9 months of age when safe foods and appropriate mouth toys are introduced for biting and chewing. It seems to be integrated by the brain between 9 and 12 months when children are actively taking bites of and chewing foods.

A newborn's transverse tongue reflex is stimulated when touch is given to either side of the baby's tongue. This causes the baby's tongue to move toward touch and eventually food. Lateral tongue movement is ultimately needed to place and collect food in the mouth for chewing and swallowing. A baby begins to gain control over this reflex between 6 and 8 months when learning to chew and manage safe foods. It becomes integrated by the brain between 9 and 24 months as the child purposefully manipulates food within and throughout the mouth.

In a newborn, the gag response is elicited on back 1/2 to 3/4 of the baby's tongue (not the front of the tongue or the baby could not breastfeed). During a gag response, the baby's mouth opens wide; head moves backward; and the soft palate, larynx and diaphragm rise. This response seems to be a protective mechanism to keep a baby from swallowing items that are too large. Babies gain control over this reflex between 4 and 6 months. By 6 to 9 months a baby's gag is on the back 1/3 of the tongue. In most people the gag continues throughout life on the back 1/4 of the tongue. The gag response is likely meant to keep people from swallowing foods that are too large and have not been chewed and managed properly.

In the previous section of this chapter, we learned a fetus has a hand-mouth connection beginning around 17 to 20 weeks of gestation. This process is carried forward via three hand-mouth reflexes seen in the newborn (i.e., palmomental, Babkin and grasp). Hands and mouths seem to work together throughout life.

Full-term newborns have a palmomental response, so when the baby's palm receives touch the mentalis muscles (below the lower lip) contract. These muscles evert the lower lip which is particularly important in breastfeeding. The palmomental response can be seen into adulthood in some people.

The Babkin response occurs when you gently press the base of a baby's palm which causes the baby's mouth to open, eyes to close, and head to move forward getting the baby ready to feed. This reflex is integrated by the brain around 3 to 4 months of age when an infant should be practiced at breastfeeding and/or bottle-feeding.

The grasp response occurs when a finger is placed into a newborn's palm. The baby's grasp tightens as the baby sucks. This reflex seems to be integrated by the brain around 8 months of age when the baby is eating safe and appropriate hand-held foods.

6.4 Breastfeeding versus bottle-feeding

Breastfeeding is biologically normal and far superior to bottle-feeding for mouth and airway development, particularly if the baby is fed in a laid-back position which helps the jaw move and grow forward (Fig. 6.4). Bottle-feeding began when mothers could not breastfeed their babies for some reason (e.g., mothers were ill or working outside the home). It's a medical way of feeding a baby and a very different process than breastfeeding.

Breastfed babies open their mouths wide using a full and graded jaw excursion which assists in jaw development. Those who are bottle-fed open the mouth just enough for a particular bottle nipple. Breastfed babies extend the tongue over the lower lip to grasp the mother's breast and pull it deeply into the baby's mouth. Bottle-fed babies extend the tongue over the lower gum when sucking [10, 39, 80-83].

When the mother's nipple and breast are drawn deeply into the infant's mouth, the broad "U" palate shape is maintained [10, 84, 85]. Neither bottle nipples nor pacifiers can help with this process. In fact, they likely contribute to the narrowing of the palate and nasal areas which ultimately may make healthy nose breathing difficult.

Breastfed babies use the front of the tongue to hold and cup the mother's breast as the baby's lips seal against the breast for a sustained latch. If a baby is fed with a rounded bottle nipple, the tongue may cup around it. Tongue cupping is essential for normal swallowing and ultimately speech production. Tongue humping and bunching are never normal.

In breastfed babies, the front of the tongue and lower jaw move together in an up-down motion with minimal effort (a precursor to jaw movement used throughout life). There is also little cheek motion if the breastfed baby has adequate sucking pads, while bottle-fed babies have more cheek and lip movement than breastfed babies. This may be one reason babies can bottle-feed when they have difficulty breastfeeding. Cheeks and lips tend to move as a unit in bottle-feeding, while breastfeeding requires graded and dissociated movement of the jaw elevator and depressor muscles, as well as the mentalis muscles that evert the lower lip [56].

Babies who are breastfed have more mentalis and masseter muscle movement than bottle-fed children. As previously mentioned, the mentalis muscles evert (protrude) the lower lip. The masseter muscles elevate (raise) the jaw. Exclusively breastfed babies have more sucking movements with more and longer pauses than bottle-fed babies, while bottle-fed babies have fewer sucking movements and shorter pauses than breastfed babies.

Breastfeeding requires significant dissociation (one part moving separately from another) and grading (each part moving just enough for the activity). As previously mentioned, the mouth seems to move as a unit during bottle feeding. Therefore, bottle-feeding appears to be a less sophisticated feeding process than breastfeeding [39, 84, 86-91].

Breastfeeding encourages good suck-swallow-breathe synchronization, and alternating breasts stimulates and exercises both sides of the baby's face, head and body. One study demonstrated breastfeeding improves later developing feeding skills such as open cup-drinking and chewing [43]. Breastfeeding also seems to be more similar to open cup feeding than it is to be bottle-feeding [87, 92-95].

Additionally, breastfeeding can be done in any position recommended by an International Board Certified Lactation Consultant (Fig. 6.5). There are balanced pressures (e.g., intraoral, nasal, sinus, middle ear, pharyngeal, laryngeal, etc.) during the breastfeeding process, while bottle-feeding and pacifier-use likely involve forces that may negatively impact mouth and airway development [10, 81, 82].

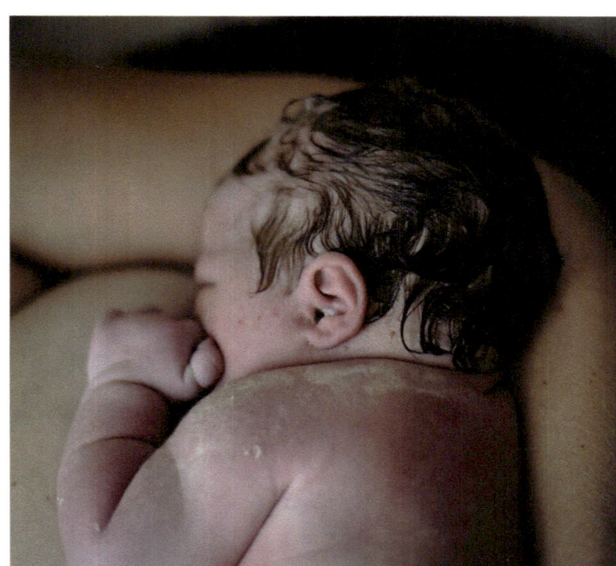

Fig. 6.4 Baby breastfeeding in laid-back position immediately after birth and breast crawl (Photo by Phelicia Cyrus with parent permission).

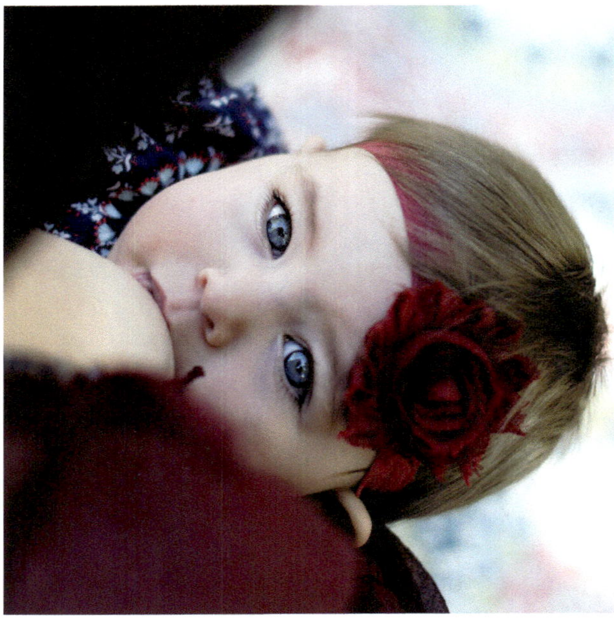

Fig. 6.5 Breastfeeding can be done in any position (Photo by Phelicia Cyrus with parent permission).

Relatively recent research suggests babies are belly feeders, so the laid-back breastfeeding position may be the most natural position [96-98]. This position also encourages the development of postural (core) control and forward jaw growth.

In recent times, many babies spend inordinate amounts of time on their backs and in containers (e.g., car seats, infant seats, swings, etc.). While back to sleep is the recommended sleeping position in many countries, babies are meant to experience a variety of intentional and supervised body positions (e.g., belly time, side-lying, baby wearing, etc.) to develop good postural (core) control which is the basis for gross motor (e.g., rolling, sitting, crawling and walking) and fine motor (e.g., eating, drinking, speaking, hand-use and vision-use) skill development [99-115].

Gravity is a constant force that can push the jaw and tongue backward into retraction and inhibit overall body development if babies spend an excessive amount of time on their backs, particularly when awake. Therapists and other professionals are seeing significant disruptions in children's physical and motor development which seems related to excessive swaddling, use of containers and time on the back. These include increases in plagiocephaly, brachycephaly and torticollis, as well as delayed feeding, speech, vision and hand development.

Children who breastfeed are healthier overall than bottle-fed babies [10, 116]. Breastfed children have fewer upper and lower respiratory, middle ear and digestive problems (e.g., gastroesophageal reflux and gastrointestinal issues) likely because breast milk has antibacterial qualities that can counteract

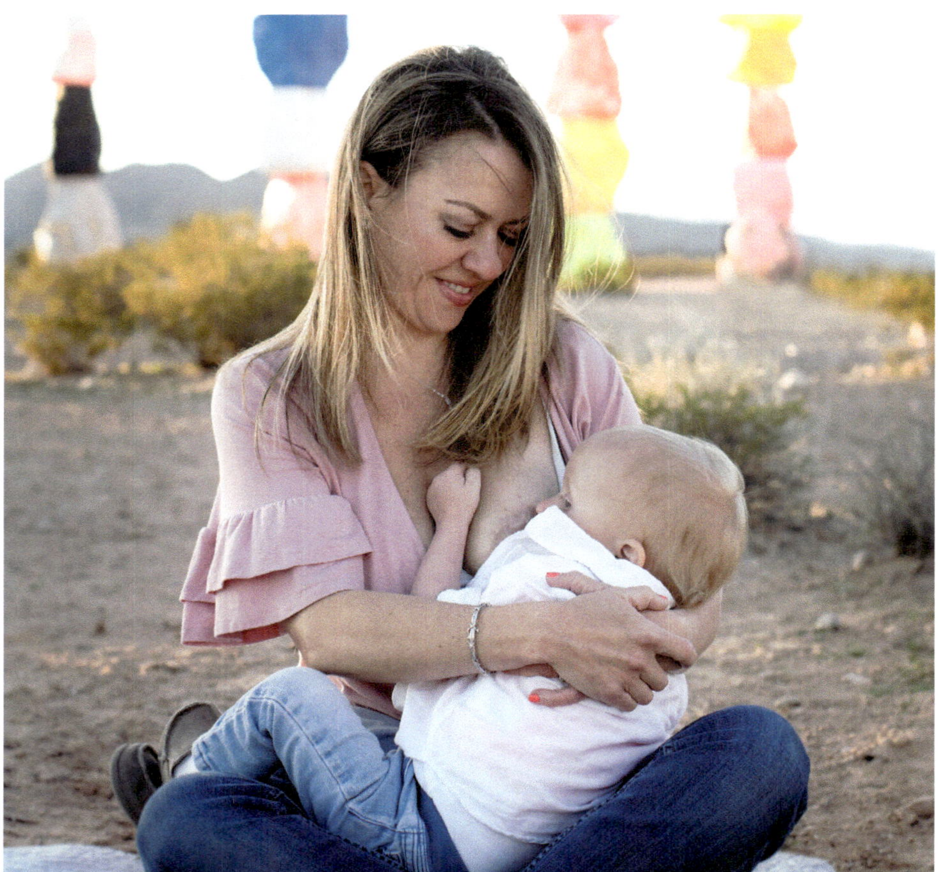

Fig. 6.6 Breastfeeding is convenient, even in the desert (Photo by Phelicia Cyrus with parent permission).

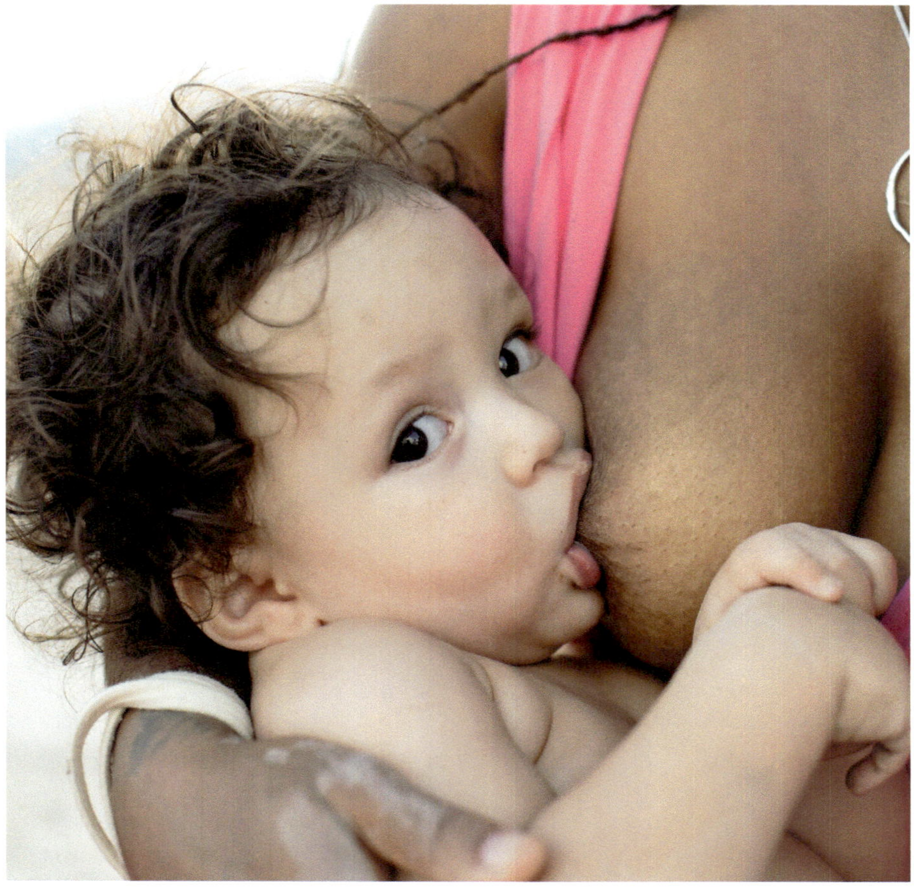

Fig. 6.7 Breastfeeding continues as other feeding skills are introduced (Photo by Phelicia Cyrus with parent permission).

infection [117-122]. They also have better face, jaw, palate, tooth, speech and cognitive development [10, 66, 123-130].

As previously mentioned, breastfed babies can be fed in any position because of the equalized pressure throughout the system during breastfeeding (Fig. 6.6). However, bottle-fed babies should be fed in a fairly upright position beginning at birth (e.g., a 45-degree angle to the horizon or Earth). This is important because the Eustachian tubes in newborns and young children are relatively horizontal. These tubes extend from the nasopharynx to the middle ear space. They ventilate and equalize pressure in the middle ear. They can also drain fluid from the middle ear. If a baby is bottle-fed lying on the back, fluid may go into the Eustachian tubes and middle ear space causing ear problems. Therefore, paced baby-led bottle-feeding is recommended [131].

In paced baby-led bottle feeding:

- The baby is placed upright with the ear above the mouth (e.g., head and body at a 45-degree angle to the horizon)
- The bottle nipple is rolled into the baby's mouth when the baby opens the mouth to feed
- The bottle is also positioned horizontally, so the baby sucks the liquid from the bottle without the help of gravity
- The parent may tip the bottle nipple upward slightly when the baby naturally takes breaks between sucking bursts.

A slow-flow bottle nipple is typically used during paced baby-led bottle feeding, and parents respond to their baby's body language (e.g., ready to eat, take a break or when full) [50, 51, 131, 132]. However, some practitioners attempt to match bottle nipple flow with the mother's breast milk flow if a breastfed baby is supplemented with bottle-feeding.

There are many baby bottles on the market. This probably reflects manufacturers' attempts to create a bottle similar to the mother's breast. To date, this has not been accomplished.

6.5 Feeding from 6 months to 2 years (a critical learning period)

Children develop most of their feeding skills used throughout life between 6 months and 2 years of age (Fig. 6.7). Therefore, feeding skills need to be introduced on time for children to remain on track in feeding and mouth development. In many Westernized cultures, based on European civilization, parents begin feeding babies with a spoon or open cup,

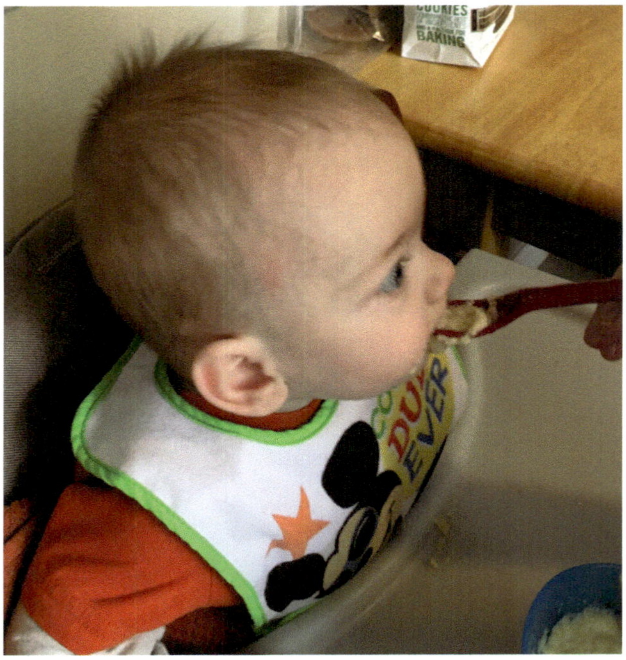

Fig. 6.8 Six-month-old learning spoon-feeding (Photo with parent permission).

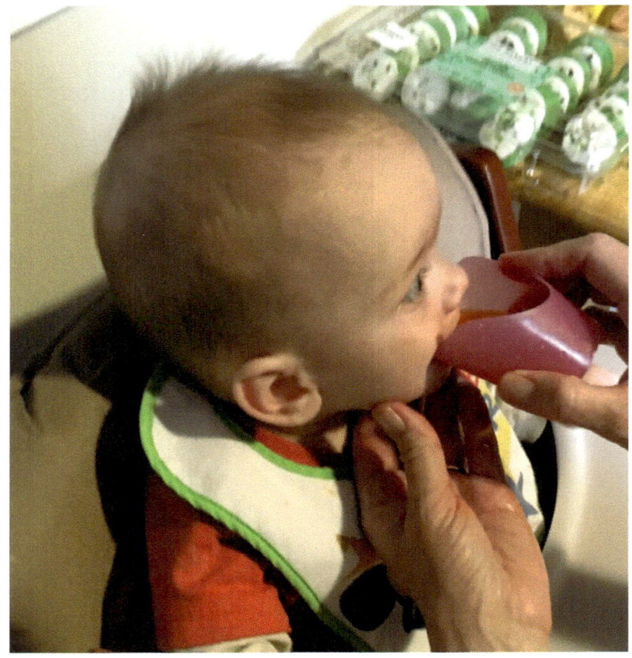

Fig. 6.9 Six-month-old learning open cup-drinking (Photo with parent permission).

while other utensils or hands may be used in different cultures. The information in this section of the book is primarily based on the only known longitudinal study on typical feeding development completed by Suzanne Evans Morris [55]. However, other references were used as well [46, 50, 51, 56, 133-137].

The properly developing 6- to 7-month-old child opens the mouth for a small, relatively flat, baby spoon in a graded manner (i.e., just enough for the spoon to go into the mouth). If given a spoon, a 6-month-old will likely explore it throughout the mouth in a discriminative way. Between 6 and 8 months, a child's upper lip clears the spoon. And, between 6 and 12 months, the child's lower lip moves inward as the spoon is removed, particularly if some food is left on the lower lip (Fig. 6.8). Between 9 and 21 months, the child's lower lip moves inward with the top teeth removing food from the bottom lip. Around 9 to 10 months of age, a child holds, bangs and imitates stirring with a spoon. Self-feeding with a spoon occurs between 12 and 14 months, scooping occurs between 15 and 18 months and, by 24 months, a child eats with a spoon in an adult-like manner.

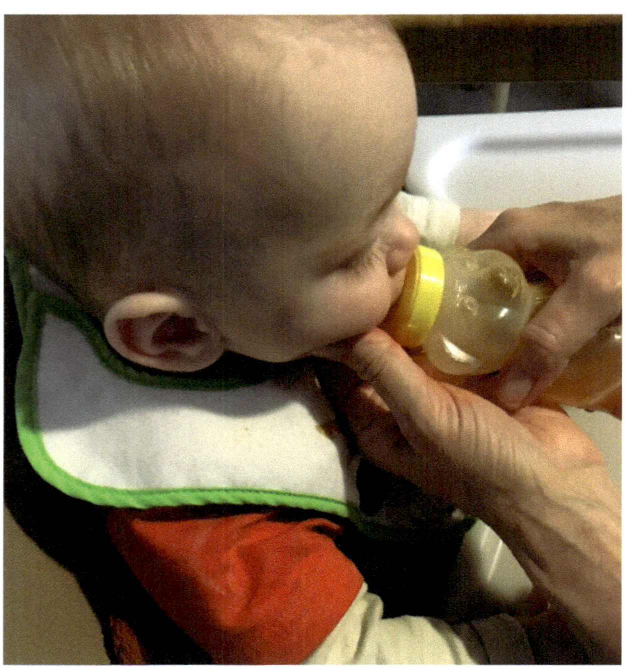

Fig. 6.10 Six-month-old learning proper straw-drinking (Photo with parent permission).

As previously mentioned, open cup-feeding is similar to breastfeeding based on the literature. Therefore, open cup-drinking (with the cup held by an adult) is a natural process for the 6-month-old child [43]. The open cup should be placed on the front inner lip borders and not into the lip corners which hyperextends the jaw (Fig. 6.9). However, between 6 and 8 months, the child can take 1 to 3 sucks from the open cup demonstrating increased jaw stability. By 12 months, the child can hold an open, recessed lid or handled cup and drink with only a small amount of spillage. The recessed lid cup reduces spilling because the lid fits inside the open cup with liquid coming through a hole or holes in the depressed lid. However, some recessed lid cups (e.g., WOW or 360 cups) may be too difficult for a young child. Between 9 and 15 months, a child can drink more than 3 consecutive suck-swallows from an open or appropriate recessed lid cup. Yet, the child may continue to bite on the open cup rim for jaw stability between 11 and 24 months. By 24 months, a child can drink from an open cup in an adult-like manner without spillage.

Around 6 months of age, straw-drinking may also be introduced (Fig. 6.10). Proper straw-drinking can be taught using a squeezable bottle made to hold food or liquid (e.g., sauce, honey, etc.). The straw is usually made of small plumbing or refrigerator tubing meant to carry water and is fitted into the bottle top. Either thin liquid, such as breast milk, or a thickened liquid, such as breast milk mixed with infant cereal, can be placed into the straw bottle.

Appropriate purees thinned with water may also be placed into the straw bottle as a baby is ready for the introduction of these complementary foods (e.g., pureed vegetables or fruits). The parent squeezes the liquid to the top of the straw away from the baby's face and mouth. A very small length of the straw is placed just on the baby's lips for the baby to suck. If the baby's lips do not round on the straw, carefully applied cheek support can be used as cheeks activate lips. Children can learn to drink properly and on their own from a straw (with the straw placed centrally just on the lips) between 6 and 12 months of age.

Teaching proper straw-drinking at an early age (where the straw is only placed on the lips, not the tongue) gives the parent and child a non-spill drinking option and can help avoid tongue thrust swallow (which is never normal in this author's opinion). However, improper straw use (where the straw is placed on the tongue when drinking) seems to encourage tongue thrust swallow.

Lip closure when swallowing properly managed foods and liquids can begin as early as 8 months of age. Mature swallow initiation (tongue tip to the alveolar ridge behind the top front teeth) is observed intermittently with appropriate foods and liquids beginning around 11 to 12 months of age. Spouted (sippy) cups, pouch foods and pacifiers are not recommended as they block the tongue from correctly initiating the mature oral phase swallow and likely encourage tongue thrust swallow. Bottle weaning usually occurs between 12 and 15 months of age as bottle nipples may also impede the mature oral phase swallowing process.

Finger feeding begins around 6 months of age. Between 6 and 8 months, a baby picks up soft, safe, food pieces with a fist and can hold a soft baby cookie (Fig. 6.11). A child can pass food from one hand to the other around 8 to 9 months. Between 9 and 12 months, a child begins to pick food up with the thumb and fingers and can finger feed. A toddler can pick up food with the thumb and index finger and place food pieces into bowls between 12 and 15 months.

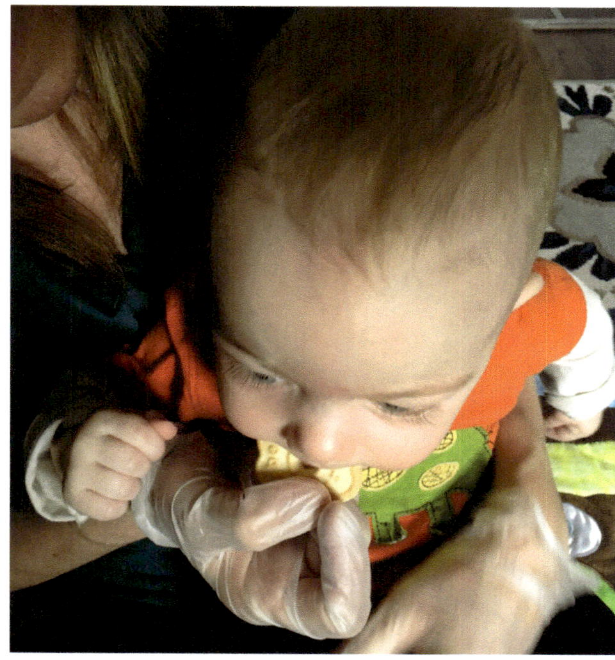

Fig. 6.11 Six-month-old learning to bite on a soft cookie (Photo with parent permission).

Taking bites of food and chewing are essential processes for tooth and jaw development. This is one reason appropriate food textures need to be introduced on time, and there are now safe feeders to help parents with this process. Around 6 months of age,

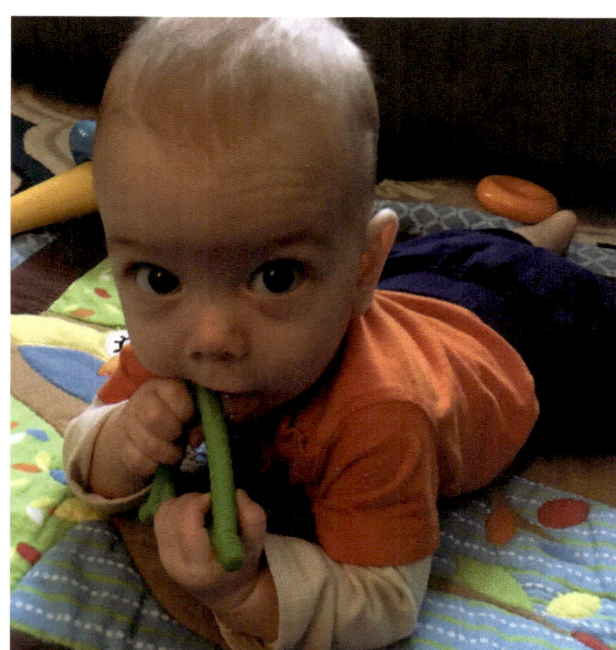

Fig. 6.12 Six-month-old biting, chewing and discriminatively mouthing appropriate toy (Photo with parent permission).

the child's jaw movements begin to match the shape and size of food when taking safe bites and chewing safe foods. The lips and cheeks begin to contract to keep food in place on the side where food is positioned. Between 6 and 9 months, a child uses an up-down biting and munching pattern on a soft cookie, a diagonal rotary chewing pattern on the side where food is placed, and a rolling and shifting motion of the tongue toward the side gums where food is located. Up-down biting and munching is used on a hard cookie between 6 and 19 months. The lip corner and cheek move inward on the side where the child is chewing between 8 and 11 months. The cheeks control and move food between 8 and 18 months. A child uses a skillful bite on a soft cookie between 7 and 12 months and on a hard cookie between 11 and 24 months. The child can also transfer food from the center of the tongue to both sides of the mouth between 7 and 12 months and move the tongue independently of the jaw to manipulate food between 12 and 36 months. The tongue moves food from one side of the mouth to the other between 21 and 36 months, and a child can chew with closed lips by 24 months.

Primary tooth eruption, between 6 and 33 months of age, accompanies biting and chewing development. These complimentary processes seem to help teeth erupt on time, in a proper sequence, and fully formed. Based on clinical observation, children who do not discriminatively mouth as well as bite and chew on appropriate items and foods frequently do not have typical tooth eruption. Children are born with a phasic bite response. Therefore, they often gently bite and chew on their fingers and appropriate toys in preparation for the introduction of foods (Fig. 6.12). Babies go through a period of generalized mouthing (placing hands or appropriate mouth items at the front of the mouth for biting and exploration) from birth until 5 or 6 months of age. They also do this in utero. Around 5 or 6 months of age, they begin the very important process of discriminative mouthing (exploring fingers and appropriate toys or foods throughout the mouth). During this time, they use the mouth like a third hand for exploration which provides the oral discrimination they need for eating, drinking and ultimately speaking.

6.6 Conclusion

Feeding development begins in utero. A child should have adult-like feeding skills by age 2 years if the child remains on track in feeding development as described in this chapter. The development of good postural control is needed for fine motor skill development such as feeding. Simultaneously, children develop speech using the same musculature with different pressures and motor plans than feeding. If parents and professionals use literature-based, criterion-referenced information such as found in this chapter, they can help children develop the best possible mouth and airway development needed for good eating, drinking and speaking.

REFERENCES

1. Gaultier C, Guilleminault C. Genetics, control of breathing, and sleep disordered breathing: A review. Sleep Med 2001; 2(4): 281-95.
2. Guilleminault C, Huang Y. From orofacial dysfunction to dysmorphism and the onset of pediatric OSA. Sleep Med Rev 2018; 40: 203-14.
3. Diewert VM. Development of human craniofacial morphology during the late embryonic and early fetal periods. Am J Orthod 1985; 88(1): 64-76.
4. Som PM, Naidich TP. Illustrated review of the embryology and development of the facial region, part 1: Early face and lateral nasal cavities. Am J Neuroradiol 2013; 34(12): 2233-40.
5. University of Minnesota Duluth (n.d.). Cleft lip & palate. CSD 2230. Lecture retrieved from http://www.d.umn.edu/~mmizuko/2230/cleft.htm.
6. Premkumar S. Textbook of craniofacial growth. India: JP Brothers Medical Publishing; 2011.
7. Enlow DH, Moyers RE. Handbook of facial growth. 2nd ed. New York: W.B. Saunders Company; 1982.
8. Miller JL, Sonies BC, Macedonia C. Emergence of oropharyngeal, laryngeal, and swallowing activity in the developing fetal upper aerodigestive tract: An ultrasound evaluation. Early Hum Dev 2003; 71(1): 61-87.
9. Upledger JE. A brain is born: Exploring the birth and development of the central nervous system. Berkeley, CA: North Atlantic Books; 1996.
10. Page DC. (2003). "Real" early orthodontic treatment: From birth to age 8. Funct Orthod. Spring-Summer 2003; 20(1-2): 48-54, 56-8.
11. Acevedo AC, da Fonseca JAC, Grinham J, Doudney K, Gomes RR, de Paula LM, Stanier P. Autosomal-dominant ankyloglossia and tooth number anomalies. J Dent Res 2010; 89(2): 128-32.
12. Ballard JL, Auer CE, Khoury JC. Ankyloglossia: assessment, incidence, and effect of frenuloplasty on the breastfeeding dyad. Pediatrics 2002; 110(5): e63.
13. Coryllos E, Genna CW, Salloum AC. Congenital tongue-tie and its impact on breastfeeding. Breastfeeding: Best for Mother and Baby. American Academy of Pediatrics 2004; Summer: 1-6.
14. Defabianis P. Ankyloglossia and its influence on maxillary and mandibular development. (A seven year follow-up case report). Funct Orthod 2000; 17(4): 25-33.
15. Forlenza GP, Black NMP, McNamara EG, Sullivan SE. Ankyloglossia, exclusive breastfeeding, and failure to thrive. Pediatrics 2010; 125(6): e1500-4.
16. Griffiths DM. Do tongue ties affect breastfeeding? J Human Lact 2004, 20(4): 409-14.
17. Guilleminault C, Huseni S, Lo L. A frequent phenotype for paediatric sleep apnoea: short lingual frenulum. ERJ Open Res 2016; 2(3): 00043-2016.
18. Haham A, Marom R, Mangel L, Botzer E, Dollberg S. Prevalence of breastfeeding difficulties in newborns with a lingual frenulum: A prospective cohort series. Breastfeed Med 2014; 9(9): 438-41.
19. Han SH, Kim MC, Choi YS, Lim JS, Han KT. A study on the genetic inheritance of ankyloglossia based on pedigree analysis. Arch Plast Surg 2012; 39(4): 329-32.
20. Klockars T, Pitkäranta A. Inheritance of ankyloglossia (tongue-tie). Clin Genet 2009; 75(1): 98-9.
21. Queiroz Marchesan I. Lingual frenulum: classification and speech interference. Int J Orofacial Myology 2004 Nov; 30: 31-8.
22. Martinelli RL, Marchesan IQ, Gusmão RJ, Rodrigues A, Berretin-Felix G. Histological characteristics of altered human lingual frenulum. Int J Pediatr Child Health 2014; 2: 6-9.
23. Messner AH, Lalakea ML. The effect of ankyloglossia on speech in children. Otolaryngo Head and Neck Surg 2002; 127(6): 539-45.
24. Messner AH, Lalakea ML, Aby J, Macmahon J, Bair E. Ankyloglossia: incidence and associated feeding difficulties. Arch Otolaryngol Head Neck Surg 2000; 126(1): 36-9.
25. Pransky SM, Lago D, Hong P. Breastfeeding difficulties and oral cavity anomalies: The influence of posterior ankyloglossia and upper-lip ties. Int J Pediatr Otorhinolaryngol 2015; 79 (10): 1714-7.
26. Ricke LA, Baker NJ, Madlon-Kay DJ, DeFor TA. Newborn tongue-tie: Prevalence and effect on breast-feeding. J Am Board Fam Pract 2005; 18(1): 1-7.
27. Genna CW. The influence of anatomic and structural issues on sucking skills. In: C.W. Genna (Ed.), Supporting sucking skills in breastfeeding infants (3rd ed.). Woodhaven, NY: Jones and Bartlett Learning; 2017: 209-267.
28. Hazelbaker AK. Tongue-Tie: Morphogenesis, impact, assessment, & treatment. Columbus, OH: Aiden & Eva Press; 2010.
29. Farronato G, Cannalire P, Martinelli G, Tubertini I, Giannini L, Galbiati G, Maspero C. Cleft lip and/or palate: review. Minerva Stomatol 2014; 63(4): 111-26.
30. Fraser FC. The genetics of cleft lip and cleft palate. Am J Hum Genet 1970; 22(3): 336-52.
31. Mossey PA, Little J, Munger RG, Dixon MJ, Shaw WC. Cleft lip and palate. Lancet 2009; 374(9703): 1773-85.
32. Murray JC. Gene/environment causes of cleft lip and/or palate. Clin genet 2002; 61(4): 248-56.
33. Parker SE, Mai CT, Canfield MA, Rickard R, Wang Y, Meyer RE, Anderson P, Mason CA, Collins JS, Kirby RS, Correa A; National Birth Defects Prevention Network. Updated National Birth Prevalence estimates for selected birth defects in the United States, 2004-2006. Birth Defects Res A Clin Mol Teratol 2010; 88(12): 1008-16.
34. Paul T, Brandt RS. Oral and dental health status of children with cleft lip and/or palate. Cleft Palate Craniofac J 1998; 35(4): 329-32.
35. Ranta R. A review of tooth formation in children with cleft lip/palate. Am J Orthod Dentofacial Orthop 1986; 90(1): 11-8.
36. Vanderas AP. Incidence of cleft lip, cleft palate, and cleft lip and palate among races: A review. Cleft Palate J 1987; 24(3): 216-25.
37. Zucchero TM, Cooper ME, Maher BS, Daack-Hirsch S, Nepomuceno B, Ribeiro L, et al. Interferon regulatory factor 6 (IRF6) gene variants and the risk of isolated cleft lip or palate. N Engl J Med 2004; 351(8): 769-80.
38. Kent RD. Motor control: Neurophysiology and functional development. In: A.J. Caruso and E.A. Strand (Eds.), Clinical management of motor speech disorders in children. New York: Thieme Medical Publishers; 1999: pp. 29-71.
39. Genna CW, Sandora L. Breastfeeding: Normal sucking and swallowing. In: C.W. Genna (Ed.), Supporting sucking skills in breastfeeding infants (3rd ed.). Woodhaven, NY: Jones and Bartlett Learning; 2017: pp. 1-48.

40. Hall KD. Pediatric dysphagia resource guide. San Diego, CA: Singular Publishing, 2001.
41. Thach BT. Maturation and transformation of reflexes that protect the laryngeal airway from liquid aspiration from fetal to adult life. Am J Med 2001; 111(Suppl 8A): 69S-77S.
42. Thach BT. Maturation of cough and other reflexes that protect the fetal and neonatal airway. Pulm Pharmacol Ther 2007; 20(4): 365-70.
43. Silveira LM, Prade LS, Ruedell AM, Haeffner LS, Weinmann, AR. Influence of breastfeeding on children's oral skills. Rev Saude Publica 2013; 47(1): 37-43. [Article in English, Portuguese]
44. Bagdade JD, Hirsch J. Gestational and dietary Influences on the lipid content of the Infant buccal fat pad. Proc Soc Exp Biol Med 1966; 122(2): 616-9.
45. Jackson IT. Anatomy of the buccal fat pad and its clinical significance. Plast Reconstr Surg 1999; 103(7): 2061-3.
46. Morris SE, Klein MD. Pre-Feeding skills: A comprehensive resource for mealtime development. (2nd ed.). Austin, TX: Pro-Ed; 2000.
47. Racz L, Maros TN, Seres-Sturm L. Structural characteristics and functional significance of the buccal fat pad (corpus adiposum buccae). Morphol Embryol 1989; 35(2): 73-7.
48. Ramsay DT, Hartmann PE. Milk removal from the breast. Breastfeed Rev 2005; 13(1): 5-7.
49. Tostevin PMJ, Ellis H. The buccal pad of fat: A review. Clin Anat 1995; 8(6): 403-6.
50. Bahr D. Nobody ever told me (or my mother) that! Everything from bottles and breathing to healthy speech development. Arlington, TX: Sensory World; 2010.
51. Bahr D. Feed your baby and toddler right: Early eating and drinking skills encourage the best development. Arlington, TX: Future Horizons; 2018.
52. Bosma JF. Maturation of function of the oral and pharyngeal region. Am J Orthod 1963; 49(2): 94-104.
53. Bosma JF. Oral and pharyngeal development and function. J Dent Res 1963; 42(1): 375-80.
54. Fayoux P, Marciniak B, Devisme L, Storme L. Prenatal and early postnatal morphogenesis and growth of human laryngotracheal structures. J Anat 2008; 213(2): 86-92.
55. Morris SE. A longitudinal study of feeding and prespeech skills from birth to three years (unpublished research study). VA: New Visions; 2003.
56. Bahr DC. Oral motor assessment and treatment: Ages and stages. Boston, MA: Allyn and Bacon; 2001.
57. Bosma JF. Anatomy of the infant head. Baltimore, MD: Johns Hopkins University Press; 1986.
58. Gola R, Cheynet F, Guyot L, Sauvant J, Richard O. Etiopathogenesis of nasal obstruction in children. Orthod Fr 2000; 71(2): 143-52. [Article in French]
59. Neskey D, Eloy JA, Casiano RR. Nasal, septal, and turbinate anatomy and embryology. Otolaryngol Clin North Am 2009; 42(2): 193-205.
60. Lundberg JO. Nitric oxide and the paranasal sinuses. Anat Rec (Hoboken) 2008; 291(11): 1479-84.
61. Lundberg JO, Weitzberg E. Nasal nitric oxide in man. Thorax 1999; 54(10): 947-52.
62. Schedin U, Norman M, Gustafsson LE, Herin P, Frostell C. Endogenous nitric oxide in the upper airways of healthy newborn infants. Pediatr Res 1996; 40(1): 148-51.
63. Cook CD, Sutherland JM, Segal S, Cherry RB, Mead J, McIlroy MB, Smith CA. Studies of respiratory physiology in the newborn infant. III. Measurements of mechanics of respiration. J Clin Invest 1957; 36(3): 440-8.
64. Fisher JT, Mortola JP, Smith JB, Fox GS, Weeks S. Respiration in newborns: development of the control of breathing. Am Rev Respir Dis 1982; 125(6): 650-7.
65. Vyas H, Milner AD, Hopkin IE. Intrathoracic pressure and volume changes during the spontaneous onset of respiration in babies born by cesarean section and by vaginal delivery. J Pediatr 1981; 99(5): 787-91.
66. Montagu A. Touching: The human significance of the skin. (3rd ed.). New York, NY: Harper & Row Publishers; 1986.
67. Love RJ, Webb WG. Neurology for the speech-language pathologist. (3rd ed.) Boston, MA: Butterworth-Heinemann; 1996.
68. Morris SE, Klein MD. Pre-Feeding skills: A comprehensive resource for feeding development. Tucson, AZ: Therapy Skill Builders; 1987.
69. Samuels M, Samuels N. The well baby book: A comprehensive manual of baby care, from conception to age four. New York: Summit Books; 1991.
70. Tuchman DN, Walter RS. Disorders of feeding and swallowing in infants and children: Pathophysiology, diagnosis, and treatment. San Diego: Singular Publishing Group; 1994.
71. Stevenson RD, Allaire JH. The development of normal feeding and swallowing. Pediatr Clin North Am 1991; 38(6): 1439-53.
72. Oetter P, Richter EW, Frick SM. M.O.R.E.: Integrating the mouth with sensory and postural functions (2nd ed.). Hugo, MN: PDP Press, Inc; 1995.
73. Lau C. Development of Suck and Swallow Mechanisms in Infants. Ann Nutr Metab 2015; 66 Suppl 5(0 5): 7-14.
74. Gewolb IH, Vice FL. Maturational changes in the rhythms, patterning, and coordination of respiration and swallow during feeding in preterm and term infants. Dev Med Child Neurol 2006; 48(7): 589-94.
75. Kelly BN, Huckabee ML, Jones RD, Frampton CM. The first year of human life: Coordinating respiration and nutritive swallowing. Dysphagia 2007; 22(1): 37-43.
76. Mathew OP, Clark ML, Pronske ML, Luna-Solarzano HG, Peterson MD. Breathing pattern and ventilation during oral feeding in term newborn infants. J Pediatr 1985; 106(5): 810-3.
77. Rogers B, Arvedson J. Assessment of infant oral sensorimotor and swallowing function. Ment Retard Dev Disabil Res Rev 2005; 11(1): 74-82.
78. Lau C, Kusnierczyk I. Quantitative evaluation of infant's nonnutritive and nutritive sucking. Dysphagia 2001; 16(1): 58-67.
79. Da Costa SP, Van Den Engel-Hoek L, Bos AF. Sucking and swallowing in infants and diagnostic tools. J Perinatol 2008; 28(4): 247-57.
80. Genna CW. Supporting sucking skills in breastfeeding infants (3rd ed.). Woodhaven, NY: Jones and Bartlett Learning; 2017.
81. Page DC. How to promote & provide functional jaw orthopedics. Funct Orthod 2001 Spring; 18(1): 22-30.
82. Page DC. The new dental-medical renaissance. Medically efficacious functional jaw orthopedics. Funct Orthod 1999 Jan-Mar; 16(1): 16-22, 24-5.
83. Nizel AE. Nursing bottle syndrome: rampant dental caries in young children. Nutrition News 1975; 38: 1-7.
84. Elad D, Kozlovsky P, Blum O, Laine AF, Po MJ, Botzer E, Dollberg S, Zelicovich M, Sira LB. Biomechanics of milk extraction during breast-feeding. Proc Natl Acad Sci USA 2014; 111(14): 5230-5.

85. Jacobs LA, Dickinson JE, Hart PD, Doherty DA, Faulkner SJ. Normal nipple position in term infants measured on breastfeeding ultrasound. J Hum Lact 2007; 23(1): 52-9.
86. Geddes DT, Kent JC, Mitoulas LR, Hartmann PE. Tongue movement and intra-oral vacuum in breastfeeding infants. Early Hum Dev 2008; 84(7): 471-7.
87. Gomes CF, Trezza E, Murade E, Padovani CR. Surface electromyography of facial muscles during natural and artificial feeding of infants. J Pediatr (Rio J) 2006; 82(2): 103-9.
88. Inoue N, Sakashita R, Kamegai T. Reduction of masseter muscle activity in bottle-fed babies. Early Hum Dev 1995; 42(3): 185-93.
89. Moral A, Bolibar I, Seguranyes G, Ustrell JM, Sebastiá G, Martínez-Barba C, Ríos J. Mechanics of sucking: comparison between bottle feeding and breastfeeding. BMC Pediatr 2010; 10:6.
90. Miller JL, Kang SM. Preliminary ultrasound observation of lingual movement patterns during nutritive versus non-nutritive sucking in a premature infant. Dysphagia 2007; 22(2): 150-60.
91. Nyqvist KH, Färnstrand C, Eeg-Olofsson KE, Ewald U. Early oral behaviour in preterm infants during breastfeeding: an electromyographic study. Acta Paediatr 2001; 90(6): 658-63.
92. Yilmaz G, Caylan N, Karacan CD, Bodur I, Gokcay G. Effect of cup feeding and bottle feeding on breastfeeding in late preterm infants: a randomized controlled study. J Hum Lact 2014; 30(2): 174-9.
93. Gupta A, Khanna K, Chattree S. Cup feeding: an alternative to bottle feeding in a neonatal intensive care unit. J Tropical Pediatr 1999; 45(2): 108-10.
94. Abouelfettoh AM, Dowling DA, Dabash SA, Elguindy SR, Seoud IA. Cup versus bottle feeding for hospitalized late preterm infants in Egypt: a quasi-experimental study. Int Breastfeed J 2008; 3:27.
95. Marinelli KA, Burke GS, Dodd VL. A comparison of the safety of cupfeedings and bottlefeedings in premature infants whose mothers intend to breastfeed. J Perinatol 2001; 21(6): 350-5.
96. Colson SD, Meek JH, Hawdon JM. Optimal positions for the release of primitive neonatal reflexes stimulating breastfeeding. Early Hum Dev 2008; 84(7): 441-9.
97. Colson S. Maternal breastfeeding positions: have we got it right? Pract Midwife 2005; 8(10); 24, 26-7.
98. Colson S. Maternal breastfeeding positions: have we got it right? (2). Pract Midwife 2005; 8(11): 29-32.
99. Chizawsky LL, Scott-Findlay S. Tummy time! Preventing unwanted effects of the "Back to Sleep" campaign. AWHONN Lifelines 2005 Oct-Nov; 9(5): 382-7.
100. Dudek-Shriber L, Zelazny S. The effects of prone positioning on the quality and acquisition of developmental milestones in four-month-old infants. Pediatr Phys Ther 2007; 19(1): 48-55.
101. Graham JM Jr. Tummy time is important. Clinical Pediatr (Phila) 2006; 45(2): 119-21.
102. Graham JM Jr, Gomez M, Halberg A, Earl DL, Kreutzman JT, Cui J, Guo X. Management of deformational plagiocephaly: repositioning versus orthotic therapy. J Pediatr 2005; 146(2): 258-62.
103. Graham JM Jr, Kreutzman J, Earl D, Halberg A, Samayoa C, Guo X. Deformational brachycephaly in supine-sleeping infants. J Pediatr 2005; 146(2): 253-7.
104. Hollier L, Kim J, Grayson BH, McCarthy JG. Congenital muscular torticollis and the associated craniofacial changes. Plast Reconstr Surg 2000; 105(3): 827-35.
105. Hutchison BL, Hutchison LA, Thompson JM, Mitchell EA. Plagiocephaly and brachycephaly in the first two years of life: a prospective cohort study. Pediatrics 2004; 114(4): 970-80.
106. Koren A, Reece SM, Kahn-D'angelo L, Medeiros D. Parental information and behaviors and provider practices related to tummy time and back to sleep. J Pediatr Health Care 2010; 24(4): 222-30.
107. Laughlin J, Luerssen TG, Dias MS; Committee on Practice and Ambulatory Medicine, Section on Neurological Surgery. Prevention and management of positional skull deformities in infants. Pediatrics 2011; 128(6): 1236-41.
108. Miller LC, Johnson A, Duggan L, Behm M. Consequences of the "back to sleep" program in infants. J Pediatr Nurs 2011; 26(4): 364-8.
109. Persing J, James H, Swanson J, Kattwinkel J; American Academy of Pediatrics Committee on Practice and Ambulatory Medicine, Section on Plastic Surgery and Section on Neurological Surgery. Prevention and management of positional skull deformities in infants. American Academy of Pediatrics Committee on Practice and Ambulatory Medicine, Section on Plastic Surgery and Section on Neurological Surgery. Pediatrics 2003; 112(1 Pt 1): 199-202.
110. Wen LM, Baur LA, Simpson JM, Rissel C, Flood VM. Effectiveness of an early intervention on infant feeding practices and "tummy time:" a randomized controlled trial. Arch Pediatr Adolesc Med 2011; 165(8): 701-7.
111. Zachry AH, Kitzmann KM. Caregiver awareness of prone play recommendations. Am J Occup Ther 2011; 65(1): 101-5.
112. Bly L. Motor Skills Acquisition in the First Year: An Illustrated Guide to Normal Development. USA: Psychological Corporation; 1994.
113. Saint-Anne Dargassies S. Neurological development in the full-term and premature neonate. New York: Excerpta Medica; 1977.
114. Vulpe SG. Vulpe assessment battery – Revised: Developmental assessment, performance analysis, individualized programming for the atypical child. New York: Slosson Educational Publications; 1994.
115. Johnson-Martin NM, Attermeier SM, Hacker BJ. The Carolina curriculum for infants & toddlers with special needs (3rd ed.). Baltimore, MD: Paul H. Brookes Publishing Company, 2004.
116. Saarinen UM, Kajosaari M. Breastfeeding as prophylaxis against atopic disease: prospective follow-up study until 17 years old. Lancet 1995; 346(8982): 1065-9.
117. Aniansson G, Alm B, Andersson B, Håkansson A, Larsson P, Nylén O, Peterson H, Rignér P, Svanborg M, Sabharwal H, et al. A prospective cohort study on breast-feeding and otitis media in Swedish infants. Pediatr Infect Dis J 1994; 13(3): 183-8.
118. Barlow B, Santulli TV, Heird WC, Pitt J, Blanc WA, Schullinger JN. An experimental study of acute neonatal enterocolitis--The importance of breast milk. J Pediatr Surg 1974; 9(5): 587-95.
119. Watkins CJ, Leeder SR, Corkhill RT. The relationship between breast and bottle feeding and respiratory illness in the first year of life. J Epidemiol Community Health 1979; 33(3): 180-2.
120. Speer CP, Schatz R, Gahr M. Function of breast milk macrophages. Monatsschr Kinderheilkd 1985; 133(11): 913-7. [Article in German]
121. Cummings NP, Neifert MR, Pabst MJ, Johnston RB Jr. Oxidative metabolic response and microbicidal activity of

human milk macrophages: effect of lipopolysaccharide and muramyl dipeptide. Infect Immun 1985; 49(2): 435-9.
122. Queiroz VA, Assis AM, da Costa R Júnior H. Protective effect of human lactoferrin in the gastrointestinal tract. Rev Paul Pediatr 2013; 31(1): 90-95. [Article in English, Portuguese]
123. Bertrand FR. The relationship of prolonged breast feeding to facial features. Cent Afr J Med 1968; 14(10): 226-7.
124. Broad FE. The effects of infant feeding on speech quality. N Z Med J 1972; 76(482): 28-31.
125. Broad FE. Further studies on the effects of infant feeding on speech quality. N Z Med J 1975; 82(553): 373-6.
126. Hoefer C, Hardy MC. Later development of breast fed and artificially fed infants. JAMA 1929, 92(8): 615-9.
127. Horwood LJ, Ferguson DM. Breastfeeding and later cognitive and academic outcomes. Pediatrics 1998; 101(1): E9.
128. Palmer B. The influence of breastfeeding on the development of the oral cavity: A commentary. J Hum Lact 1998; 14(2): 93-8.
129. Pottenger FM, Krohn B. Influence of breast feeding on facial development. Arch Pediatr 1950; 67(10): 454-61.
130. Rey J. Breastfeeding and cognitive development. Acta Paediatr Suppl. 2003; 92 (442): 11-8.
131. West D, Marasco L. The breastfeeding mother's guide to making more milk. Columbus, OH: McGraw Hill; 2008.
132. Satter E. Child of mine: Feeding with love and good sense, Revised. Boulder, CO: Bull Publishing Company; 2000.
133. Morris SE. Developmental implications for the management of feeding problems in neurologically impaired infants. Semin Speech Lang 1985; 6(4): 293-315.
134. Stevenson RD, Allaire JH. The development of normal feeding and swallowing. Pediatr Clin North Am 1991; 38(6): 1439-53.
135. Matsuo K, Palmer JB. Anatomy and physiology of feeding and swallowing: normal and abnormal. Phys Med Rehabil Clin N Am 2008; 19(4): 691-707.
136. Mennella JA, Reiter AR, Daniels LM. Vegetable and fruit acceptance during infancy: Impact on ontogeny, genetics, and early experiences. Adv Nutr 2016; 7(1): 211S-219S.
137. Bahr D, Johanson N. A family-centered approach to feeding disorders in children (birth to 5-years). SIG 13 Perspectives on Swallowing and Swallowing Disorders (Dysphagia) 2013; 22(4): 161-71.

7

Introducing solid foods to infants

Gill Rapley

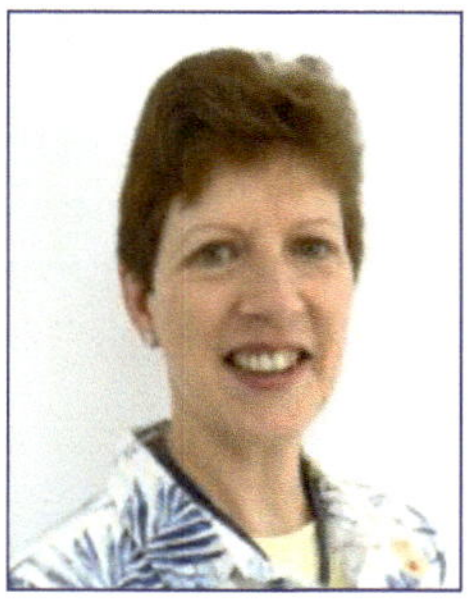

7.1 Introduction

As explained in chapter 6, breastfeeding has a major part to play in optimizing the early development of the orofacial complex. But what happens when the infant begins to need other foods? Might the way in which those are presented – and therefore the way in which they are eaten – have similar implications for facial growth? The answer is: almost certainly – and it has implications for many other areas of development as well. This chapter considers just how important the way solid foods are introduced may be for a child's long-term health.

7.2 Complementary feeding and weaning

For the first six months of life, the only food the vast majority of infants need is breastmilk. Avoiding any other food or drink during this period – that is, breastfeeding exclusively – is associated with the best health outcomes [1], including optimal development of the facial bone structure and musculature [2]. During these early months, the infant draws on the stores of key nutrients – notably iron – laid down during fetal life, to supplement those available from breastmilk. However, from about six months onwards these stores begin to decline, meaning that some expansion of the diet is needed [3]. This expansion is termed "complementary feeding".

The purpose of complementary foods is, as the name suggests, to *complement* breastmilk, not to replace it [4]. They are intended to fill the micronutrient gap in the infant's diet, while at the same time acquainting the infant with an increasingly wide range of flavors and textures. Amounts ingested are expected to remain small for several months, with breastfeeding providing the majority of the infant's nourishment until the first birthday, and continuing until age two, or beyond.

The change from milk feeds to family meals is sometimes referred to as "weaning". However, this term is ambiguous. It is commonly defined in one of two ways: as the introduction of solid food or as the cessation of breastfeeding. In reality, weaning is an extended period of time encompassing both these events, from the first taste of solid food to the last breastfeed [5]. In contexts in which infant formula replaces breastmilk, the end of weaning can be understood to mean the last formula feed.

Gill Rapley, PhD
Canterbury Christ Church University, Canterbury, Kent, UK

Email: gill@rapleyweaning.com

7.3 The development of chewing

The average full-term newborn infant has innate reflexes that enable him or her to feed at the breast or from a bottle, drawing in liquid food and swallowing it. Feeding from a bottle relies mainly on suction, whereas feeding at the breast exercises the muscles of the jaw, tongue and palate in more complex ways [2]. In the early months non-liquids are spontaneously expelled from the mouth by the extrusion or "tongue thrust" reflex, but by four months this reflex is disappearing, and the position of the infant's larynx allows more space within the oral cavity [6], such that the infant can "mouth" pieces of food when they are held up to his or her lips. However, the infant is still not able to bite or chew; therefore, he or she cannot manage "solid" foods except in semiliquid form, using an adapted sucking action.

By six months the situation is very different. At this age, infants have developed a range of oral motor skills that allow them to manage foods of varying textures. Infants are able to "munch" food with an up-and-down movement of the lower jaw and are beginning to use their tongue in a lateral manner, enabling them to move food to the sides of the mouth for chewing [7]. Between six and nine months, infants develop the ability to collect together a bolus of food on the tongue and move it deliberately to the back of the mouth for swallowing, independently of the sucking movement.

Infants are commonly described as needing to "learn" to chew, via the use of semisolid "transitional" foods fed to them by spoon. Indeed, clearing a spoon with the top lip is seen by some as a key feeding skill, preceding the development of chewing. In fact, there is no evidence to support this notion. Biting, chewing and swallowing appear spontaneously, as part of an infant's natural development [7], whereas spoons and pureed foods are the chosen attributes of specific cultural groups [8].

7.4 A historical perspective

The age of introduction of complementary foods has varied enormously over time and differs across the world, even today. However, while tradition in some cultures dictates that infants should be given small tastes of one or more foods when they are only a few days or weeks old, the idea of routinely giving foods other than milk before the child himself or herself can grasp them is a relatively modern one. Infants spontaneously begin to reach out for food and take it to their mouth at approximately the same age as they begin to chew, that is, at around six months [9]. This is – coincidentally (or not?) – the age at which, we now know, they are just beginning to need small additions to their diet. Thus, it seems infants can be relied upon to initiate this change themselves, at the point where they need to. Indeed, archeological evidence indicates that thousands of years ago, infants were routinely chewing tough foods from around six months [10]. As Gabrielle Palmer points out, in prehistoric times a breastfeeding mother would have had no reason to coax her baby to eat or drink anything other than breastmilk; the transition to other foods would have happened naturally, at the child's instigation [11]. That the human race has survived thus far is a testament to the reliability of this process.

The move to giving complementary foods to children younger than six months has been linked to the Industrial Revolution, which significantly altered the role of women [11-13]. When mothers began to undertake industrial and factory work, they were necessarily separated from their infants for long periods, so a replacement for breastmilk had to be found. Initially, this took the form of broths, gruels or "paps" but, for slightly older babies, it became common to grind and/or sieve other foods into a semisolid form, so they could be fed by spoon. The increasing medicalization of infant care meant that these practices were encouraged by doctors and other "experts", many of whom produced their own patented formulas. It was not long before an industry emerged to relieve hard-pressed mothers of the need to make their own infant food, quickly normalizing the use of commercial "baby food" and encouraging its continued use long after the child had begun to chew.

7.5 The conventional approach

For most of the last century, it has been the norm, at least in the UK and USA, to begin complementary feeding with spoon-fed purees, an approach that still predominates today. The most common first food is cereal or rice, quickly followed by fruits and/or vegetables, either as individual flavors or in combinations of two or three. The infant then progresses to blended meals, containing meat or fish as well as vegetables, and cereal-fruit combinations. These may be home-cooked or – increasingly – consist of commercially prepared jars or pouches. From around six or seven months the infant is offered "finger foods", such as toast, rusks and fruit, to pick up and eat with his or her hands, while continuing to be spoon fed by his or her caregivers. As the infant matures, the food is presented mashed rather than pureed and he or she is encouraged to begin holding the spoon himself or herself. Independent feeding is not normally expected before about one year, and the majority of the infant's food may continue to be mashed for several more months.

Typically, in the early months of the conventional approach, the infant is fed separately from the rest of the family and eats different food. The parent (or other caregiver) decides what each spoonful will consist of and how rapidly the next one will be presented – and, by implication, how quickly the baby will process each mouthful. If the baby does not comply readily, persuasion and/or distraction techniques, such as rhymes, counting ("One more for Grandma") and games of airplanes or trains, are employed to coax him or her to open his or her mouth so that the spoon can be inserted. Following the guidance of health professionals, the parent gradually increases the amount of food the infant is expected to eat at each meal and regulates the frequency of breastfeeding (or amount of formula offered) accordingly.

7.6 Baby-led weaning

Baby-led weaning (also known as BLW) is an approach to complementary feeding in which the infants set the pace for the transition from milk feeds to family foods [14]. Infants are the ones who choose when they will have their first taste of solid food, what they will eat at each meal, how quickly they will eat it and when they will stop eating. They sit at the family table and are offered healthy foods from among those the rest of the family are eating, in shapes, sizes and textures that lend themselves to easy grasping, handling and chewing. There is no coaxing, praise or trickery to persuade them to eat – indeed, no pressure for them to engage with the food at all unless they wish to.

Baby-led weaning gives the infants time to explore food, both before they decide to take their first mouthful and at each mealtime thereafter. Using all their senses, they quickly learn to link appearance and odor with taste and texture. This allows them to recognize familiar foods, to anticipate taste and to predict how a new food is likely to behave in their mouth. This, in turn, enhances their ability to choose foods according to their appetite and to manage a variety of textures safely and efficiently. They are also able to watch their parents eating food that looks the same as theirs – and may even be handed food from their plates. This enables the infants to copy their parents' eating behaviors, while increasing their confidence that what they have been offered is both edible and safe.

The baby-led approach likens moving on to solid foods to other developmental milestones, such as rolling over, walking and talking, all of which occur at a time determined by the infants – as long as the necessary opportunities are provided. The theory is underpinned by the fact that typical six-month-old infants are interested in their surroundings and keen to mimic what they see others doing. They spontaneously reach out for objects that interest them – including food – and take them to their mouth. When infants are allowed to experiment in this way, they learn what is edible and what isn't and – eventually – that eating assuages feelings of hunger.

Baby-led weaning differs from the conventional approach most obviously in the consistency and presentation of the food, and in where the agency and control over feeding lie, but it is not just about finger foods or who does the feeding. The baby-led approach centers on respecting infants' abilities, their maturity and their appetite. It allows them to begin eating when they are developmentally ready to do so, to eat only what they need, and to control the pace at which solid foods take over from milk feeds.

The theory of BLW rests on the fact that infants are born able to feed themselves. Although we talk about mothers breastfeeding their babies, the mother's role is, in reality, simply to make her breast available; it's the baby who does the feeding. It makes no sense that infants should cease to be able to meet their own nutritional needs, at the point when they begin to require additional foods. Our insistence, in recent times, on spoon feeding and purees stems from a belief – fueled by commercial interests – that the need for complementary foods precedes the ability to chew. Now that research has established a new timeline, in which the expansion of the diet and the development of chewing *coincide*, there seems no justification for overriding the infant's innate motivation and abilities. All we need to do is to prepare healthy food, in a format that the babies can handle, and then share it with them.

7.7 Disadvantages of spoon feeding and purees

The conventional approach to the introduction of complementary foods has a number of disadvantages for the infant. Parent-led mealtimes commonly offer little or no opportunity to examine and explore the food, or to taste it before taking a mouthful. The food itself varies little in appearance, so the flavor of each spoonful cannot be reliably anticipated – and combined purees make it impossible for the baby to enjoy preferred flavors while rejecting disliked ones. The infant is usually the only person eating, fed by a single caregiver, so he or she has little opportunity to witness, or be part of, family mealtime interaction. There are also biophysical ramifications, in that pureed foods require little or no chewing. This means that each mouthful can be swallowed almost instantly – a response that is further encouraged if the next spoonful is already being proffered.

When infants are first introduced to spoon feeding their default mechanism for taking the food from the spoon is to suck [15]. This tends to propel the food to the back of the mouth, allowing it to be swallowed quickly. Thus, spoon feeding of pureed food fosters the continuation of an immature suck-swallow action, bypassing the need to engage the muscles of mastication. If this action is perpetuated beyond the point at which chewing should be happening, there may be consequences for both food acceptance [16] and facial growth [17].

Rapid swallowing permits shorter mealtimes. This may be an advantage for the hard-pressed parent, but it is generally accepted that eating rapidly – at any age – tends to outstrip the brain's ability to sense fullness. At the same time, a focus on the next mouthful allows the infant little opportunity to indicate satiety, even once he or she has become aware of it. Lack of mouth time also reduces the contact of the food with salivary enzymes, thereby shortening what may be a key part of the digestive process. Spoon feeding, therefore, incurs a risk of both overfeeding and undernutrition.

The picture is no better when the food contains lumps. The infant's natural inclination to suck food from a spoon – reinforced by previous experience with purees – means that the food tends to be directed towards the back of the mouth, necessitating a complex series of movements to bring it forward and sideways to the gums, to enable it to be chewed (and to avoid choking). Therefore, spoon feeding tends to make chewing more difficult than it needs to be and may even make eating less safe, as well as less pleasurable. Finally, pureeing involves the destruction of cell walls, a process that is known to increase the proportion of free sugars in the food, which may have immediate consequences for oral health, as well as encouraging an ongoing preference for sweetened foods.

It has been suggested that a lack of agency during eating may be frustrating – or even threatening – for the infant, and that being spoon fed could itself engender dislike of mealtimes [18]. If this is so, then much of what has been termed "food refusal" may, in fact, be *feeding* refusal. It is possible that spoon feeding, coupled with a lack of opportunity to examine what is offered and the homogenous appearance and texture of pureed foods, may have as great an influence on the development of food preferences in infancy as do individual food flavors themselves.

7.8 Advantages of self-feeding and graspable foods

Research into the longer-term benefits of baby-led weaning is growing. It has been shown to be associated with a longer period of exclusive breastfeeding and, in the toddler years, with less chance of picky eating and a greater enjoyment of food [19, 20]. There are also indications that it may help to reduce the risk of overeating and enhance overall nutrition [21-23]. Crucially, it has been shown to be at least as safe as the conventional approach [19, 24, 25]. Moreover, although the available evidence is largely anecdotal, many practitioners believe that the opportunity to chew a variety of textures from six months of age enhances the development of oral motor skills and fosters optimal growth of the orofacial complex, with implications for speech, respiratory health and the avoidance of malocclusion. But the benefits of BLW extend well beyond eating itself.

Infants learn about the world around them through their senses. Self-feeding with graspable foods offers unique opportunities for multisensory learning and exploratory play by providing access to materials that are texturally different from those likely to be available outside of mealtimes [26]. Therefore, it promotes the development of a wide range of fine motor skills. While the potential effects of this have yet to be studied, many parents and some healthcare practitioners report enhanced hand-eye coordination and fine motor skills among infants who have been introduced to solid foods this way.

Allowing the infant to feed herself frees the parent to eat alongside their child. This, in turn, leads to some valuable subsidiary benefits of shared mealtimes, such as the development of social skills and language [27] and the acquisition of table manners and use of cutlery, as well as wider cultural learning [28]. Parents who have implemented a baby-led approach report the absence of mealtime battles and pride in their child's confident approach to, and enjoyment of, food. They comment on the child's ability to act autonomously and to make healthy choices. And they value the chance to prepare one meal for everyone to eat together – often choosing to make improvements to the whole family's diet as a result.

7.9 Conclusion

Self-feeding from around six months of life, with chewable foods, fits with our knowledge of how infants develop and with existing research into the nutritional aspects of complementary feeding. It is likely that it has always been practiced by some parents (or has simply occurred spontaneously, especially in larger families), but it is only since the emergence of a supporting theory that the approach has had a name, enabling it to be discussed and researched.

Available evidence suggests that BLW works for the majority of babies [29, 30], that it may have benefits for many aspects of infant health, growth and development, and that it promotes relaxed and enjoyable family mealtimes. In the last eighteen years, awareness of the approach has exploded across social media and the Internet [June 16th, 2021: 6,300,000 Google results for "baby-led weaning"], such that it is now recognized worldwide as a feasible and rational alternative to the conventional way. Evidence, surely, that the proof of the pudding is in the way it is eaten.

REFERENCES

1. Kramer MS, Kakuma R. Optimal duration of exclusive breastfeeding. Cochrane Database Syst Rev 2012; 2012(8): CD003517.
2. Palmer B. The influence of breastfeeding on the development of the oral cavity: a commentary. J Hum Lact 1998; 14(2): 93-8.
3. Butte NF, Lopez-Alarcon MG, Garza C. Nutrient adequacy of exclusive breastfeeding for the term infant during the first six months of life. Geneva: WHO; 2002.
4. World Health Organization and UNICEF. Global Strategy for Infant and Young Child Feeding. Geneva: WHO; 2003.
5. Sellen DW, Smay DB. Relationship between subsistence and age at weaning in "preindustrial" societies. Hum Nat 2001; 12(1): 47-87.
6. Delaney AL, Arvedson JC. Development of swallowing and feeding: prenatal through first year of life. Dev Disabil Res Rev 2008; 14(2): 105-17.
7. Naylor AJ. Infant oral motor development in relation to the duration of exclusive breastfeeding. In: Naylor AJ and Morrow A. (eds.) Developmental Readiness of Normal Full Term Infants to Progress from Exclusive Breastfeeding to the Introduction of Complementary Foods: Reviews of the Relevant Literature Concerning Infant Immunologic, Gastrointestinal, Oral Motor and Maternal Reproductive and Lactational Development. Washington (DC): Wellstart International and the LINKAGES Project Academy for Educational Development; 2001: 21-26.
8. Stevenson RD, Allaire JH. The development of normal feeding and swallowing. Pediatr Clin North Am 1991; 38(6): 1439-53.
9. Illingworth RS, Lister J. The critical or sensitive period, with special reference to certain feeding problems in infants and children. J Pediatr 1964; 65(6): 839-48.
10. Corruccini RS. An epidemiologic transition in dental occlusion in world populations. Am J Orthod 1984; 86(5): 419-26.
11. Palmer G. Complementary Feeding: Nutrition, Culture and Politics. London: Pinter & Martin; 2011.
12. Boyd KL. Darwinian dentistry Part 1: an evolutionary perspective on the etiology of malocclusion. J Am Orthod Soc 2011; 11(6): 34-9.
13. Boyd KL. Darwinian dentistry part 2: early childhood nutrition, dentofacial development and chronic disease. J Am Orthod Soc 2012; 12(2): 28-32.
14. Rapley G, Murkett T. Baby-led Weaning: Helping Your Baby to Love Good Food. London: Vermilion; 2008.
15. Wickenden M. The development and disruption of feeding skills in babies and young children. In: Southall A and Martin C. (eds.). Feeding Problems in Children. 2nd ed. Abingdon, Oxon: Radcliffe Publishing Ltd.; 2010: 7-28.
16. Northstone K, Emmett P, Nethersole F; ALSPAC Study Team. The effect of age of introduction to lumpy solids on foods eaten and reported feeding difficulties at 6 and 15 months. J Hum Nutr Diet 2001; 14(1): 43-54.
17. Lieberman DE, Krovitz GE, Yates FW, Devlin M, St. Claire M. Effects of food processing on masticatory strain and craniofacial growth in a retrognathic face. J Hum Evol 2004; 46(6): 655-77.
18. Rapley G. Starting solid foods: does the feeding method matter? Early Child Dev Care 2016; 188(8): 1109-23.
19. Taylor RW, Williams SM, Fangupo LJ, Wheeler BJ, Taylor BJ, Daniels L, Fleming EA, McArthur J, Morison B, Erickson LW, Davies RS, Bacchus S, Cameron SL, Heath A-L M. Effect of a Baby-Led Approach to Complementary Feeding on Infant Growth and Overweight: A Randomized Clinical Trial. JAMA Pediatr 2017; 171(9): 838-46.
20. Fu X, Conlon CA, Haszard JJ, Beck KL, von Hurst PR, Taylor RW, Heath A-LM Food fussiness and early feeding characteristics of infants following Baby-Led Weaning and traditional spoon-feeding in New Zealand: An internet survey. Appetite 2018; 130:110-16.
21. Brown A, Lee MD. Early influences on child satiety-responsiveness: the role of weaning style. Pediatr Obes 2015; 10(1): 57-66.
22. Townsend E, Pitchford NJ. Baby knows best? The impact of weaning style on food preferences and body mass index in early childhood in a case-controlled sample. BMJ Open 2012; 2(1): e000298.
23. Rowan H, Lee M, Brown A. Differences in dietary composition between infants introduced to complementary foods using Baby-led weaning and traditional spoon feeding. J Hum Nutr Diet 2019; 32(1): 11-20.
24. Dogan E, Yilmaz G, Caylan N, Turgut M, Gokcay G, Oguz MM. Baby-led complementary feeding: Randomized controlled study. Pediatr Int 2018; 60(12): 1073-80.
25. Brown A. No difference in self-reported frequency of choking between infants introduced to solid foods using a baby-led weaning or traditional spoon-feeding approach. J Hum Nutr Diet 2018; 31(4): 496-504.
26. Goldschmied E, Jackson S. People Under Three: Young Children in Day Care. 2nd ed. London: Routledge; 2004.
27. Shutts K, Kinzler KD, DeJesus JM. Understanding infants'

and children's social learning about foods: previous research and new prospects. Dev Psychol 2013; 49(3): 419-25.

28. Fieldhouse P. Food and Nutrition: Customs and Culture. London: Chapman & Hall Ltd.; 1995.

29. Lakshman R, Clifton EA, Ong KK. Baby-Led Weaning-Safe and Effective but Not Preventive of Obesity. JAMA Pediatr 2017; 171(9): 832-33.

30. Wright CM, Cameron K, Tsiaka M, Parkinson KN. Is baby-led weaning feasible? When do babies first reach out for and eat finger foods? Matern Child Nutr 2011; 7(1): 27-33.

8 Good oral habits since day one

Pía Villanueva B. and Hernán Felipe Palomino V.

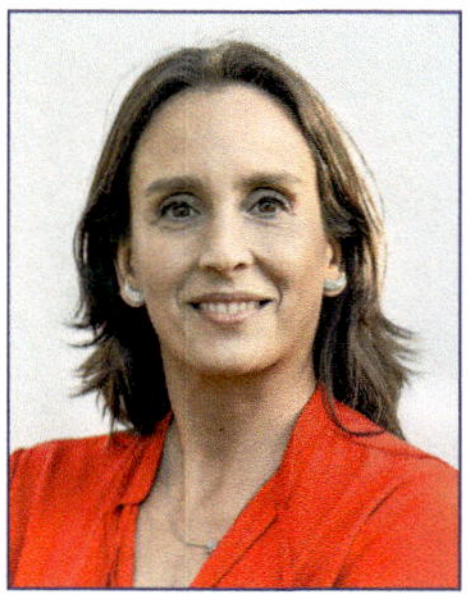

8.1 Introduction

Speech language pathology (*fonoaudiología*, logopedia) is celebrating its 50th anniversary in Chile. At present, our students are trained in five main areas: Children's Language, Audiology, Orofacial Motor Skills, Voice and Adult Language. In Orofacial Motor Skills we have multiple refinement options in which the professional speech language pathologists can deepen their knowledge and clinical practices in neonatology, labio-velo-palatine cleft, dentomaxillary anomalies, snoring and apnea, temporomandibular joint (TMJ) dysfunction and facial paralysis, among others. In the great majority of these patients, we can find a common factor: the presence of oral habits that perpetuate, increase or, in some cases, are causal factors of the treated pathology [1].

In order to contribute to the prevention of myofunctional orofacial disorders and to avoid the occurrence and establishment of oral habits, our efforts in the last 15 years have been aimed at changing the mentality of the clinical professional – speech pathologists, dentists, preschool educators – changing the focus from "evaluation and treatment of bad oral habits" to "prevention of dysfunctions and early stimulation of appropriate oral habits".

Working with children, parents, preschool educators, nurses, pediatricians and dentists, toward the opportune incorporation of favorable oral habits, we can promote this concept that is not generally considered within the care of children under 3 years of age, and its favorable consequence in the evolution of nutrition, speech development, growth and development of the maxillofacial complex.

We have worked hard in the development of a protocol to measure the incorporation of oral habits, as well as to monitor the functions of breathing, swallowing and speech in children, so that it can be applied in any area in which the child develops, as well as by the clinical professionals who serve in this area.

8.2 Protocol of appropriate incorporation of oral habits

Habits are unconscious repetitions of an act that begins as a conscious response to a functional, dysfunctional or parafunctional need of the individual. For the act of sucking, we can associate the physiological purpose of feeding. However,

Pía Villanueva B., MD, SLP
Professor, Universidad de Chile; Faculty of Medicine, Speech, Language & Hearing Science Department, Santiago, Chile

Email: piavilla@uchile.cl

Hernán Felipe Palomino V.
Universidad de Chile; Faculty of Medicine, Human Genetics Program, Institute of Biomedical Sciences (ICBM), Santiago, Chile

some children perpetuate the act in response to an emotional need, so the habit of sucking (fingers, objects, lips) develops.

Among the favorable habits, we can include nasal breathing, which not only favors clean, moist and filtered air intake, but also ensures the necessary myofunctional balance for adequate growth and maxillofacial development, with the sagittal, vertical and transverse stimulation of the tongue, as well as the opposite force of the cheeks and lips.

Considering that evaluations in Orofacial Myology detect pathologies in different stages of the growth and development of the subject, the protocols must also be associated with the needs of evaluation throughout the life cycle and, according to the degree of progress of the pathology, prevention, interception and treatment.

It is important to work in multi-professional informed teams to be able to solve orofacial pathologies. However, as the science progresses and we

Table 8.1 Protocol for inclusion of aproppiate oral habits (PIAOH)
Record Sheet **Prof. Pía Villanueva B., Chile**

Name: .... Date of Birth: .... Age: ....

Who applied the protocol

Name: .... Relation with the child: .... Institution: ....

1. NASAL HYGIENE AND NASAL PERMEABILITY CONSERVATION

1.1. Detection of functional nasal permeability

	right nostril	left nostril	
			Assessment date: ....
PeNaF	☐	☐	
PeNaF	☐	☐	Assessment date: ....
	Referred to ENT if the result is (+)		ENT Diagnosis /Procedure

1.2. Nasal Hygiene teaching

	present	absent
Air cycle management: mouth-nose	☐	☐
Parents: use of one hand	☐	☐
Child: use of both hands	☐	☐

2. EARLY DETECTION OF STRUCTURAL ALTERATION IN PHONOARTICULATORY ORGANS

	present	absent
Obstruction in the airways		
– Enlarged tonsils	☐	☐
– Nasal bridge deviation	☐	☐
– Enlarged nasal turbinates	☐	☐
Mechanical or structural impairments		
– Altered sublingual frenulum - ankiloglossia	☐	☐
– Craniofacial malformations	☐	☐
– Dentomaxillary anomalies	☐	☐

3. EARLY INCLUSION OF CONSISTENCIES, POSTURE AND FOOD UTENSILS

Stage	*Consistencies*	*Postures*	*Utensils*	*Movement*
0-4 months	liquid	face-up or semi- seated	mother breast or bottle	anteroposterior lingual
4-6 months	liquid	semi- seated	cup	oral games
6-10 months	mashed	sitting in a high chair with support	spoon	vertical lingual/vertical labial
10-12 months	chopped	sitting in a high chair without support	glass by the feeder	labial backwards
12-18 months	chopped	family chair with support	blunt fork	wrist action when the child eats alone
18-24 months	chopped or whole	family chair without support	glass	lingual-mandibular independence

know more about the triggers of each pathology, that an informed team must work together on procedures for the prevention of concomitant factors [2].

The Protocol for Inclusion of Appropriate Oral Habits (PIAOH) aims to contribute to the prevention of organic, functional and, in some cases, also psycho-emotional alterations, associated with bad oral habits (Table. 8.1) [3].

For the efficient application of the PIAOH one must manage the typical characteristics of the child's orofacial development, in order to sustain the appropriate incorporation of corresponding consistencies, postures, utensils and hygiene habits, which guarantee the morphological maintenance of the orofacial structures and functions and nasal breathing.

8.2.1 Maxillofacial aspects to be included in the health examination of children

A newborn has many orofacial features that favor nasal breathing and breastfeeding, such as a retruded mandible, a large tongue that occupies the entire oral cavity, and fatty pads that make up the walls of the mouth and cheeks. This orofacial environment, in conjunction with the rugae on the palate, allows for an efficient extraction of breast milk. The high position of the larynx, as well as the contact between the base of the tongue and the uvula, allows almost exclusively nasal breathing and offers a fantastic system of protection of the upper airway against aspiration events.

As a result of breastfeeding, the jaw begins to grow down and forward, producing the first physiological mandibular advance [4]. In addition, since the child can support his or her head, the laryngeal descent can occur and the reabsorption of the fatty pads of the cheeks begins, all factors that increase the intraoral space. During all this time the baby presents protrusive lingual movements and generates sounds as an oral expression. Feeding is through breastfeeding or formula in bottle.

At about six months of age, the larynx descends again, because the child is already able to keep an upright spine and spends most of the time with his or her head in an upright position and can remain seated. It is advisable to start using the high chair, initially with support and then gradually remove the support in order to promote motor control of the child's head and face. The lips and tongue acquire greater control and the anterior bilabial and vowel speech sounds appear. At this stage of the maxillofacial development, pediatricians suggest the incorporation of the first porridge and the use of a spoon. The child is already able to hold a toy in his or her hands and move it, and so is also capable of self-feeding and tearing food.

If the spoon and self-feeding are part of the life of the child, at nine months, the upper lip can be lowered and is able to drag the contents of the spoon into the mouth. This favors the symmetrical bilabial production of the sounds that the child has already begun to make.

When the child begins to walk, and the first deciduous molars erupt between 10 to 12 months of age, the first physiological mastication begins. It is necessary to incorporate new consistencies that favor mastication. At the same time, the child can produce vocalic, nasal, velar, bilabial sounds and begins to produce the first meaningful words and holophrases.

At 18 months of age, the child is neurologically prepared to demonstrate a soft closing of the lips and movements of lingual elevation during swallowing and speech, events that will be delayed as long as the child continues to be fed with utensils that keep the tongue low, such as milk bottles, sipping cups, suck/twist/squeeze food containers, or maintain suction habits of pacifiers, objects or fingers [5]. Therefore, the incorporation of a real cup or a narrow-mouth bottle is proposed at this time. At this time, it is also appropriate to chop the food to stimulate and increase control of chewing, and to feed the child at the family table in a chair with a cushion or a lift, eliminating the baby high chair.

If the child uses utensils, and if the child's posture during feeding and the incorporation of consistencies have been adequate, then at 24 months the child is able to share the same foods as the parents. At this time, the child is also able to present a soft closing of the lips at rest and during swallowing, without spillage of food during chewing and swallowing, and presents an articulation of bilabial sounds with symmetrical participation of the lower and upper lips. Regarding to lingual movements, the appearance of the second molar ensures the second physiological rise of the occlusion and the consequent increase in vertical intraoral space. Thus, the lingual protrusion will be replaced by the anterior third of the tongue at rest, in swallowing, and in the production of speech sounds with non-vibrating lingual elevation, such as / t /, / d /, / l /. These steps constitute the establishment of lingual-mandibular independence [3].

Nasal breathing, the correct inclusion of food consistencies, the progression of the positions in which the children are fed, as well as the inclusion of feeding utensils, favor the development of hard and soft tissues of the oral and nasal cavities, as well as the development of chewing, swallowing and speech functions [6].

If we promote early detection and adequate management of poor nasal hygiene, unnecessary bottle feeding, habitual suction of fingers or objects (like pacifiers) as well as the early detection of anatomical orofacial alterations, such as a short lingual frenulum, we will prevent the establishment of parafunctional oral habits, dentomaxillary anomalies and orofacial dysfunctions [7].

8.2.2 National evidence in Chile

Through joint projects between professionals and researchers in speech language pathology, dentistry, orthodontics, maxillo-facial surgery, genetics and pediatrics, we have conducted studies regarding the factors just mentioned.

We know that lingual interposition between teeth, produced by an anterior tongue thrust, modifies the tongue's axis with a consequent development of an anterior or lateral dental open bite, depending on the place of force. There could be a persisting lingual thrust at rest, affecting also swallowing and, in Chilean Spanish, frequently affecting the production of the speech sounds / s /, / t / and / d /, and in more severe cases, affecting the speech sounds / n /, / ñ / and / ch /. Although lingual interposition is related to an anterior open bite, it is also a sign of lingual dysfunction or parafunction. An anterior tongue thrust was reported in 84-95% of cases with dentomaxillary anomalies and in 33% of children with normal occlusion [8]. An interesting aspect was that lingual interposition was present regardless of the type of malocclusion (deep bite, open bite or cross bite).

Regarding finger sucking, we can mention that it causes maxillary compression and the consequent increase in the vertical dimension of the palate. This is the reason why we studied nasal permeability (nasal breathing) and its behavior in children with severe maxillary compression who would undergo orthopedic treatment by Rapid Palatal Expansion (RPE), since the palate is part of the "floor" of the nose. It was shown that all the children with severe maxillary compression had their tongue in a low resting position, a retruded mandibular position, oral breathing, as well as an increase in nasal resistance during breathing. After the RPE, the children showed an increase in the palatal transverse dimension and a decrease in the vertical dimension of the palate, with a consequent decrease in nasal resistance, which directly improved clinical nasal permeability [9].

Regarding the incorporation of utensils, as well as consistency and habits of nasal and oral hygiene, we conducted a survey of two different social realities [10]. One group of parents, who answered the survey, lived in an isolated rural area of Chile and belonged to a low socioeconomic status. These parents reported maintaining breastfeeding and the most favorable patterns of incorporation of "utensils, consistencies and postures in the diet". Basically, they were following traditions that are passed from generation to generation, because it is the mother who cares for her children. Moreover, the economic situation motivates the use of adult utensils as soon as possible, without incorporating accessory utensils (such as sipping cups or plastic spoons) that may be expensive and are not for sale in this geographical area.

The parents in the urban area, who answered the survey, and who belong to a high sociocultural level, tended to stop breastfeeding early and replace it with bottle formula and to use accessory utensils such as sipping cup, small plastic spoons or containers that squeeze out the food. These parents were more likely to delegate feeding to caregivers who were often unaware of the importance of modifying food consistencies, postures and utensils. Regarding oral hygiene, both groups of parents reported having being informed by the dentist about the proper techniques to use, while regarding nasal hygiene, neither group reported having received any formal instruction on how to efficiently cleanse the nose [10].

This is why the PIAHO (*Protocolo de Incorporación Apropiada de Hábitos Orales*, in Spanish) was created and tested. The protocol consists of three evaluation and stimulation items, where the health professional, parent or educator can simply record the findings, while also keeping track of progress as changes are implemented [3].

The first item on the PIAHO is the maintenance of nasal hygiene and patency, which assesses the ability of the children and/or their parents to perform an efficient nasal hygiene technique; it records the ease of breathing, the use of one or two hands in handling objects, and finally creates a plan of what parents and children should learn and implement. Functional nasal patency is also measured by the PeNaF test (*Permeabilidad Nasal Funcional*, in Spanish) [11], the results of which are recorded before and after efficient nasal hygiene. Functional nasal patency is therefore monitored for two months prior to requesting an ENT (Ear, Nose and Throat) evaluation if the results remain altered.

The second item on the PIAHO is related to the early detection of organic alterations in orofacial structures through an intra- and extra-oral clinical evaluation. In this section of the protocol the parents and educators find an observation guide manual and photos to compare, and if they detect any anomalies it is suggested to refer the child to a specialist for confirmation of the observed feature and its timely management.

The third on the PIAHO is about the proper incorporation of food textures and consistencies, utensils and postures during early feeding. A diagram is shown to the parents in which the child's skills are identified according to each of these characteristics and thus the profile of the child's eating skills can be determined. For example, if a 4-year-old child is still fed with a baby bottle and smooth porridge, while sitting on his mother's lap and using a small plastic spoon, then that child meets the skills of a 6 months old in terms of food consistency and use of a utensil, but the level of a 4 months old in terms of feeding posture [12].

8.3 If we lose the battle

If, for lack of information or lack of adherence to early stimulation, we lose the battle of prevention and a poor oral habit is established, we, the clinicians, must be aware of it and inform the parents, or other adults caring for the child, that oral habits are unfavorable for the correct maxillofacial development. A poor oral habit is a behavior that may start as a conscious action, but, when repeated frequently, it becomes unconscious and chronic and it interferes with the neuromuscular balance, thus altering the growth and normal development of the maxillofacial complex. This is due to the fact that the forces of the agonist muscles are prevented from exercising their action, while the force of the antagonist muscles increases in intensity, thus producing a deformation or malocclusion. The magnitude of this deformation or malocclusion will then depend on several factors and among them the age at which the habit begins to manifest itself, the frequency, intensity and duration of the stimuli. In practice, damage may be caused by how early in life the habit is established, how much time is spent while the habit occurs (in hours or minutes), how frequently it occurs (every 5 min or once a day) and with what intensity it occurs (especially important for thumb sucking). These habits can cause not just eating issues, but also structural, functional and facial aesthetic alterations, which may result in emotional issues, and even suggest learning problems, which may interfere with interpersonal relationships.

8.4 Conclusion

To evaluate oral habits, it is necessary for the participation of a multidisciplinary team, which includes among others: a dentist, a pediatrician, an ENT, a psychologist, a speech pathologist, a teacher and the parents. The earlier the oral habit is detected, the less damage it causes, so early detection (possibly at birth) is an important goal to pursue. It is therefore important that teachers and parents are educated on the issue of oral habits and eating habits, so they can observe the child directly during the day to request the most appropriate referral and make the anamnesis more informative. This will allow us to perform treatments with efficient results ensuring the best quality of life.

REFERENCES

1. De Barbieri Z, et al. Fonoaudiología 40 años de historia. Ed. Esc de Fonoaudiología: Universidad de Chile, 2012.
2. Susanibar F, Marchesan I, Parra D, Dioses A. Tratado de Evaluación de Motricidad Orofacial. Madrid: Ed. EOS. 627-36, 2014.
3. Villanueva P. PIAHO: una herramienta para la prevención de hábitos orales deletéreos (protocolo de incorporación apropiada de hábitos orales). Rev. CEFAC 2014; 16(4): 1326-39. [Article in Spanish]
4. Condori Quispe WW, Ayca Castro IR. Relation between maternal and artificial lactation with mandibular growth in children from age 0 to 6 months of age attended at the Health Center La Esperanza, Tacna-2017. Revista Odontológica Basadrina 2019; 3(1): 15-9.
5. Morris SE, Klein MD. Pre-Feeding Skills: A comprehensive resource for feeding development. Arizona: Therapy Skill Builders, 2000.
6. Marchesan I. Antecedentes clínicos en Motricidad Orofacial. Sao Paulo: Pulso Ed. 238-252, 2013.
7. Marchesan I. Tratamento da Degluticao. Sao Paulo: Pulso ed: 239-246, 2005.
8. Villanueva P, Palomino HM, Arancibia C, Lagos X, Navarrete M. Disfunciones linguales en pacientes con maloclusión. Odontología Chilena 2002; 50: 23-8.
9. Palomino HM, Villanueva P, Lagos X, Illanes A. Expansión palatina rápida y respiración bucal. Rev Chil Fonoaud 2002; 3: 99-113.
10. Villanueva P. Lecture: Chilean Reality in Orofacial Motricity: clinical and basic evidence. At Meeting of CMOL (Comunidad de Motricidad Orofacial Latinoamericana). Lima. April 2013.
11. Villanueva P, Niño De Zepeda A, Lizana ML, Fernández MA, Palomino HM. Eficiency in Detection of Functional Nasal Permeability: Clinical Test Report. Rev Chil Ortod 2008; 25: 98-106.
12. Villanueva P. Deglución atípica: implicancias ortodóncicas. Rev Chil Ortod 2005; 22: 92-9.

9 Physiological weaning and psychological weaning

Rita De Angelis

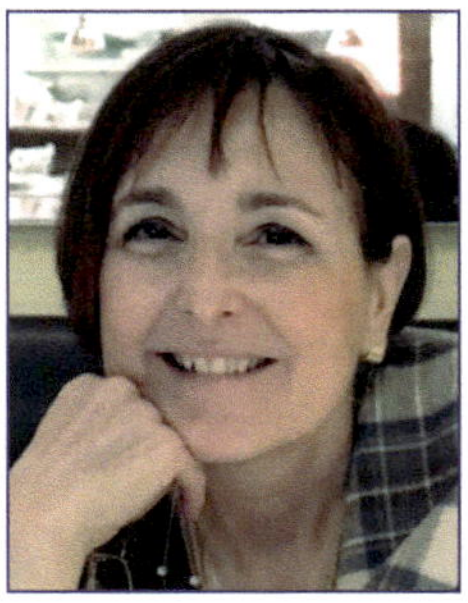

9.1 Introduction

The term weaning refers to the passage from an exclusively milky diet to an adult diet, diversified from an organoleptic point of view and methods of administration. Currently, weaning does not indicate separation from the breast, but rather the introduction of foods other than milk, usually semisolid.

Feeding the child in the first year of life has remained limited to breastfeeding for many centuries, while changing profoundly in the second half of the last century, as a result of new socioeconomic and cultural factors.

On the one hand, guiding the feeding of the infant has slowly moved from traditional family figures to the figure of the pediatric specialist. Furthermore, the food industry has created freeze-dried and homogenized ready to use products that can be easily administered to infants, earlier and earlier in life.

The figure of the pediatrician fits into this picture, almost acting as a hinge in the refinement of knowledge about the child's digestive physiology and the industry that proposes increasingly safer and specifically designed products. The advance in weaning practices is also linked to the new role of women in society and in the workplace, which has led consequently to the rapid decline in incidence and duration of breastfeeding. In the USA, in the 1950s, solid foods were introduced in 88% of cases within the first 3 months of life; in the 1960s, 82% of infants ate solid foods in the second month of life. Very strong promotion of these products succeeded in creating guilt feelings in mothers who did not use them. These attitudes have also had repercussions in Europe, albeit more conservatively.

The progressive advance of weaning has reached a plateau in recent years and, in some cases, a reversal of the trend, as some potential risks have been highlighted in the premature introduction of foods other than milk into the child's diet. These risks can range from possible intolerances due to the gut metabolism limits of the infant's organism, to sensitization to heterologous proteins, to potential dietary imbalance, with excessive introduction of calories, fats, sugars and salt, leading to a tendency towards obesity, tooth decay, changes in taste, hypertension and other metabolic disorders later in life.

Currently, a period of weaning between the 5th and 7th month is recommended by all pediatric schools. It is precisely at this age that some maturing

Rita De Angelis, MD
Medical Surgeon
Specialist in Pediatrics
Specialist in Puericulture
Pediatrician ASL Rome 2 (1985-2022)
Scientific Committee FIMP, Rome, Italy (until 2022)

Email: rita.deangelis.pediatra@gmail.com

phenomena linked to weaning are being completed, such as the maturation of the intestine and the anatomo-neuro-functional modifications of the oropharynx [1].

Until the 3rd month of life, the child is oriented towards the function of sucking: the structure of the mouth (small and elongated) and the reflexes (cardinal points) lead to the localization of the nipple and its squashing, while expelling solid foods from the pharynx and spitting, as defense mechanisms protecting the respiratory tract from food inhalation.

Between the 4th and 8th month after birth, the tongue stretches, the muscles that allow chewing movements and the lip closure around the spoon and cup also mature. Salivation increases considerably, the extrusion reflex disappears and finally the dentition process begins; the *drinking* child turns into an *eating* child.

Last but not least, the psychomotor maturation of the children allows them a safe control of the head at 3 months, then the acquisition of the sitting position with support by the 6th month, and finally without support by the 8th month. This position allows the child to no longer need to take food while being in the mother's arms but to sit alone in front of the mother, *with the dish that separates them,* to have a different relationship with the person who feeds the child, and more suitable for intake of semisolid food. Thus, the child gains greater independence, learns to coordinate the movements of the hand to and from the mouth, initially in the absence of food, then aimed at self-feeding, and learns to communicate acceptance or rejection of the food [2].

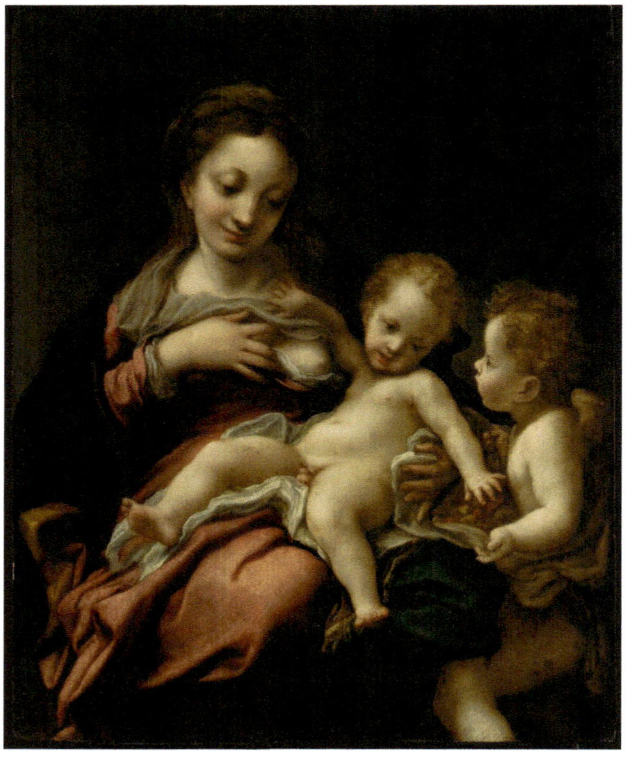

Fig. 9.1 Nursing Madonna with an angel by Correggio.

9.2 The psychological development of the child

Every human has a long way to go before becoming autonomous. A human has many potentials that must "unfold" little by little, and it is a very slow path that must reach a "psychological birth" after many months of "contact" with the mother. The birth of the human being takes place in a continuum, where the growth process goes from the biological to the mental [3].

In the first month of life, children are attentive to sensations that come from within their bodies, and a state of absolute narcissism (physiological autism) prevails, their life is based on the sensations and satisfactions of their needs, and they are invested in "myself" [4]. A new stage follows, in which there is a vague awareness that the fulfillment of one's own needs cannot come from within but from some external entity (this is the beginning of the symbiotic phase). That awareness manifests itself with following one's gaze or turning towards the breast.

From the second month onwards, there is a *symbiosis* (fusion with the mother in which the "I" is not yet differentiated from the "non-I"), in which children behave as if they and their mothers were an omnipotent system, a dual unity with oceanic sensations without boundaries. The autistic shell cracks and a new protective shelter against the stimuli begins to form, which envelops the symbiotic orbit of the dyad mother-child.

In the first semester of life, the dependence on the mother is absolute and, if basic needs are satisfied, then the children develop desires, trust, the ability to wait and memories. The development moves from feelings to perceptions of oneness (through the mother's body language and her eyes), and from individual perceptions to affections, and then thinking.

In the first part of the symbiotic phase (between the 2nd and the 4th month), the formation of one's *self* takes place, along with the sense of self as an individual, forming a foundation. The self is constituted by the contribution of innate potentials and the environment (the mother) that act on them as facilitators or pathogens. If there is no creation of confidence or trust in the first 3-4 months, then self-esteem in adulthood will be missing or lacking.

The second part of the symbiosis (4-6 months) is more rational: it is emblematic of the representation that Correggio makes of it in the painting "*La Ma-*

donna del Latte" (The Mother and the Milk) (Fig. 9.1) which, as Goethe says in his "Italian Journey", should have been called "The Weaned Jesus ". The Infant Jesus is represented with one hand on his Mother's breast, representing the ongoing contact with his mother, while the other hand is reaching out towards the pear, symbol of the breast, offered by an Angel.

The first sign that the child begins to be able to *lose* is making objects fall to the ground: "the game of dropping objects begins around 5 months and continues until 12-13 months".

Separation also depends on the mother and from how much she is able to facilitate the separation process. The Madonna by Correggio has a "facilitating" expression. Unlimited giving during the period of symbiosis and knowing how to mitigate this gratification of needs facilitate the separation process [5].

The mother's physical presence in the same bed or in the room delays normal dyad separation-individualization, a process that takes place at the end of the first year. When symbiotic connections with the mother are maintained and the child physically does not lose them, he/she has less need to symbolize them. This excessive presence exerts an inhibiting or delaying action on the formation of symbols and on the development of an imaginative life.

The Transitional Object (TO) is created on the basis of a continuum that goes from the holding situation in the mother's arms to the "blankie" (favorite blanket or rag), and the common element is the sensation. What matters for the child is the fact that his/her mother held him/her in her arms and that this holding in her arms took place in a "good" and comfortable manner.

It is in being "held in mom's arms" that the child develops the feeling of his/her own boundaries, and this is the origin of the first concepts related to the body. The first feeling of himself/herself seems to be based on tactile sensation, and she will begin to "feel himself/herself " and that in reality he/she will be.

The TO is what the child feels sensorially in the early days of breastfeeding, such as the feeling of the blanket or the sheet in which he/she was wrapped, or the contact with the mother's robe, all this is stored and, at psychological birth, when there is detachment or separation by the loss of the mother for a few hours, there is reparation and comfort through the TO. The child uses those sensations, evokes the happy lost sensations and invents the first symbol: his/her **transitional object** that represents the lost union; it is the thing that stands for the person.

At 10-15 months the child manipulates everything, "experiments", and the facilitating environment is very important, like a smile that consents, welcomes, participates. The child wants to check on mom and be able to say: "I'll find you later", but he/she also lives the drama: "to remain one with you" or to venture into the world.

From 18-20 months up to 3 years of age is the period of object knowledge or complex cognitive functions. Memory is fervid, imagination and fantasy are no longer in or about the body but also about the outside world. Memory makes it possible to no longer need the real person (the mother), she is within the child, the child has internalized her and nostalgically evokes her. The need becomes desire: the mental level has been reached.

9.3 Practical advice for weaning

At about 6 months it's time to introduce the first baby food: vegetable stock (carrot, chard, lettuce, potato, eggplant). Starting with about half a cup of vegetable broth (150 g), adding 1-2 tablespoon of vegetable puree, 2 tablespoons of cream of wheat or semolina (gluten if tolerated), 1/2 freeze-dried chicken, veal, lamb and beef, 1 teaspoon of extra virgin olive oil. Fruit apple, pear, banana, plum one-quarter cup (60 g) homogenized x 2/day.

When the child eats all the food, we can also introduce the second one for dinner.

Around 8-9 months, new foods and new flavors are introduced:

- tomatoes, first in vegetable broth then as a dry tomato sauce
- parmesan cheese, 1 teaspoon
- chicken, turkey, in addition to beef, veal and lamb (fresh meat 15 g steamed and then blended) or 40 g blended
- ham 15 g, ricotta or cottage cheese 20 g (once a week)
- fish (4 times a week): cod, sea bass, sea bream, wild salmon
- citrus fruits, apricot, peach
- legumes with rice or pasta to make as a single dish (twice a week)
- egg starting with a teaspoon per day for 2-3 days and then 1 whole egg once a week
- At 12 months: honey
- At 15 months: whole egg 1-2 times a week
- At 3 years: free diet
- cocoa and chocolate – dried fruit, almonds, nuts, hazelnuts, pine nuts – red berries: strawberries, raspberries.

REFERENCES

1. Gaddini De Benedetti R. Dal biologico al mentale. Roma: Lombardo Editore, 1984.
2. Gaddini E. La frustrazione come fattore della crescita normale e patologica. In: Scritti. Milano: Raffaello Cortina Editore, 1989.
3. Mahler M, Pine F, Bergman A. The Psychological Birth of the Human Infant. New York: Basic Books, 1975.
4. Winnicott DW. L'osservazione dei bambini piccoli in una situazione prefissata. In: Dalla pediatria alla psicoanalisi. Firenze: Martinelli editore, 1975, 1991 (pp. 66-87).
5. Gaddini De Benedetti R. Il processo maturativo. Studi sul pensiero di Winnicott. Padova: CLEUP, 1985.

10 Learning to eat for a lifetime

Simonetta Di Paola

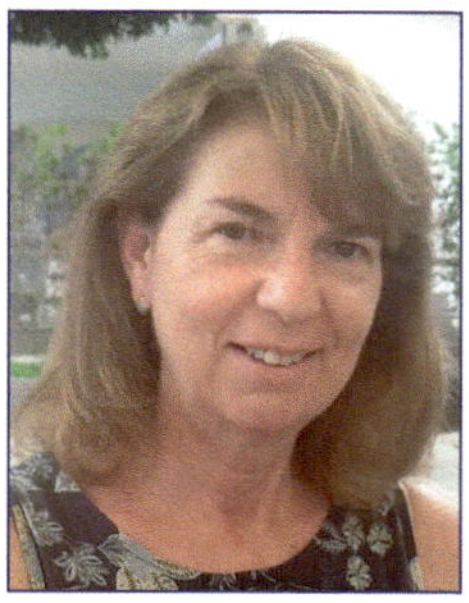

10.1 Introduction

Nutrition has a decisive role in the child's survival and therefore in the life of the future person. Thus, for a healthy and balanced growth of newborns, it is important to pay particular attention to their meal, not only knowing what to do but also (and above all) how to do it, thanks to the precious advices of the medical specialists.

The reality in which we have been immersed for so long is defined as "a society in movement", with men and women called to fill many roles, performing at their best and with less and less time available. Haste never produces positive effects in any kind of "approach with the other", including in a community, being that the family or in the workplace, and often produces communication gaps between sender and receiver.

In the private sphere, with the family as the first educational agency, it is hoped that there will be the necessary attention and care taken to create individuals "in line" that, once they grow up, they will fully enter a society that promises to offer its members "a better world"; "world" is intended as a maximum expression of values and knowledge. Indeed, school programs speak of the integral formation of children as future citizens, where they are expected to be educated in absolute values and to be instructed through notions, in appropriate ways and terms for the interests of that age range.

In recent years, as a result of various social changes, slowly but inexorably, different family models have surfaced. Regardless of any family model considered, parents will nevertheless have the task of attentively raising their children, of being able to interpret their requests especially during the early childhood period (0-3 years), thus respecting their development or their sensitive periods, bearing in mind that the physical and psychological growth of an individual does not respect an established timeline but follows absolutely personal paths and timelines.

In any case, it is well documented that the lack of parental attention, perhaps due to inexperience or lack of time or because the topic is underestimated, will produce over time *real damages to the child's soul*, man or woman of the future. These are damages that children will carry with them forever, irremediably changing their personality along with interpersonal and intrapersonal relationships. Such damages will affect their whole life, their choices. This means that if the parents pay attention to the needs of their children in due time, they will not find themselves having to recover or correct later on, what they have not previously done.

Simonetta Di Paola
Educator specialized in the Montessori Method
Former director of the early childhood education facility at the Conferenza Episcopale Italiana (CEI), Rome, Italy

Email: simonadipaola@libero.it

In this regard, it has been noticed that for a long while the hospitals, pediatricians and obstetricians have been committed to organizing pre- and post-partum courses, aimed at promoting better knowledge and therefore tranquility to the parents. As we know, these meetings deal with topics such as labor, childbirth, pain management, couple's psychological approach in dealing with this delicate moment, transition from couple to parental couple, management of the newborn in terms of breastfeeding, bathing, soothing and much more.

However, after this first intense period and although continuously informed and possibly supported by the pediatrician, the parents find themselves living a daily life "discovering the child's world", a discovery that requires great attention, presence and sensitivity. The relationship understood as "connection" and "communication" with the mother has been present since the child was in her womb. From the first months after birth onwards, through daily gestures, solid relational bases will be established between mother and child.

10.2 Mealtime

In early childhood, among the daily gestures full of *meanings*, mealtime is certainly to be considered as probably the most important meaningful time. Behind "a healthy meal", obviously there is more than just an aseptic respect for medical prescriptions indicating exact quantities of milk or food, which then become a single meal during weaning (around 5-6 months). There must be, above all, the predisposition and the mother's attempts to make her child perceive the ever increasing harmony between them, which develops day after day. Understanding the needs and requests of the child at any stage of development is crucial, even when the child is going through the developmental phase of language *comprehension*, and before the child can express himself/herself through language. During this phase, the child can only use non-verbal communication modalities, such as crying, tantrums, or throwing objects and food, which, if not properly perceived, can be easily misunderstood.

Mealtime is one of those exclusive moments of great intimacy and communication between mother and child [1]. Therefore, it needs to be managed very carefully, with a healthy affective-emotional predisposition free of fears and insecurities, where the child will be absolutely able to perceive and discriminate positive or negative feelings. Through an adequate management of mealtime, solid foundations will establish ever stronger relations with the mother while the establishment of proper behaviors are acquired for life. Mealtime should be considered as "time to sit at the table", not just as a meal or "time for to feed oneself" but as a time of sharing, considering the table the place where family and loved ones meet to be together. In a society like ours, where everything moves faster and faster, loved ones need to dialogue, to discover themselves, to have time for breaks in a long day full of commitments for everyone.

The social aspect has certainly changed, but the harmonious development of an individual has always remained the same and it is therefore necessary to respect the times set by our biological clock. Nourishment for the human being, therefore, does not mean only "feeding" but it also has a relational and symbolic meaning. During the first months of life, the child is dependent on the mother's breast, the relationship with the mother is absolutely exclusive and important for the child's psychic development. Overall, time for breastfeeding and meals is fundamental in the life of every child, not only for immediate physical and psychological health, but also for future health. In fact, an adequate approach to food will be crucial in adolescence and adulthood. Therefore, it is necessary to emphasize to parents that it is not only important the quality of the food or the diets prescribed by pediatricians, but – even more so – it's important the way it is offered.

It is important to inform parents, to make them think about how to approach this delicate moment. For the adequate psychological development of children, it is crucial to dedicate the right time. Let them eat calmly and make them feel "in company". Speak to them in a low voice, informing them about what is happening. The nourishment of the small child is linked to a slow but incessant path, moving towards the achievement of his/her own autonomy and the conquest of skills and self-esteem. For this to happen in the best way possible, it will be necessary for the parents to consciously cross the fundamental phases of this journey with their own child.

10.3 Breastfeeding phase

In compliance with medical recommendations, whether breastfeeding or bottle-feeding, before beginning this activity it is advisable to let the baby know, in a low voice, smiling, that he/she is about to drink milk. It's best to sit on a chair with armrests or on a comfy chair, to be able to rest the arm, which cradles the child's head, on the armrest and to keep the feet well resting on the ground.

If the bottle is used, it must be kept in an oblique position in relation to the child, to avoid swallowing air. During feeding, it is important to try to catch the baby's gaze. To facilitate this contact, it is helpful to speak in a low voice, explaining to the child what you are doing and what he/she is doing. The same routine, with the necessary differences, must also be implemented with breastfeeding. This behavior will stimulate an ever stronger bond, based on the child's trust in the mother.

Moreover, attention must be paid to the way the child ingests milk. If the child drinks quickly, it is useful to take breaks for a few moments, and to check if the baby bottle has a teat hole that it is adequately wide. When the children have finished feeding, it is good to hold them in the parent's arms, making them assume the vertical position near the parent's shoulder, rubbing or gently patting their back, in order to facilitate the emission of air that they may have ingested while sucking.

10.4 Weaning

At around 5-6 months of age, the child faces a second development *crisis* (in its original meaning of turning point): weaning or crisis of objectification. The first crisis is birth. It is appropriate to give the right meaning to the term "crisis" which must not be understood in a negative sense, but only as a "time of change" of the child's tension towards the achievement of new balances.

Babies still need to be helped. They are fed and feeding is a vital need for them. Therefore, it is necessary for the parents to take the baby in the parent's arms respecting the baby's rhythms.

The timing of spoon feeding

From the beginning of spoon feeding, it is important not only to pay attention to the feeding mechanism, but also on how to present "mealtime".

Therefore, before feeding the children, parents must have nearby a table with a tablecloth, a small bowl, a teaspoon and possibly even a table centerpiece with flowers. It is important to pay attention to the environment surrounding the child. In fact, within the development of a child there is "love for the environment" (from 0 to 6 years) and the subsequent one called "about order" (from 5-6 months to 3 years). The child is naturally attracted to everything that surrounds him.

While presenting the food, a very few words may be spoken with great tenderness, e.g.: "here is the *apple!!!*" and the word "*apple!!!*" will be repeated. The spoon will be brought with the new food to the child's mouth, waiting for his/her reaction.

If the baby shows he/she likes it, the parent will proceed with the feeding, otherwise it is preferable to interrupt with that food, to then repeat the offering in the following days without ever insisting.

When the 6- to 7-month-old child is held in his/her parent's arms to eat, he/she must be held in a position that keeps the head more raised. It is no longer necessary to use the position used for breastfeeding. The way the mother relates to the child and the tools used during feeding will remain as indicated above. Parents have to dedicate a lot of time to the children; parents must not hurry the children, because it is an activity that favors their psychic development.

10.4.1 Weaning phase from 6-7 to 11 months

As the first tooth appear, nature prepares the child to eat foods other than breast milk. At this stage, the child can sit, and can be placed on a chair of his/her size, with armrests and have a small table available.

The mother sitting on a low stool, will position herself in front of her child, will feed the child again, but at this moment the child will be able to participate by having his/her own cup, spoon and small bowl glass or ceramic (as their use is allowed in Italy). The utensils and dishes usually avoided for safety reasons must be offered to the child in order to allow him/her to use them properly. In fact, only if a glass or ceramic plate falls and breaks, the child learns from this experience and – protected by the adult – will avoid repeating the mistake. Therefore, the child will quickly learn to use tools and objects in general the proper way. The concept of repetition of error is part of the Montessorian pedagogical philosophy, of great value and well known all over the world by other educators since the 1900s [2-4]. The child will be able to put into practice his/her first conquest of autonomy, since coming down from the arms of the adult is a conquest of self-esteem, autonomy and independence. At the beginning it is important to allow children to even eat with their hands, offering them some fruit or bread cut into appropriate pieces. It is essential to allow this activity, because the children who touch the fruit, or bread, carry out a sensory activity of discovery.

10.4.2 Phase "of the exercise of affirmation of one's inner capacities, of one's own awareness"

From 12 to 13 months onwards, that is, when the child has learned to walk and is autonomous, to stimulate his/her motor development more and more, we can offer the children small activities, such as setting a table, bringing glasses, in order to making them participate in the small daily gestures, where obviously the "ritual" of food is included.

10.4.3 Towards the 24 months

Approaching the 24 months, we must set ourselves the objective of stimulating and increasing the conquest of the child's autonomy. Therefore, it will be proposed at home, and eventually in the nursery and then kindergarten, to participate in the ritual of lunch, of setting and clearing, of cleaning, following as a model what he/she saw or better observed doing up to then, from his/her mother [5]. It is important to underline that children can be encouraged to start using:

- plain-colored tablecloths;
- napkins of various colors (which they will have to learn to fold, the size of the tea napkin);
- ceramic dinner plates (from a fruit plate size with a diameter of 20 cm);
- soup bowls (type of ceramic bowl, with a diameter of about 18 cm);
- drinking glasses (4.7 cm diameter and 6.5 cm height);
- small glass pitchers (from 0.5 L to 0.25 L);
- spoons (sizes from dessert to coffee) and finally stainless steel forks (from fruit size on or between 13 to 16 cm);
- small cups or glasses or ceramic bowls with a diameter of about 10.5 cm;
- serving ladles with a diameter of about 6 cm and a handle length of about 12 cm;
- serving spoons and forks adult size, bowl capacity with a diameter of about 22 cm, serving plate (only the size of a regular adult plate), straw bread basket (about 15 cm width and 7 cm height).

The use of the aforementioned objects is recommended even if for many years the disposable cutlery, glasses and plastic plates have entered fully into kitchens, school cafeteria and catering. It would be desirable to use them as little as possible in order not to expose individuals to toxicity, for prevention and, as described above, for pedagogical reasons, especially in the school environment.

In fact, disposable plastic objects have been subjected to numerous tests to guarantee consumers the suitability. For instance, in Italy, participants to courses regarding the Hazard Analysis Critical Control Point (HACCP) are informed that although there are only a few materials and objects in contact with food (MOCA in Italian) [6], there are many substances used to produce them (Italian Legislative Decree 193/07). For this reason, specific legislation was implemented to protect the health of consumers. In fact, European directives approved the EC Framework Regulation 1935/2004 and the most recent 2016/1416, where it has been expressly stated that materials and objects in contact with food, in order not to be harmful to the health of the users, must feature specific and recognizable labels.

It has been noted, above all in the school environment, that disposable plastic silverware, even if they have been produced in compliance with the regulations in force on this subject, can break during use and that some fragments of the same cannot be identified with the naked eye. These fragments may mix with the food, putting in serious danger the person eating. In fact, some cases of suffocation have been reported for this reason.

Coming back to the importance of using traditional cutlery, plates and glasses in the school setting, it must be considered that if the child is suitably followed, in the event of one of these objects being broken, he/she will be able to verify that the consequences of not following instructions or not paying attention are that a damage occurred. Therefore, in order not to repeat the mistake, next time the child will be more careful. Through the event memory the behavior will autocorrect itself. This experience, very pleasing to children, will make them responsible and able to participate completely.

Children will live with enthusiasm, in ways and terms appropriate to the age group, the intimate great joy of discovery the dimensions of sociality and conviviality. Mealtime, if wisely managed within the family and at school, always respecting the age group, will help the child not only to discover the taste of the various foods offered, but will learn the most polite table manner to keep for the rest of his/her life. In addition, they finally become more careful and better master their own movements, which will increasingly be refined over time [7-8].

As a preventative measure, since breastfeeding in infancy, mothers are advised to clean their babies' gums and tongue with a moistened gauze to avoid milk stagnation in the mouth. Subsequently, with the eruption of the first deciduous tooth, it is desirable that the oral hygiene ritual is also introduced after meals both at home and at school, from nursery school onwards.

It is important to remember that in the small child there is a being who is rich in great energies, who needs to express himself/herself psychologically, when offered the opportunity through an interesting activity for such a sensitive period of the developmental stage [9].

At that point, we will all have the honor of witnessing the magical moment in which the child will be immersed in an activity exhibiting "concentration". In carrying out the proposed activity, including eating and related activities, while respecting the development plan, we will see the child abstracting from everything that surrounds him/her. He/she will only be committed to performing the task entrusted to him/her in the best possible way.

REFERENCES

1. Montessori e il vostro bambino. Un manuale per i genitori – Presentazione di Renato Dulbecco a cura di Elena Dompè – Roma: Edizioni Opera Nazionale Montessori, 1999 – Original Title: "Montessori and Your Child: A Primer for Parents by Terry Malloy, 1974, Published by Schocken Books; pp. 50-51 & pp. 74-75.
2. Montessori M. Il bambino in famiglia. Milano: Garzanti Elefanti, quinta ristampa gennaio 2010. Capitoli: L'educazione nuova, pp. 41-50; Del mio metodo in generale, pp. 53-66.
3. Montessori M. La mente del bambino Milano: Garzanti Elefanti, quinta ristampa settembre 2010. Capitoli: IX – Cure da prendersi all'inizio della vita, pp. 100-110; XIX – Contributo sociale del bambino: normalizzazione, pp. 200-206; XX – La costruzione del carattere è una conquista, pp. 207-213.
4. Montessori M. Il segreto dell'infanzia. Milano: Garzanti Elefanti, sesta ristampa ottobre 2010. Parte Seconda, Capitoli: XVIII – L'educazione del bambino, pp. 145-156; XIX – La ripetizione dell'esercizio, pp. 157-159.
5. Indicazioni nazionali per il curricolo della scuola dell'infanzia e del primo ciclo d'istruzione – Capitoli: Cultura, scuola, persona – La scuola nel nuovo scenario; Per una nuova cittadinanza; Per un nuovo umanesimo – (Periodico multimediale per la scuola italiana a cura del Ministero dell'Istruzione, dell'Università e della Ricerca – Anno LXXXVIII – Annali della Pubblica Istruzione: Numero speciale 2012 – Le Monnier), pp. 7-11.
6. Direttive Europee: Regolamento quadro CE 1935/2004 (MOCA QUADRO) e più recente 1416/2016. Per ultimo inserito anche il D.Lgs. 29/2017 disciplina sanzionatoria per la violazione degli obblighi dei regolamenti MOCA, GMP e altri.
7. La Cura dell'Anima in Maria Montessori – L'educazione morale, spirituale e religiosa dell'infanzia – AA.VV. a cura di Leonardo de Sanctis – Roma: Fefè Editore – Prima Edizione, 2011; pp. 115-117.
8. Le ricette di Maria Montessori cent'anni dopo – AA.VV. a cura di Leonardo de Sanctis – Roma: Fefè Editore, 2013; pp. 17-23.
9. Formae mentis. Saggio sulla pluralità dell'intelligenza – Universale Economica Feltrinelli/Saggi – Traduttore: L. Sosio – Original Title: "Frames of Mind, The Theory of Multiple Intelligences by Howard Gardner – New York: Basic Books, Inc. – Seconda Edizione 2013 – Capitolo 10 – Le intelligenze personali, pp. 341-349; Lo sviluppo dell'intelligenze personali, pp. 349-350; Il neonate; pp. 351-352; Il bambino da due a cinque anni; pp. 353-356.

Section 3 Food and the stomatognatic system

11 Microbiota and feeding

Valentina Prete

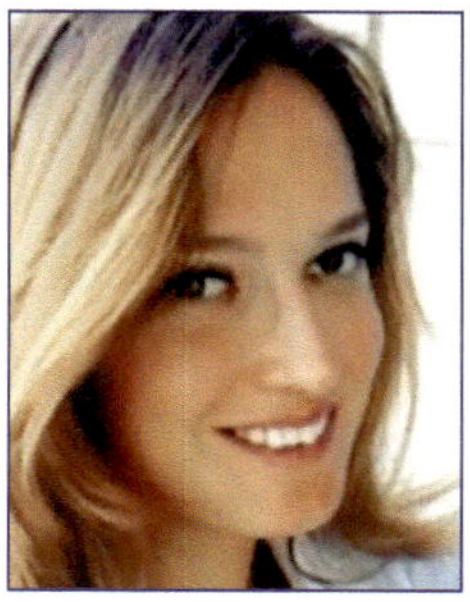

11.1 Oral cavity and resident microbial species

The oral cavity, or mouth, constitutes an ecosystem formed by distinct microbial habitats very different from each other. They reside between the teeth, in the gingival sulcus, on the tongue, cheek, lips, hard palate and soft palate. The oral microbiota still differs continuing along the tonsils, the pharynx, the esophagus and beyond, the Eustachian tube, the middle ear, the trachea and beyond, the nasal passages and the sinuses. We therefore define the human *oral microbiome* as all the microorganisms found on or in the human oral cavity and its adjoining extensions.

The oral microbiome is the complex microbial community that resides in the human oral cavity. It is estimated that out of about 500 to 700 species resident in the oral cavity, only half can be cultivated anaerobically through classical microbiological techniques, the remainder being identified by molecular methods based on RNA16s cloning studies [1].

It is important to correctly define the human microflora of the healthy oral cavity before understanding the role of bacteria in oral diseases. Currently it is possible to consult the Human Oral Microbiome Database (HOMD) in which species and phenotypes, present in the oral cavity, have been reported. All this information in the database is publicly available online (www.homd.org).

The ecosystem within the oral cavity is unique, it is the result of interactions between components such as oral fluids and oral microorganisms with soft and hard tissue structures of the oral cavity. The soft structures are represented by the mucous membranes while the hard surface is represented by the teeth. Both soft and hard tissue structures influence the distribution of microbes in the mouth.

The oral cavity represents a host environment that has characteristics that support the constitution and growth of a great diversity of microbes; the mucosa of the cheek, the tongue, the gingival fissure and the surface of the tooth provide sites with different physicochemical and nutritional microorganisms that allow the adherence and growth of selective microorganisms.

In a healthy subject and with good hygiene, a balance is normally established between the numerous bacterial species present in the oral ecosystem and the defense systems of the organism. Table 11.1 shows the bacterial species prevalent in the oral cavity.

It is possible that the cultivable organisms so far studied can only be a relatively small component of some oral communities known to us. Therefore, un-

Valentina Prete, MD, PhD
Policlinico A. Gemelli, Rome, Italy

Email: valentina.prete@unicatt.it

Table 11.1 Bacterial species prevalent in the oral cavity of healthy individuals

Gram-positive	Gram-negative
Actinomyces	*Actinobacillus*
Arachnia	*Bacteroides*
Bacterionema	*Capnocytophaga*
Bifidobacterium	*Eikenella*
Lactobacillus	*Fusobacterium*
Micrococcus	*Haemophilus*
Peptostreptococcus	*Leptotrichia*
Propionibacterium	*Moraxella*
Rothia	*Neisseria*
Streptococcus	*Selenomonas*
Treponema	*Simonsiella*
	Veillonella
	Wolinella

derstanding the composition of the oral microbial community of a healthy subject, as opposed to the disease, is a crucial objective in the study of microbiology, and can open new horizons regarding not only oral health as an entrance portal for the gastrointestinal (GI) tract, but also for the respiratory tract [2].

11.2 Alterations of the resident microbial flora and related oral pathologies

The oral cavity is characterized by a very intense bacterial dynamism and proliferation, which occurs in the various districts of the oral cavity and continues along the digestive tract through the entire human body. The food introduced daily, remains in the mouth the time necessary for chewing and to be mixed with saliva, thus reaching a consistency that can be pushed along the digestive tract, passing through the stomach and the intestinal tract. The moist environment that characterizes the oral cavity promotes bacterial proliferation: the microorganisms that colonize an area of the oral cavity have a significant probability of spreading on contiguous surfaces of the epithelium in neighboring sites. It has been shown that oral microorganisms cause several oral infectious diseases, including caries (cavities), periodontitis (gingival disease), endodontic (root canal) infections, alveolar osteitis and tonsillitis. Oral bacteria are responsible for systemic diseases [3], including cardiovascular disease, stroke [4], diabetes [5] and pneumonia [6].

The etiological cause of infections caused by microorganisms, such as caries, periodontitis, otitis media and other infections, are now recognized as being caused by specific microbial species or by the biofilm produced by pathogenic microbes [1]. In the oral cavity, polymicrobial species producing biofilms coexist, mainly covering the surfaces of the teeth, prostheses (when present), gums and tongue [7]. It is likely that many of the individual groups of bacteria that make up these communities cannot survive outside of it because of the metabolic interdependencies that are created between bacteria. Initial adhesion invariably implies the binding of bacteria to the components of saliva that are absorbed by the surfaces of the oral cavity. The interaction between bacteria and the salivary components takes place in several main mechanisms that include a process of agglutination (clumping of particles), subsequent adhesion of bacteria to the salivary films, and microbial nutrition using substrates present in the saliva [8, 9]. The ability of the first colonizing bacteria to express more adhesions probably confers an important selective advantage with respect to those bacteria which have less versatility in the receptor recognition.

All the main diseases of oral tissues derive from polymorphic etiology. Dental caries is one of the most common chronic and multifactorial diseases affecting the human population. The lesions of dental caries are due to relatively acid-resistant organisms: species of *Streptococcus*, *Lactobacilli*, *Actinomyces*, *Prevotellae* and occasionally *Candida* yeasts. The appearance of a cavity lesion is determined by the coexistence of two main factors: acidophilic microorganisms and carbohydrates derived from the diet. The development of caries, due to an ecological imbalance of the stable oral microbiome as oral microorganisms, form dental plaque on tooth surfaces, causing the carious process. Biofilm formation appears to be influenced by large-scale changes in protein expression over time, and under genetic control cariogenic microorganisms produce lactic, acetic and propionic acids, which are a product of carbohydrate metabolism [10]. Infections of the roots and the pulp of teeth are also polymicrobial and the periodontal lesions contain hundreds of different bacterial phyla [2].

11.3 Formation and composition of the microbiota in various phases of human life

During the growth and development of the individual, the composition of the microbiota changes considerably. Major changes occur in the first year of life, where the definitive concentration of microbiota takes place and remains so throughout the entire life span [11].

It is believed that the initial microbial exposure is important in defining what the composition of the microbiota will be in adulthood, in fact the initial communities can act as a direct source of protective or pathogenic bacteria very early in life. The factors that can influence the composition of the microbiota are certainly the type of birth (natural or cesarean), the way in which newborns are fed (breastfed or using artificial milk) [12], treatment with drugs (prolonged use of antibiotics) [13], the external environment, eating habits and lifestyle [14].

The host-microbiota interaction is strongly conditioned by environmental factors, the host's genetic structure and the integrity of its immune system, both local and systemic. Although the microbiota remains constant in the healthy adult individual, alterations in the composition of the microbiota may occur following endogenous or exogenous events. Different pathologies can determine a significant change in the composition of the intestinal microbiota, as subjects with metabolic pathologies present a remarkable variation in the bacterial species that constitute the microbiota itself [15, 16].

Unhealthy eating habits represent one of the main factors in the variation of the intestinal microflora, therefore it is important not to underestimate both the role of the alimentation, through which it is possible to modulate the composition of the microbiota that is forming, and the role of other factors that influence the definitive composition, i.e., genetic and functional environmental factors. As far as possible it is therefore appropriate to know how to modulate and correct those elements that may have any negative repercussions on the development and composition of the microbiota itself.

The relationship between human beings and their oral microflora begins shortly after birth and lasts a lifetime. Breast milk is the optimal source for infant nutrition, as it promotes immune defenses and gastrointestinal function. It is known that breastfeeding constitutes a vector of the microbial community present in breast milk, which in turn is influenced by factors such as the age of mother, the external-geographical environment, and the use of antibiotics [17]. The first colonizing bacteria are either *aerobic* or *anaerobic facultative bacteria,* that is bacteria that makes ATP in both aerobic respiration when oxygen is present, or anaerobic breathing when oxygen is not available. These facultative aerobic-anaerobic bacteria are first of all *Streptococci*, then *S. salivarius.* Anaerobic bacteria are scarce: *Veillonelle* (coccus Gram-negative, from the 2nd day of life), *Fusobacteria* (from the 3rd-4th month), *Peptostreptococcus* (after the 5th month).

Around the 6th-7th month the first teeth appear, and the first occlusal relationship is established. In the following months important anatomical changes occur, such as increased mobility of the jaw and the first exposure to more consistent foods. It is important that even in these early stages of life, during early infancy, there is a thoughtful choice of foods to be introduced into the daily feeding routine of a child. Studies reported in the literature document how massive changes in the composition of the microbiota occur within the first 3 years of life, while beyond this period of life the microbiota tends to assume a composition very similar to that of the adult [18].

The habit of mothers to put their children to sleep with a bottle containing milk and sugar or honey, sweet herbal teas, chamomile, with the aim of calming and facilitating children's sleep, is an incorrect food choice. The nocturnal intake of these substances (sugars) affects the composition of the oral microbiota, while prolonged exposure of baby teeth to sugars favors the appearance of the carious process.

After the first six months of life, with the beginning of the weaning period, the diversification of the diet and the introduction of solid foods, a further differentiation of microorganisms occurs. Thus, the typical composition of adulthood is created, characterized by two main phyla: *Bacteroidetes* and *Firmicutes*.

The composition of the intestinal microbiota in adulthood remains almost unchanged. Changes of the intestinal bacterial flora, from a qualitative and quantitative point-of-view, can make the organism more vulnerable to pathogenic bacteria. In other words, this state of dysbiosis is determined by an alteration of the resident bacterial flora.

11.4 Oral microbiota and intestinal microbiota, dysbiosis and consequences

Although it is known that the oral cavity and the intestine both belong to the alimentary system, it is generally less known that their well-being is closely linked. The human microbiome plays a fundamental role in the existence of the individual, to the point of influencing many physiological functions such as the development of the human being, its physiology, immunity and, of course, nutritional level. Although the composition of human microbiology has received considerable attention in recent years, the precise mechanisms by which these microbial communities mediate disease and restore and maintain health remain a subject of study. However, recent studies have shown that different chronic diseases of the mouth and GI tract are associated with alterations in the composition of the microbiome called "dysbiosis" [4].

The alteration of the intestinal balance was observed especially in relation to the intake of broad-spectrum antibiotics. The latter can cause a reduction of the sensitive microflora (in particular of anaerobic microorganisms). A qualitative and quantitative change of the microbial species can reduce the fermentative and metabolic capacity of the microbiota [19].

Different bacterial species coexist in the intestine; when an alteration of the composition of the intestinal microbiota occurs, some bacteria can exert a noxious action for example *Staphylococcus, Clostridium, Pseudomonas* counteract the protective action of *Lactobacillus, Bifidobacterium* and *Eubacterium* [20]. Many studies underline the fundamental role of the diet in the composition of the microbial flora from the first months of life, others are based on the observation of different eating habits in the adult subject and how these can bring about considerable modifications in the composition of the intestinal microbiota in the long term [21].

It is known that intestinal microbiota is involved in the pathogenesis of Inflammatory Bowel Disease (IBD), mainly in Crohn's disease and in ulcerative colitis. Subjects suffering from these inflammatory pathologies have localized symptoms in the GI tract. Recent studies have also shown an increase in the frequency of alteration of the oral microbiota in these patients with IBD.

Alterations in the composition of the oral microbiota (alterations in the gums, tongue, saliva) have been found in subjects with IBD. At the same time patients who present pathologies such as: ulcerative colitis, Crohn's disease, or other diseases involving the intestine, present a greater risk of periodontitis or inflammatory states in the oral cavity. The saliva microbiota of patients with IBD are predominant in the following bacteria: *Streptococcus, Prevotella, Neisseria, Hemophilus, Veillonella.* This close correlation has been the object of study in recent times, and the hypotheses advanced so far show that oral and intestinal inflammation are connected by a complex system of reciprocal repercussions at both inflammatory and microbiological levels [22].

In a woman, alterations of the oral microbiota have been found following hormonal changes, which can be caused by the consumption of birth control pills or in the physiological state of pregnancy. In the second case, studies reported in literature show that women with premature birth have a higher percentage of the following microbial species: *Bacteroides forsythus, Porphyromonas gingivalis, Aggregatibacter actinomycetemcomitans, Treponema denticola, Fusobacterium nucleatum, Campylobacter rectus, Peptostreptococcus micros, Prevotella nigrescens* and *Prevotella* [4, 23].

Alterations in the composition of the oral microbiota have also been found in subjects suffering from diabetes mellitus. Diabetes represents a serious disorder in glucose metabolism with severe hyperglycemia and insulin insufficiency. The relationship between dental caries and diabetes mellitus is complex. Children and adolescents with type 1 diabetes often receive diets that limit the intake of carbohydrate-rich foods, while for adults with type 2 diabetes, which is often associated with obesity and intake of foods rich in calories and carbohydrates, in addition to limiting simple carbohydrates, a low-calorie diet is recommended. In subjects suffering from diabetes mellitus, a reduction in salivary flow and a mutation of *Streptococcus mutans* has been reported [24]. To prevent inflammation and dysbiosis in the oral cavity, it is essential to prevent the onset of diseases of the oral cavity, taking care of hygiene, diet, lifestyle, and limit the use of antibiotics that can cause alterations of the oral cavity influencing its composition and functionality.

11.5 Microbiota and food

Foods are what we choose to introduce into our body through the GI tract, to feed ourselves. The metabolic effects that the substances contained in the foods have on the various organs and tissues, after digestion and absorption, are fundamental for the state of health and well-being of the individual. The correct, diversified and balanced diet preserves the microbiota, and furthermore guarantees an abundant microbial diversity, in which more geo-genus and families (phyla) are present and proliferate.

A healthy diet must never be restrictive, and the choices must fall into the existing food categories by varying the frequency of food intake as much as possible. An omnivorous choice is always advisable and, whenever possible, based on time and time constraint it is best to have five small meals: breakfast, snacks, lunch, snack and dinner, in order to favor digestion times, absorption and metabolism.

This complex of good habits, which should be acquired in childhood and practiced lifelong, favors not only the adhesion to a correct nutrient intake (in quality and quantity), but also favors the defense of the health of the microbiota. On the contrary, not respecting the "timing" of meals and the variety of food choices, over time can promote the appearance of obesity, metabolic syndrome, diabetes and gastrointestinal disorders [25].

The intestinal microbiota performs an important metabolic function: it integrates the host's metabolism in many aspects and allows the microbiota to be identified as a metabolically active organ, responsible for the digestion of different nutrients, which otherwise would not be modifiable and assimilated by our organism. The microflora can influence the energy balance of the host organism. Through the fermentative processes, the intestinal bacteria draw the necessary energy from sugars and proteins. An important metabolic function of the intestinal microflora is the fermentation of the non-digestible dietary residue and the endogenous mucopolysaccharides produced by the intestinal epithelium. The transformation of non-digestible polysaccharides of the diet, such as cellulose, hemicellulose, pectins, gums or non-digestible starch, occurs by bacterial enzymes that transform the material derived from foods into volatile carbon dioxide, hydrogen sulfide and Short-Chain Fatty acids (SCFA). The final product of the bacterial metabolism is the SCFA: acetic acid, butyric acid and propionic acid, which exert a powerful trophic and energetic action in the intestinal lumen and stimulate proliferation and differentiation of skin epithelial cells. Acetic acid is reabsorbed by the intestinal wall and poured back into the peripheral circulation where it is used as an energy substrate by the various tissues including the adipose tissue for lipogenesis. Butyric acid is the energy source for the same intestinal cells, while propionic acid is reabsorbed in the intestine and used by the liver as a gluconeogenic substrate [26]. The result of this complex and autonomous metabolic activity of the microbiota is the recovery of energy and absorbable substrates for the host, but also the supply of energy and nutritional products for the growth and proliferation of the same resident bacterial species. The synthesis of fatty acids, defined as saccharolytic fermentation, causes an acidification of intestinal pH, which represents an efficient defense system against pathogenic microorganisms and furthermore favors the growth proliferation and differentiation of the epithelial intestinal cells. A diet poor in fibers and in complex starches, not only results in a low production of SCFA, but it can be implicated in the high incidence of neoplastic and inflammatory pathologies of the colon, at least in Western populations [15, 27-29].

The intestinal microbiota also plays an important role in lipid metabolism, influencing cholesterol homeostasis and regulating the composition of bile. For example, some bacteria of the genus *Bacteroides* suppress the inhibition of lipoprotein lipase in adipocytes, with consequent storage of triglycerides in adipose tissue.

The bile acid metabolism is instead mainly responsible for the bile which promotes the deconjugation of bile acids with consequent reduced reabsorption and greater elimination of cholesterol [30]. Protein metabolism is guaranteed by microbial enzymes in association with host enzymes. Proteases produced by proteolytic microbial groups hydrolyze proteins to amino acids and simple peptides, which represent an important source of nitrogen, although not the only one, for the entire microbiota. Protein hydrolysis by *Clostridium, Bacteroides, Propioniobacterium, Fusobacterium, Streptococcus* and *Lactobacillus* results in the production of peptides which are then assimilated by the microbiota. Amino acids not assimilated by some bacteria will be used by others.

The intestinal bacterial microflora is also involved in the metabolism of micronutrients, in particular by vitamins. The synthesis of vitamins B and K is one of the main functions of the intestinal microbiota, the bacteria present in the colon synthesize vitamin K and most of the B complex vitamins: biotin, cobalamin, folate, nicotinic acid, pantothenic acid, pyridoxine, riboflavin and thiamine.

The microbial flora present in the intestine performs important functions: contributes to the biochemical processes of the organism, promotes the assimilation helping the digestion's absorption and peristalsis, and acts as a defense mechanism protecting the intestinal barrier from any pathogens. The nutritional health of the individual depends very much on a correct intestinal functioning, as the intestine performs essential functions in digestion and absorption, along with exclusion and elimination of ingested substances. The composition of the microorganisms present in the intestine affects not only proper digestion but also the individual's immune system.

11.6 Smoking and alcohol: consequences for oral health

The bacterial load present in cigarettes is transferred to the oral cavity during tobacco aspiration, some bacteria can survive the tobacco burning process and remain in the oral cavity: for example, *Bacillus spp.* and *Clostridium spp.* Thus, in smokers, an altered homeostasis of the oral microbiota has been found, where commensal species are added to new bacterial species introduced from the outside.

Because of the various types of samples used to study the oral microbiome and the known variation in microbial communities in different parts of the oral cavity [31], the comparison between studies is difficult.

There are several potential mechanisms through which smoking can alter the oral microbiota, including: increased acidity of saliva [32], decreased oxygen with the consequent proliferation of anaerobic bacteria, effects normally due to antibiotics [33], mucosal adherence, and the host's immune response against local infections [34]. Smoking intrinsically promotes an oral ecosystem more favorable to pathogens, thus increasing the risk of an oral disease such as periodontitis.

It has been observed that the composition of the oral microbiome of ex-smokers does not differ from that of non-smokers; this result is very promising as it is a valid indication that the smoking-related changes of the oral microbiome are not permanent. As it has been observed with other smoking-related health changes, smoking cessation clearly remains the best practice for restoring a healthy phenotype [35].

In association with smoking, excessive alcohol consumption, in addition to damaging the oral mucosa, contributes to increasing acetaldehyde concentrations in saliva, resulting in an increase in mycetes (for example, *Candida albicans*) and an increase in the relative proportion of the Gram-positive compared to Gram-negative. Impurities, contaminants, fermentation and distillation products can cause changes in the oral environment, compromising existing bacterial species.

Oral microbiota can affect the tumorigenic properties of alcohol through the overproduction of acetaldehyde starting from ethanol through the easy induction of the expression in bacteria of alcohol-metabolizing enzymes.

Regular but moderate consumption of red wine does not lead to substantial alterations in the composition of the oral microbiota, but alcohol abuse and consumption in association with smoking, on the other hand, leads to an alteration in terms of stability and richness of the oral bacterial component, in addition to negative repercussions not only on oral health but on the body in general [36].

11.7 The environment and individual choices affect the composition of the microbiota

It is important to take care of one's health as the human body is a complex organism and its maximum efficiency is obtained through the close correlation and function of every vital organ, a concept known since the days of ancient medicine. Now we have to consider a full-fledged organ that lives and performs vital functions within the human body, which is its microbiome. Different microbial species characterize different body districts and live as commensal species, the alteration determines a state of dysbiosis with negative consequences on the district and on human health.

Therefore, health, understood in its totality, must preserve every vital component of man, eukaryotic and bacterial cells. The total integrity of the individual (*in toto*) must be preserved by the smallest fundamental unit, the microbial cell. Conscious choices influence and preserve the state of health, and such choices are conditioned by exogenous factors such as: external environment, social and economic status, eating habits, hygienic state.

Some choices can be easily modified, while others require a commitment, and it is not always possible to change the starting situation. Discordant choices affect a different microbiotic composition of the individual. Subjects with different eating habits have different profiles and different macrobiotic positions [37]. The main explanation of these different bacterial profiles would be due to the different food choices and habits, even hygienic ones, which, unfortunately, are dictated by economic resources not easily comparable.

REFERENCES

1. Dewhirst FE, Chen T, Izard J, et al. The human oral microbiome. J Bacteriol 2010; 192(19): 5002-17.
2. Jenkinson HF, Lamont RJ. Oral microbial communities in sick-ness and in health. Trends Microbiol 2005; 13(12): 589-95.
3. Seymour GJ, Ford PJ, Cullinan MP, Leishman S, Yamazaki K. Relationship between periodontal infections and systemic disease. Clin Microbiol Infect 2007; 13 Suppl 4: 3-10.
4. Sudhakara P, Gupta A, Bhardwaj A, Wilson A. Oral dysbiotic communities and their implications in systemic diseases. Dent J (Basel) 2018; 6(2): 10.
5. Yamashita M, Okubo H, Kobuke K, et al. Alteration of gut microbiota by a Westernized lifestyle and its correlation with insulin resistance in non-diabetic Japanese men. J Diabetes Investig 2019; 10(6): 1463-70.
6. Awano S, Ansai T, Takata Y, et al. Oral health and mortality risk from pneumonia in the elderly. J Dent Res 2008; 87(4): 334-9.
7. Colombo APV, Tanner ACR. The role of bacterial biofilms in dental caries and periodontal and peri-implant diseases: A historical perspective. J Dental Res 2019; 98(4): 373-85.
8. Scannapieco FA. Saliva-bacterium interactions in oral microbial ecology. Crit Rev Oral Biol Med 1994; 5(3-4): 203-48.
9. Hegde MN, Attavar SH, Shetty N, Hegde ND, Hegde NN. Saliva as a biomarker for dental caries: A systematic review. J Conserv Dent 2019; 22(1): 2-6.
10. Struzycka I. The oral microbiome in dental caries. Pol J Microbiol 2014; 63(2): 127-35.
11. Cheng J, Palva AM, de Vos WM, Satokari R. Contribution of the intestinal microbiota to human health: from birth

to 100 years of age. Curr Top Microbiol Immunol 2013; 358: 323-46.
12. Munyaka PM, Khafipour E, Ghia JE. External influence of early childhood establishment of gut microbiota and subsequent health implication Front Pediatr 2014; 2: 109.
13. Jernberg C, Löfmark S, Edlund C, Jansson IK. Long-term impacts of antibiotic exposure on the human intestinal microbiota. Microbiology 2010; 156(Pt 11): 3216-23.
14. Kashtanova DA, Popenko AS, Tkacheva ON, et al. Association between the gut microbiota and diet: Fetal life, early childhood, and further life. Nutrition 2016; 32(6): 620-7.
15. Baothman OA, Zamzami MA, Taher I, Abubaker J, Abu-Farha M. The role of Gut Microbiota in the development of obesity and Diabetes. Lipids Health Dis 2016; 15: 108.
16. Clemente JC, Ursell LK, Parfrey LW, Knight R. The impact of the gut microbiota on human health: an integrative view. Cell 2012; 148(6): 1258-70.
17. Biagi E, Aceti A, Quercia S, et al. Microbial community dynamics in mother's milk and infant's mouth and gut in moderately preterm infants. Front Microbiol 2018; 9: 2512.
18. Yatsunenko T, Rey FE, Manary MJ, et al. Human gut microbiome viewed across age and geography. Nature 2012; 486(7402): 222-7.
19. Gallo A, Passaro G, Gasbarrini A, Landolfi R, Montalto M. Modulation of microbiota as treatment for intestinal inflammatory disorders: An uptodate. World J Gastroenterol 2016; 22(32): 7186-202.
20. Zou S, Fang L, Lee MH. Dysbiosis of gut microbiota in promoting the development of colorectal cancer. Gastroenterol Rep (Oxf) 2018; 6(1): 1-12.
21. David LA, Maurice CF, Carmody RN, et al. Diet rapidly and reproducibly alters the human gut microbiome. Nature 2014; 505(7484): 559-63.
22. Said HS, Suda W, Nakagome S, et al. Dysbiosis of salivary microbiota in inflammatory bowel disease and its association with oral immunological biomarkers. DNA Res 2014; 21(1): 15-25.
23. Davenport ES. Preterm low birthweight and the role of oral bacteria. J Oral Microbiol 2010; 2: 5779.
24. Latti BR, Kalburge JV, Birajadar SB, Latti RG. Evaluation of relationship between dental caries, diabetes mellitus and oral microbiota in diabetics. J Oral Maxillofac Pathol 2018; 22(2): 282.
25. Gletsu-Miller N, McCrory MA. Modifying eating behavior: novel approaches for reducing body weight, preventing weight regain, and reducing chronic disease risk. Adv Nutr 2014; 5: 789-91.
26. Chambers ES, Preston T, Frost G, Morrison DJ. Role of gut microbiota-generated short-chain fatty acids in metabolic and cardiovascular health. Curr Nutr Rep 2018; 7(4): 198-206.
27. den Besten G, van Eunen K, Groen AK, Venema K, Reijngoud DJ, Bakker BM. The role of short-chain fatty acids in the interplay between diet, gut microbiota, and host energy metabolism. J Lipid Res 2013; 54(9): 2325-40.
28. Vrieze A, Holleman F, Zoetendal EG, de Vos WM, Hoekstra JB, Nieuwdorp M. The environment within: how gut microbiota may influence metabolism and body composition. Diabetologia 2010; 53(4): 606-13.
29. Festi D, Schiumerini R, Eusebi LH, Marasco G, Taddia M, Colecchia A. Gut microbiota and metabolic syndrome. World J Gastroenterol 2014; 20(43): 16079-94.
30. Joyce SA, Shanahan F, Hill C, Gahan CG. Bacterial bile salt hydrolase in host metabolism: Potential for influencing gastrointestinal microbe-host crosstalk. Gut Microbes 2014; 5(5): 669-74.
31. Segata N, Haake SK, Mannon P, et al. Composition of the adult digestive tract bacterial microbiome based on seven mouth surfaces, tonsils, throat and stool samples. Genome Biol 2012; 13: R42.
32. Kanwar A, Sah K, Grover N, Chandra S, Singh RR. Long-term effect of tobacco on resting whole mouth salivary flow rate and pH: an institutional based comparative study. Eur J Gen Dent 2013; 2: 296-9.
33. Macgregor ID. Effects of smoking on oral ecology. A review of the literature. Clin Prev Dent 1989; 11: 3-7.
34. Brook I. The impact of smoking on oral and nasopharyngeal bacterial flora. J Dent Res 2011; 90: 704-10.
35. Wu J, Peters BA, Dominianni C, et al. Cigarette smoking and the oral microbiome in a large study of American adults. ISME J 2016; 10(10): 2435-46.
36. Homann N, Tillonen J, Meurman JH, et al. Increased salivary acetaldehyde levels in heavy drinkers and smokers: a microbiological approach to oral cavity cancer. Carcinogenesis 2000; 21(4): 663-8.
37. Avershina E, Storrø O, Øien T, Johnsen R, Pope P, Rudi K. Major faecal microbiota shifts in composition and diversity with age in a geographically restricted cohort of mothers and their children. FEMS Microbiol Ecol 2014; 87(1): 280-90.

12

Food and periodontal diseases

Antonio D'Addona and Paolo De Angelis

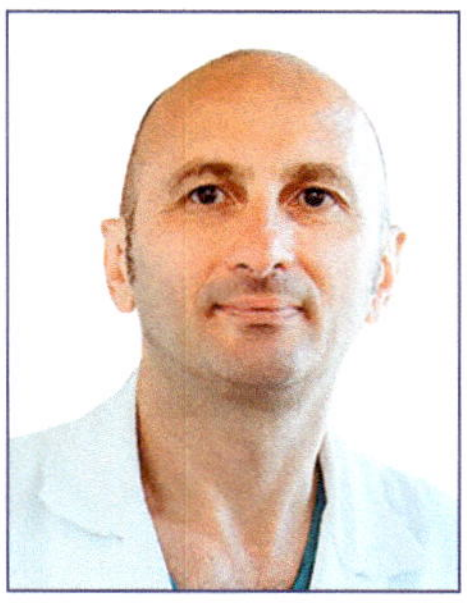

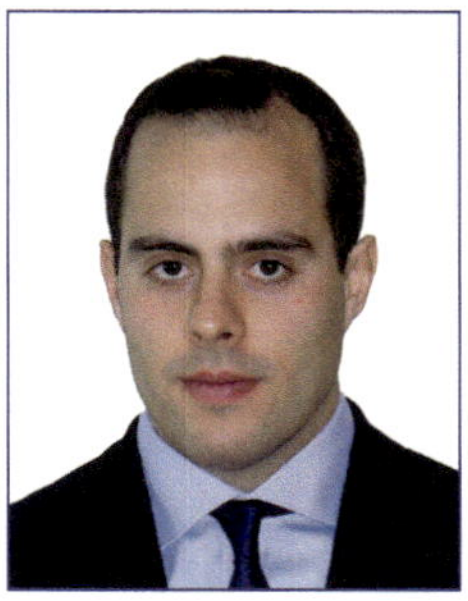

Periodontitis is a common chronic inflammatory disease affecting 10-15% of the developed world's population. It involves the supporting structures of the teeth and, if not recognized and correctly managed, it leads to tooth loss [1, 2]. Periodontitis can cause several consequences and progressively reduces chewing function, impairs aesthetics and causes disability, which may lead to social inequality, a reduced quality of life and significant impacts on public health costs [3]. Chronic periodontitis is a multifactorial disorder, however, and microbial dental plaque biofilms are considered the main etiological factor [4]. The overgrowth of biofilms, especially in the subgingival area, with the emergence of periodontal pathogens, is a necessary but often insufficient condition for the development of periodontitis [5], because other local and systemic factors have important modifying roles in its pathogenesis [4].

The role of risk factors should be carefully considered because they are able to change the susceptibility or resistance of individuals to the disease [5]. Systemic risk factors for periodontal disease include behaviors such as smoking, medical conditions (i.e., poorly controlled diabetes, obesity, stress, osteopenia), and inadequate dietary consumption of calcium and vitamin D [5]. There is overwhelming evidence that both smoking and types 1 and 2 diabetes are important risk factors for the severity of periodontal tissue loss and the progression of the disease [4]. For these reasons, it seems reasonable to try to eliminate or modify these risk factors as part of the management of periodontal disease. Although some risk factors, such as race or genetics, cannot be changed, knowing all the risk factors for each person provides a means to target interventions.

Furthermore, the population in Western countries is shifting toward higher proportions of older people [1], and aging is associated with declines in mental and physical health, as well an increased risk of chronic diseases, including atherosclerosis, cancer, diabetes and periodontitis [6]. Aging is also associated with elevations in systemic markers of inflammation [6]. This will result in more people with periodontal disease, further reinforcing the need for its successful management to reduce its global burden [1].

In the USA, chronic diseases account for seven out of ten deaths each year [6], with estimates indicating that nearly 25% of adults have multiple chronic condi-

Antonio D'Addona, DDS
Professor, Department of Head and Neck and Sensory Organs, Division of Oral Surgery and Implantology, Fondazione Policlinico Universitario A. Gemelli IRCCS, Università Cattolica del Sacro Cuore, Rome, Italy

Email: antonio.daddona@policlinicogemelli.it

Paolo De Angelis, DDS
Department of Head and Neck and Sensory Organs, Division of Oral Surgery and Implantology, Fondazione Policlinico Universitario A. Gemelli IRCCS, Università Cattolica del Sacro Cuore, Rome, Italy

Email: dr.paolodeangelis@gmail.com

tions with healthcare costs of about 75% of healthcare expenditures. This percentage increases among older adults, reaching almost 95% of expenses [6]. Periodontitis has been clearly recognized as a risk factor for various systemic diseases where low-grade inflammation within the peripheral circulation is associated with the etiology of that disease or its progression. In literature, these associations have been demonstrated repeatedly between periodontitis and type 2 diabetes [5] and cardiovascular and cerebrovascular disease [6, 7]. Furthermore, cross-sectional and prospective epidemiological studies have shown that periodontitis increases the risk of poor glycemic control in patients with diabetes mellitus, as well as diabetes complications and associated morbidity. Successful periodontal interventions also improve glycemic control in patients with type 2 diabetes [3].

The etiopathogenesis of the periodontal disease relates to the subgingival plaque biofilm, and tissue destruction appears to be largely mediated by an abnormal host response to specific bacteria and their byproducts [2]. Acute inflammation can be considered a protective response of our body; however, chronic and non-resolving inflammation is destructive and plays a key role in a number of chronic diseases [1]. The aberrant response, which is observed in the periodontal disease, fails to remove the causative pathogens and is characterized by hyperinflammation and prolonged release of neutrophil proteolytic enzymes, pro-inflammatory mediators and Reactive Oxygen Species (ROS) [7].

Diet and nutrition are generally categorized as modifiable lifestyle risk factors for the development of this disease. In Latin, diet means a "way of living," and this is a broad and complex field which only recently has received attention within scientific literature in relation to chronic diseases of humans. Diet influences the inflammatory status, arguably, as strong as or stronger than bacterial deposits, and until recently, the mechanisms underpinning those effects were poorly understood [8]. Good nutrition and other healthy lifestyle indicators, such as maintaining normal weight and engaging in the recommended level of exercise have also shown to reduce the risk for developing several other chronic diseases like coronary heart disease and stroke.

Recently, obesity and low levels of physical activity were found to be significantly associated with the risk of periodontitis [9]. Obesity is an emerging major public health problem because the prevalence of obesity and overweight has tripled since the 1980s [5]. Several studies over the last decade showed a link between being overweight or obese and having increased levels of periodontitis, yet it is not clear whether obesity affects the oral flora. Haffajee and Socransky [10] hypothesized that the overgrowth of *T. forsythia* may occur in periodontally healthy individuals who are obese, putting them at risk for the initiation and progression of periodontitis. In another study, Goodson et al. [11] observed higher levels of *Selenomonas noxia* in the saliva of overweight women, higher than in non-obese women. However, more studies are required to analyze and understand these differences [5].

Other studies found that obese individuals are more often prone to develop infections of various types (including postoperative and nosocomial infections) than are people of normal weight [12]. The reasons which lead obese people to be more susceptible to infection include the role played by adipose tissue in inflammation and immunity. This role is confirmed by the fact that a variety of pro-inflammatory and anti-inflammatory mediators are produced by adipose tissue, and an increase of the inflammatory response can be found in obese individuals. The adipocytes in centrally located adipose tissue act as critical sites for the generation of inflammatory responses and mediators. In addition, the examination of adipose tissue in obese individuals shows an increased number of macrophages, which may also contribute to the inflammatory mediators produced by adipose tissue. However, in patients affected by periodontal disease, an increase in inflammatory mediators was observed with and without obesity.

Recently, Saxlin and collaborators [13, 14] demonstrated associations between obesity, serum lipid levels, and the cytokines tumor necrosis factor (TNF)-α and interleukin (IL)-6. Physical activity may protect against excessive inflammatory response in periodontitis by decreasing the risk of elevated IL-1 and C-reactive protein. However, the specific molecular and cellular mechanisms are not yet clear, and further studies are needed to unravel the mechanisms which may provide targets for prevention or treatment [5].

Food intake can also affect the development of dental plaque biofilms. Although dental plaque is made up of a large variety of bacterial species, the colonization follows a pattern: adhesion of initial colonizers to the acquired pellicle, followed by secondary colonization through interbacterial adhesion. Animal studies have shown that diet may be important in the development of gingivitis [15, 16]. Studies in humans have demonstrated that subjects on a high-carbohydrate diet developed gingivitis compared to subjects on a low-carbohydrate diet. An increase in dietary sucrose has been associated with a greater accumulation of plaque and evidence of gingivitis in humans [17, 18].

However, the prevalence of periodontitis seems to have remained virtually constant during the past

3,000 years in Great Britain, despite considerable changes in the oral environment. In an isolated community (Isla Grande, Colombia) with no dental services and a low education level, a Community Periodontal Index of Treatment Needs (CPITN) score of 1 (presence of bleeding on probing [BOP]) was found in only 18% of subjects, and 11% presented with Probing Depths (PDs) ≥ 5 mm (CPITN = 4.28). To the best of our knowledge, there are no studies on the periodontal and oral microbiologic conditions in subjects without access to oral hygiene measures or a modern diet [19].

The onset and progression of periodontitis is influenced by the balance between the microbial challenge and the host response. In this respect, nutrition may be of great importance since it has been implicated in several inflammatory diseases and conditions, including cardiovascular diseases, type 2 diabetes, rheumatoid arthritis and inflammatory bowel disease, all of which have been associated with periodontitis [20].

There are six major nutrient classes: carbohydrates, fats, minerals, protein, vitamins and water. These nutrient classes can be categorized as either macronutrients (needed in relatively large amounts) or micronutrients. Micronutrients are dietary compounds, such as vitamins, minerals, trace elements, amino acids, Poly-Unsaturated Fatty Acids (PUFA) that are required only in small quantities (micrograms or milligrams per day) by living organisms and are essential for optimal health, proper growth and metabolism [20]. Researchers have found evidence that macronutrients and micronutrients modulate pro-inflammatory and anti-inflammatory cascades, which influence a person's baseline inflammatory status. The functionality of nutrients in human biology extends beyond that of being fuel for energy production and cofactors in metabolism, to acting as molecular cues that are capable of modulating gene and protein expression at a molecular level [7].

Diets containing a lot of complex carbohydrates are generally healthy, whereas those rich in refined carbohydrates can be more associated with chronic inflammation. Exaggerated postprandial surges in glucose (and triglycerides) result from high calorie diets, especially from diets containing refined and processed foods rich in glucose and lipids that can be absorbed rapidly into the bloodstream. High glucose and lipid levels may generate ROS overcoming endogenous antioxidant systems and, as a result, causing oxidative stress. Postprandial dysmetabolism seems to have a role in causing inflammation. Multiple elevations in glucose levels can lead to the development of chronic inflammatory pathologies, such as coronary artery disease. The excess tissue glucose and triglyceride levels exceed the capacity of the Krebs cycle and electron transporters on the inner mitochondrial membranes to generate adenosine triphosphate.

Electron leakage leads to the single electron reduction of molecular oxygen, thus forming superoxide (O_2^-) and, further downstream, ROS. The term "meal-induced inflammation" has been introduced for describing the postprandial oxidative stress which has been linked with recorded increases in CRP and pro-inflammatory cytokines. Excess glucose derived from over nutrition through insulin metabolism leads to the formation of free fatty acids and the formation of triglycerides within adipocytes. Insulin production in response to excess carbohydrate levels also decreases the breakdown of fat (lipolysis) within adipose tissue, increasing adiposity. The adipose tissue is described in literature as an endocrine organ capable of secreting adipocytokines, such as TNF, IL-6, IL-1, adiponectin and leptin.

These adipocytokines also trigger ROS production in inflammatory cells via the nicotinamide adenine dinucleotide phosphate oxidase (that is, the enzyme complex that generates functional superoxide radicals from oxygen and glucose) and redox-sensitive gene transcription factors, such as nuclear factor-kappa β (NF-κB) and activating protein-1 (AP-1), further enhancing inflammatory cascades and oxidative stress. Oxidative stress can cause a reduced pancreatic β-cell function and intracellular antioxidant capacity and lead to the development of insulin resistance. Thus, chronic hyperglycemia-induced oxidative stress over time causes insulin resistance, further elevating plasma glucose levels. Chronic hyperglycemia is also associated with the production of Advanced Glycation End-products (AGEs) by nonenzymatic glycation of proteins, which, on binding to their surface receptor for AGEs, trigger further ROS and pro-inflammatory sequelae by various cells [7].

Inflammation can also be linked to saturated fats which are connected to the aforementioned mechanisms and are associated with high caloric intake from refined carbohydrates and oxidative stress. Additionally, diet-induced hyperlipidemia causes oxidative stress and downstream inflammation, and lipoproteins formed by liver hepatocytes can be converted to free fatty acids within the circulation and taken up by adipocytes, thus acting as a source of pro-inflammatory adipokines. Furthermore, under conditions of oxidative stress, lipid peroxidation arises triggering NF-κB activation and other related pathways. NF-κB transcribes several pro-inflammatory cytokines [7].

Several studies in literature identified the role of

oxidative stress in the pathobiology of chronic periodontitis. Increased levels of biomarkers for tissue damage, induced by ROS have been observed in periodontitis patients, and in response to oxidative stress, antioxidant enzymes appear locally upregulated in inflamed periodontal tissues and in gingival crevicular fluid and seem to be correlated inversely with pocket depth. Furthermore, extracellular antioxidant scavengers are depleted both individually, as well as in terms of Total AntiOxidant Capacity (TAOC), and tissue damage is a direct consequence from oxidative stress and an indirect consequence via activation of redox-sensitive gene transcription factors like NF-κB, which, in turn, leads to downstream pro-inflammatory cytokine/chemokine production [2].

In a study by Chapple et al., a strong and consistent inverse association between serum vitamin C concentrations and the prevalence of periodontitis was found [2]. The protective effects of vitamin C seems related to maintaining tissue homeostasis through its function in collagen synthesis and therefore maintenance of the structural integrity of the connective tissues as well as its role as a radical scavenger. Vitamin C also seems able to antagonize C-reactive protein-mediated chemotaxis and phagocytosis of inflammatory cells in ascorbate deficient monkeys [21]. Such vitamin C functions are not related to its radical scavenging activities and are likely to reduce the transit time of inflammatory/immune cells within the tissues and therefore potentially decrease the likelihood of tissue damage due to extracellular ROS release. The results for bilirubin are intriguing because it is generally seen as a powerful antioxidant, with significant inverse relations between serum levels demonstrated in atherosclerosis and coronary artery disease. These reports are consistent with the inverse association of serum bilirubin with the prevalence of periodontitis in the present study and may reflect inhibition of common pro-inflammatory pathways. Low vitamin C intake has been clearly connected with an increased risk of tooth loss and edentulous patients may have lower serum vitamin C concentrations. Data from studies in literature have shown reduced plasma TAOC in periodontitis patients outlining the presence of an inverse correlation between serum antioxidant concentrations and periodontitis prevalence. Low serum antioxidant concentrations could be the result of periodontal inflammation or could be a risk factor for periodontitis, or indeed both, and the results of the present cross-sectional study are consistent with all the above explanations.

Chapple et al. [22] have demonstrated that some of the reduction in plasma TAOC in periodontitis arises secondarily to the oxidative stress induced by periodontal inflammation. Taken together, these findings may have significant implications for periodontitis as a risk factor for diseases such as stroke, cardiovascular disease and type 2 diabetes, which have low-grade systemic inflammation implicated in their pathogenesis. Longitudinal studies are needed to ascertain whether successful periodontal therapy reduces both the oxidative and nonoxidative inflammatory burden within the peripheral vasculature and whether serum antioxidant concentrations are true risk factors for periodontitis. If confirmed, intervention studies involving antioxidant approaches would be indicated to determine the potential for reducing the risk of periodontitis [2].

The clinician during the diagnostic phase should try to look beyond the oral cavity and identify all the factors that can potentially help to reach the treatment goal of prevention or management of periodontal disease and, thereby, possibly improving general health [5].

REFERENCES

1. Milward M, Chapple I. The role of diet in periodontal disease. Clin Dent Health 2013; 52: 18-21.
2. Chapple IL, Milward MR, Dietrich T. The prevalence of inflammatory periodontitis is negatively associated with serum antioxidant concentrations. J Nutr 2007; 137(3): 657-64.
3. Chapple IL, Wilson NH. Manifesto for a paradigm shift: periodontal health for a better life. Br Dent J 2014; 216(4): 159-62.
4. Albandar JM. Global risk factors and risk indicators for periodontal diseases. Periodontol 2000 2002; 29: 177-206.
5. Genco RJ, Borgnakke WS. Risk factors for periodontal disease. Periodontol 2000 2013; 62(1): 59-94.
6. Reynolds MA. Modifiable risk factors in periodontitis: at the intersection of aging and disease. Periodontol 2000 2014; 64(1): 7-19.
7. Chapple IL. Potential mechanisms underpinning the nutritional modulation of periodontal inflammation. J Am Dent Assoc 2009; 140(2): 178-84.
8. Chapple IL, Griffiths HR, Milward MR, Ling MR, Grant MM. Antioxidant micronutrients and oxidative stress biomarkers. Methods Mol Biol 2017; 1537: 61-77.
9. Al-Zahrani MS. Increased intake of dairy products is related to lower periodontitis prevalence. J Periodontol 2006; 77(2): 289-94.
10. Haffajee AD, Socransky SS. Relationship of cigarette smoking to attachment level profiles. J Clin Periodontol 2001; 28(4): 283-95.
11. Goodson JM, Groppo D, Halem S, Carpino E. Is obesity an oral bacterial disease? J Dent Res 2009; 88(6): 519-23.
12. Falagas ME, Kompoti M. Obesity and infection. Lancet Infect Dis 2006; 6(7): 438-46.

13. Saxlin T, Suominen-Taipale L, Leiviska J, Knuuttila M, Ylostalo P. Role of serum cytokines tumour necrosis factor-alpha and interleukin-6 in the association between body weight and periodontal infection. J Clin Periodontol 2009: 36: 100-5.
14. Saxlin T, Ylostalo P, Suominen-Taipale L, Aromaa A, Knuuttila M. Overweight and obesity weakly predict the development of periodontal infection. J Clin Periodontol 2010: 37: 1059-67.
15. Carlsson J, Egelberg J. Local effect of diet on plaque formation and development of gingivitis in dogs. II. Effect of high carbohydrate versus high protein-fat diets. Odontol Revy 1965; 16: 42-9.
16. Egelberg J. Local effect of diet on plaque formation and development of gingivitis in dogs. I. Effect of hard and soft diets. Odontol Revy 1965; 16: 31-41.
17. Sidi AD, Ashley FP. Influence of frequent sugar intakes on experimental gingivitis. J Periodontol 1984; 55: 419-23.
18. Pfister W, Sprössig M, Gängler P, Mirgorod M. Bacteriological characterization of gingivitis-inducing plaque depending on different sugar levels of the diet. Zentralbl Bakteriol Mikrobiol Hyg A 1984; 257(3): 364-71 [Article in German].
19. Baumgartner S, Imfeld T, Schicht O, Rath C, Persson RE, Persson GR. The impact of the stone age diet on gingival conditions in the absence of oral hygiene. J Periodontol 2009; 80(5): 759-68.
20. Van der Velden U, Kuzmanova D, Chapple IL. Micronutritional approaches to periodontal therapy. J Clin Periodontol 2011; 38 Suppl 11: 142-58.
21. Alvares O, Altman LC, Springmeyer S, Ensign W, Jacobson K. The effect of sub-clinical ascorbate deficiency on periodontal health in nonhuman primates. J Periodontal Res 1981; 16: 628-36.
22. Chapple IL, Brock GR, Milward MR, Ling N, Matthews JB. Compromised GCF total antioxidant capacity in periodontitis: cause or effect? J Clin Periodontol 2007; 34(2): 103-10.

13 Food and dental malocclusion: epidemiology, epigenetics and prevention

Sabina Saccomanno, Lucia Bovicelli, Stefano Saran, Vincenzo Quinzi, Giuseppe Marzo and Licia Coceani Paskay

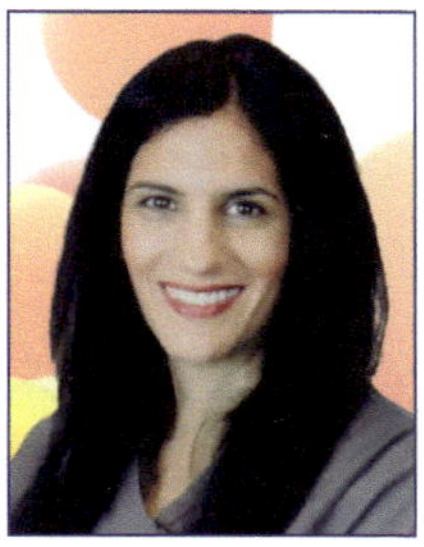

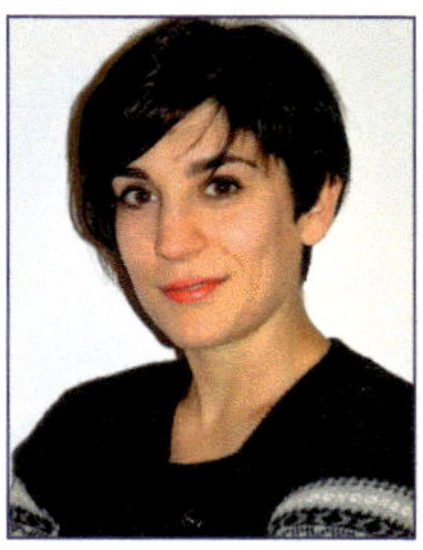

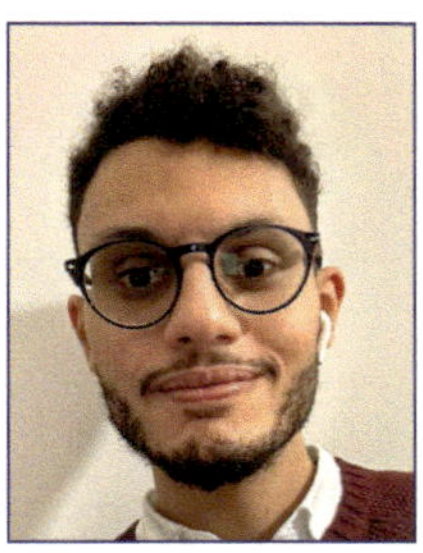

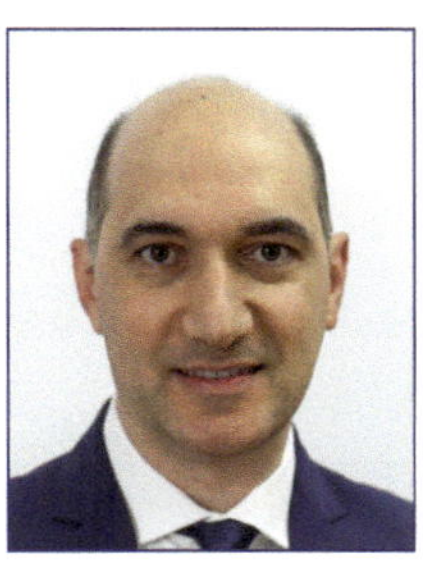

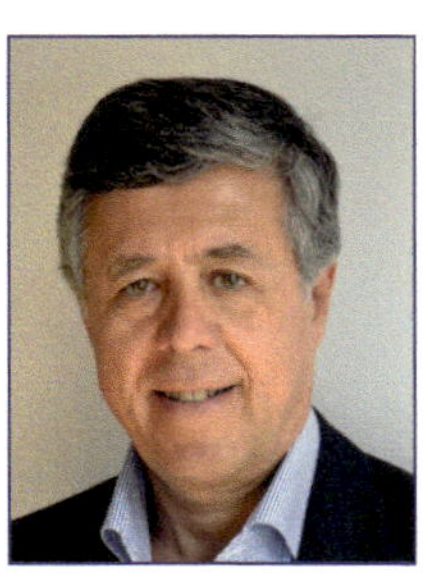

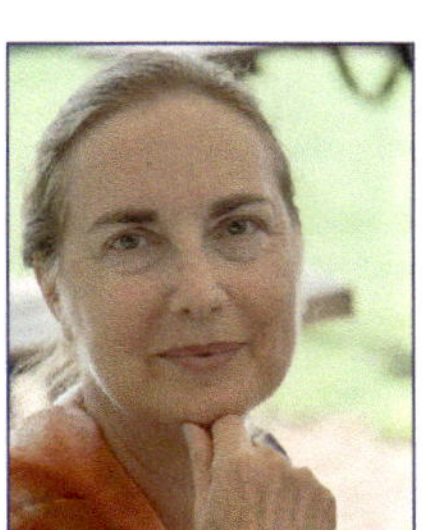

13.1 Introduction

Although a malocclusion refers to teeth, the forces playing a role in its development start to emerge at birth, with the ability of the baby to breastfeed, which is the precursor activity to develop all the sensory-motor skills later needed in weaning and in regular chewing and swallowing. The prevention of a malocclusion, therefore, begins at birth, continues through weaning and it is maintained through a lifetime.

How is a malocclusion defined? For the sake of stability and function, teeth come in contact in a very specific way called *occlusion*. *Malocclusion* means the upper and lower teeth, or the dental arches, are not properly lined up in a horizontal (Class I, II, III) or vertical (open bite, anterior cross bite, overbite or deep bite), or transverse (posterior cross bite) reciprocal relationship, or present excessive spaces (missing teeth, diastema) or reduced space (crowding) (Figs. 13.1, 13.2 and 13.3).

Sabina Saccomanno, DDS
Department of Life, Health and Environmental Sciences, University of L'Aquila, L'Aquila, Italy

Email: sabinasaccomanno@hotmail.it

Lucia Bovicelli, DDS
Private Practice

Stefano Saran, DDS
Department of Human Sciences, Innovation and Territory, School of Dentistry, Postgraduate of Orthodontics, University of Insubria, Varese, Italy

Vincenzo Quinzi, DDS
Department of Life, Health and Environmental Science, University of L'Aquila, L'Aquila, Italy

Giuseppe Marzo, MD
Director of Post Graduate School of Orthodontics
Department of Life, Health and Environmental Science, University of L'Aquila, L'Aquila, Italy

Licia Coceani Paskay, MS, CCC-SLP
Speech-Language Pathologist, Private Practice
Los Angeles, USA

Email: lcpaskay@gmail.com

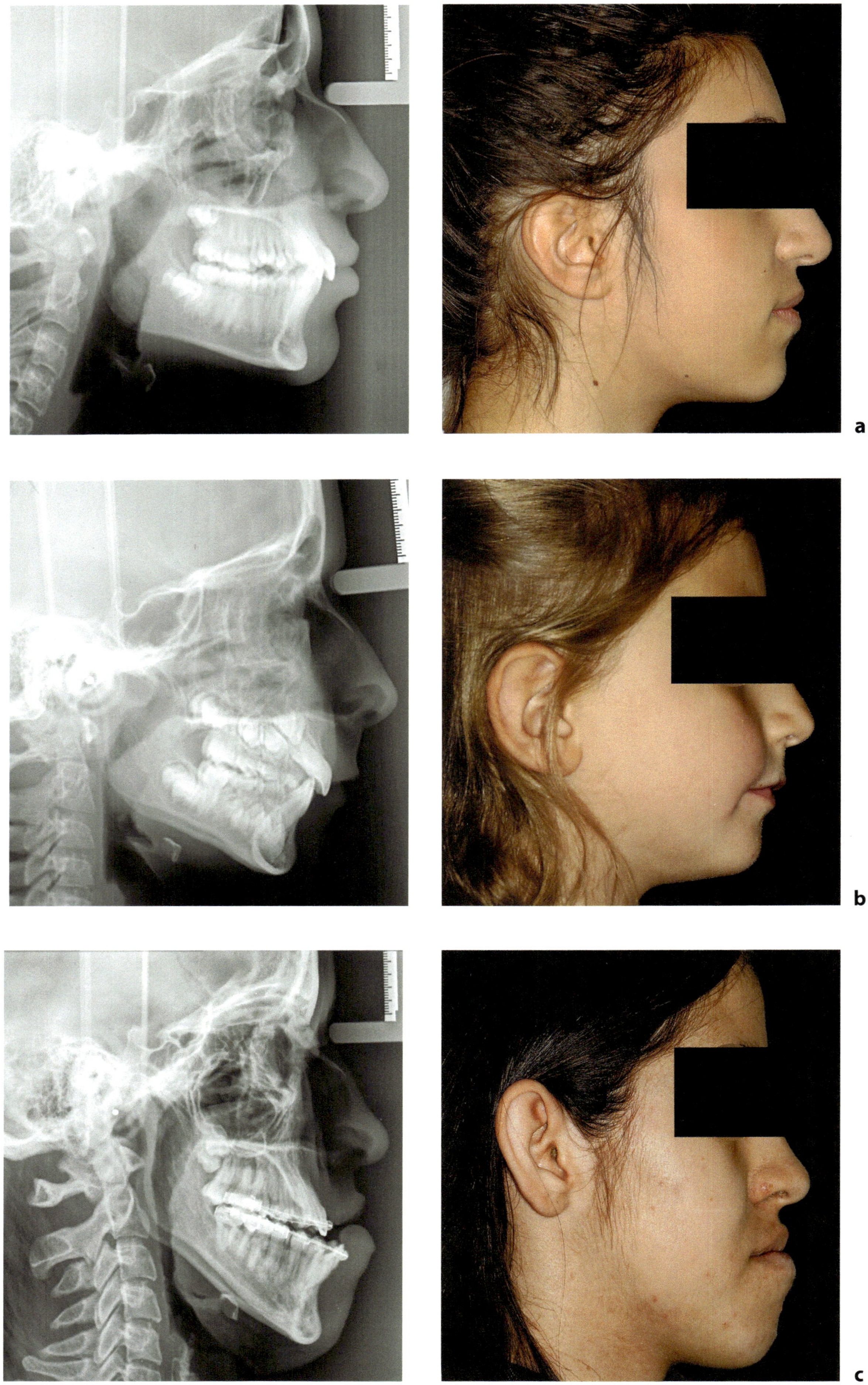

Fig. 13.1 Sagittal discrepancies from a skeletal standpoint: Class I (**a**), Class II (**b**) and Class III (**c**).

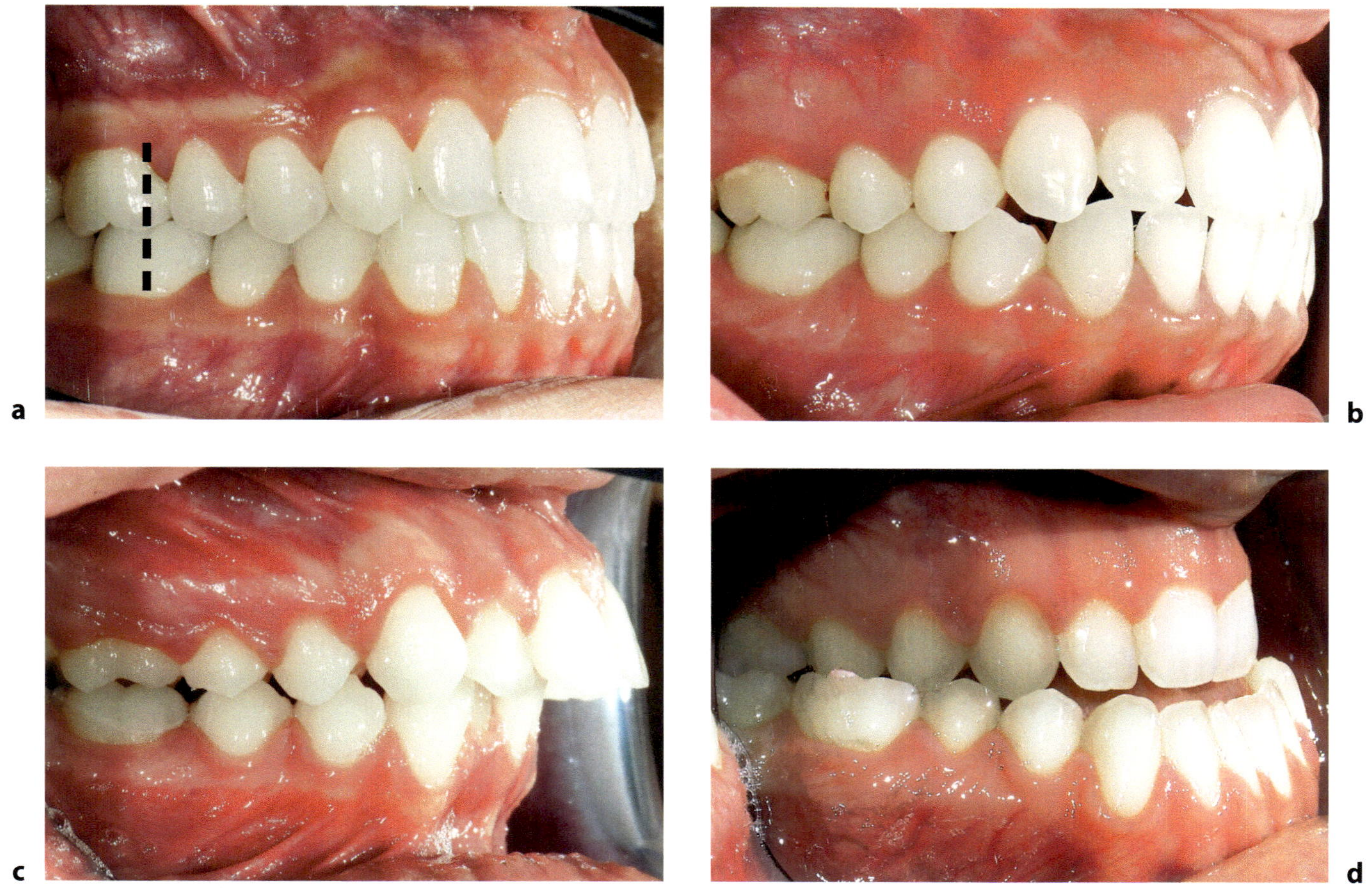

Fig. 13.2 Classification of occlusions according to Angle: normal (**a**), Class I malocclusion (**b**), Class II malocclusion (**c**) and Class III malocclusion (**d**).

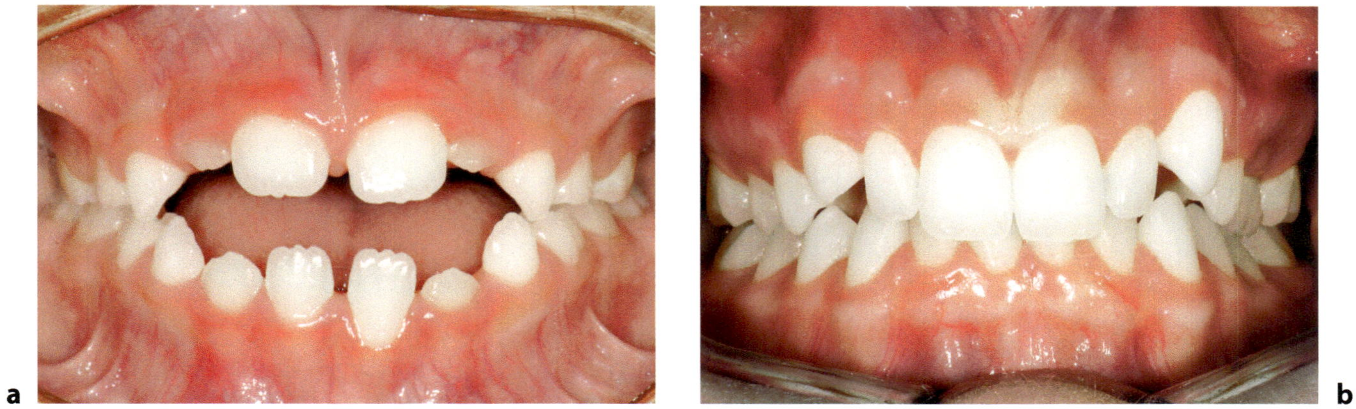

Fig. 13.3 Open bite: front view (**a**); deep bite: front view (**b**).

13.2 How is malocclusion established?

Like any alteration affecting an individual's health, the causes that contribute to the establishment of a malocclusion are both genetic and environmental (epigenetic). Let us consider for now the so-called "Habsburg's chin," that is, the protruding chin (a Class III malocclusion, with a prognathic mandible) which was a typical characteristic of the royal Habsburg family, so much so that it was widespread among family members and in others related to them, across more than seven centuries. The presence of a markedly prognathic mandible was therefore linked to a genetic malformation that often recurred, due to the fact that noble families tended to marry relatives.

As clinicians, this teaches us to carefully observe the family components of our patients and to evaluate the origin of traits that may occur in the younger generations (progeny). There is no doubt that the *genetic* factor is difficult to counter with therapy (without very early intervention) as it is determined by the DNA of the individual. But again, it's the *epigenetic* factors, especially related to poor nasal breathing, food consumption and eating practices, that influence the various *expressions* of that genetic heritage. For more details on these subjects, we suggest the readers refer to chapters 1, 6 and 7 of this book.

13.3 Epidemiology of malocclusion

A systematic review by Alhammadi et al. [1], shows that globally, in permanent dentition, the global distributions of Class I (the least severe), Class II and Class III malocclusions were 74.7% [31–97%], 19.56% [2–63%] and 5.93% [1–20%], respectively. The study indicated that Class I malocclusions are mostly present in African populations; Class II have a higher prevalence in Caucasian subjects compared to other groups [1-4]; while Asian, Arabian and African subjects, on the other hand, are more likely to have Class III malocclusions [1, 3, 5-8].

Geographical differences are also observed regarding the overjet. The decreased overjet, or the inversion of the anterior bite, has a much lower prevalence in the general population than the increased overjet, but shows a relatively greater presence in South American and West Asian countries.

The Chinese population appears to have a higher incidence of Class III malocclusion compared to Caucasians, while the incidence of Class II malocclusion is quite similar to that reported in Caucasians [9]. Among all ethnic groups, the Chinese and the Malaysian populations show the highest prevalence of Class III malocclusion [10].

Indian subjects seem to follow the prevalence of Caucasian malocclusion, in fact they are more likely to have a Class II malocclusion than other Asian populations, while their Class III prevalence is lower [6]. Among all ethnic groups, the Indian population shows the lowest prevalence for Class III malocclusions [10].

Class I malocclusion, which is the least severe of the malocclusions, is the most common occlusal model among Nigerian adolescents [11]. According to a study conducted on a group of adolescents in Tanzania, it was noted that some of the recorded malocclusion traits were relatively mild deviations from a normal occlusion, which did not require orthodontic treatment [12]. As a group, Africans showed the highest prevalence of Class I malocclusion and open bite in permanent and mixed dentition [1]. The presence of more natural and textured and less industrialized foods within the traditional African diet probably helps the development of a better dental occlusion, with a lower incidence of severe malocclusions.

About 20% of the North American populations have deviations from the ideal relationship of dental occlusion. Already, in 1998, Profit et al. [13] documented that in Mexican Americans incisive teeth irregularity and severe Class II and III malocclusions were more common, and deep bite and open bite were less prevalent, when compared to the rest of the US population.

A study by Corruccini et al. [14] conducted on older (originally nomadic) and younger (stabilized and rationed) Australian aborigines, tested the trend of correlation between the variation in dental occlusion and industrialized or modernized lifestyle habits, currently defined as *epigenetic* influence. Although there were significant differences in the traits of the incisive relationship, in the misalignment of the teeth and in the relative width of the dental arches, these are minimal when compared to other studies conducted on populations subjected to Western-style food for a generation.

Apart from genetic factors such as tooth size, some of the reasons for these structural changes may concern epigenetic influences, including concomitant differences in diet or chewing habits, partial sampling depending on tooth retention, or fluoride in water reserves.

There are many characteristics present in the older generations that are often not observed in the newer ones: genetic studies on twins are enlightening in this sense. One brother develops periodontal disease, the other does not. Why not? We cannot overlook an important factor: the environment.

13.4 Epigenetics and the human face

With the term *environment* we refer not only to the environment in the strict sense, and therefore to the interactions of pollutants or incorrect habits, but also as a whole series of behaviors and lifestyles (epigenetics) that can change the physical structure (genetics) of the individual. Already in the second half of the 19th century, the physiologist Claude Bernard spoke of "the function that creates the organ". Therefore, the organ, genetically determined, develops and defines itself thanks to the function it performs. In the case of the craniofacial growth and development, the intricate relationships between bones (structure) and soft tissues (function), at histological, biological and functional levels are well explained by Moss [15-18].

Let's start from the origins, from prehistory. The best-preserved elements in vertebrate fossils are the teeth, so paleoanthropologists studying the shape and the wear of the dental elements, the mineral component, the presence of stable isotopes, have traced back the history of dental occlusion starting from the hominid diet. Through the observation of the dental elements one can infer the diet of an individual, as well as important changes in human teeth, which have been noticed while studying food changes in prehistoric times. Let's consider the famous skull of Lucy the hominid, where the molars, including the third, are large, well-represented and all erupted. As the human species evolved, up to modern man, the molars are now reduced in size, the third molar is often small, appears late and often does not erupt at all. Why did this happen? The answer is probably the diet.

The diet has changed over the millennia, as foods are now finely chopped, minced, sliced and cooked, so they are softer, including tough meat and fibrous vegetables. The molar size has reduced as well as the mandibular length which often, therefore, does not allow the eruption of the third molar.

Anthropological research on teeth has revealed how all skulls in the history of humanity had an incisive "head-to-head" occlusion, just like primates. The American anthropologist Charles Loring Brace, a specialist in the evolution of the hominids' teeth, associated the appearance of the dental overbite, i.e., the vertical superposition ratio of incisors, to the diffusion of the tools used for feeding [19]. Brace's concept was later confirmed by Zink and Lieberman [20] who estimated that by using better tools to modify food (slicing meat and pounding roots) hominids reduced the masticatory force by 12% and improved the ability to chew meat by 41%.

Teeth are quite mobile, and just like orthodontic appliances, the orofacial functions are able to determine dental movements: just think of the favorable role of chewing or the deleterious action of parafunctions such as thumb sucking or bruxing on the growth and development of the craniofacial structure. According to Brace's hypothesis, the observed occlusal modification is attributable to the anthropological change of functions, in particular that of the use of the incisors, which hominids used to grasp and tear apart hard and rubbery foods, such as meat, while today this function is largely dependent on the use of tools: knives are used to slice and dice food, while forks are used to bring it to the mouth.

According to Brace, proof of his hypothesis came by examining the teeth of a young aristocrat, dating from the Song dynasty (960 to 1279 AD), at the Shanghai Museum of Natural Sciences. The young man's occlusion presented a peculiar dental overbite. According to Brace, since overbites started to appear around 1600 in the West and several centuries earlier in the East, a probable reason for that subject's malocclusion seemed to be the use of chopsticks for eating, as opposed to finger food (or use of spoons) eaten by the less affluent population. Chopsticks became established among the common people in what is now China and Japan during the eighth-ninth century [21, 22].

Other studies suggest that during the Japanese Medieval and Edo periods, the craniometry of the Japanese population seems to have changed. Craniometric studies indicate a discrepancy in the length of the dental arches and in the size of the teeth, with an evident reduction in facial width and a consequent increase in the incidence of malocclusion, in particular the appearance of alveolar prognathism [23]. The cause of the craniofacial changes that emerged in the Japanese population was probably multifactorial, with a marked functional component.

In the Middle Ages, mostly in Europe and Asia, there was a change in nutrition thanks to the development of a new culinary culture with a consequent reduction in chewing activity, such as: the introduction of different cooking methods, the introduction of new crops in local agriculture [24, 25] and the use of chopsticks and utensils at the table. Bee Wilson [26] also explored how tools have shaped food culture and changed the evolution of our mouth. The relationship between the dental arches has been modified by the way we eat, and the forks have contributed to the transition from a "head-to-head" occlusion to a structure similar to that of a box with the lid snugly overhanging, a characteristic of the ideal occlusion according to modern orthodontics.

The appearance of the overbite has paved the way for the resulting occlusal deviations, such as Class II dental malocclusions, which in the past were not present, but have proliferated along with the introduction of forks at the table [27]. Both chopsticks and forks presume that the food has been prepared already in small morsels, easier to chew and swallow, but also chopped food cooks more thoroughly and it is more tender.

Over the centuries, it seems that the advent of utensils at the table and the consistency of food are linked to changes in our craniofacial and occlusal conformation. However, other factors may also play a role in this structural and functional modification, such as the nutrients now readily available for consumption, and the type of diet in general, which has changed along with the civilization over centuries, with a notable acceleration since the Industrial Revolution [24, 28-31]. Weston A. Price [32] travelled all over the world in the 30's to document the "degeneration" of the human face and dental occlusion due to modern, industrialized food and especially sugar. Although some of his conclusions are still quite controversial, his extensive photographic documentation showed the very rapid changes to humans features due to people's type of food eaten and their eating practices.

In light of all this, in orthodontics, in addition to considering the chewing function, it cannot be forgotten that the craniofacial district performs other life preserving functions such as breathing and swallowing. To give an example, the *adenoid facies* is the term used to indicate a child with a long face (lower third of the face), narrow nostrils, dark circles under the eyes, a maxillary transverse contraction, often an increased overjet and a habitual open mouth posture. These skeletal characteristics are typical of patients suffering from hypertrophic (enlarged) adenoids and forced to breathe with their mouth open. The flow of air through a habitually open mouth, over time, causes a posterior mandibular rotation contributing to the elongation of the face, narrowing of the nasal cavities (due to the lack of nasal airflow and swelling of the nasal mucosa) and consequent contracted palate (due to a low habitual, compensatory posture of the tongue). The function creates the organ, even for us orthodontists. It is all the oro-nasal-facial functions or dysfunctions that impact occlusion and the growth and development of the orofacial complex [24, 31]. D'Onofrio [33] reported a nice summary of the impact of orofacial muscle functions on occlusion.

But how can eating behaviors affect us so closely in our clinical practice? There are numerous *in vivo* studies conducted on rats, pigs and rabbits, investigating the effects of diet changes from suckling to weaning to chewing regular foods on facial bones and chewing muscles, induced by a diet consisting of solid foods vs. diets with soft foods or powdered foods [34-40]. The results of Katsaros et al. [36] show how a diet with solid pellets induces, at the level of the median suture of the palate, an intense cell proliferation, hypertrophy, differentiation of mesenteric cells into chondrocytes, while, on the contrary, a "soft" diet seems to even block the cellular differentiation at the sutural level. The negative effect of the soft/liquid diet during weaning and after, on the palatal suture, cannot be completely reversed even after rats are allowed to resume a regular hard pellet diet [37].

Studies on animal models, show the impact of suckling and weaning on orofacial and cranial bone growth and development, which is something that has been observed in humans as well. However, while mammals have no choice but to suckle to stay alive and grow, humans have developed some alternatives.

13.5 Feeding practices influence growth and development of the face and mouth

13.5.1 What happens in humans from day one?

Just like all mammals, there is a built-in set of reflexes and functions in human babies, having the sole purpose to allow breastfeeding in which breathing and swallowing are well coordinated to safely allow both. During breastfeeding, the newborn establishes the appropriate nasal breathing pattern coordinated with swallowing. Swallowing happens at the end of a peristaltic wave-like action of the tongue that eventually spreads to the soft palate, lifting it during swallowing, closing the nasal cavities and allowing milk to flow into the oropharynx and esophagus (Fig. 13.4).

The tongue serves to create both positive pressure (given by the pressure of the tongue on the nipple) and negative pressure (which is created after the

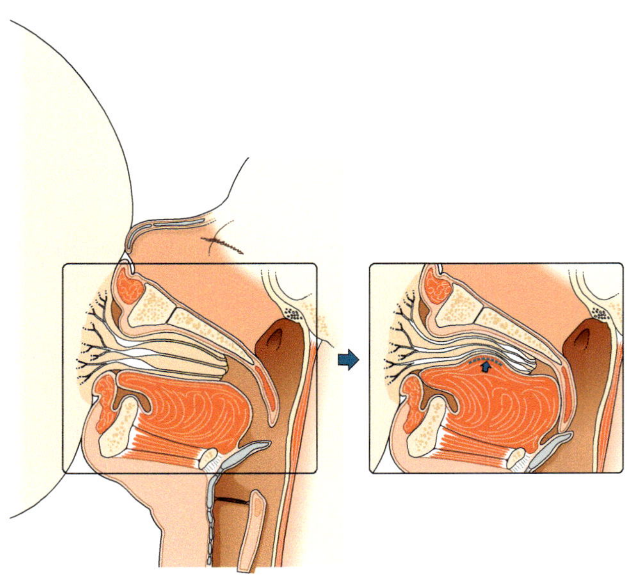

Fig. 13.4 During breastfeeding, the newborn establishes the appropriate nasal breathing pattern coordinated with swallowing. The breast nipple is flattened against the palate by the tongue, the lips are flanged, the epiglottis and the soft palate seal the oral cavity, the tongue moves in a wave-like pattern expressing the milk and triggering the swallow reflex.

contraction of the posterior portion of the tongue on the palate), which has the function of keeping the nipple in the mouth and favoring the exit of milk from the mammary glandular ducts to the nipple. Meanwhile, the lips flange on the breast's areola, stimulating the whole perioral musculature.

Suction stimulates the development of the nearby structures, and the mandible grows and consequently creates the intraoral space. The tongue can now move in all three planes of space, forward, backward, upward and expands laterally counterbalanced by the cheeks, and can follow the jaw in the processes of lowering and raising. Moreover, Palmer indicated that breastfeeding, by activating all the orofacial muscles, has an additional, preventative effect on pediatric sleep apnea [41].

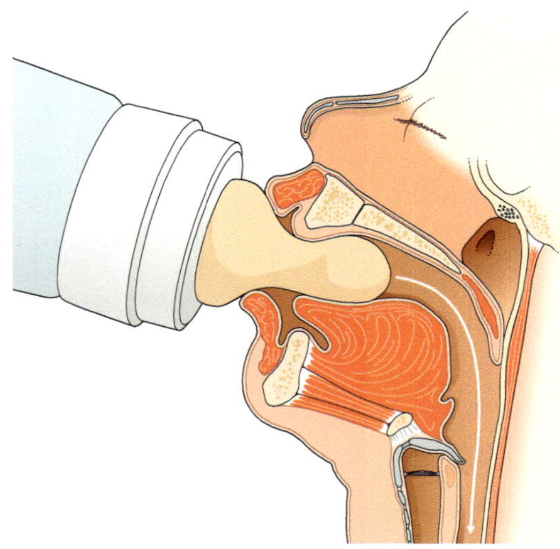

Fig. 13.5 Orofacial mechanics of bottle feeding: little to no involvement of the lips, little contact between the tongue and the palate, often the milk flow triggers a tongue thrust to control it.

13.5.2 How does artificial breastfeeding differ?

Here too we have a teat, which over time has been developed into more and more ergonomic shapes, created to assist physiological breastfeeding as much as possible. The bottle nipple, which is kept inside the oral cavity thanks to the hermetic closure of the lips, the tongue holds the teat pressed against the palate, the lateral margins rest on it like a spoon [42].

The tongue no longer makes a peristaltic and upward movement, which is crucial for palatal development, but, instead, a piston movement, moving back and forth to squeeze the milk out of the teat toward the back of the mouth. There is less overall muscular involvement in bottle feeding as it's easier than expressing milk from a breast.

In bottle feeding as well, nasal breathing briefly stops during the swallowing act, as the vocal folds close to prevent spillage of liquid in the larynx, the epiglottis closes the larynx and the back of the tongue "sits" on top of the larynx, to allow the flow of liquid into the esophagus (Fig. 13.5).

The WHO recommends exclusive breastfeeding for at least the first 6 months of the baby's life [43]. Maintaining breastfeeding at least until the incisors appear allows the newborn to maintain physiological nasal breathing ensuring that, at a zero cost, one of the fundamental functions of the craniofacial district, which is breathing, contributes to a correct growth pattern.

Breastfeeding is made possible and is maintained in the newborn thanks to fundamental orofacial neurological reflexes that persist in the infant for at least 4/6 months:

- *Rooting reflex*: this reflex allows the baby to find and grasp the nipple.
- *Suction/swallow reflex*: after the baby opens his/her mouth and the milk touches the lip area, the baby sucks the milk in and then the swallow reflex takes over.
- *Tongue thrust reflex*: when the lips are touched, the baby's tongue is pushed out of the mouth. This reflex allows the newborn to be fed with the breast or bottle but not through a spoon.
- *Gag reflex*: it is activated in the newborn if an object, a spoon or a solid food slip back into the mouth, and the tongue spits it out.

These reflexes are one of the reasons why babies up to 4/6 months are not ready to receive solid foods. However, given the importance of breastfeeding in the development of chewing muscles, breathing and orofacial bones development, whenever possible, children should be allowed to breastfeed for at least one year, even while weaning.

After 4/6 months (a period that generally coincides with the eruption of the first lower incisors), these orofacial reflexes tend to disappear and give way to the swallowing reflex which consolidates. At this point, the baby is ready to receive solid food and must be encouraged to "hold and bite". That is, the child alone must be able to grab food, explore it and bite it with the lower incisors — the first teeth to appear. At this age, spontaneously, babies bring to the mouth anything they grab with their hands [42].

In the early stages of weaning, the mandible is propelled forward to touch the upper jaw and thus promote the eruption of the incisors by biting the gingiva covering the erupting teeth. In the months following the appearance of the incisors, the canines

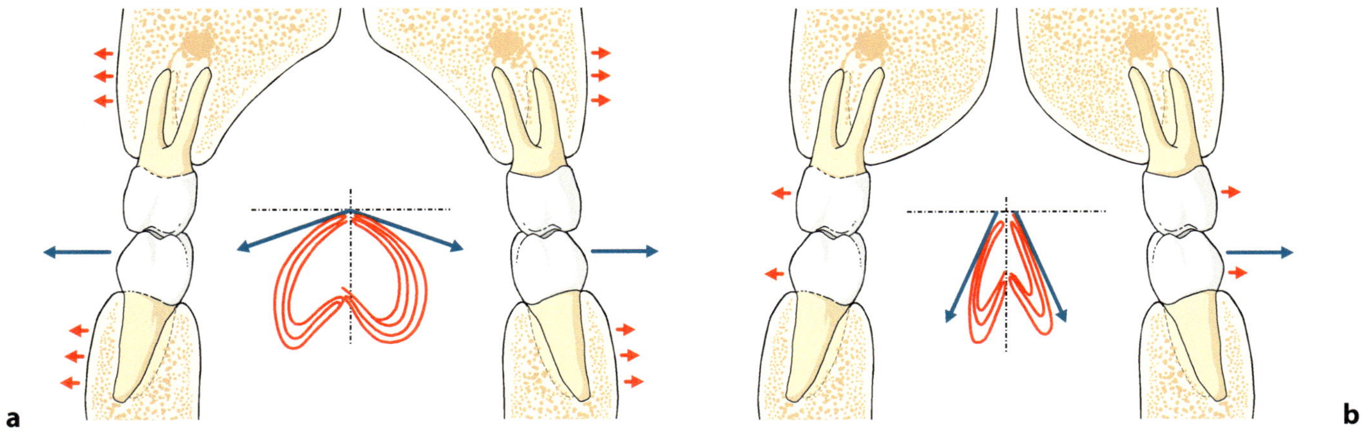

Fig. 13.6 In the presence of powerful muscles and regular consistency foods, an "attritional" occlusion develops with stimulation of the growth processes in a transversal sense (**a**). Conversely, in the presence of weaker muscles and soft foods, the maintenance of a "non-attritional" occlusion inhibits stimulation of transverse growth (**b**).

and the first molars erupt until the deciduous dentition is completed at age two. Babies tend to mouth various objects to assist the eruption of the teeth, and this could be a good time to introduce 6-month-old babies to hard foods that they can gnaw on and use as teething toys and explore various consistencies and flavors.

At that point, regular foods should be offered to the baby/toddler to promote good chewing habits for the future. Readers can find further details regarding breastfeeding, bottle feeding and weaning in chapters 6, 7, 8, 9 and 10. Limme et al. [44], highlights how, in the presence of powerful muscles and regular consistency foods, an "attritional" occlusion develops with stimulation of the growth processes in a transverse sense (Fig. 13.6a). Conversely, in the presence of weaker muscles and soft foods, the maintenance of a "non-attritional" occlusion inhibits stimulation of transverse growth (Fig. 13.6b).

Activating a good chewing function from 18 months or sooner — to reach by 2.5-3 years an alternating bilateral chewing pattern — is the key factor in the transverse development of the jaws. Granted that we do have a "preferential or dominant side" for chewing, just like we have eye dominance, or foot dominance, still, why is bilateral alternating chewing important?

Planas [45] already stressed the importance of bilateral chewing: the occlusal plane develops more harmoniously if chewing is alternated. If chewing was unilateral, we would have variations at the occlusal, mandibular, maxillary and condylar levels. From the working side we could probably observe a raised occlusal plane, a shorter mandible, a more developed maxillary in a transverse sense and a more hypertrophic condyle. On the balancing side, the situation will be reversed.

13.6 Food consistency and craniofacial development

How important is the consistency of food in craniofacial development? Very important, as anthropological and studies with animal models have indicated [20, 36, 37, 46].

The mandibular movements happen in all three planes of space. It is common experience that to chew soft food, such as bread (the soft part, not the crust), the prevailing movements are the opening and closing the mouth. Minimal chewing movements occur, the tongue squeezes the food against the palate and the saliva soaks up the food, making it ready to be swallowed. In fact, in the first periods of weaning, where only the incisors are present, the child mostly performs a mandibular protrusion and elevation movement.

As the posterior teeth appear, mandibular movements also become more complex. The presence of large surfaces and molar sliding surfaces allow the mandible to move to the right and the left. The molars are teeth that can grind (*comminute)* fibrous foods, such as meat or celery. The lateral movements are stimulated above all by the shredding and grinding of consistent foods. The lateral movement allows the selective grinding of the deciduous teeth (baby teeth), eventually facilitating the change from deciduous to permanent teeth.

Moreover, every time food is crushed by the teeth, a proprioceptive stimulation of the periodontal ligament is induced, which, together with the muscular strength, proportionally becomes more intense with the greater consistency of the chewed food, thus stimulating the growth of the craniofacial region and the dental eruption. From this perspective, the frequent eruption delays, dental crowding and reduced transverse diameter of the maxillary bones can be seen as a direct consequence of an increasingly civilized and "soft" diet. In addition to chewing, in relation to the orthodontic disorders present in the population, several authors observed how most of them are due to dysfunctional breathing, swallowing, lingual posture, parafunctions, and nocturnal sleep and habits [47-53].

13.7 Conclusion

Apart from the impact of food on malocclusion there are several basic functions playing a part as variables on malocclusion, such as breathing, chewing, salivating and swallowing that are modulated by the neurosensory-motor system, the sympathetic and parasympathetic systems and by the enteric nervous system. And, of course, humans have been eating hard textured foods for millennia, which has been determining our facial growth and development, dental occlusion [54] and some studies even suggested that chewing seems to increase cognitive performance [55, 56].

Only in the last two centuries has the texture of food and its preparation drastically impacted the way food is consumed and therefore an optimal dental occlusion, overtime, has become a malocclusion of epidemic proportion. Hard textured food is still the best option in adulthood to increase and preserve the physiological parameters of proper chewing, muscle coordination and changes in chewing sides [57]. Malocclusion is not a destiny, and it can be changed through prevention, education, early intervention and an appropriate diet.

REFERENCES

1. Alhammadi MS, Halboub E, Fayed MS, Labib A, El-Saaidi C. Global distribution of malocclusion traits: A systematic review. Dental Press J Orthod 2018; 23 (6): 40.e1-40.e10.
2. Petroviç D, Vukiç-Culafi B, Iviç S, Djuriç M, Milekiç B. Study of the risk factors associated with the development of malocclusion. Vojnosanit Pregl 2013; 70(9): 817-23.
3. Joshia N, Hamdanb AM, Fakhouric WD. Skeletal malocclusion: a developmental disorder with a life-long morbidity. J Clin Med Res 2014; 6(6): 399-408.
4. Lux CJ, Dücke B, Pritsch M, Komposch G, Niekusch U. Occlusal status and prevalence of occlusal malocclusion traits among 9-year-old schoolchildren. Eur J Orthod 2009; 31(3): 294-9.
5. Bazzini E, Ciapponi E, Tomatis F, Garattini G. Valutare la prevalenza dei differenti tratti malocclusivi attraverso una revisione della letteratura. Il Dentista Moderno 2016; 3: 84-104. [Article in Italian]
6. Soh J, Sandham A, Chan YH. Occlusal status in Asian male adults: prevalence and ethnic variation. Angle Orthod 2005; 75(5): 814-20.
7. Borzabadi-Farahani A, Borzabadi-Farahani A, Eslamipour F. Malocclusion and occlusal traits in an urban Iranian population. An epidemiological study of 11- to 14-year-old children. Eur J Orthod 2009; 31(5): 477-84.
8. Josefsson E, Bjerklin K, Lindsten R. Malocclusion frequency in Swedish and immigrant adolescents – Influence of origin on orthodontic treatment need. Eur J Orthod 2007; 29(1): 79-87.
9. Lew KK, Foong WC, Loh E. Malocclusion prevalence in an ethnic Chinese population. Aust Dent J 1993; 38(6): 442-9.
10. Hardy DK, Cubas YP, Orellana MF. Prevalence of angle class III malocclusion: A systematic review and meta-analysis. Open Journal of Epidemiology 2012; 2(4): 75-82.
11. Onyeaso CO. Prevalence of malocclusion among adolescents in Ibadan, Nigeria. Am J Orthod Dentofacial Orthop 2004; 126(5): 604-7.
12. Rwakatema DS, Nganga PM. Prevalence of malocclusion among 12-15-year-olds in Moshi, Tanzania, using Bjork's criteria. East Afr Med J 2006; 83(7): 372-9.
13. Proffit WR, Fields HW Jr, Moray LJ. Prevalence of malocclusion and orthodontic treatment need in the United States: estimates from the NHANES III survey. Int J Adult Orthodon Orthognath Surg 1998; 13(2): 97-106.
14. Corruccini RS, Townsend GC, Brown T. Occlusal variation in Australian aboriginals. Am J Phys Anthropol 1990; 82(3): 257-65.
15. Moss ML. The functional matrix hypothesis revisited. 1. The role of mechanotransduction. Am J Orthod Dentofacial Orthop 1997; 112(1): 8-11.
16. Moss ML. The functional matrix hypothesis revisited. 2. The role of an osseous connected cellular network. Am J Orthod Dentofacial Orthop 1997; 112(2): 221-6.
17. Moss ML. The functional matrix hypothesis revisited. 3. The genomic thesis. Am J Orthod Dentofacial Orthop 1997; 112(3): 338-42.
18. Moss ML. The functional matrix hypothesis revisited. 4. The epigenetic antithesis and the resolving synthesis. Am J Orthod Dentofacial Orthop 1997; 112(4): 410-7.
19. Brace CL, Montagu A. Human Evolution: An Introduction to Biological Anthropology. Macmillan, 1977.
20. Zink KD, Lieberman DE. Impact of meat and Lower Palaeolithic food processing techniques on chewing in humans. Nature 2016; 531(7595): 500-3.
21. Ishiki H. Why the Japanese use chopsticks? Otsuki-shoten, Tokyo, 1987. [Article in Japanese]
22. Kaifu Y. Changes in the pattern of tooth wear from prehistoric to recent periods in Japan. Am J Phys Anthropol 1999; 109(4): 485-99.
23. Ohsako M. Temporal Changes in Maxillary Alveolar Profile Angle and Inclination of Incisor in Japan. Anthropological Science 2000; 108(4): 387-406.
24. Boyd K, Saccomanno S, Lewis CJ, Coceani Paskay L, Quinzi V, Marzo G. Myofunctional therapy. Part 1: Culture, industrialisation and the shrinking human face. Eur J Paediatr Dent 2021; 22(1): 80-1.
25. Nagayama H. History of Japanese dietary. Kawade-shobo, Tokyo, 1998. [Article in Japanese]
26. Wilson B. Consider the Fork: A history of how we cook and eat. Basic Books, a member of the Perseus Books Group, New York, 2013.

27. Peck S, Peck H. Orthodontic aspects of dental anthropology. Angle Orthod 1975; 45(2): 95-102.
28. Corruccini RS. An epidemiologic transition in dental occlusion in world populations. Am J Orthod 1984; 86(5): 419-26.
29. Di Chiara A. La differente incidenza delle malattie dentali e delle alterazioni maxillofacciali tra popolazioni tradizionali e civilizzate. Estratto da "Evoluzione del rapporto dinamico-funzionale tra occlusione e ATM" di S. Dettori e A. Confaloni Mercurio Editore, 2001. [Article in Italian]
30. Lieberman DE. The Evolution of the Human Head, Belknap Press of Harvard University Press, 2011, pp. 276–277.
31. Boyd KL, Saccomanno S, Coceani Paskay Hv L, Quinzi V, Marzo G. Maldevelopment of the cranio-facial-respiratory complex: A Darwinian perspective. Eur J Paediatr Dent 2021; 22(3): 225-9.
32. Price WA. Nutrition and Physical Degeneration. 8th Edition, 23rd Printing. Price-Pottenger Nutrition Foundation Editor, Lemon Grove, CA, USA. 2009
33. D'Onofrio L. Oral dysfunction as a cause of malocclusion. Orthod Craniofac Res 2019; 22 Suppl 1(Suppl 1): 43-8.
34. Bond LE, Mayerl CJ, Stricklen BM, German RZ, Gould FDH. Changes in the coordination between respiration and swallowing from suckling through weaning. Biol Lett 2020; 16(4): 20190942.
35. Campbell-Malone R, Crompton AW, Thexton AJ, German RZ. Ontogenetic changes in Mammalian feeding: insights from electromyographic data. Integr Comp Biol 2011; 51(2): 282-8.
36. Katsaros C, Zissis A, Bresin A, Killaridis S. Functional influence on sutural bone apposition in the growing rat. Am J Orthod Dentofacial Orthop 2006; 129(3): 352-7.
37. Mavropoulos A, Odman A, Ammann P, Killaridis S. Rehabilitation of masticatory function improves the alveolar bone architecture of the mandible in adult rats. Bone 2010; 47(3): 687-92.
38. Takasu H, Matsunaga T, Morita T, Hiraba K, Kuroki K, Saito K, Fujiwara T, Goto S. Changes in masseter muscle fibers by liquid diet rearing in rabbits and recovery by chewing of solid diet. Arch Oral Biol 2019; 108: 104548.
39. Kawai N, Sano R, Korfage JAM, Nakamura S, Kinouchi N, Kawakami E, Tanne K, Langenbach GEJ, Tanaka E. Adaptation of rat jaw muscle fibers in postnatal development with a different food consistency: an immunohistochemical and electromyographic study. J Anat 2010; 216(6): 717-23.
40. Ulgen M, Baran S, Kaya H, Karadede I. The influence of the masticatory hypofunction on the craniofacial growth and development in rats. Am J Orthod Dentofacial Orthop 1997; 111(2): 189-98.
41. Palmer B. Snoring and sleep apnoea: how it can be prevented in childhood. Breastfeed Rev 2006; 14(2): 11-4.
42. Bahr D. Feed Your Infant and Toddler Right: Early Eating and Drinking Skills Encourage the Best Development. Future Horizons Publisher, Arlington TX, 2018.
43. https://www.who.int/health-topics/breastfeeding#tab=tab_1
44. Limme M, Rozencweig G. La fonction modèle la forme et la forme conditionne la fonction Entretien avec Michel Limme. Orthod Fr 2013; 84(3): 211-20. [Article in French]
45. Planas P. Rehabilitación neuro-oclusal (RNO). Ediciones Científicas y Técnicas. Universidad Católica Boliviana, 1994. [Spanish]
46. Silvester CM, Kullmer O, Hillson S. A dental revolution: The association between occlusion and chewing behaviour. PLoS One 2021; 16(12): e0261404.
47. Sfondrini MF, Ferrante F, Sala G, Gandini P, Scribante A. Deglutizione atipica, anomalie occlusali e alterazioni posturali: esiste una correlazione? Dental Cadmos 2019; 87 (1): 8-21. [Article in Italian]
48. Botero-Mariaca P, Sierra-Alzate V, Rueda ZV, Gonzalez D. Lingual function in children with anterior open bite: A case-control study. Int Orthod 2018; 16(4): 733-43.
49. Verrastro AP, Stefani FM, Rodrigues CR, Wanderley MT. Occlusal and orofacial myofunctional evaluation in children with anterior open bite before and after removal of pacifier sucking habit. Int J Orthod Milwaukee 2007; 18(3): 19-25.
50. Green S. Case history: improved maxillary growth and development following digit sucking elimination and orofacial myofunctional therapy. Int J Orofacial Myology 2013; 39: 45-53.
51. Cheynet F. TMJ, eating and breathing. Rev Stomato Chir Maxillofac Chir Orale 2016; 117(4): 199-206. [Article in French]
52. Pirelli P. Respirazione orale e sviluppo craniofacciale: importanza dell'approccio interdisciplinare. Mondo Ortodontico 1996; 21: 265-275. [Article in Italian]
53. Quinn GW. Airway interference syndrome. Clinical identification and evaluation of nose breathing capabilities. Angle Orthod 1983; 53(4): 311-9.
54. Tyszkowski M. Is There a Relationship between Nutrition, Facial Development, and Crowding of the Teeth? Int J Orthod Milwaukee 2016; 27(1):15-7.
55. Hirano Y, Onozuka M. Chewing and cognitive function. Brain Nerve 2014; 66(1): 25-32. [Article in Japanese].
56. Bergdahl M, Habib R, Bergdahl J, Nyberg L, Nilsson LG. Natural teeth and cognitive function in humans. Scand J Psychol 2007; 48(6): 557-65.
57. Tonni I, Riccardi G, Piancino MG, Stretti C, Costantinides F, Paganelli C. The influence of food hardness on the physiological parameters of mastication: A systematic review. Arch Oral Biol 2020; 120: 104903.

14 The many benefits of chewing

Licia Coceani Paskay

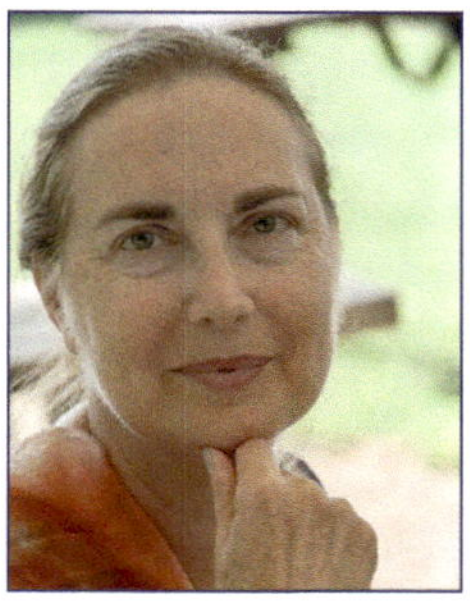

14.1 Introduction

The body works economically using the same function for more than one purpose. For instance, breathing provides not only oxygen but it's involved in aiding the peristaltic movement of the intestines and pumping the spinal fluid. Similarly, chewing is involved in more than simple smashing of foods to be swallowed. Chewing is a complex function that implies exertion of forces, in a rhythmical fashion, involving multiple structures.

No other part of the body is as hard as the teeth in the mouth because no other part of the body is design to withstand such a pressure and wear for our entire lives. Whenever the food eaten is soft and does not require adequate chewing, the teeth lose some of their purpose. But the structures dependent on teeth are also subjected to changes. The mandibular and maxillary bones, in which the teeth are embedded, change according to the force applied on the teeth.

14.2 Chewing and epigenetics

One concept that can guide diagnostics and therapy is the fact that the bony and dental structures of the face and mouth develop around soft tissue organs (tongue and eyes) that are determined genetically while bone and dentition are also influenced epigenetically. In other words, while our eyes or our tongue have a determined size, stable in time, harder structures such as the maxilla or the mandible or the dental arches, are influenced by stimuli applied. Presence of habitual mouth breathing influences the position of the tongue and of the mandible and the activation of facial, lingual and chewing muscles. All these muscular activations, or lack of, allow communication with the underlining bones informing them, via the bone periosteum, of pressures or pulling. The bone responds by absorbing some bone or by apposing more bone tissue. Therefore, it's function that drives the growth and development of the face. Harmonious functions promote harmonious growth and development.

14.3 Development of chewing

The chewing function is complex and begins at birth. It's promoted by breast feeding, is refined during weaning, and can be influenced positively or negatively at any point in life. From birth, the growth and development of muscles,

Licia Coceani Paskay, MS, CCC-SLP
Speech-Language Pathologist, Private Practice
Los Angeles, USA

Email: lcpaskay@gmail.com

later needed for chewing, is well documented although mostly through animal models. For instance, a study by Suzuki et al. shows that an important component of chewing muscles, the Myosin Heavy Chains (MHC) intensify especially in the temporalis muscles, as baby mice are weaned from milk into an adult like hard food [1]. Similar findings are reported by Okubo et al., where the MHC becomes more evident in the anterior digastric muscle, which also changes position as the baby mice are weaned from milk to regular food [2]. Maejima et al. confirmed that the muscles of the tongue change during the shift between sucking milk and eating regular food, with the tongue becoming stronger and contracting faster during chewing of hard food pellets, which is due to the increased presence of MHC [3].

And yet, when that natural transition between breastfeeding and eating regular adult-like food is altered by the artificial introduction of softer food consistencies animal models are indicators that once the weaning is done with soft foods the correct chewing may never be recovered [4]. Mavropoulos et al. indicated that the alveolar bone architecture in rats, after cessation of growth, was influenced by early feeding practices [5]. The rats that were weaned directly to hard food pellets fared better than the ones who received soft food during initial weaning and were switched to regular hard food pellets a few weeks later. A later introduction of harder consistency did not allow the rats' bone to catch up to the level of the rats weaned with hard food. A similar conclusion was reached by Katsaros et al. [6].

Morquette et al., Westberger and Kolta, Lund and Kolta indicated that trigeminal feedback circuits promote the development of the chewing pattern and the neurological central pattern generator for chewing [7-9]. The trigeminal connections activated during chewing modulate the neuro-occlusal circuits, stimulate saliva production, bolus control, triggering swallowing, with the trigeminal (V) in connection (plexus) with the facial (VII) and glossopharyngeal (IX) cranial nerves. The trigeminal connections also predispose the alimentary system by way of the trigeminal (V), vagus (X) and hypoglossus (XII) cranial nerves.

These connections can be crucial in devising a prevention and treatment plan.

14.4 Prevention across a lifetime

In terms of prevention, the knowledge of the impact of epigenetic factors (factors in the internal and external environment that influence our lives), the studies on animal models, the recent trove of studies on the impact of neuroplasticity and the application of the "Nudge Theory" (making it easier for people to make the right decisions) suggest that changes in the cultural approach to breathing nasally, breastfeeding, weaning and eating would make many small changes in behavior that over time promote better chewing and better health. Breast feeding should be encouraged and promoted. Political will is needed to help women worldwide to have the time and the opportunity to breastfeed their babies as long as possible (see the WHO recommendations on breast feeding).

Weaning should include more hard food selected by babies spontaneously. Letting them munch and suck on a hard dinner roll or on a piece of meat or fruit, clearly under supervision, would stimulate the hand mouth reflex, allow the baby to explore textures and flavors and exercise the chewing function. A successful model is the "Baby-led Weaning" (see chapter 7) which, although it sounds like a new concept, it has been adopted by mothers for eons worldwide. Unfortunately, companies selling baby food have a strong interest and strong political lobbies to fan terror in mothers who are afraid their babies are going to choke on food unless it's ground or blenderized. However, principles of neuroplasticity dictate that what babies learn in their first year or so of life becomes engrained for the rest of their lives. Babies weaned with soft food will always prefer soft food.

There are profound implications regarding weaning techniques and impact of food preparation on adult chewing. Most fast food is high in carbohydrates because they are easy to chew, often requiring no chewing at all, and therefore more likely to be swallowed in big chunks as opposed to being comminuted thoroughly. Reduced chewing implies reduces salivation and it's the ptyalin in the saliva that begins the breaking down of the carbohydrate chains, facilitating a further breaking down by the stomach (Fig. 14.1). Reduced chewing causes consumption of large amounts of calories in very short time, bypassing the production of ghrelin, which signals satiety, which is released about 20 minutes from the beginning of eating.

14.5 Chewing and digestion

Chewing provides a powerful signal to the entire alimentary system, from the mouth to the intestine. In fact, a study by Kimura et al. analyzed chewing and subsequent swallowing and digestion in a sample of 60 residents of nursing homes, of which 30 of them were fed via gastric tube (g-tube) or nasogastric tube (ng-tube) [10]. The bypassing of chewing, swallowing and the production of saliva, even in

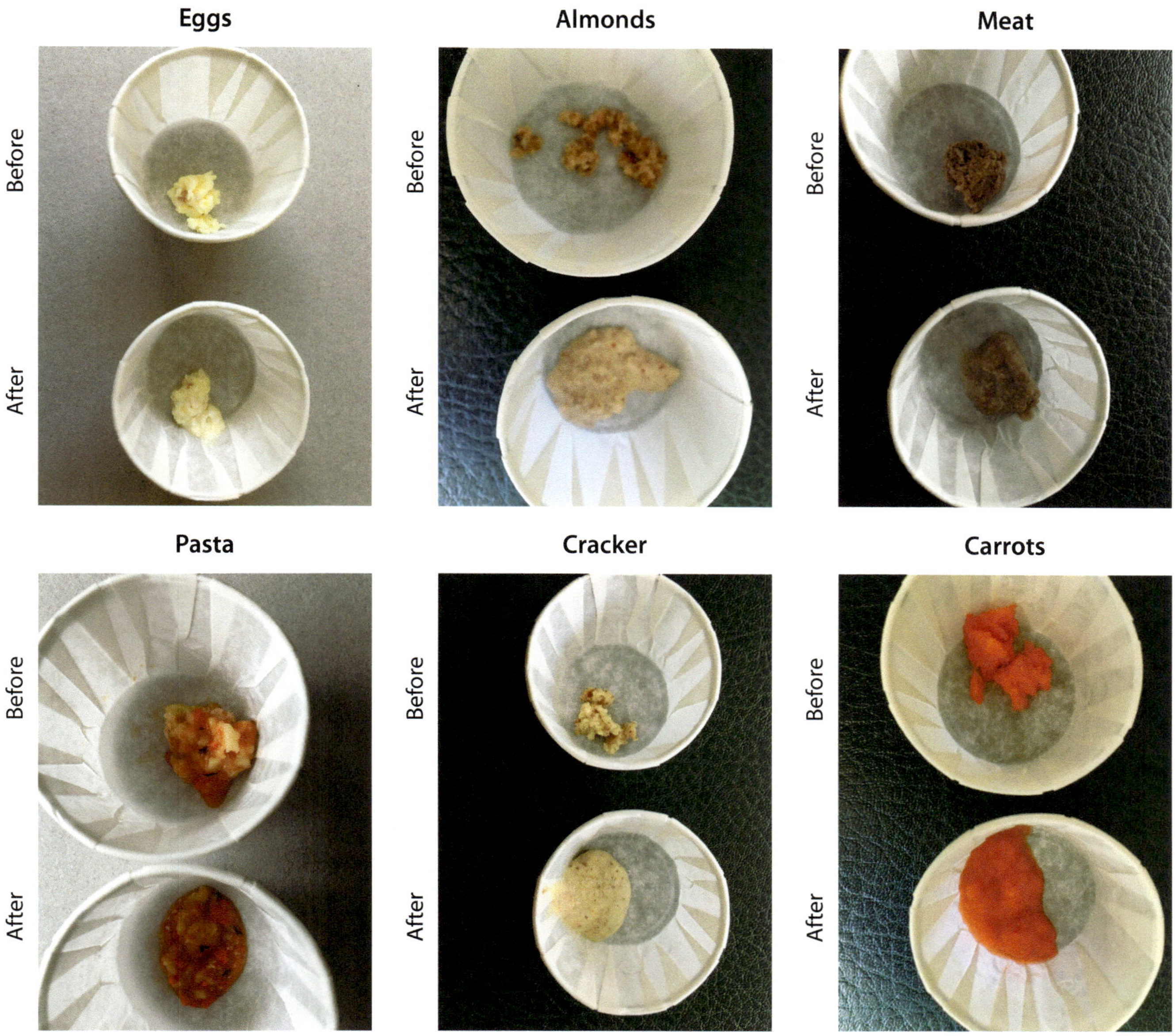

Fig. 14.1 These *before and after* images feature various foods for chewing training, ranging from "soft" (eggs) to "hard" (almonds), from "fibrous" (meat) to "sticky" (pasta), and from "dry" (cracker) to "juicy" (carrots). Before training, the food boluses tend to be dry, poorly cohesive, with little saliva coating. After training, regardless of the consistency and texture, the bolus should look and feel the same before swallowing, soupy and with very tiny food particles. However, meat tends to retain some of its fibrousness while fruit and veggie morsels require swallowing the juice first.

presence of food delivered parenterally, affected gastric motility, digestion and salivary production by decreasing the autonomic system input. Clearly, even if humans are very adaptable, never in history the body has been able to get food that did not pass through the mouth. Therefore, the signals coming (or not coming) from the mouth are intimately connected to the rest of the alimentary system. A similar result was reached by Lunding et al. when he compared 14 patients with dyspepsia vs. 14 normal subjects [11]. The patients with dyspepsia were asked to eat clear soup with or without also chewing flavorless chewing gum (sham chewing) and spitting the saliva not to interfere with the results. Clearly those patients with dyspepsia had more disturbed gastric motility compared with the healthy subjects, but those patients who were allowed to chew gum showed an improved gastric motility, compared with those who only drank the clear soup without additional sham chewing.

14.6 Benefits of "sham" chewing

Sham chewing, in other words, is able to trick the brain into activating the alimentary system, activation that does not happen the same way when we drink clear liquids, or we receive food via g-tube or ng-tube.

Over 200 peer reviewed studies at the time of this writing analyzed the many applications of chewing gum just after surgery to prevent post-operative ileus, a delay in return of bowel function that is often a deadly complication of surgery. While gum chewing pre-operatively is either not recommended for various reasons or has been found to have no influence on the surgery's outcome, more studies support the use of chewing gum post-surgery, especially after colorectal surgery [12, 13], cesarian [14], liver resection [15] , laparoscopic colectomy surgery [16], appendectomy [17] and even orthopedic surgery [18] to improve gastrointestinal function [19].

14.7 Chewing and the brain

There are connections between chewing and cognitive skills that only recently have been gaining attention for their wide implications. An article by Ono et al. reports that chewing, by reducing stress in animals and in humans, maintains the cognitive function of the hippocampus and the prefrontal cortex, crucial neurological striations in the formation of memory [20]. Conversely, reduced mastication is an epidemiological risk factor for development of dementia in humans as it impacts the hippocampus, causing functional and morphological changes to its neurons. Another promising article by Kawanishi et al. suggested that, in rats, chewing solid food could be effective for the rehabilitation of sensorimotor and learning/memory dysfunctions induced by cerebral infarction [21].

Although focusing on very specific features of chewing, such as masseters activation, jaw movement, biting and unilateral or bilateral clenching, many studies suggest interesting aspects of chewing as a rhythmical activity that promotes bilateral Middle Cerebral Artery blood flow velocity (MCAv) [22, 23], activation of the bilateral sensorimotor cortex, supplementary motor area, dorsolateral prefrontal cortex and posterior parietal cortex [24]. Chewing gum has also been implicated in attention, reduction of sleepiness and increase of alertness [25].

Biting and clenching, which may be part of taking in morsels of food or holding a larger chunk of food, could be also happening in isolation, as they have powerful neuro connections with stress reduction, not only documented in animal models but it's a common experience with people under stress clenching their teeth, biting pens and pencils, or chewing gum [26-28].

14.8 Chewing and saliva

Proper chewing requires proper salivation, which is a neurologically mediated by the cranial nerves V, VII and XII activating the various salivary glands: sublingual, submandibular, parotid and all the tiny salivary cells scattered around the oral cavity. It's not by chance that the salivary glands are innervated by the same cranial nerves that regulate muscles involved in chewing (facial, masticatory, soft palate, etc.), as mastication stimulates saliva production. Some medications, radiotherapy after tumor resection, some atrophic diseases may cause various degrees of changes in the quantity and quality of saliva, commonly referred as xerostomia, or *dry mouth*. Xerostomia causes difficulty in chewing and swallowing as it does not assist the bolus formation, but it could also be a consequence of reduced chewing, due to the many neuro connections involving the salivary glands. The connections between saliva and chewing starts during weaning. Elewa et al. reported how the salivary glands of baby goats (kids) also increase their output during the transition from sucking milk to eating regular hard food [29].

14.9 Conclusion

Food for thoughts regarding the new industry of high caloric and high protein liquids sold as substitutes for meals. There is a time and a place for liquid food, but not in daily life. This is also food for thought for patients with dysphagia, in which the first sign of aspiration is met with immediate changes in the food consistency, usually by pureeing everything, when more emphasis should be placed on sham chewing, and then optimizing regular food chewing, to recover the muscle coordination, strength and timing necessary to swallow in safety [30-32].

REFERENCES

1. Suzuki K, Abe S, Kim HJ, et al. Changes in the muscle fibre properties of the mouse temporal muscle after weaning. Anat Histol Embryo 2007; 36(2): 103-6.
2. Okubo K, Abe S, Usami A, et al. Changes in muscle-fiber properties of the murine digastric muscle before and after weaning. Zoolog Sci 2006; 23(12): 1079-84.
3. Maejima M, Abe S, Sakiyama K, et al. Changes in the properties of mouse tongue muscle fibres before and after weaning. Arch Oral Biol 2005; 50(12): 988-93.
4. Fujishita A, Koga Y, Utsumi D, Nakamura A, Yoshimi T, Yoshida N. Effects of feeding a soft diet and subsequent rehabilitation on the development of the masticatory function. J Oral Rehabil 2015; 42(4): 266-74.
5. Mavropoulos A, Odman A, Ammann P, Kiliaridis S. Rehabilitation of masticatory function improves the alveolar bone architecture of the mandible in adult rats. Bone 2010; 47(3): 687-92.
6. Katsaros C, Zissis A, Bresin A, Kiliaridis S. Functional influence on sutural bone apposition in the growing rat. Am J Orthod Dentofacial Orthop 2006; 129(3): 352-7.
7. Morquette P, Lavoie R, Fhima MD, Lamoureux X, Verdier D, Kolta A. Generation of the masticatory central pattern and its modulation by sensory feedback. Prog Neurobiol 2012; 96(3): 340-55.
8. Westberg KG, Kolta A. The trigeminal circuits responsible for chewing. Int Rev Neurobiol 2011; 97: 77-98.
9. Lund JP, Kolta A. Generation of the central masticatory pattern and its modification by sensory feedback. Dysphagia 2006; 21(3): 167-74.
10. Kimura Y, Nomura M, Sawada Y, Muraoka N, Kohno N, Ito S. Evaluation of the effects of mastication and swallowing on gastric motility using electrogastrography. J Med Invest 2006; 53(3-4): 229-37.
11. Lunding JA, Nordström LM, Haukelid AO, Gilja OH, Berstad A, Hausken T. Vagal activation by sham feeding improves gastric motility in functional dyspepsia. Neurogastroenterol Motil 2008; 20(6): 618-24.
12. Vergara-Fernandez O, Gonzalez-Vargas AP, Castellanos-Juarez JC, Salgado-Nesme N, Sanchez-Garcia Ramos E. Usefulness of gum chewing to decrease postoperative ileus in colorectal surgery with primary anastomosis: A randomized controlled trial. Rev Invest Clin 2016; 68(6): 314-8.
13. Liu Q, Jiang H, Xu D, Jin J. Effect of gum chewing on ameliorating ileus following colorectal surgery: A meta-analysis of 18 randomized controlled trials. Int J Surg 2017; 47: 107-15.
14. Yenigul NN, Aydogan Mathyk B, Aslan Cetin B, Yazici Yilmaz F, Ayhan I. Efficacy of chewing gum for improving bowel function after cesarean sections: a randomized controlled trial. J Matern Fetal Neonatal Med 2020; 33(11): 1840-5.
15. Jang SY, Ju EY, Kim DE, et al. First flatus time and xerostomia associated with gum-chewing after liver resection. J Clin Nurs 2012; 21: 2188-92.
16. Asao T, Kuwano H, Nakamura J, Morinaga N, Hirayama I, Ide M. Gum chewing enhances early recovery from postoperative ileus after laparoscopic colectomy. J Am Coll Surg 2002; 195: 30-2.
17. Ngowe MN, Eyenga VC, Kengne BH, Bahebeck J, Sosso AM. Chewing gum reduces postoperative ileus after open appendectomy. Acta Chir Belg 2010; 110: 195-9.
18. Karmali S, Jenkins N, Sciusco A, John J, Haddad F, Ackland GL, POM-X Study Investigators. Randomized controlled trial of vagal modulation by sham feeding in elective nongastrointestinal (orthopaedic) surgery. Br J Anaesth 2015; 115(5): 727-35.
19. Short V, Herbert G, Perry R, et al. Chewing gum for postoperative recovery of gastrointestinal function. Cochrane Database Syst Rev 2015; (2): CD006506.
20. Ono Y, Yamamoto T, Kubo KY, Onozuka M. Occlusion and brain function: mastication as a prevention of cognitive dysfunction. J Oral Rehabil 2010; 37(8): 624-40.
21. Kawanishi K, Koshino H, Toyoshita Y, Tanaka M, Hirai T. Effect of mastication on functional recoveries after permanent middle cerebral artery occlusion in rats. J Stroke Cerebrovasc Dis 2010; 19(5): 398-403.
22. Zhang M, Hasegawa Y, Sakagami J, Ono T, Hori K, Maeda Y, Chen YJ. Effects of unilateral jaw clenching on cerebral/systemic circulation and related autonomic nerve activity. Physiol Behav 2012; 105(2): 292-7.
23. Hasegawa Y, Ono T, Hori K, Nokubi T. Influence of human jaw movement on cerebral blood flow. J Dent Res 2007; 86(1): 64-8.
24. Iida T, Kato M, Komiyama O, et al. Comparison of cerebral activity during teeth clenching and fist clenching: a functional magnetic resonance imaging study. Eur J Oral Sci 2010; 118(6): 635-41.
25. Hodoba D. Chewing can relieve sleepiness in a night of sleep deprivation. Sleep Res Online 1999; 2(4): 101-5.
26. Hori N, Lee MC, Sasaguri K, Ishii H, Kamei M, Kimoto K, Toyoda M, Sato S. Suppression of stress-induced nNOS expression in the rat hypothalamus by biting. J Dent Res 2005; 84(7): 624-8.
27. Gómez FM, Ortega JE, Horrillo I, Meana JJ. Relationship between non-functional masticatory activity and central dopamine in stressed rats. J Oral Rehabil 2010; 37(11): 827-33.
28. Koizumi S, Minamisawa S, Sasaguri K, Onozuka M, Sato S, Ono Y. Chewing reduces sympathetic nervous response to stress and prevents poststress arrhythmias in rats. Am J Physiol Heart Circ Physiol 2011; 301(4): H1551-8.
29. Elewa YH, Ichii O, Otsuka S, Hashimoto Y, Kon Y. Structural changes of goat parotid salivary gland: pre- and post-weaning periods. Anat Histol Embryol 2014; 43(4): 265-72.
30. Felício CM, Couto GA, Ferreira CL, Mestriner Junior W. Reliability of masticatory efficiency with beads and correlation with the muscle activity. Pro Fono 2008; 20(4): 225-30.
31. Clark HM. Food for thought. Therapeutic exercise in dysphagia management: philosophies, practices, and challenges. Perspectives on Swallowing and Swallowing Disorders 2005; 14(2): 24-7.
32. de Felício CM, de Oliveira MM, da Silva MA. Effects of orofacial myofunctional therapy on temporomandibular disorders. Cranio 2010; 28(4): 249-59.

15 Promote chewing to prevent choking in children and adults

Licia Coceani Paskay and Sabina Saccomanno

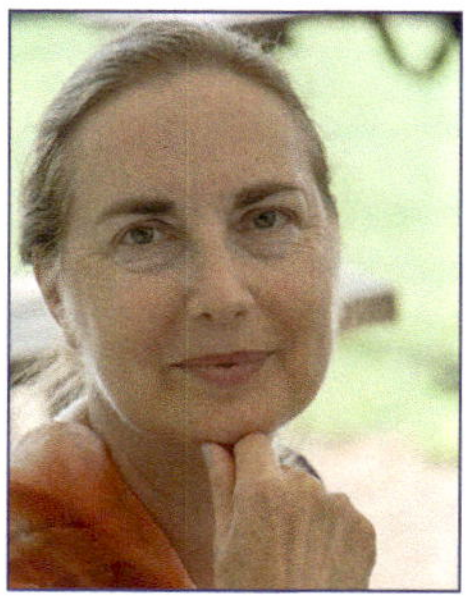

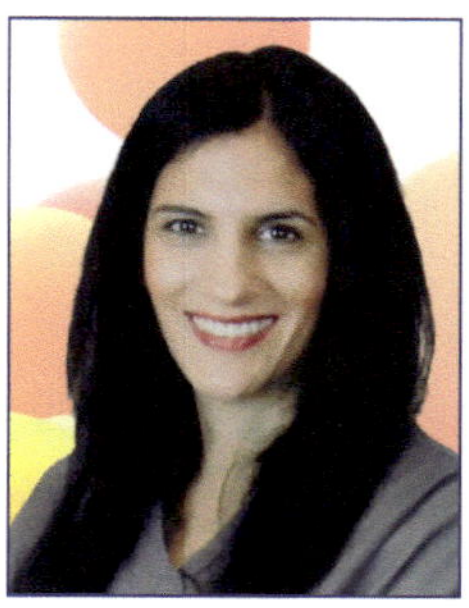

15.1 Introduction and epidemiology of choking

Choking is the blockage or hindrance of respiration by a foreign-body obstruction in the internal airway, including the pharynx, hypopharynx and trachea. Airway obstruction can be fatal if it leads to serious impairment of oxygenation and ventilation [1]. The risk of dying by choking during a lifetime is about 1 in 3,100 compared to the chance of being killed by a wasp or a bee sting (1 in about 54,000) or being attacked by a dog (1 in about 132,000) [2]. Choking is a serious but somewhat underestimated and haphazardly prevented, although according to the National Safety Council (NSC), in the USA, choking is the 4th leading cause of unintentional deaths and two-thirds of choking deaths happened in people over 75 [3]. Also, in the USA, of +76,000 deaths from choking, in adults over 65, (or 6.5% of deaths) were classified as food choking [4] while in the San Diego County alone most choking deaths were due to meat and 45% of those episodes happened at home [5]. Even in the UK the situation is not any better: in London, in the calendar year of 2016 there were 159 mean number of choking episodes per day, requiring an ambulance response, with the majority of victims being either very young (age 0-4) or very old (age 90+) and a spike in cases on Sundays at lunch time [6].

Children choke too, although the reasons and mechanics are usually different. Dentures, distractions, alcohol, fatigue, malocclusions, some neurological, neuromuscular or psychiatric diseases, may contribute to an increased risk of choking in adults. Choking deaths also depend on traditional or cultural foods and on specific circumstances in which they are consumed: Birthday party foods such as cake but also alcohol consumption can often lead to choking [7]; and a study in Italy identified fish bones as the most common occurrence of choking [8]; sticky mochi rice cakes, very popular in Japan, are also among the types of foods most often involved in choking episodes in adults [9]; nuts and seeds commonly eaten for "Autumn day" in Spain [10] and hot dogs consumed daily in the USA [1] are also involved in choking episodes often with fatal consequences.

Choking episodes in children may be underreported, like adult episodes, as only those which cause either a visit to the ER or death are usually recorded and counted for statistical purposes. Therefore, the true occurrence of choking is virtually unknown. Choking episodes in children, rightly so, are very upsetting to

Licia Coceani Paskay, MS, CCC-SLP
Speech-Language Pathologist, Private Practice
Los Angeles, USA

Email: lcpaskay@gmail.com

Sabina Saccomanno, DDS
Department of Life, Health and Environmental Sciences, University of L'Aquila, L'Aquila, Italy

Email: sabinasaccomanno@hotmail.it

parents who often are not familiar with the concept that coughing is the natural lifesaving mechanisms preventing choking. Often after a significant episode of choking, the parents resort to softer, more fluid types of foods, but in doing so the whole chewing system, comprises dental occlusion, musculature, temporomandibular joint (TMJ), and the tongue, etc., which become less than optimal with long term consequences.

However, choking is real: the CDC, in 2011 estimated that about 66 to 77 children younger than 10 die from choking on food each year in the United States [11] and over 10,000 ER visits annually can be attributed to choking on food among children aged 14 years and younger. The situation is not any better in other comparable countries: in Canada for every choking fatality in children there are 110 children who are treated at hospitals' ERs and Australia recorded that 19% of child fatalities in the age range between 0 and 14 were caused by "foreign body aspiration" [12]. In the European Union each year, an estimated 400 children (14 years or younger) die from choking while each year an estimated 50,000 children (14 years or younger) have a choking episode. In Europe, 1 in 5 childhood choking injuries involve industrial products, such as plastic and metal parts, coins and toys [13].

15.2 Choking hazards: food and non-food

According to the American Academy of Pediatrics [1], man-made items are most likely to cause choking in kids. Man-made objects that are usually the cause of choking episodes are: coins, beads, balloons, little toys or parts of toys. Man-made foods are usually also industrialized foods, which include hard candies, hot dogs, marshmallows or other soft confections, popcorn, cake, chewing gum or small pieces of meat. However, that begs the question: which natural foods are more risky and conducive to possible choking? Nuts, seeds and dry fruits are only dangerous when given at an inappropriate age (in children younger than 4) and in excessive amount (a pinch or a handful as opposed to a single one at the time). Also, air-way size foods such as grapes, cherry tomatoes, apple chunks or carrots are only dangerous when they are too big to be chewed, not properly cut, prepared or chewed. In other words, risk in food can be classified based on the characteristics of the food:

- Bites are too big (hamburgers, sandwiches, cake)
- Round and slippery (candies, jellies)
- Cylindrical and cut into rounds (carrots, grapes, hotdogs, little sausages)
- Hard (candies, some meat)
- Dry or sticky (PB sandwich, muffins, dry fruits)
- Fibrous or stringy (some veggies, pizza cheese, cured ham)
- Compressible (marshmallows, popcorn, hotdogs)
- Mixed texture or requiring more chewing (mixed salad, beef, snack bars).

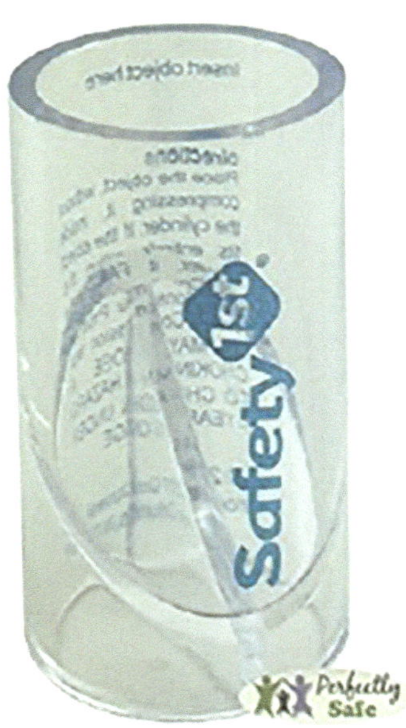

Fig. 15.1 Safety 1st Small Objects Choking Tester®.

Often parents do not know how to determine if something (object of food piece) is a choking hazard for their babies and toddlers. Designed by the Consumer Product Safety Commission [14], Safety 1st Small Objects Choking Tester® is a simple device to determine if an object is too small or too big to be safely placed in the mouth [15]. It has approximately the same size of a toddler's airway and if an object fits entirely inside this Choking Tester, then it's a choking hazard to a child and it should be disposed accordingly (Fig. 15.1).

15.3 How and why we choke

How did we get to this point, in which so many children (and adults) end up in the ER and even die choking? What happened to our ability to manipulate foods in our mouths and instinctively determine if we can swallow or not, that bite of food? The answer is quite complex and can be found in fields such as anthropology, history, culture, capitalism and advertisement, to name a few. Humans have been eating rough and tough food for hundreds of thousands of years and the proof is in the craniofacial bones and teeth left behind [16, 17]. Babies were only breastfed and weaned with "adult food" until the Industrial Revolution and we know from animal model studies [18-23] that these two practices account for the epigenetic expression of the optimal genetic phenotype, guiding growth, development and maintenance of the splancnocranium (bones of the face).

Epigenetics is the influence of the environment, including eating practices, that impacts functions and ultimately the shape and size of the facial bones and the effectiveness of muscles that are responsible for chewing, swallowing and even protective mechanisms [24-30]. Humans learned to process food more efficiently, getting a huge evolutionary advantage over other animals, even primates. By simply slicing meat and pounding roots and tubers, hominids would have improved their ability to chew meat into smaller particles by 41% and decreased masticatory force requirements by an additional 12% [31].

Conversely, in the last 200 years, since the Industrial Revolution and with an acceleration post World War II and the industrialization of food, the so called "Westernized" populations have been experiencing less breastfeeding, a widespread use of baby food often passed the weaning period, an explosive increased use of "fast food" and an increased bypassing of chewable foods in favor of foods in the form of smoothie, slushes, pureed, gelatinized, etc. [32]. This phenomenon is now permeating even cultures that may still rely mostly on traditional hunter-gather type of foods.

15.4 The many benefits of chewing

Pureed foods are also ubiquitous in nursing homes where debilitated elderly receive pureed food that requires no effort to eat but it does not contribute to the maintenance of the oral manipulation/chewing/swallowing system necessary to prevent dysphagia. The issue of dysphagia is complex but even in patients who are fed through gastric or nasogastric tubes, sham chewing or chewing gum has been documented as being beneficial and reducing dyspepsia associated with drastic changes in feeding [33, 34]. In children and in adults chewing devices such as MyoMunchee® [35] or silicone wafers or rubber tubes (Figs. 15.2-15.5) may be beneficial to restore muscle tone and coordination.

What is involved in chewing? Anatomically and physiologically speaking, chewing is a very complex function requiring the fine-tuned interaction of the:

- Sensory motor system (olfactory, visual, auditory, gustatory, proprioceptive, etc.)
- Central pattern generators (breathing, chewing, swallowing)
- Cranial nerves (I, II, V, VII, VIII, IX, X, XI, XII)
- Muscles and fascia
- TMJ
- Dental occlusion
- Salivary glands.

Just the musculature involved in chewing, and the individual innervation, is remarkable:

- Masseters muscles - paired - V
- Temporalis muscles - paired - V
- Pterygoid muscles - paired - V
- Suprahyoid muscles - paired V, VII and XII
- Infrahyoid muscles - paired XII and cervical plexus (part of XII)
- Intrinsic tongue muscles - 3 paired + vertical - XII
- Extrinsic tongue muscles - paired - XII
- Palatoglossus muscles - paired - X
- Facial muscles - paired and unpaired (orbicularis oris and mentalis) - VII
- Soft palate muscles - paired and unpaired uvula - Pharyngeal plexus IX, X, XII.

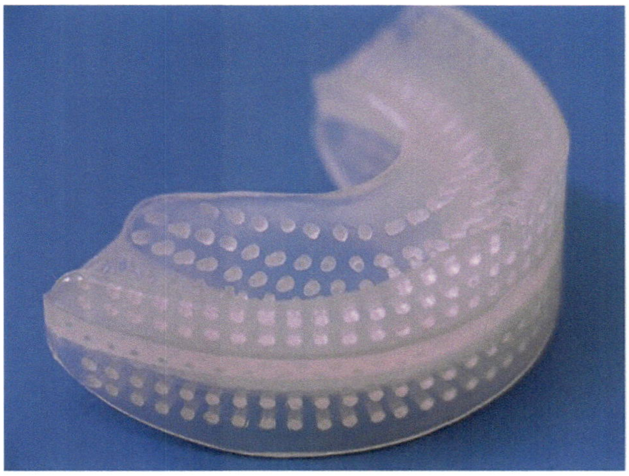

Fig. 15.2 Myo Munchee.

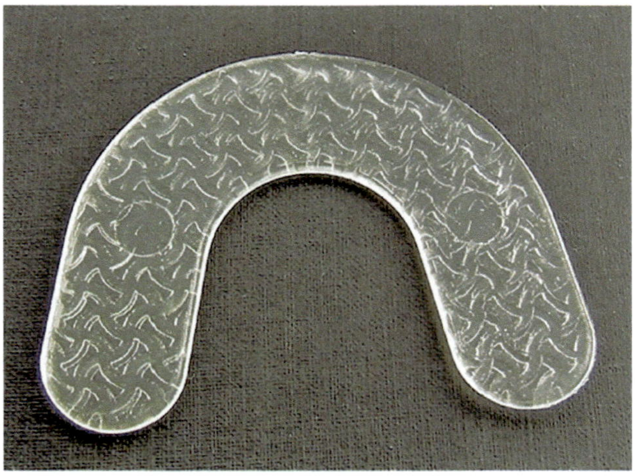

Fig. 15.3 Silicone wafer courtesy Therabite.

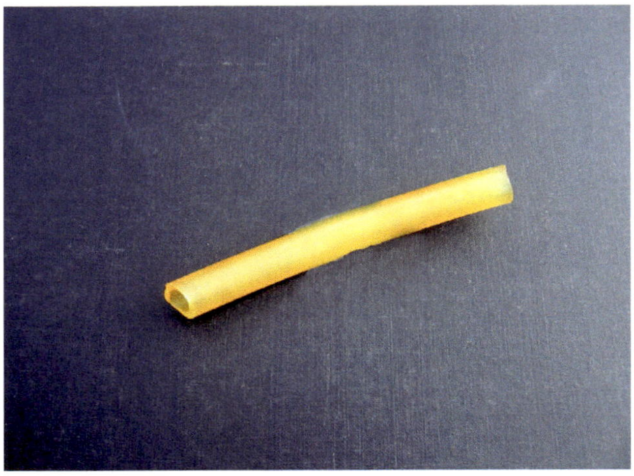

Fig. 15.4 Rubber tube 1 cm diameter.

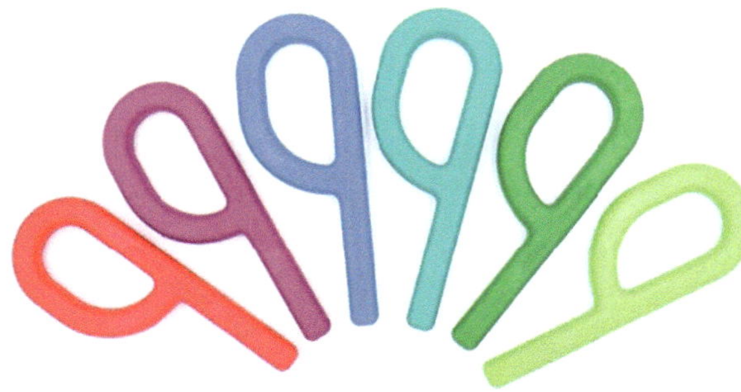

Fig. 15.5 Silicone chewing Ps for easy gip.

15.5 Risk factors

Given the amazing complexity inherent in chewing it's easy to understand that sometimes things can go wrong. Health conditions, age and eating habits have a lot to do with the risk of choking. Some of the predisposing or co-occurring conditions for choking are:

- Neurological, neuromuscular or psychiatric diseases
- Dysphagia
- Breathing conditions or diseases, i.e., sleep apnea or mouth breathing
- Excessive use of alcohol, drugs, and risky behaviors (such as timed hotdog eating contests)
- Use of certain medications
- Certain surgeries (especially intraoral or to the pharynx-larynx structures)
- Allergic reactions
- Distractions and rushing while eating.

From a strictly oral perspective, choking episodes can occur in the presence of:

- Teeth-related factors like pain or tooth instability
- Severe malocclusion or missing several teeth
- Being edentulous (having no teeth)
- Unsteady, unsuitable dental items (crowns, prosthesis, etc.).

Dental prosthesis, especially full dentures, can make it difficult to sense whether food is fully chewed before it is swallowed. If dentures fit poorly or hurt, individuals wearing them might not bother to chew their food or may not wear them at all thus being unable to properly chew their food. There are many studies that suggest connections between poor oral/occlusal health and difficulty chewing and swallowing and even accidental swallowing of oral prosthetic elements [36-38]. Orthodontic appliances may also pose a choking risk [39-41].

A tongue-tie, or restricted lingual frenum or ankyloglossia, by virtue of restricting the tongue movement can reduce or prevent tongue lateralization and elevation, making it harder for individuals to break down food properly and safely, adversely impacting bolus collection and reducing the ability to clear the oral cavity from food residues. A tongue tie in newborn and babies is known to negatively affect breastfeeding, causing coughing, gagging, spitting, agitation and increase the risk of failure to thrive. A timely diagnosis and usually a surgical release with a laser can ensure optimal tongue movement and food bolus gathering [42-44].

Among groups of people (children and adults) who are more at risk for choking are those who present physical or neurological disabilities. Their difficulties range from:

- The inability to communicate, problems in chewing, swallowing or protective mechanisms
- Decreased or absent protective airway reflexes
- Impacted oral motor skills due to generalized or localized hypotonia or hypertonia
- Gastroesophageal reflux disease (GERD)
- Seizures
- Dysphagia
- Certain medications
- Impulsivity
- Need for feeding assistance.

15.6 Preventing choking

Although not all choking episodes are fatal, unfortunately they can still result in a perforation of the mediastinum, infections, aspiration pneumonia (ab ingestis), a need for invasive surgeries, and psychological trauma (PTSD) often resulting in food aversion, which can be quite dramatic in children. Therefore, it is imperative for the healthcare professionals to teach proper chewing and to make parents and caregivers aware of strategies to reduce the risk of choking in children, adults and people of all ages who have special needs.

A review of recommendations to prevent choking from food, coming from several international organizations can be summarized in the following 10 points:

For Children:

1) Breastfeed as long as possible (ideally over a year)
2) Introduce different textures and flavors during weaning, under supervision
3) Adopt the "baby-led weaning" techniques [45]
4) Teach children the proper consistency of well chewed food: regardless of what is chewed it should end up in the mouth like a thick blended veggie soup
5) Cut any little fruit or veggie (grapes, cherry tomatoes, olives, etc.) lengthwise and not into small rounds
6) Teach and remind children not to talk with their mouth full. Model the correct behavior too.
7) Teach and remind children not to run, play, scream, laugh or "stuff" their mouths while eating
8) Provide a quiet and unhurried environment during meals
9) Prevent distractions such as video games, TV and play stations
10) Model the correct behavior and chew something crunchy every day.

Clearly, it's important to follow common-sense supervision of toddlers and young children to prevent choking with non-food objects, especially those that have food-like qualities in appearance and scent (small erasers, play clay, dollhouse toys, etc.). Keeping children away from small objects such as buttons, beads, large pills, pebbles and even balloons remains a priority in preventing choking.

In adults and elderly, 10 simple strategies to prevent choking can be the following:

1) Eat slowly and let the saliva soak the food until the bolus has a soupy consistency
2) Practice mindful chewing to identify small changes in texture and to identify extraneous objects such as seeds, dirt, plastic fragments, etc.
3) Cut the meat into small bites and chew them thoroughly
4) Avoid distractions and physical movements during meals (no TV, computers, walking or talking)
5) Cut hotdogs and sausages and round veggies or fruit lengthwise and not into round thick slices.
6) Be mindful that dentures reduce oral sensitivity needed to find smaller extraneous items such as little bones
7) Excessive alcohol may impair oral sensitivity and motor performance
8) Chew well foods that are sticky such as rice, wafers, peanut butter and avoid hard candies
9) Supervise the meals of anybody with neurological or psychiatric issues
10) Don't try to answer quickly or avoid laughing with your mouth full.

15.7 Education

For people with sensory-motor or neurological disorders, the following strategies may be helpful in preventing choking:

1) Organize a meal or snack when the person is alert and/or when not fatigued, from physical activity or from lack of sleep
2) Always optimize posture for eating, maintaining as much as possible, hips, knees and feet at 90 degrees for stability of the torso that in turn helps stabilize orofacial structures for safe eating
3) For those who have reduced oral sensory awareness, when appropriate, start the meal with some "alerting" foods and drinks, such as spicy and/or sour taste, crunchy textures, lemonade, carbonated water or ice chips
4) Visual input with a mirror at mealtime can help individuals to see when they have chewed to the proper consistency and placed the right amount of food in the mouth
5) Certain foods may not be appropriate at any age: popcorn, cherries with pits, sunflower seeds, nuts of any kind, hard or sticky candies, watermelon with seeds, grapes, small cheese cubes, peanut butter or chewing gum.

For non-food items, some precautions are similar to those suitable for children: keeping away small objects remains the priority for preventing choking. Whenever possible such items should locked in cabinets, especially those that smell and look like food (cake decorations, erasers, large pills, toys, etc.).

Health care professionals, teachers and, of course, parents are the best persons to teach strategies and proper thorough chewing to prevent choking. Educational flyers and brochures may be available in multiple language from major health organizations including foodsafety.gov [46].

When prevention fails and a choking episode is happening, the abdominal thrust (also called the Heimlick Maneuver) may be the best immediate solution to that emergency. Classes on how to properly and safely perform the abdominal thrust are available almost anywhere and, in many professions (speech pathologists, teachers, dentists, restaurateurs, etc.), it is mandatory to attend classes and learn how to save peoples' lives.

REFERENCES

1. From the American Academy of Pediatrics-Policy Statement-Prevention of Choking Among Children-Committee on Injury, Violence, and Poison Prevention. Pediatrics. March 2010, Volume 125, Issue 3.
2. https://injuryfacts.nsc.org
3. https://www.nsc.org/home-safety/safety-topics/choking-suffocation
4. Wu WS, Sung KC, Cheng TJ, Lu TH. Associations between chronic diseases and choking deaths among older adults in the USA: a cross-sectional study using multiple cause mortality data from 2009 to 2013. BMJ Open 2015; 5(11): e009464.
5. Dolkas L, Stanley C, Smith AM, Vilke GM. Deaths associated with choking in San Diego county. J Forensic Sci 2007; 52(1): 176-9.
6. Pavitt MJ, Nevett J, Swanton LL, Hind MD, Polkey MI, Green M, Hopkinson NS. London ambulance source data on choking incidence for the calendar year 2016: an observational study. BMJ Open Respir Res 2017; 4(1): e000215.
7. Matsubayashi T, Ueda M. Suicides and accidents on birthdays: Evidence from Japan. Soc Sci Med 2016; 159: 61-72.
8. Data from the San Filippo Neri Hospital, Rome, Italy, 2017-2018.
9. Kiyohara K, Sakai T, Nishiyama C, et al. Epidemiology of Out-of-Hospital Cardiac Arrest Due to Suffocation Focusing on Suffocation Due to Japanese Rice Cake: A Population-Based Observational Study From the Utstein Osaka Project. J Epidemiol 2018; 28(2): 67-74.
10. Lluna J, Olabarri M, Domènech A, Rubio B, Yagüe F, Benítez MT, Esparza MJ, Mintegi S; en representación del Comité de Seguridad y Prevención de Lesiones No Intencionadas en la Infancia de la Asociación Española de Pediatría. [Recommendations for the prevention of foreign body aspiration]. An Pediatr (Barc) 2017; 86(1): 50.e1-50. e6. [Article in Spanish].
11. https://www.cdc.gov/nutrition/infantandtoddlernutrition/foods-and-drinks/choking-hazards.html
12. https://www.cps.ca/documents/position/preventing-choking-suffocation-children
13. http://dontchoke.ubc.ca/about/references/
14. https://www.cpsc.gov/Business--Manufacturing/Business-Education/Business-Guidance/Small-Parts-for-Toys-and-Childrens-Products
15. Safety 1st Small Objects Choking Tester®: https://www.childproofadvice.org/product/small-objects-choke-tester/
16. Corruccini RS. An epidemiological transition in dental occlusion in world population. Am J Orthod 198; 86: 419-26.
17. Corruccini RS, Townsend GC, Richard LC, Brown T. Genetics and environmental determinants of dental occlusal variation in twins of different nationality. Hum Biol 1990; 62(3): 353-67.
18. Mavropoulos A, Odman A, Ammann P, Killaridis S. Rehabilitation of masticatory function improves the alveolar bone architecture of the mandible in adult rats. Bone 2010; 47(3): 687-92.
19. Katsaros C, Zissis A, Bresin A, Killaridis S. Functional influence on sutural bone apposition in the growing rat. Am J Orthod Dentofacial Orthop 2006; 129(3): 352-7.
20. Okubo K, Abe S, Usami A, Agematsu H, Nakamura H, Hashimoto M, Ide Y. Changes in muscle-fiber properties of the murine digastric muscle before and after weaning. Zoolog Sci 2006; 23(12): 1079-84.
21. Maejima M, Abe S, Sakiyama K, Agematsu H, Hashimoto M, Tamatsu Y, Ide Y. Changes in the properties of mouse tongue muscle fibers before and after weaning. Arch Oral Biol 2005; 50(12): 988-93.
22. Suzuki K, Abe S, Kim HJ, Usami A, Iwanuma O, Okubo H, Ide Y. Changes in the muscle fibre properties of the mouse temporal muscle after weaning. Anat Histol Embryol 2007; 36(2): 103-6.
23. Elewa YH, Ichii O, Otsuka S, Hashimoto Y, Kon Y. Structural changes of goat parotid salivary gland: pre- and post-weaning periods. Anat Histol Embryol 2014; 43(4): 265-72.
24. Hallgrimsson B and Hall B. Epigenetics: Linking Genotype and Phenotype in Development and Evolution. Berkeley and Los Angeles; University of California Press, 2011.
25. Francis RC. Epigenetics: How environment shapes our genes. WW Norton, London, 2011.
26. Lieberman D. The evolution of the human head. Belknap Harvard, Cambridge, Massachusetts, 2011.
27. Moss ML. The functional matrix hypothesis revisited. 1. The role of mechanotransduction. Am J Orthod Dentofacial Orthop 1997; 112(1): 8-11.
28. Moss ML. The functional matrix hypothesis revisited. 2. The role of an osseous connected cellular network. Am J Orthod Dentofacial Orthop 1997; 112(2): 221-6.
29. Moss ML. The functional matrix hypothesis revisited. 3. The genomic thesis. Am J Orthod DentofaciL Orthop 1997; 112(3): 338-42.
30. Moss ML. The functional matrix hypothesis revisited. 4. The epigenetic antithesis and the resolving synthesis. Am J Orthod DentofacIAL Orthop 1997; 112(4): 410-7.
31. Zink KD, Lieberman DE. Impact of meat and Lower Palaeolithic food processing techniques on chewing in humans. Nature 2016; 531(7595): 500-3.
32. Boyd KL. Darwinian dentistry part 2: early childhood nutrition, dentofacial development and chronic disease. J Am Orthodont Soc 2012; 12(2): 28-32.
33. Kimura Y, Nomura M, Sawada Y, Muraoka N, Kohno N, Ito S. Evaluation of the effects of mastication and swallowing on gastric motility using electrogastrography. J Med Invest 2006; 53(3-4): 229-37.
34. Lunding JA, Nordström LM, Haukelid AO, Gilja OH, Ber-

stad A, Hausken T. Vagal activation by sham feeding improves gastric motility in functional dyspepsia. Neurogastroenterol Motil 2008; 20(6): 618-24.
35. https://myomunchee.com
36. Qin H, Qing H, Hu N, Zhu H, Wang J. An All-Zirconia Crown Discovered 2 Years Following Aspiration. J Prosthodont 2018; 27(6): 492-5.
37. Maroulakos G, Voulgarelis S. Impending total airway collapse involving a maxillary removable partial denture: A clinical report. J Prosthet Dent 2018; 120(5): 642-4.
38. Abusamaan M, Giannobile WV, Jhawar P, Gunaratnam NT. Swallowed and aspirated dental prostheses and instruments in clinical dental practice: a report of five cases and a proposed management algorithm. J Am Dent Assoc 2014; 145(5): 459-63.
39. Handa A, Handa JK. Accidental Ingestion of a Foreign Body of Orthodontic Origin - A Review of Risks, Complications and Clinical Recommendations. Int J Orthod Milwaukee 2016; 27(1): 41-4.
40. Park JH, Owtad P, Milde B. Incident management guidelines for an ingested orthodontic object. 2013. Int J Orthod Milwaukee 2013; 24(3): 45-9.
41. Umesan UK, Ahmad W, Balakrishnan P. Laryngeal impaction of an archwire segment after accidental ingestion during orthodontic adjustment. Am J Orthod Dentofacial Orthop 2012; 142(2): 264-8.
42. Haham A, Marom R, Mangel L, Botzer E, Dollberg S. Prevalence of breastfeeding difficulties in newborns with a lingual frenulum: a prospective cohort series. Breastfeed Med 2014; 9(9): 438-41.
43. Dollberg S, Marom R, Botzer E. Lingual frenotomy for breastfeeding difficulties: a prospective follow-up study. Breastfeed Med 2014; 9(6): 286-9.
44. Martinelli RL, Marchesan IQ, Gusmão RJ, Honório HM, Berretin-Felix G. The effects of frenotomy on breastfeeding. J Appl Oral Sci 2015; 23(2): 153-7.
45. Rapley G, Murkett T. Baby-Led Weaning: Helping Your Baby to Love Good Food. Vermillion-Ebury Publishing, England, 2008.
46. https://www.foodsafety.gov/risk/children/index.html

16

Loss of chewing, edentulism and food

Paolo Francesco Manicone and Paolo De Angelis

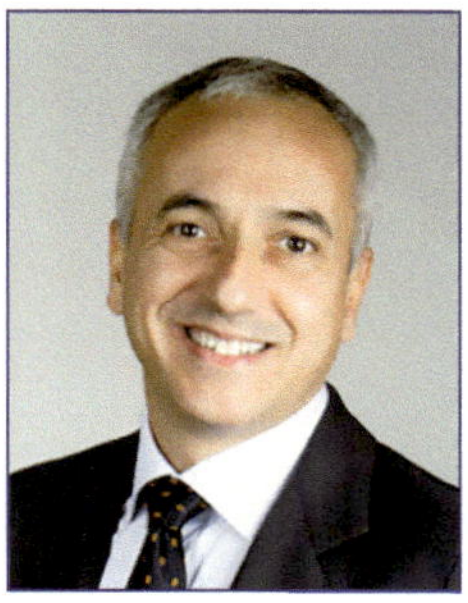

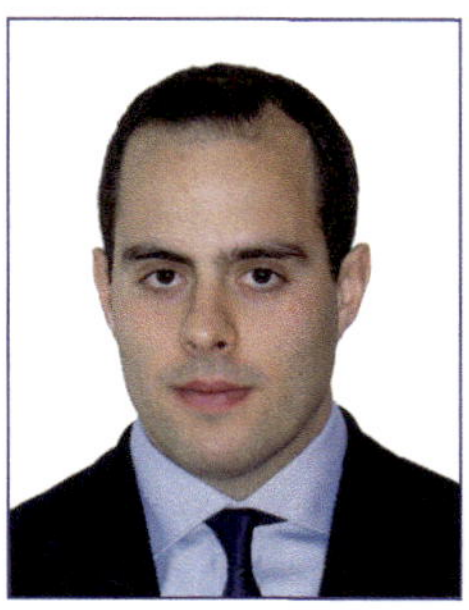

The oral processing of food is based on three main functions: oral manipulation of the food bolus, mastication (chewing) and swallowing [1]. Chewing food can be considered the first step in the digestion process because it promotes food breakdown (also called comminution), increasing the overall surface area of the resulting particles, while saliva is produced to moisten and lubricate the food, along with any liquid released from the food itself [2-4]. The primary role of mastication is to transform the food into a bolus ready to be swallowed and processed further in the digestive system. Mastication and swallowing are both controlled by a specific Central Pattern Generator (CPG), which receives extensive sensory information from the oral cavity about bolus changes in the mouth. Importantly, safe swallowing relies on these sensory inputs [1, 4]. This is not only an essential process to meet nutritional requirements, but also it imparts enjoyable sensations that fulfill a basic human need [3, 5, 6]. To be safe, the food bolus should be smooth, pliable and cohesive [7], because smoothness and plasticity help to ensure harmless sliding through the pharyngeal walls and esophagus, while cohesiveness is required to avoid bolus scattering, which can contribute to aspiration of food particles into the airways [3, 4, 7]. By continuously analyzing sensory information on the bolus state, the CPG can decide either to continue mastication, for further food comminution, or to stop chewing and control lingual forces and movements to propel the bolus into the pharynx, thus starting deglutition [1]. Among the factors analyzed are particle size distribution, lubrication and the cohesive forces between food fragments [1]. The deglutition process can be ideally represented as a three-phase model consisting of an oral phase, a pharyngeal phase and an esophageal phase [8]. However, the exact state of the food bolus and the conditions required to initiate the deglutition process are still not fully understood [4].

Over the years, changes in oral health status can result in a reduced number of teeth and functional tooth units (pairs of opposing teeth), causing an impairment of masticatory function in patients, who may experience further consequences in their general health and Oral Health-Related Quality of Life (QoL) (OHRQoL) [9-11]. A negative impact on OHRQoL may also be due to poor speech, pain and dissatisfaction with appearance [11]. Edentulism (partial or total loss of

Paolo Francesco Manicone, DDS
Professor, Department of Head and Neck and Sensory Organs, Division of Oral Surgery and Implantology, Fondazione Policlinico Universitario A. Gemelli IRCCS, Università Cattolica del Sacro Cuore, Rome, Italy

Email: paolofrancesco.manicone@unicatt.it

Paolo De Angelis, DDS
Department of Head and Neck and Sensory Organs, Division of Oral Surgery and Implantology, Fondazione Policlinico Universitario A. Gemelli IRCCS, Università Cattolica del Sacro Cuore, Rome, Italy

Email: dr.paolodeangelis@gmail.com

teeth) is consistently shown to increase with age, and the aging of the population, in both developed and developing countries, is occurring as a result of both a reduction in birth and mortality rates and a longer life expectancy [12]. Age-related systemic diseases, drug consumption and hyposalivation can make it difficult to maintain an adequate level of oral hygiene among the elderly [13]. However, an increased life-expectancy would not be a significant achievement without the addition of quality to those added years, because food intake and nutrition are crucial factors contributing to the QoL [14, 15].

QoL of Life is difficult to define because it is a subjective and dynamic concept based on an individual's internal frame of reference, understanding or perceived life experience [16]. Currently, different instruments, such as scales and questionnaires, are used to assess QoL, but there is still a lack of consensus about its exact definition and appropriate measurement methods [16]. However, QoL can be considered as the result of both medical and non-medical factors such as age, gender, social class and cultural background, which all play an important role in the perception of health. It has been reported that people with chronic disabling disorders can perceive their QoL as being as good as that of healthy individuals because poor health and/or the presence of disease does not necessarily correlate with poor QoL. Adaptive capacity and personal characteristics appear to influence a patient's response to a disease [17].

Tooth loss occurs as a result of dental caries, periodontal disease, trauma, neoplastic disease, developmental disorders and environmental factors [18]. Tooth loss due to caries and periodontal diseases remains prevalent worldwide despite the increasing number of older adults retaining their natural teeth for longer in life, due to prevention campaigns, changed patterns of dental awareness and earlier treatments [19]. This trend applies in particular in the Western countries with higher socioeconomic statuses [13]. Over the years, the prevalence of total edentulism has decreased, while a rising rate of partially edentulous patients can be observed. Probably, in the future, this condition will be most frequently observed only among economically deprived populations and the elderly [13]. Caries and periodontitis are the most prevalent oral diseases and they usually do not cause symptoms in the early stages [17]. This might be explained because the clinical indicators of caries or periodontal disease are not strongly associated with OHRQoL [17]. However, these are chronic and progressive diseases that lead to tooth loss if not treated adequately; multiple tooth loss will presumably cause functional impairment and ultimately affect QoL [17].

The relationship between masticatory performance and the number of occluding pairs of teeth seems to be linear [20]. However, it can be argued that the number of teeth is not the only factor to consider, because the arrangement of teeth, as well as the number and types of occluding pairs of teeth, seem to be more related to the masticatory potential [10]. Furthermore, the perceived ability to chew foods is closely associated with the number of natural teeth remaining as well as the number of occluding pairs of teeth [13].

The evaluation of the masticatory function can be performed using a variety of subjective and objective methods [21, 22]. Among the subjective methods, interviews and questionnaires have been developed to assess the self-perceived chewing function and patients' satisfaction about chewing [22]. Regarding objective methods, the masticatory performance – defined as the particle size distribution of food particles after a given number of chewing strokes [23] – is assessed by analyzing the degree of breakdown of natural foods or standardized artificial foods after a given number of chewing cycles [22]. The subsequent sieving process has gradually been replaced over the years and now the chewed particles are scanned, and the average size is calculated using a software program [24]. For example, carrots, peanuts, almonds, Brazilian nuts, chickpeas (gram), soybeans, coffee beans all have been used as natural test foods. Examples of modified natural foods include colored chewing gum and colored paraffin wax [25]. Some of these methods are based on colorimetric measurements [24]. The silicone-based materials such as Optosil®, Optocal Plus® and Cuttersil® have been used as artificial test foods. Some of the advantages of using artificial test foods include that there is no need to dissolve them in water; they can be stored longer without losing their properties; they present more reproducible physical properties (i.e., size, shape and toughness); there is an absence of seasonal variation in texture; there is a possibility to incorporate all of the characteristics of real food [25, 26]. However, it should be remembered that being artificial, these are not foods that we are used to eating and therefore it is questionable whether or not their particles, produced at the moment of swallowing, correspond to the actual particle sizes that people would normally swallow [25]. Objective measurements might be preferred because they have been considered as more reliable indicators of masticatory performance, but they are time-consuming and require special instruments [10]. On the other hand, subjective methods are simple, informative and convenient for evaluation of large sample populations [10].

Any oral disease that affects the number, structure or positioning of teeth is supposed to have an impact on chewing and, in turn, on a person's systemic health, as it is known that nutrient deficiencies are associated with a variety of diseases, especially in the elderly population [21, 27]. An unbalanced diet related to a masticatory deficiency can affect systemic health because, although some nutrients are essential, the excessive intake of other components may be harmful to health [19]. Furthermore, the number of teeth present was associated with the onset of disability and mortality in old age and seems to be a risk indicator for early mortality and cardiovascular mortality [28-30]. There are many factors that can potentially influence food choices, such as drinking coffee or tea, smoking, aging, loss of taste, psychological status, socioeconomic status, cultural beliefs and personal preferences [13]. The physical ability to bite and chew a wide variety of foods of different textures and nutritional values is the principal benefit provided by the teeth [27]. Whether humans need to masticate their food or not, for the absorption of nutrients in the gastrointestinal tract, is a topic not well studied, but impaired mastication is known to affect food choice adversely, leading to the favoring of the selection of an unbalanced diet as well as decreased enjoyment of food [7, 13]. Harder and more coarse foods such as fruits, vegetables and meats, which are typically major sources of vitamins, minerals and proteins, come to be regarded as either difficult or nearly impossible to chew. Subjects with an incomplete dentition – and thus a reduced masticatory performance – also use more chewing strokes to prepare the food for swallowing than do subjects with a complete natural dentition [25]. People with a reduced masticatory ability may also use home processing approaches to soften foods such as longer cooking times, which can alter the nutritional value of foods by degrading and reducing the bioavailability of essential nutrients (such as vitamin C, thiamin and folates) or by producing trans-fatty acids [19]. Consequently, a tendency to favor softer, more processed foods develops. Soft but nutritious fruits such as raspberries, strawberries, grapes and tomatoes may also be avoided by those people who wear dentures due to prosthetic problems resulting from these foods' seeds lodging under their prostheses [19]. Furthermore, a different number of chewing cycles is required for the various foods, ranging for example from 17 for cake to 63 for carrot [31]. Dry (bread or bagels) and hard products require more chewing cycles before swallowing, probably because more time is required to break the food down and to add enough saliva to form a cohesive bolus [31]. In fact, subjects with less saliva need to chew dry food products more. Consequently, more saliva, a higher maximum bite force and better masticatory performance are correlated with a smaller number of chewing cycles [31].

From a nutritional point of view, lower levels of vitamin C, vitamin A and calcium are most frequently observed in edentulous individuals; dietary fibers are inadequate as well as proteins, folates and iron. The major sources of these nutrients are fruits, vegetables, meats, nuts, seeds, dairy products, breads and cereals. Two additional changes in nutrient intake, due to variations in diet among edentulous individuals, include an increase in the percentage of total calories obtained from fat and an increase in the amount of cholesterol and saturated fatty acids consumed [19].

Furthermore, some authors have also suggested a direct impact of poor mastication on the digestive process [1, 7, 19]. Up to date, the consequences of inadequate mastication on food digestion and absorption have not been frequently explored in the literature, probably because of ethical limitations [19]. Studies conducted on animals have shown outcomes that seem to be species-specific [19]. Gastrointestinal disturbances may be caused by a masticatory deficiency and provoke symptoms such as diarrhea and constipation, especially in the elderly. Patients should be informed of the consequences of losing their teeth and reducing their masticatory performance [19]. Furthermore, public health prevention programs should raise awareness about oral health and help all patients to receive the care they need.

The aim of a prosthetic rehabilitation is to restore impaired mastication by replacing missing teeth; the latter can be achieved through Fixed (FDP) or Removable (RDP) Dental Prostheses [22]. However, it is not clear what is the minimum number of teeth that should be saved or restored to guarantee satisfactory oral functionality [10]. Prosthodontics can provide a range of increasingly complex treatments depending on the severity of the disease, but sometimes a complete rehabilitation may be not possible or even undesirable due to physical and mental conditions, inadequate oral hygiene maintenance and financial restrictions [10]. It should also be noted that the compulsion to save or replace every missing tooth may lead to overtreatment [32]. The rate and state of oral disease in a patient should be balanced as part of a benefit-to-risk ratio prior to choosing a treatment procedure, because every prosthodontic intervention carries a certain benefit-to-risk ratio that should be preoperatively assessed [18]. The general treatment goal largely shifted after 1992, from the restoration of a complete dental arch to providing sufficient mastication [10]. The "Shortened Dental Arch" (SDA) is a minimally invasive approach that has been advocated for a wide range of partially edentulous patients, such as middle-aged and elderly adults with a history of compromised systemic and oral health [18]. This concept was first introduced by Käyser in 1981 by observing that there is sufficient adaptive capacity to maintain oral function in SDA when at least four occlusal units are left [32]. The SDA concept can be seen as a way of providing a suboptimal but still acceptable level of oral function [17].

In patients with absence of posterior molar support, providing a Partial Removable Dental Prosthesis (PRDP) is one of the means available to restore both function and aesthetics. In a study conducted by Wallace et al., the chewing capacity of patients fitted with prosthesis designed according to the SDA principles was equivalent to that of patients fitted with PRDP [13]. It should be considered that patients need time to adapt both functionally and psychosocially to the use of a removable prosthesis, and some may never achieve this goal even if the prosthesis satisfies all objective criteria regarding fit, quality and appearance [32].

In fact, a high rate of patients with SDA rehabilitated using a RPD may be dissatisfied with the latter because, while SDA can initially affect oral comfort, its use is still acceptable to some patients, and it is controversial to suggest that providing distal-extension RPD could significantly enhance oral comfort [32]. Moreover, there is still conflicting evidence on the benefits of replacing missing teeth by removable prosthesis in terms of influence on dietary intake or nutrition [33]. However, there is a lack of general perspective on the effects of tooth loss and denture status on QoL and OHRQoL: the relationship with oral health rehabilitation still needs to be investigated in order to understand whether using a removable prosthesis can improve QoL of those who experience a considerable loss of teeth [33]. In a study conducted by McGrath et al., patients who claimed that they had experienced considerable tooth loss (i.e., those having fewer than 20 teeth), but who did not have recourse to wear dentures, were among those with the poorest OHRQoL in the population, after controlling sociodemographic factors [33]. However, the acceptance of dental extraction and replacement of teeth with conventional removable dentures, either partial or complete, has diminished; furthermore, as previously mentioned, the ability to adapt to complete replacement dentures in old age is also uncertain [17]. This can lead to an increased demand for dental implant-retained restorations and other costly forms of treatment with a high burden of maintenance [17].

An alternative solution, when conventional *mandibular* dentures are not accepted, is the use of mandibular overdentures supported by two implants. Mandibular overdentures have been extensively studied and selected, for the vast majority of patients, as the first treatment of choice when compared to the lack of stability and comfort of a conventional denture. On the contrary, there exists a lack of consensus for *maxillary* overdentures. Maxillary overdentures have been shown to be a favorable treatment option for patients with persistent complaints of retention and stability. However, while two endosseous implants are generally considered to provide sufficient support to a mandibular overdenture, the number of implants needed to support a maxillary overdenture is still not clear, even though the presence of at least four implants seems to be associated with a higher implant life rate [34]. Implant-supported restorations are predictable treatment solutions, but different technical and biological complications can occur, and periodical follow-up visits should be scheduled for the purpose of patient monitoring. Furthermore, the use of implant-supported prostheses requires patient enrollment in a strict maintenance program tailored to the individual risk of biological complications such as peri-implantitis.

In conclusion, it seems reasonable to suggest that the application of the SDA approach is acceptable, particularly in older adults. Furthermore, given the rising burden of chronic disease in the aging population, coupled with its negative impact on QoL, preventive strategies aimed at reducing tooth loss need to be reinforced because most oral diseases share common risk factors. National health programs should consider actively working to counteract these factors through disease prevention and health promotion initiatives.

REFERENCES

1. Peyron MA, Gierczynski I, Hartmann C, Loret C, Dardevet D, Martin N, Woda A. Role of physical bolus properties as sensory inputs in the trigger of swallowing. PLoS One 2011; 6(6): e21167.
2. Engelen L, Fontijn-Tekamp A, van der Bilt A. The influence of product and oral characteristics on swallowing. Arch Oral Biol 2005; 50(8): 739-46.
3. Peyron MA, Mishellany A, Woda A. Particle size distribution of food boluses after mastication of six natural foods. J Dent Res 2004; 83(7): 578-82.
4. Mishellany A, Woda A, Labas R, Peyron MA. The challenge of mastication: preparing a bolus suitable for deglutition. Dysphagia 2006; 21(2): 87-94.
5. Christine Sandra Flynn. The particle size distribution of

solid foods after human mastication: a thesis presented in partial fulfilment of the requirements for the degree of Doctor of Philosophy in Food Technology at Massey University, Auckland, New Zealand (2012).
6. Pocztaruk Rde L, Frasca LC, Rivaldo EG, Fernandes Ede L, Gavião MB. Protocol for production of a chewable material for masticatory function tests (Optocal - Brazilian version). Braz Oral Res 2008; 22(4): 305-10.
7. Mishellany-Dutour A, Renaud J, Peyron M-A, Rimek F, Woda A. Is the goal of mastication reached in young dentates, aged dentates and aged denture wearers? Br J Nutr 2008; 99(1): 121-8.
8. Chen J, Khandelwal N, Liu Z, Funami T. Influences of food hardness on the particle size distribution of food boluses. Arch Oral Biol 2013; 58(3): 293-8.
9. Sierpińska T, Gołebiewska M, Długosz JW. The relationship between masticatory efficiency and the state of dentition at patients with non rehabilitated partial lost of teeth. Adv Med Sci 2006; 51 Suppl 1: 196-9.
10. Naka O, Anastassiadou V, Pissiotis A. Association between functional tooth units and chewing ability in older adults: a systematic review. Gerodontology 2014; 31(3): 166-77.
11. Bortoluzzi MC, Traebert J, Lasta R, Da Rosa TN, Capella DL, Presta AA. Tooth loss, chewing ability and quality of life. Contemp Clin Dent 2012; 3(4): 393-7.
12. Rodrigues SM, Oliveira AC, Vargas AM, Moreira AN, E Ferreira EF. Implications of edentulism on quality of life among elderly. Int J Environ Res Public Health 2012; 9(1): 100-9.
13. Wallace S, Samietz S, Abbas M, McKenna G, Woodside JV, Schimmel M. Impact of prosthodontic rehabilitation on the masticatory performance of partially dentate older patients: Can it predict nutritional state? Results from a RCT. J Dent 2018; 68: 66-71.
14. Bessadet M, Nicolas E, Sochat M, Hennequin M, Veyrune JL. Impact of removable partial denture prosthesis on chewing efficiency. J Appl Oral Sci 2013; 21(5): 392-6.
15. Lamy M, Mojon P, Kalykakis G, Legrand R, Butz-Jorgensen E. Oral status and nutrition in the institutionalized elderly. J Dent 1999; 27(6): 443-8.
16. Mack F, Schwahn C, Feine JS, Mundt T, Bernhardt O, John U, Kocher PT, Biffar R. The impact of tooth loss on general health related to quality of life among elderly Pomeranians: results from the study of health in Pomerania (SHIP-O). Int J Prosthodont 2005; 18(5): 414-9.
17. Gerritsen AE, Allen PF, Witter DJ, Bronkhorst EM, Creugers NH. Tooth loss and oral health-related quality of life: a systematic review and meta-analysis. Health Qual Life Outcomes 2010; 8: 126.
18. Bowley J. Minimal intervention prosthodontics: current knowledge and societal implications. Med Princ Pract 2002; 11 Suppl 1: 22-31.
19. N'gom PI, Woda A. Influence of impaired mastication on nutrition. J Prosthet Dent 2002; 87(6): 667-73.
20. van der Bilt A, Olthoff LW, Bosman F, Oosterhaven SP. The effect of missing postcanine teeth on chewing performance in man. Arch Oral Biol 1993; 38(5): 423-9.
21. Kim BI, Jeong SH, Chung KH, Cho YK, Kwon HK, Choi CH. Subjective food intake ability in relation to maximal bite force among Korean adults. J Oral Rehabil 2009; 36(3): 168-75.
22. Liang S, Zhang Q, Witter DJ, Wang Y, Creugers NH. Effects of removable dental prostheses on masticatory performance of subjects with shortened dental arches: A systematic review. J Dent 2015; 43(10): 1185-94.
23. Bates JF, Stafford GD, Harrison A. Masticatory function – a review of the literature. III. Masticatory performance and efficiency. J Oral Rehabil 1976; 3(1): 57-67.
24. Tarkowska A, Katzer L, Ahlers MO. Assessment of masticatory performance by means of a color-changeable chewing gum. J Prosthodont Res 2017; 61(1): 9-19.
25. Fontijn-Tekamp FA, van der Bilt A, Abbink JH, Bosman F. Swallowing threshold and masticatory performance in dentate adults. Physiol Behav 2004; 83(3): 431-6.
26. Khoury-Ribas L, Ayuso-Montero R, Rovira-Lastra B, Peraire M, Martinez-Gomis J. Reliability of a new test food to assess masticatory function. Arch Oral Biol 2018; 87: 1-6.
27. Hutton B, Feine J, Morais J. Is there an association between edentulism and nutritional state? J Can Dent Assoc 2002; 68(3): 182-7.
28. Padilha DM, Hilgert JB, Hugo FN, Bós AJ, Ferrucci L. Number of teeth and mortality risk in the Baltimore Longitudinal Study of Aging. J Gerontol A Biol Sci Med Sci 2008; 63(7): 739-44.
29. Tu YK, Galobardes B, Smith GD, McCarron P, Jeffreys M, Gilthorpe MS. Associations between tooth loss and mortality patterns in the Glasgow Alumni Cohort. Heart 2007; 93(9): 1098-103.
30. Holm-Pedersen P, Schultz-Larsen K, Christiansen N, Avlund K. Tooth loss and subsequent disability and mortality in old age. J Am Geriatr Soc 2008; 56(3): 429-35.
31. Engelen L, Fontijn-Tekamp A, van der Bilt A. The influence of product and oral characteristics on swallowing. Arch Oral Biol 2005; 50(8): 739-46.
32. Armellini D, von Fraunhofer JA. The shortened dental arch: a review of the literature. J Prosthet Dent 2004; 92(6): 531-5.
33. McGrath C, Bedi R. Can dentures improve the quality of life of those who have experienced considerable tooth loss? J Dent 2001; 29(4): 243-6.
34. Raghoebar GM, Meijer HJ, Slot W, Slater JJ, Vissink A. A systematic review of implant-supported overdentures in the edentulous maxilla, compared to the mandible: how many implants? Eur J Oral Implantol 2014; 7 Suppl 2: S191-201.

17 Masticatory function: assessment possibilities and connections with temporomandibular disorders

Marco Antônio Moreira Rodrigues da Silva,
Ana Maria Bettoni Rodrigues da Silva and Laís Valencise Magri

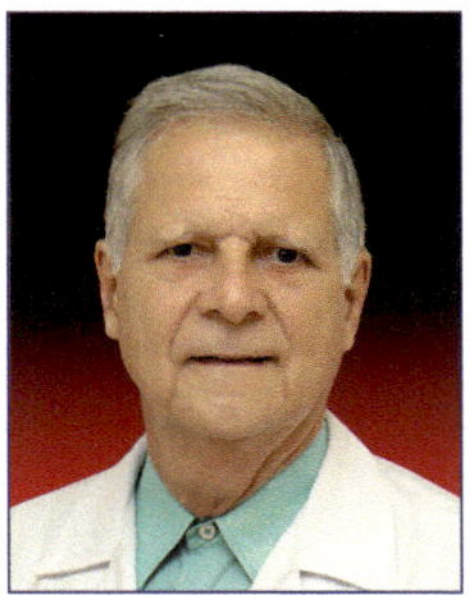

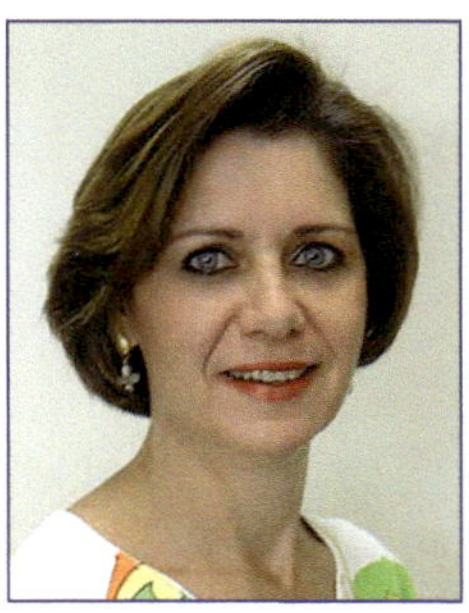

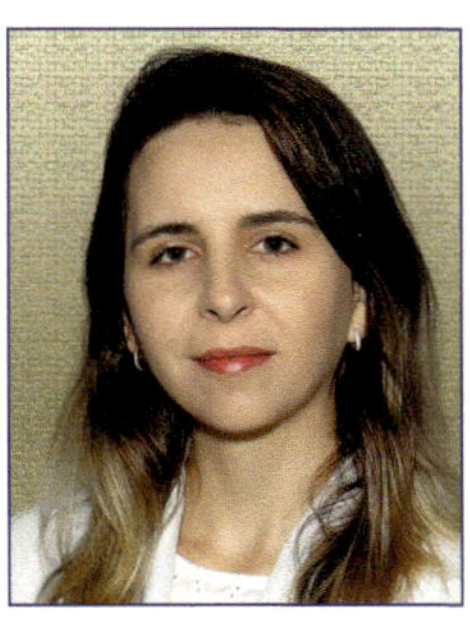

17.1 Assessment of the masticatory muscles

17.1.1 Surface electromyography

The Surface Electromyography (SEMG) of the masticatory muscles is part of the quantitative assessment of patients in Odontology, and other health areas today. This type of examination can provide quantitative data regarding surface muscles, with minimum distress on the patient, and without invasive procedures. The diagnosis of alterations in the stomatognathic system, and the evaluation of the effects of therapies that can benefit the treatment, reduce the disagreement among multiple clinical examinations. Electromyography can be used to aid in a deeper understanding of muscular changes in patients with severe temporomandibular disorder (TMD), and to control the production of occlusal splints [1]. The influence of occlusal conditions in stomatognathic function may also be assessed by electromyography [2].

The SEMG permits checking and quantifying the muscular balance, both among muscles on the sides of the body (symmetry), and between pairs of muscles with possible effect of lateral deviation of the jaw (torque) [1, 3]. Beside that, a quantitative assessment of the muscular contraction patterns during standardized dynamic activities allows us to evaluate the muscular coordination [3, 4], both before and after the modification of occlusal surfaces [1]. The SEMG is a low cost, non-invasive method, applicable in research, and in dental clinical practice for qualitative and quantitative assessments of the muscles of the head and neck. Since the SEMG does not evaluate the muscular fibers directly, a well-standardized protocol must be used, thus removing (or reducing) biological and technical artifacts [5]. In fact, the thickness of the hypoderm, the functional relationship between different muscles, instrumental noise, the position of the electrodes in relation to the muscular fibers, and the motor point may al influence the electromyographic signal. Taking into consideration these technical characteristics, a proper SEMG evaluation must only be performed with a reproducible protocol, using standardized/normalized potentials to minimize most biological and technical noise [1-5].

Marco Antônio Moreira Rodrigues da Silva, DDS, MD, PhD; Ana Maria Bettoni Rodrigues da Silva, DDS, MD, PhD; Laís Valencise Magri, DDS, MD, PhD
Department of Restorative Dentistry, School of Dentistry of Ribeirão Preto, São Paulo University, Ribeirão Preto, São Paulo, Brazil

Email: marco@forp.usp.br; anabettoni@usp.br; laisvm@forp.usp.br

Asymmetry is a common aspect of the human being. Both the structure and the morphology of the paired organs differ on both right and left sides of the body [2]. Morphological assessments of craniofacial asymmetry have become a usual part of characterizing not only health individuals, but also unhealthy ones. The evaluation of functional asymmetry of the craniofacial complex generally involves observing the pattern of movement of the jaw, and the activity of masticatory muscles [1-5]. The pattern in contraction of the paired muscles can be investigated through surface electromyography [6].

The SEMG implies a diagnostic device to identify and record electric potentials in skeletal muscular fibers [2]. Thus, it is possible to know when and how a muscle is activated, and after that, one can determine how the coordination of different muscles involved in the movement is established [7]. The SEMG system is composed of electrodes that capture the electric potentials (activity) of the muscle contracted (input information phase); an amplifier that processes a small electrical signal (processing phase); and a decoder that permits graphic visualization and/or audio output, which will allow a complete analysis of the data (output information phase) [6].

The analysis of the electromyographic data can be done through indexes, among which the most used are: POC index (percental overlapping coefficient, %), torque coefficient (TC%), torsion index (TORS), asymmetry index (ASSIM), activation index (ATTIV), impact index (IMPACT). This way, POC is calculated for masseter muscles (POC MASS), temporalis muscles (POC Temp), and the average (Mean POC) on each patient.

The protocol used at the Laboratory of Research in Electromyography of the Stomatognathic System (LAPESE) at the Odontology School of Ribeirão Preto from the University of São Paulo (FORP/USP) consists in the following sequence:

Standardization: maximum voluntary contraction with 10 mm thick cotton rollers (Roeko Luna number 2, Coltene, Roeko, Germany), positioned between the second and first premolars, bilaterally, for 5 s. Maximum voluntary contraction: at maximum habitual intercuspation for 5 s.

Chewing: the habitual chew is performed with sugar-free chewing gum on the unilateral right and left for 15 s. All the electromyographic examinations are performed without changing the electrodes or position wires. A resting period of one minute is established between each test so that the patient can rest, avoiding muscle fatigue. The investigations are carried out in a single moment of evaluation, during the same session. The main analyzed variables are:

- POC (percentage overlapping coefficient) of the masseter and temporalis muscles (calculated using the Electrical Myograph Analyzer software). This is an index of muscle contraction symmetry as a function of time; it varies from 0 to 100%. When two pairs of muscles contract in perfect symmetry, POC is 100%; the normality considered is above 83% [8].
- Static SEMG: electromyographic indexes: TORS: torsion index (lateral displacement force component of the jaw); ASSIM: asymmetry index (relation between working and balance sides); ATTIVE: activation index (relation between masseter and anterior temporalis); IMPACT: impact index (system energy production).
- Dynamic SEMG: number of masticatory cycles, masticatory frequency, IMPACT (average of the total electromyographic activities calculated from the amplitude of electromyographic potentials in RMS, recorded during chewing), and SMI (neuromuscular coordination values or masticatory symmetric index).

Some authors consider SEMG an appropriate method to assess the jaw resting position, by always maintaining the correct posture of the head of the patient, in a calm and silent environment during the electromyographic examination [9, 10].

The SEMG is an examination that provides an analysis of electric activity of the muscles, and it can be employed for the stomatognathic muscular system. The SEMG has been used in several scientific studies, and it complements the evaluation of patients with musculoskeletal distresses, such as TMD and other orofacial pain. Its execution demands proper criteria and training, to ensure trustworthy outcomes that can be compared. Added to other clinical evaluations, the SEMG has been shown to be of great value to monitor the action or functional alterations of the muscles.

17.1.2 Bite force

Bite force is a quantitative test of the power of compression of the stomatognathic system, which enables the evaluation and comparison of aspects related to the neuromuscular coordination, level of contraction of the muscles, and alterations that may harm the functionality of this system [11, 12]. Bite force measurement is performed using a device called dynamometer, through which the maximum molar occlusal force is obtained. Bite force contributes to the diagnostics of masticatory function [12, 13]. The measurement of the bite force allows the quantification of masticatory potential through the contraction of chewing muscles reflected on other anatomic components such as teeth and bones, along with the neuromuscular control of the central nervous system [11-13].

Variables such as age and gender influence significantly the bite force. A previous study has demonstrated that women present an average of 30% stronger bite force in comparison with men, and that children present reduced values when compared to adults, besides having a smooth trend of reduced strength while aging [12].

The occlusal condition is another important aspect in interpreting bite force, as further dental losses are related to the reduction of muscular contraction, and to the higher miscoordination of masticatory movements [14]. In this sense, the reestablishment of the occlusal system through oral rehabilitation is highly important in terms of the maximum molar force gain, and masticatory potential. Recent studies have demonstrated that patients rehabilitated with implant-supported teeth presented an increase in bite force and masticatory potential, with results similar to those in the control group after three months of rehabilitation procedure [15, 16].

The craniofacial morphology influences the muscular capacity of the stomatognathic system, and consequently the bite force. Individuals with brachyfacial profiles show higher muscular tonicity, along with shorter and more resistant fibers, which leads to superior values in tests of bite force [17, 18]. However, craniofacial morphology does not influence masticatory efficiency and the ability to chew, because higher forces do not mean better function, considering that several other aspects are involved in chewing, such as movement coordination, speed, time, number of repetitions and others [17].

Related to chronic TMD, a painful musculoskeletal condition, there is no consensus in the scientific literature towards the maximum molar bite force, since some studies have found more reduced values in comparison with controls [11, 13], and others have not reported any difference [19, 20]. The presence of pain in masticatory muscles during orofacial function can lead to alterations in the measurement of bite force. Kogawa et al. [11] emphasize the possible differences among TMD diagnoses, thus painful conditions in muscles may manifest higher impairment of bite force than articular conditions and studies many times do not present standardization about TMD diagnosing methodologies, and instrumental measurement of bite force.

According to one study by Palinkas et al. [21], sleeping bruxism does not change the thickness of masticatory muscles and bite force. So, the impairment of bite force in TMD and in sleeping/vigilant bruxism is not completely elucidated, as studies point out controversial outcomes. Therefore, more studies with these sleeping/vigilant populations are needed to identify subgroups of patients who indeed presented altered values due to the presence of a pathology, and not an individual variability of gender or age.

In summary, bite force measurement helps the assessment of the functional capability of the stomatognathic, and it can be influenced by a series of factors, including gender, age, occlusal condition, and the presence of disorders that affect this system (TMD, musculoskeletal painful syndromes, intra-articular pathologies, systemic conditions and other factors). It is important to highlight that bite force must not be analyzed in isolation, and it does not represent by itself a better or worse function, as it is only a quantitative variable of force. Added to other evaluations, bite force measurement contributes to a better understanding of the functional aspect of specific populations, in terms of possible variations.

17.1.3 Pressure pain threshold (pain sensitivity)

Sensitivity to pain of masticatory muscles is a parameter used to diagnose various orofacial myofunctional conditions, such as TMD. The most used technique is based on measuring the Pressure Pain Threshold (PPT), with the aid of a compression algometer, through which the patient reports to the researcher the moment at which the pressure applied by the device becomes painful [22, 23]. In research, the use of this device ensures more objective clinical results when compared to the subjective evaluation by palpation [23, 24]. Some studies have already shown good accuracy and precision of the algometer to test the sensitivity to pain in patients with TMD [24, 25].

The reliability of measurements of the PPT is associated to the following factors: application speed of the compression stimulus, size of the algometer tip, state of muscular contraction, reaction time of the patient and the examiner, and degree of subjectivity while reporting pain. It is relevant to say that variations in PPT are also related to gender, age and group of muscles assessed, besides the presence or absence of some musculoskeletal pain syndrome [22-25].

Pain in the orofacial region, especially in masticatory muscles and in the region of the temporomandibular joint (TMJ), can impair those functions linked to mandibular mobility, such as chewing. In the presence of pain, muscular compensations and/or reduction in the amplitude of movements may occur, so that it avoids nociception, which may cause damage in the long term. Such damage is not only local, but it can also contribute to central sensitization phenomena, developing trigger points in the extratrigeminal regions and orofacial myofunctional disorders [25, 26].

In addition to quantitative measures of pain, the evaluation of sensitivity to pain through PPT has been used more and more to assess patients with symptoms of TMD. Several studies have demonstrated that the PPT has great applicability in the clinical practice and research [24, 27]. One study performed by Santos Silva et al. [23] compared the PPT values for masticatory muscles among women diagnosed with either painful and/or asymptomatic TMD. These authors have obtained a specificity of 90.8% with PPT values of 1.5 Kgf/cm^2 for masseter, 2.47 Kgf/cm^2 for anterior belly of digastric, 2.75 Kgf/cm^2 for intermediate belly, and 2.77 Kgf/cm^2 for the posterior one, defining the cutoff values that can be used in clinical evaluation of the patients. Cunha et al. [27] assessed the PPT reference value to identify arthralgia in the TMJ, and they have found that 1.36 Kgf/cm^2 represents the most accurate threshold to pain sensitivity for this joint.

Emotional factors can influence significantly the PPT of masticatory muscles, altering the sensitivity to pain in the orofacial region, and predisposing the development of painful TMD. Previous studies have demonstrated the influence of stress and anxiety over the PPT of masseter and digastric muscles, in terms of emotional variations, in patients with anxiety and stress disorders who presented reduced PPT in different facial and body locations [28, 29].

Measuring the PPT in masticatory muscles is a great contribution, but it is relevant to highlight that this must not be used and interpreted in isolation, but along with other assessments based on more reliable diagnostic criteria, such as those described in Diagnostic Criteria for Temporomandibular Disorders (DC/TMD) [30]. Slade et al. [31] stated that the PPT is a floating variable that can be altered, so it must not be used as a predictive factor for the development or permanence of a painful TMD. Greenspan et al. [32] have demonstrated that the increase in sensitivity to pain contributes to a modest increase of risk of developing TMD. This means that the modification of the PPT does not guarantee the absence of pain noticed by patients with TMD, or even the appearance of signs and symptoms. Thus, the PPT is one useful tool for evaluating masticatory muscles, that must be used prudently as a complement to other examinations of the orofacial region. Furthermore, the PPT contributes to the understanding the pain phenomenon, and the identification of myofascial trigger points.

17.2 Evaluation of the masticatory function

17.2.1 Masticatory efficiency (performance)

Masticatory efficiency is defined as appropriate chewing cycles with resulting compensatory physiological mechanisms of the sensory mechanism of teeth eruption and deterioration, developed at different ages, when the joints and the masticatory muscles are in perfect functional adaptation. Each masticatory cycle consists of several movements of the food inside the oral cavity, by the mechanical reduction of food, called comminution, and by the fluid secreted by salivary glands. These actions reduce the volume of the food, making it easier to swallow [33]. Various terms are used to refer to masticatory function, including masticatory efficiency, masticatory capability and masticatory performance [34].

There are several methods to assess masticatory efficiency. One method is the analysis with sieves of different diameters, in which food is chewed and collected after being crushed. This way, the higher the quantity of food that passes through thinner sieves, the higher the masticatory efficiency. The sieve method has been already tested and employed in many studies [35, 36]. However, the sieve methodology is not used often due to the impracticality of employing it in clinical studies, according to Santos et al. [33], who reported other alternatives, such as the measurement through a scanner of the size of the particles chewed [37], and optical scanning [38]. Moreover, the authors have described the study performed by means of visible spectrophotometry, also named the colorimetric method [33].

Another method for analyzing masticatory efficiency in chewing has been studied by many researchers, by using several methods and types of test-food [33, 35, 36, 39-43]. Despite the existing variety of methods to evaluate and assess masticatory efficiency, they are not practical in clinical practice. According to Santos et al. [33], variations in the testing material is one of the reasons for the imprecision of this method. The colorimetric method of standardized masticatory capsules presents advantages, such as reduced variability, besides being fast, simple, reproducible, low-cost and effective [33, 36].

The need to develop efficient assessment systems, to understand the masticatory function, and to determine parameters of normality, led Cazal et al. [42] to relate SEMG to the colorimetric method to determine masticatory efficiency. Researchers compared chewing electromyographic indexes of the capsules used to evaluate the masticatory efficiency according to the Analysis program: "ME-mastig", and foods of different textures (gum, raisins and peanut), which were analyzed by MAST 08 software – Differential Lissajous Electromyography Software (Ferrario VF: Laboratory of Functional Anatomy of the Stomatognathic System, Department of Human Morphology, University of Milan, Milan, Italy, 2008). The sample was composed of thirty young adults, healthy, with an average age of 23.46 years, without symptoms of TMD, confirmed by clinical examination, by the Research Diagnostic Criteria for Temporomandibular Disorders, and by the static test of electromyography (SEMG). Afterwards, dynamic tests (bilateral chewing of the compounds) were performed to determine the number of chewing cycles (CYCLES); the masticatory frequency (FREQ); the symmetric masticatory index – related to the neuromuscular coordination value during chewing (SMI); and the total electromyographic activity performed by the system during chewing, corresponding to the impact (IMPACT). According to the results obtained, the cycle and frequency were similar. Regarding SMI and IMPACT, the values found were similar to each other, and different from those of the gum. The authors have concluded that the use of masticatory capsules and the natural foods with different textures produced similar results to those of the SEMG indexes. Thus, the researchers invited the scientific community to create new studies in the area of chewing efficiency, aimed at analyzing the masticatory performance of various populations, including individuals with TMD. The authors have also concluded that the colorimetric method may be employed as a complement in the evaluation of the masticatory efficiency in several situations.

The masticatory efficiency test employed in the studies from Cazal et al. [42] consisted in using the same capsules that had been used in the Masticatory Efficiency Test, developed by the Laboratory of Pharmacotechnics of the School of Pharmaceutic Sciences of Ribeirão Preto, USP, and by using the reports from the evaluation performed at the Laboratory of Masticatory Efficiency of the Department of Pediatric Clinic, Preventive and Social Dentistry of the School of Dentistry of Ribeirão Preto (FORP/USP) [33]. These capsules are composed by granules of fuchsin produced by drip process, of approximately 1 mm of diameter. The granules are obtained by ionotropic gel setting of aqueous dispersion of pectin at 2%, which contains 50% of solids and fuchsin, in a solution of calcium chloride 1.0 M. After this preparation phase, the granules are covered with Eudragit 5% solution (Eudragit E100) in a mixture of 10% acetone solvents in absolute ethanol. Then, a portion of 250 mg of the granules is encased in each PVC capsule, set for evaluation of the masticatory efficiency (Table 17.1) [33].

Table 17.1 Basic composition of the fuchsin granules. Developed at the Laboratory of Pharmacotechnique of the School of Pharmaceutic Sciences of Ribeirão Preto (São Paulo University, Ribeirão Preto, Brazil)

Compounds	*Weight (g) – Volume (mL)*
Lactose	20.60 g
Microcrystalline cellulose	36.85 g
Amid	17.10 g
Sucrose	17.10 g
Hydrogenated oil	8.05 g
Basic fuchsin	0.16 g
Water	60 mL
Coverage substance (*Eudragit E 100% to 5% in acetone)	50 mL

* Polymeric methacrylate (Rohm Pharma GmBh, Germany).
Adapted from Santos et al. [33].

The chewing dynamic test with the capsules was carried out for a period of 20 seconds, pre-established in the protocol of evaluation of masticatory efficiency. However, for the electromyographic analysis, the period taken into consideration was 15 seconds. Before performing the test, the participants were instructed to position the capsule on the tongue and wait for the signal from the researcher to start chewing. During chewing, the granules inside the capsules were smashed, and the fuchsin liberated was proportional to the energy employed during this process. After chewing, every capsule was stored, identified and then sent for laboratory analysis [33, 42].

Evaluation of the capsules through Visible Spectrophotometry Stage was performed by a technician at the Laboratory of Masticatory Efficiency of the School of Dentistry of Ribeirão Preto at the University of São Paulo. The content of the capsules was dissolved in 5 mL of water, constantly stirred for 30 seconds. Afterwards, this solution was filtered with filter paper, and the coloring extracted was quantified in nanometers (nm) by using a UV visible spectrophotometer (Beckman DU-640) with wavelength equals to 546 nm. This way, it was possible to determine the EM, from the concentration of fuchsin extracted. The values in nanometers of absorbance found were transformed in fuchsin coloring concentration from a standard deviation, calculated by $x = (y+0.0045)/0.167$, where y corresponds to the absorbance of the solution in 546 nm, and x corresponds to the concentration of the coloring in microgram per milliliter (µg/mL). Thus, for each capsule chewed, a fuchsin concentration value (µg/mL) was obtained, which corresponds to EM. The EM values were transformed by the square root for the statistical analysis through the analysis of variance [33].

Therefore, measuring the masticatory efficiency has several applications in research and clinical practice, especially while evaluating patients with TMD, as well as in the analysis of oral rehabilitations and dental losses. Fuchsin capsules are among the most reported methods in the literature, and they provide valuable results when comparing different groups of patients.

17.2.2 Chewing electromyography

In 1949, Moyers [44] used electromyography in Odontology for the first time, specifically with regards to the chewing musculature by assessing temporalis, masseter, pterygoids, mentalis and suprahyoid muscles in individuals with a Class II malocclusion, Angle division I, in opening, closing and lateral sliding of the jaw. Moyers highlighted in his studies that the electromyographic examination is an auxiliary method to diagnose the muscular function of the stomatognathic system [44]. Starting from the 1950s, electromyography has been used as a study method, and it has contributed to explaining the performance of the facial muscles, as well as those involved in chewing, deglutition, occlusion, and phonation [1, 6, 13, 43, 45]. In 1962, Basmajian and De Luca [46] published the book "Muscles Alive – Their function revealed by Electromyography" and made kinesiologic electromyography popular.

It is important to emphasize that the lack of instruments to measure, easily and objectively, the physiologic parameters of the behavior of chewing muscles has led researchers to perform their studies with the use of electromyography in order to acquire greater information about the subject [6, 13, 43, 45, 47].

Reduction in electromyographic activity is an important factor in preventing parafunctional activities, and in the development of TMD [48]. Nonetheless, Raustia et al. [49] reported that psychological factors, such as stress or fear of pain, as well as sleeping disorders, fracture or instability of protheses, age and sex, may have an important role in the reduction of the muscular activity. However, McCarrol et al. [50] have stated that the ideal situation would be a similar SEMG activity among muscles, bilaterally, following the highest symmetry pattern possible. The bilateral balance of electromyographic activity of the masticatory muscles is important in treating TMD, although the normal behavior of the musculature presents some degree of asymmetry, even in healthy individuals.

In 2017, Silva et al. [13] investigated whether the maximum molar bite force (BF) and the electromyographic activity (SEMG) are altered in patients with TMD with abfraction lesions (AL) (fracture of the teeth) when compared to those without AL. The sample was composed of 45 patients (18-60 years old), 30 of them diagnosed having TMD (15 with AL, and 15 without it), and 15 subjects were in the control group. Bite force and SEMG were tested in masticatory muscles by way of maximum voluntary contraction (MVC) and while chewing gum. According to the results obtained, TMD patients presented diminished BF ($P < 0.001$), without differences among patients with or without AL. Electromyographic activity during MVC was similar among all groups ($P > 0.005$), despite the presence of a higher trend of muscular balance in the control group (percentage of overlapping coefficient and electromyographic index). The TMD group without AL presented a lower number of cycles and masticatory frequency. Patients with TMD, with and without AL, presented similar results in BF and SEMG.

Ferreira et al. [47] have investigated the characteristics of orofacial motor functions in patients with chronic TMD (with duration superior to 6 months), presenting considerably severe signs and symptoms. The group with TMD presented higher difficulty in chewing than the control group. The differences between groups increased when tested with hard consistency food. Besides that, while evaluating the orofacial myofunctions, patients with TMD presented impairment of appearance and posture, as well as mobility, chewing and deglutition, with noticeable differences when compared to the control group, except for breathing. Patients with TMD presented higher unilateral chewing frequency (TMD 54%; Control group = 26%), although during the electromyographic analysis in SEMG tests, chewing frequencies were similar in patients with TMD and for those in the control group. Altered coordination was found within the masseter and temporalis muscles in the TMD group, while chewing gum. Researchers have concluded that patients with chronic TMD and those presenting considerably severe symptoms have shown impairment of clinical parameters, SEMG and masticatory function, with a less precise recruitment of temporalis and masseter muscles on both the working and the balancing sides. A deficiency in deglutition and other motor orofacial functions was also observed, which must be taken into consideration while elaborating rehabilitation programs in TMD, to soften pain and to promote a long-lasting functional recovery.

17.3 Relation between masticatory function and TMD

17.3.1 TMD – New concepts

Temporomandibular disorders (TMD) refer to a set of signs and symptoms present in a painful musculoskeletal syndrome, which impair masticatory muscles, the temporomandibular joint, and structures associated to the stomatognathic system, as well as trigeminal or extratrigeminal systems. This syndrome is related to multisystemic alterations, besides those related to behavior, emotions and social interactions, known to be manifestations of irregularity in the nervous system [51, 52]. Among the main predictors of the development of TMD there are: the presence of comorbidities, non-painful orofacial symptoms (such as self-reported parafunctions), frequency of somatic symptoms, poor sleep quality, as well as genetic and epigenetic factors [52].

Epidemiological studies indicate that 75% of the population in general already presents at least one sign of TMD, and that 33% presents at least one symptom. Patients with TMD often show painful symptoms at rest and during mandibular function, with limitation and asymmetry of movement of the orofacial structures, besides popping and crackling noises of the articulations [53, 54]. TMD are frequent conditions, ranking third in prevalence of daily chronic pain, after headaches and cervicalgia (neck ache). It is estimated that these three clinical indicators of TMD (pain in the orofacial region, limitations in mandibular movements and articular noises) are present in among 5 to 50% of the population, at any moment of their lives, though not always related to the presence of any diagnosed disorder [53, 54].

According to the results of the OPPERA study (Orofacial Pain: Prospective Evaluation and Risk Assessment), TMD presents an annual incidence of 4%, which means that for each group of 100 healthy people, 4 of them will develop TMD within a year, approximately [52]. Epidemiological studies performed in the general population reveal a high prevalence of TMD signs and symptoms, ranging between 21.2% and 68.8% [54-56]. This condition strikes mostly young adults, with an average age between 20 to 40, but it may become apparent under different diagnoses throughout life [53, 54].

The TMD diagnosis is based on varied and well-defined clinical criteria. As a diagnostic tool, *Research Diagnostic Criteria for Temporomandibular Disorders* (RDC/TMD) was the first protocol introduced by Dworkin and LeResche [57] in 1992, with the aim to establish reproducible and valid clinical criteria for the TMD subtypes more commonly found in clinical practice. This protocol was translated into several languages, and it is used all over the world as a TMD/maxillofacial pain clinical research tool, applied to systemic investigations and standardizing methods with higher reliability [58]. The clinical investigation performed through RDC/TMD follows criteria from both diagnosis axes, reaching a physical diagnosis (Axis I) and a psychosocial assessment (Axis II). According to Axis I of this protocol, patients may be classified in three groups: I (myofascial pain), II (disk displacement) and III (arthralgia, osteoarthritis and osteoarthrosis) [57].

The most recent version of this protocol, the Diagnostic Criteria for Temporomandibular Disorders (DC/TMD) was released in 2014, and it has been widely used in clinical and research areas [30]. Through its use, it is possible to classify TMD in 12 categories: myalgia, local myalgia, myofascial pain, referred myofascial pain, disk displacement with reduction of intermittent locking, disk displacement with opening limitation, disk displacement without reduction of opening, degenerative disease and subluxation. Besides that, DC/TMD presents sensitivity and acceptable specificities for diagnosis of subtypes, though these values may be superior in muscular conditions in compared to those originating from the articulations [30, 59].

In conclusion, painful TMD has significant incidence and prevalence in the population, and it generates impairment in the quality of life, especially if it is directly associated to emotional factors, such as stress and anxiety. Similar to other painful chronic musculoskeletal syndromes, painful TMD has an important impact over family, social and working environment settings. In this sense, several aspects related to diagnosis, treatment, risk factors and comorbidities are studied more and more, to promote better strategies to deal with this condition.

17.3.2 Masticatory alterations in patients with TMD

Patients with TMD frequently report pain, and present limitations in mastication, which can be affected directly or indirectly by a series of factors, such as dental losses, oral rehabilitations, disk displacements, mandibular hypermobility, muscle force and facial profile among others [60, 61]. Muscular activity, coordination of movements and chewing time are influenced by the orofacial structures, by the functional/adaptive capability of the masticatory muscles and the temporomandibular joints, besides by the food's characteristics [62, 63].

Severity and perception of TMD signs and symptoms may affect the coordination of mandibular movements through conscious and unconscious mechanisms to avoid pain, thus generating altered masticatory patterns [43]. Many times, maintenance of masticatory function in adverse conditions is non-effective, contributing to the progression of painful TMD in the long term. Several studies have demonstrated that patients with TMD present different masticatory patterns from those of the control group [43, 60-65].

Among the main alterations, patients with TMD presented a higher tendency for unilateral chewing, longer chewing time and a greater number of masticatory strokes [43, 61]. Regarding masticatory efficiency, results from the scientific literature are controversial, as some present studies of patients with TMD having higher efficiency than those of the control group [43], while other have found lower efficiency [61, 66]. However, it is relevant to highlight the differences among techniques and samples studied, that might have influenced the results. A previous study has shown that the masticatory performance of individuals with disk displacement was inferior when compared to individuals from the control group, even though in cases of severe pain in the orofacial region, the performance was similar [66].

While experiencing pain, there is a natural tendency to chew the food in smaller parts and to perform more careful movements, which results in longer chewing time, higher number of strokes, resulting in masticatory efficiency being similar to healthy individuals [43, 61, 66]. Mapelli et al. [64] have observed that during chewing, patients with painful TMD recruited more muscles from the balancing side, specially the masseter, generating more functional imbalance and asymmetry in both masticatory sides. These conditions probably occurred to avoid pain and noises/displacements in joints, since chewing is a vital function related to surviving.

In this regard, Rodrigues et al. [43] found that the masticatory pattern in patients with TMD is altered, but there is no impairment or damage to the masticatory function or efficiency. Even in the presence of TMD signs and symptoms, these patients still need to chew, be it by adaptation or compensation, which in the long term can contribute to worsening of the pain [60, 65, 66].

Even if the scientific literature points to a strong association between unilateral chewing and the presence of TMD signs and symptoms [43, 47, 61, 67], the casual relation has not been demonstrated since plenty of individuals presented unilateral chewing and have not developed TMD. Other factors are more important in developing this condition, such as emotional issues and the presence of parafunctional habits. Nevertheless, alterations in such an important function like chewing may be one more factor that contributes to a painful and disordered condition and thus deserves attention in screening and in therapeutic intervention.

In summary, patients with TMD frequently complain about pain, noises and limitations in chewing, which generates compensations and altered masticatory patterns, in comparison to patients without TMD. There are many factors which should be taken into consideration while analyzing chewing, especially those related to dental/occlusal and muscular components (characteristics of masticatory muscles and facial profile). Even with these differences in chewing, it is still not clear whether patients with TMD present a worsen or diminished capable chewing.

17.3.3 Relation between TMD and chewing

TMD, being musculoskeletal conditions, often present pain or its exacerbation during orofacial functions. Among them, chewing is the one that demands the most effort from the stomatognathic system and consequently it is the most common complaint from many patients with TMD [43, 61]. Its performance is influenced by a series of variables, which can act as confounding factors in clinical and instrumental analysis, for example: age, occlusal interferences, dental losses, variables related to the examination, type of food or presence of pain, besides other conditions that can impair the muscular power of contraction, such as degenerative diseases [63].

It is known that in the presence of pain, mandibular kinetics may suffer significant alterations, affecting the mechanisms of neuromuscular control, which interfere in the activity of the masticatory muscles, and other structures associated to the stomatognathic system [60, 68]. Patients with TMD may show limitations in mandibular movements or perform them at a slower pace when compared to healthy individuals [69]. This limitation has the purpose of avoiding pain exacerbation, by taking more time to chew the food, with higher number of masticatory strokes and with more careful movements [43]. Complementary to these findings, during orofacial myofunctional assessment and therapy, patients with painful TDM frequently experience greater difficulty and decreased ability to chew, which is proportional to the intensity of pain and to the severity of TMD. That means that the greater the pain, and the more severe or chronic the pain is, the more alterations are found in the masticatory function [47].

The results of the electromyographic evaluation

of chewing are often inconsistent and controversial. Some studies have found a higher activity of the masseter and anterior temporalis muscles, associated with a lower precision of movements and an increased function during laterality of the jaw, on both working and balancing sides [43, 45, 47]. Other studies revealed reduced electromyographic activity, lower number of masticatory cycles, and lower masticatory frequency in patients with TMD in comparison to control subjects [13, 60]. Another interesting finding in these studies is the greater activation of the temporalis muscles in comparison to the masseter muscles, related to the presence of increased occlusal contact of the anterior teeth, along with changes in the mandibular kinetics, due to the presence of pain. Other signs and symptoms are usually present, such as noises of the joints, which may modify the masticatory pattern, altering or adapting the function. It is important to state that noises per se do not cause articular alterations, as they are a symptom of something else going on in the TMJ capsule [47, 60, 70].

A preferential side for chewing is indicated when the activity is performed consistently, or prevalently on the left side, or on the right side of the dental arches. It is unknown if this preference is related to an involvement of the central nervous system, or to peripheral factors, such as occlusion and type of food. In the general population, there is a higher preference for chewing on the right side, which is also found in patients with painful TMD [71, 72]. A recent study has suggested that unilateral chewing seems to be a common factor in the development of bruxism during sleep and in TMD, however it must not be directly considered a risk or casual factor [72].

Another study published in 2017 proposed an index named Masticatory Stability Index (MSI), whose purpose is to assess the stability of masticatory cycles in various conditions. The MSI was successful in differentiating patients with TMD patients from asymptomatic individuals [73]. The instrumental evaluation of chewing though the MSI and other methods, such as SEMG or fuchsin granules to measure masticatory efficiency, contribute to the clinical evaluation of this function and can provide a guide to decide which patients with TMD patients would benefit from orofacial myofunction therapy.

Thus, there is an intrinsic relation between painful TMD and alterations in masticatory functions, even though it is not possible to determine if these alterations occur because of the signs and symptoms of TMD, or if the reporting of pain and other signs and symptoms lead to these alterations. What is known so far, is that patients with TMD often complain about pain during chewing and that their masticatory standard is different from healthy individuals presenting slower mandibular movements, decreased coordination, with more masticatory strokes and longer chewing time. It is evident that this orofacial function must be evaluated thoroughly by trained professionals and, if necessary, some therapeutic interventions must be applied so that rehabilitation and chewing adaptation are proposed to patients with painful TMD.

17.4 Case report

General information: R.C.M.S., female, 41 years old, complains about pain on her face when waking up and during chewing for the last 15 years (intensity of pain: 6 at a visual analogic scale) (Fig. 17.1). Worsen-

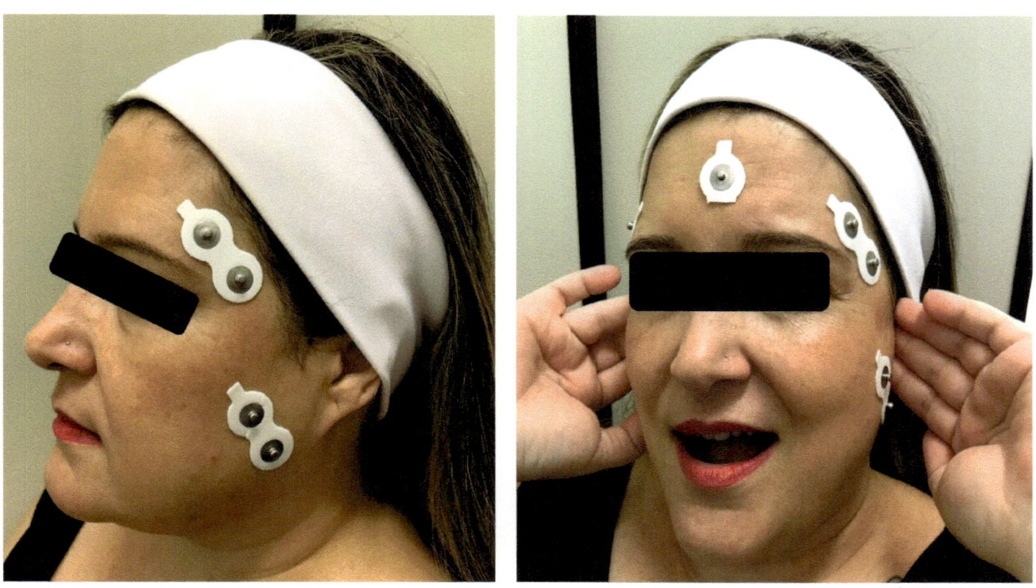

Fig. 17.1 Indication of myofascial pain sites: pre-auricular and parotid-masseteric region, limitation of mouth opening, difficulty in performing mandibular movements.

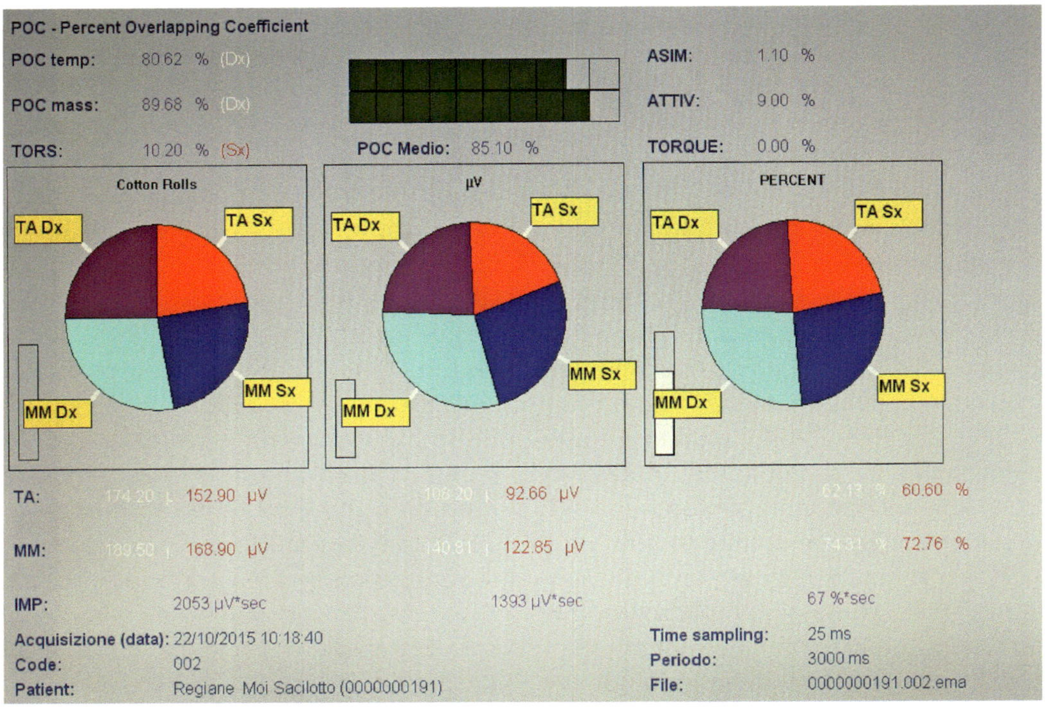

Fig. 17.2 Static surface electromyography's analysis before the interocclusal stabilizing splint, with the values of the electromyographic index, demonstrating an imbalance in the muscle activity.

ing factors: stress and anxiety. Triggering factors: chewing hard food and talking for a prolonged time. Improving factors: massage and heat pad. She reports clenching her teeth during the day and bruxing at night. She wakes up with her facial muscles rigid and in pain. She reports other oral habits: biting her lips and cheeks and biting objects (pens and others).

Clinical examination: patient experiences pain while touching bilaterally the masseter, temporal and cervical regions; she has absence of noise in the temporomandibular joints; she has limited mouth opening (active –29 mm, passive –32 mm); her reported pain on the right side of the temporalis and masseter muscles radiates to her teeth; she experiences pain

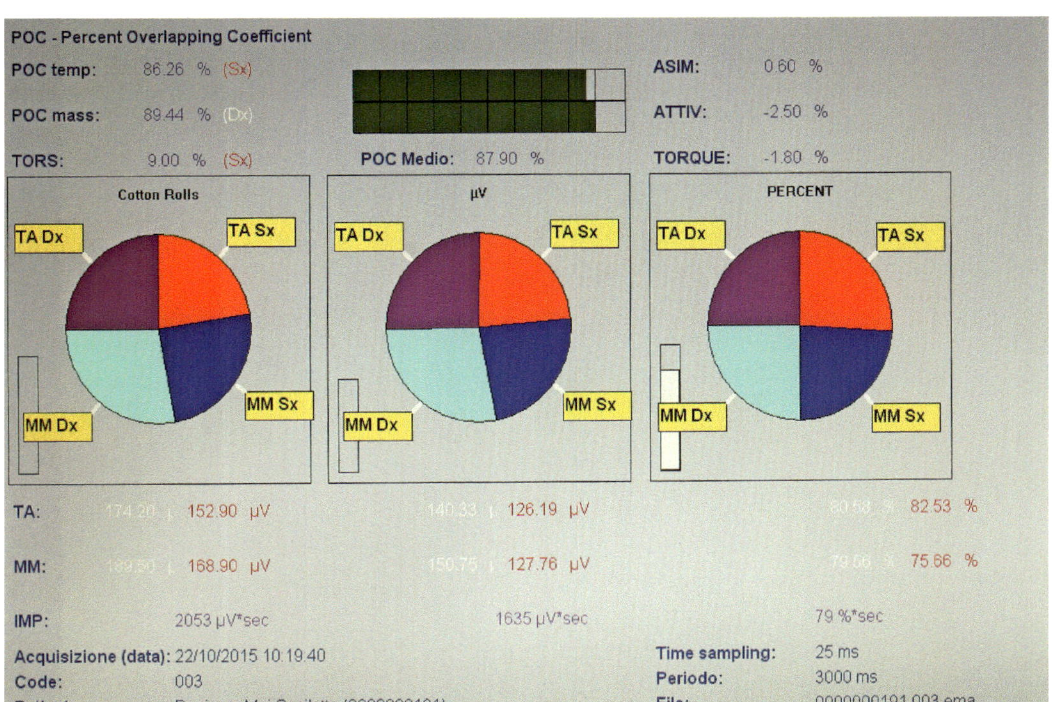

Fig. 17.3 Static surface electromyography's analysis after the stabilizing interocclusal splint, with the values of the electromyographic index, demonstrating a balance in the muscle activity when compared to the Figure 17.2.

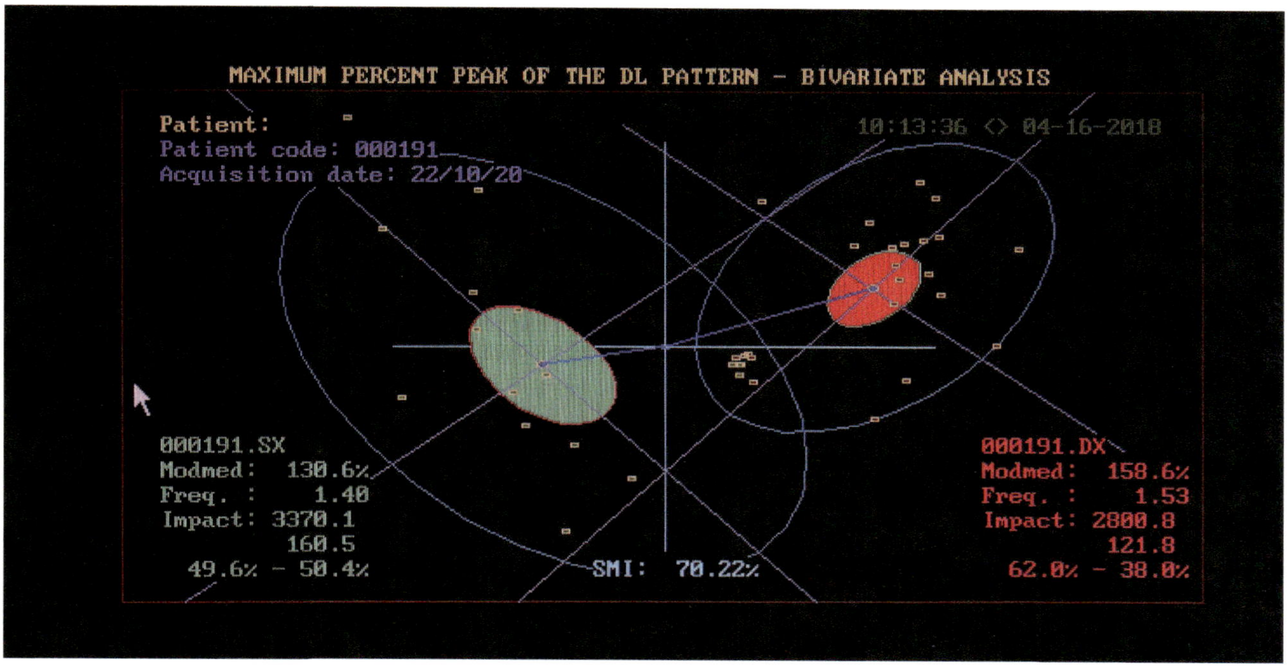

Fig. 17.4 Analysis of chewing surface electromyography, with the ellipses demonstrating the movements performed during masticatory cycles.

Table 17.2 Comparison of static electromyographic analysis on maximum voluntary contraction (initial and after treatment moments in the maximum intercuspation position): POC (Temporalis, Masseter and Mean), Asymmetry, Activity, Torque, TORS and IMPACT (electromyographic indexes)

Maximum voluntary contraction	*Initial*	*After treatment*
POC Temporalis	80.62%	86.26%
POC Masseter	89.68%	89.44%
POC Mean	85.10%	87.90%
Asymmetry	1.10%	0.60%
Activity	9.0%	2.5%
Torque	1.80%	0.0%
TORS	10.20%	9.0%
IMPACT	67%	79%

Source: own elaboration. POC: percental overlapping coefficient (%), Asymmetry: asymmetry index, Activity: activation index, Torque: torque index, TORS: torsion index, IMPACT: impact index.

Table 17.3 Analysis of the chewing electromyography for the right and left sides of the face: module, number of cycles, frequency, working and balancing side, IMPACT and SMI

Chewing EMG	*Right side*	*Left Side*
Module	149.26	82.5
Number of cycles	12	21
Frequency	1.53	1.4
Working side	62	49.6
Balancing side	38	50.4
IMPACT	11.7%	160.5%
SMI	70.22	

Source: own elaboration. IMPACT: impact index, SMI: symmetry Index.

during laterality movements and protrusion of the jaw. The diagnosis is based on the criteria described in the Diagnostic Criteria for Temporomandibular Disorders (DC/TMD): myofascial pain trigger points with referred pain.

Treatment: Training in self-awareness in controlling deleterious oral habits; applying a humid pad to the head and face 3 times a day for 20 minutes; massaging the face in circular motions; performing isotonic exercises of mouth opening and closing with tongue support on the palate, in 10 repetitions after using heat pads; use of cell phone application "*Desencoste seus Dentes*" (don't close your teeth) for learning and controlling daytime bruxism; superior rigid occlusal plate; and dry needling for trigger points of masseter and temporalis muscles.

Electromyographic evaluation: The results of SEMG analysis are summarized in Tables 17.2 and 17.3, and Figs. 17.2, 17.3 and 17.4.

REFERENCES

1. Ferrario VF, Sforza C, Tartaglia GM, Dellavia C. Immediate effect of a stabilization splint on masticatory muscle activity in temporomandibular disorder patients. J Oral Rehabil 2002; 29(9): 810-5.
2. Ferrario VF, Sforza C, Colombo A, Ciusa V. An electromyographic investigation of masticatory muscles symmetry in normo-occlusion subjects. J Oral Rehabil 2000; 27: 33-40.
3. Ferrario VF, Sforza C, Serrao G. The influence of crossbite on the coordinated electromyographic activity of human masticatory muscles during mastication. J Oral Reabil 1999; 26(7): 575-81.
4. Ferrario VF, Sforza C. Coordinated electromyographic activity of the human masseter and temporalis anterior muscles during mastication. Eur J Oral Sci 1996; 104(5-6): 511-7.
5. Lodetti G, Marano G, Fontana P, Tartaglia GM, Maria de Felício C, Biganzoli E, et al. Surface electromyography and magnetic resonance imaging of the masticatory muscles in patients with arthrogenous temporomandibular disorders. Oral Surg Oral Med Oral Pathol Oral Radiol 2014; 118(2): 248-56.
6. Botelho AL, Brochini APZ, Martins MM, Melchior MO, Silva AMBR, Silva MAMR. Avaliação eletromiográfica de assimetria dos músculos mastigatórios em sujeitos com oclusão normal. RFO 2008; 13(3): 7-12.
7. Marchiori SC, Vitti M. Eletromiografia na fala: como e por quê? In: Marquesan IQ; Zorzi J, Dias Gomes I. Tópicos em fonoaudiologia. São Paulo: Lovise 1996; 289-93.
8. Ferrario VF, Sforza C. Biomechanical model of the human mandible in unilateral clench: distribution of temporomandibular joint reaction forces between working and balancing sides. J Prosthet Dent 1994; 72(2): 169-176.
9. Arita CA. Análise eletromiográfica e eletrognatográfica da Estimulação Elétrica Transcutânea (T.E.N.S) em pacientes com dor-disfunção miofascial – efeitos sobre os valores da distância interoclusal e posição de repouso mandibular [dissertation]. Faculdade de Odontologia de Ribeirão Preto: Universidade de São Paulo, Ribeirão Preto; 2000.
10. Sgobbi de Faria CR, Bérzin F. Electromyographic study of the temporal, masseter and suprahyoid muscles in the mandibular rest position. J Oral Rehabil 1998; 25(10): 776-80.
11. Kogawa EM, Calderon JR, Lauris JRP, Araújo CRP, Conti PC. Evaluation of maximal bite force in temporomandibular disorders patients. J Oral Rehabil 2006; 33(8): 559-65.
12. Palinkas M, Nassar MS, Cecílio FA, Siéssere S, Semprini M, Machado-de-Sousa JP, et al. Age and gender influence on maximal bite force and masticatory muscles thickness. Arch Oral Biol 2010; 55(10): 797-802.
13. Da Silva AMBR, Magri LV, da Silva MAMR, Sousa Neto MD. Are the bite force and electromyographic activity altered in muscle TMD patients with abfraction lesions? Cranio 2017; 24: 1-7.
14. Gibbs CH, Anusavice KJ, Young HM, Jones JS, Esquivel-Upshaw JF. Maximum clenching force of patients with moderate loss of posterior tooth support: a pilot study. J Prosthet Dent 2002; 88(5): 498-502.
15. Meena A, Jain V, Singh N, Arora N, Jha R. Effect of implant-supported prosthesis on the bite force and masticatory efficiency in subjects with shortened dental arches. J Oral Rehabil 2014; 41(2): 87-92.
16. Al-Omiri MK, Sghaireen MG, Alhijawi MM, Alzoubi IA, Lynch CD, Lynch E. Maximum bite force following unilateral implant-supported prosthetic treatment: within-subject comparison to opposite dentate side. J Oral Rehabil 2014; 41(8): 624-9.
17. Bavia PF, Vilanova LS, Garcia RC. Craniofacial Morphology Affects Bite Force in Patients with Painful Temporomandibular Disorders. Braz Dent J 2016; 27(5): 619-24.
18. Quiudini PR Jr, Pozza DH, Pinto ADS, de Arruda MF, Guimarães AS. Differences in bite force between dolichofacial and brachyfacial individuals: Side of mastication, gender, weight and height. J Prosthodont Res 2017; 61(3): 283-9.
19. Pizolato RA, Gavião MB, Berretin-Felix G, Sampaio AC, Trindade Junior AS. Maximal bite force in young adults with temporomandibular disorders and bruxism. Braz Oral Res 2007; 21(3): 278-83.
20. Hotta PT, Hotta TH, Bataglion C, Pavão RF, Siéssere S, Regalo SC. Bite force in temporomandibular dysfunction (TMD) and healthy complete denture wearers. Braz Dent J 2008; 19(4): 354-7.
21. Palinkas M, Bataglion C, de Luca Canto G, Machado Camolezi N, Theodoro GT, Siéssere S, et al. Impact of sleep bruxism on masseter and temporalis muscles and bite force. Cranio 2016; 34(5): 309-15.
22. Jensen R, Rasmussen BK, Pedersen B, Lous I, Olesen J. Cephalic muscle tenderness and pressure pain threshold in a general population. Pain 1992; 48(2): 197-203.
23. Santos Silva RS, Conti PC, Lauris JR, da Silva RO, Pegoraro LF. Pressure pain threshold in the detection of masticatory myofascial pain: an algometer-based study. J Orofac Pain 2005; 19(4): 318-24.
24. Farella M, Michelotti A, Steenks MH, Romeo R, Cimino R, Bosman F. The diagnostic value of pressure algometry in myofascial pain of the jaw muscles. J Oral Rehabil 2000; 27(1): 9-14.
25. Więckiewicz W, Woźniak K, Piątkowska D, Szyszka-Sommerfeld L, Lipski M. The diagnostic value of pressure algometry for temporomandibular disorders. Biomed Res Int 2015; 2015: 575038.
26. Campi LB, Jordani PC, Tenan HL, Camparis CM, Gonçalves DA. Painful temporomandibular disorders and central sensitization: implications for management-a pilot study. Int J Oral Maxillofac Surg 2017; 46(1): 104-10.
27. Cunha CO, Pinto-Fiamengui LM, Castro AC, Lauris JR, Conti PC. Determination of a pressure pain threshold cut-off value for the diagnosis of temporomandibular joint arthralgia. J Oral Rehabil 2014; 41(5): 323-9.
28. Woda A, L'heveder G, Ouchchane L, Bodéré C. Effect of experimental stress in 2 different pain conditions affecting the facial muscles. J Pain 2013; 14(5): 455-66.
29. Vedolin GM, Lobato VV, Conti PC, Lauris JR. The impact of stress and anxiety on the pressure pain threshold of myofascial pain patients. J Oral Rehabil 2009; 36(5): 313-21.
30. Schiffman E, Ohrbach R, Truelove E, Look J, Anderson G, Goulet JP, et al.; International RDC/TMD Consortium Network, International association for Dental Research; Orofacial Pain Special Interest Group, International Association for the Study of Pain. Diagnostic Criteria for Temporomandibular Disorders (DC/TMD) for Clinical and Research Applications: recommendations of the International RDC/TMD Consortium Network* and Orofacial

Pain Special Interest Group†. J Oral Facial Pain Headache 2014; 28(1): 6-27.
31. Slade GD, Sanders AE, Ohrbach R, Fillingim RB, Dubner R, Gracely RH, et al. Pressure pain thresholds fluctuate with, but do not usefully predict, the clinical course of painful temporomandibular disorder. Pain 2014; 155(10): 2134-43.
32. Greenspan JD, Slade GD, Bair E, Dubner R, Fillingim RB, Ohrbach R, et al. Pain sensitivity and autonomic factors associated with development of TMD: the OPPERA prospective cohort study. J Pain 2013; 14(12 Suppl): T63-74,e1-6.
33. Escudeiro Santos C, de Freitas O, Spadaro AC, Mestriner-Junior W. Development of a colorimetric system for evaluation of the masticatory efficiency. Braz Dent J 2006; 17(2): 95-9.
34. Boretti G, Bickel M, Geering AH. A review of masticatory ability and efficiency. J Prosthet Dent 1995; 74(4): 400-3.
35. Hotta TH, Petenusci SO, Bataglion C, Matteo MAS, Suguiuti DB. Análise da eficiência mastigatória de indivíduos com dentição natural completa: estudo preliminar. J Bras Ortod Ortop Facial 2003; 8(48): 478-82.
36. Mestriner Junior W, Mazzetto MO, Felício CM, Freitas O, Spadaro ACC. Comparação da eficiência mastigatória avaliada pelo uso de um método colorimétrico nas dentições decídua e permanente. Jorn Bras de Ort e Orto Facial 2005; 10(57): 242-8.
37. Shi CS, Ouyang G, Guo TW. Comparison of food particle distribution masticated by subjects wearing complete dentures and with natural teeth. J Oral Rehabil 1990; 17(6): 611-5.
38. Mowlana F, Heath MR, Van der Bilt A, Van der Glas HW. Assessment of chewing efficiency: a comparison of particle size distribution determined using optical scanning and sieving of almonds. J Oral Rehabil 1994; 21(5): 545-51.
39. Mazzetto MO, Hotta TH, Petenusci SO, Mestriner Jr W, Yamasaki MK, De Paula MMV. Masticatory efficiency: analysis of correlation between two tests. RGO 2010; 58(3): 319-22.
40. Ribeiro JA, de Resende CM, Lopes AL, Mestriner W Jr, Roncalli AG, Farias-Neto A, Carreiro Ada F. Evaluation of complete denture quality and Masticatory efficiency in denture wearers. Int J Prosthodont 2012; 25(6): 625-30.
41. De Abreu RA, Pereira MD, Furtado F, Prado GP, Mestriner W Jr, Ferreira LM. Masticatory efficiency and bite force in individuals with normal occlusion. Arch Oral Biol 2014; 59(10): 1065-74.
42. Cazal MS, da Silva AM, Galo R, Junior WM, da Silva MA. Comparison of dynamic electromyographic analysis of masticatory capsules with materials of different textures. Cranio 2015; 23: 1-7.
43. Rodrigues CA, Melchior MO, Magri LV, Mestriner Jr W, Mazzetto MO. Is the masticatory function changed in patients with temporomandibular disorder? Bras Dent J 2015; 26(2): 181-5.
44. Moyers RE. Temporomandibular muscle contraction patterns in Angle Class II, division 1 malocclusions; an electromyographic analysis. Am J Orthod 1949; 35(11): 837-57.
45. De Felício CM, Ferreira CL, Medeiros AP, Rodrigues Da Silva MA, et al. Electromyographic indices, orofacial myofunctional status and temporomandibular disorders severity: A correlation study. J Electromyogr Kinesiol 2012; 22(2): 266-72.
46. Basmajian, JV; De Lucca, CJ. Muscles alive: their function revealed by eletromyography. Baltimore: Williams and Wilkins; 1962.
47. Ferreira CL, Machado BC, Borges CG, Da Silva MAMR, Sforza C, et al. Impaired orofacial motor functions on chronic temporomandibular disorders. J Electromyogr Kinesiol 2014; 24(4): 565-71.
48. Grubwieser G, Flatz A, Grunert I, Kofler M, Ulmer H, Gausch K, Kulmer S. Quantitative analysis of masseter and temporalis SEMGs: a comparison of anterior guided versus balanced occlusal concepts in patients wearing complete dentures. J Oral Rehabil 1999; 26: 731-6.
49. Raustia AM, Salonen MA, Pyhtinen J. Evaluation of masticatory muscles of edentulous patients by computed tomography and electromyography. J Oral Rehabil 1996; 23(1): 11-6.
50. McCarrol RS, Naeije M, Kim YK, Hansson TL. The immediate effect of splint-induced changes in jaw positioning on the asymmetry of submaximal masticatory muscle activity. J Oral Rehabil 1989; 16: 163-70.
51. Ohrbach R, Dworkin SF. The Evolution of TMD Diagnosis: Past, Present, Future. J Dent Res 2016; 95(10): 1093-101.
52. Slade GD, Ohrbach R, Greenspan JD, Fillingim RB, Bair E, Sanders AE, et al. Painful Temporomandibular Disorder: Decade of Discovery from OPPERA Studies. J Dent Res 2016; 95(10): 1084-92.
53. Scrivani SJ, Keith DA, Kaban LB. Temporomandibular disorders. N Engl J Med 2008; 359(25): 2693-705.
54. De Leeuw R, Klasser GD. Orofacial Pain: Guidelines for Assessment, Diagnosis, and Management. 5ª Ed. Quintessence: Charlotte, 2013.
55. Gonçalves DA, Dal Fabbro AL, Campos JA, Bigal ME, Speciali JG. Symptoms of temporomandibular disorders in the population: an epidemiological study. J Orofac Pain 2010; 24(3): 270-8.
56. Progiante PS, Pattussi MP, Lawrence HP, Goya S, Grossi PK, Grossi ML. Prevalence of Temporomandibular Disorders in an Adult Brazilian Community Population Using the Research Diagnostic Criteria (Axes I and II) for Temporomandibular Disorders (The Maringá Study). Int J Prosthodont 2015; 28(6): 600-9.
57. Dworkin SF, LeResche L. Research diagnostic criteria for temporomandibular disorders: review, criteria, examinations and specifications, critique. J Craniomandib Disord 1992; 6(4): 301-55.
58. Kim YK, Kim SG, Im JH, Yun PY. Clinical survey of the patients with temporomandibular joint disorders, using Research Diagnostic Criteria (Axis II) for TMD: preliminary study. J Craniomaxillofac Surg 2012; 40(4): 366-72.
59. List T, Jensen RH. Temporomandibular disorders: Old ideas and new concepts. Cephalalgia 2017; 37(7): 692-704.
60. De Felício CM, Mapelli A, Sidequersky FV, Tartaglia GM, Sforza C. Mandibular kinematics and masticatory muscles SEMG in patients with short lasting TMD of mild-moderate severity. J Electromyogr Kinesiol 2013; 23(3): 627-33.
61. De Felício CM, Melchior MO, Silva MAMR, Celeghini RMS. Masticatory performance in adults related to temporomandibular disorder and dental occlusion. Pro-Fono Rev 2007; 19(2): 151-8.
62. Hatch JP, Shinkai RS, Sakai S, Rugh JD, Paunovich ED. Determinants of masticatory performance in dentate adults. Arch Oral Biol 2001; 46(7): 641-8.
63. Mioche L, Bourdiol P, Monier S. Chewing behaviour and bolus formation during mastication of meat with different textures. Arch Oral Biol 2003; 48(3): 193-200.
64. Mapelli A, Zanandréa Machado BC, Giglio LD, Sforza C, De Felício CM. Reorganization of muscle activity in pa-

tients with chronic temporomandibular disorders. Arch Oral Biol 2016; 72: 164-71.

65. Tartaglia GM, da Silva MAMR, Bottini S, Sforza C, Ferrario VF. Masticatory muscle activity during maximum voluntary clench in different research diagnostic criteria for temporomandibular disorders (RDC/TMD) groups. Man Ther 2008; 13(5): 434-40.
66. Peroz I, Tai S. Masticatory performance in patients with anterior disk displacement without reduction in comparison with symptom-free volunteers. Eur J Oral Sci 2002; 110(5): 341-4.
67. Ratnasari A, Hasegawa K, Oki K, Kawakami S, Yanagi Y, Asaumi JI, et al. Manifestation of preferred chewing side for hard food on TMJ disc displacement side. J Oral Rehabil 2011; 38(1): 12-7.
68. Lobbezoo F, Van Selms MK, Naeije M. Masticatory muscle pain and disordered jaw motor behaviour: Literature review over the past decade. Arch Oral Biol 2006; 51(9): 713-20.
69. Bakke M, Hansdottir R. Mandibular function in patients with temporomandibular joint pain: a 3-year follow-up. Oral Surg Oral Med Oral Pathol Oral Radiol Endod 2008; 106(2): 227-34.
70. Tartaglia GM, Lodetti G, Paiva G, De Felicio CM, Sforza C. Surface electromyographic assessment of patients with long lasting temporomandibular joint disorder pain. J Electromyogr Kinesiol 2011; 21(4): 659-64.
71. Diernberger S, Bernhardt O, Schwahn C, Kordass B. Self-reported chewing side preference and its associations with occlusal, temporomandibular and prosthodontic factors: results from the population-based Study of Health in Pomerania (SHIP-0). J Oral Rehabil 2008; 35(8): 613-20.
72. Yalçın Yeler D, Yılmaz N, Koraltan M, Aydın E. A survey on the potential relationships between TMD, possible sleep bruxism, unilateral chewing, and occlusal factors in Turkish university students. Cranio 2017; 35(5): 308-14.
73. Pimenta Ferreira CL, Zago M, de Felício CM, Sforza C. An index for the evaluation of 3D masticatory cycles stability. Arch Oral Biol 2017; 83: 124-9.

18 Relationship between myofunctional therapy and nutrition

Joy L. Moeller

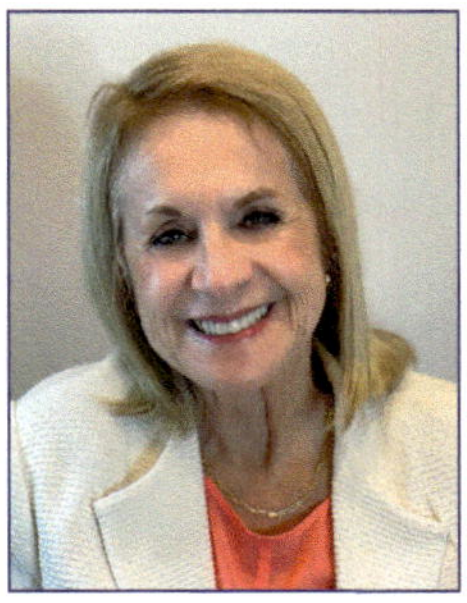

18.1 What is myofunctional therapy?

Myofunctional Therapy (MT) is the neurologic re-education of the orofacial muscles. It is a rehabilitation therapy program designed to re-pattern stomatognathic functions, such as chewing, swallowing and breathing. This is accomplished through the use of therapeutic techniques and positive behavioral modification. The dynamics of chewing alone may help to guide the growth to develop in an ideal manner, as therapy allows the brain to develop new neural pathways to the muscles through repetition and time, which is commonly known as neuroplasticity. Repetition of the therapeutic techniques will increase the strength, tone and coordination of the stomatognathic muscles, and because the muscles influence the bones to which they are attached, they help to develop facial symmetry. The purposes of these exercises are to:

- Recover and improve muscle tone and dyskinetic muscle function
- Re-acquire correct posture: Lips, tongue, and jaw rest posture as well as head and neck posture
- Re-educate functions (swallowing, chewing and breathing)
- Reduce and eliminate habits such as thumb sucking, pacifier use, nail biting, lip or hair sucking or biting, tongue sucking, leaning and others using awareness and behavior modification.

In the United States, MT includes breathing education as well as chewing and proper swallowing to assist in the treatment of myofunctional disorders. New clinical studies are showing that breathing education must be included in the treatment of patients with sleep disorders [1]. Myofunctional therapists look at the volume of air, the correct muscles to use such as the diaphragm, and nasal breathing as opposed to mouth breathing. In order to attain optimal results, MF therapists work collaboratively with ENTs, Allergists, Osteopathic Physicians, Orthodontists and other allied health care professionals.

Awareness and elimination of oral habits must be addressed conjointly with the myofunctional pathology [2]. Myofunctional therapists will look at the *cause* of nail biting, thumb sucking, bruxism, lip biting or licking, chewing on pens or pencils and many other noxious habits that people develop because of a myofunctional disorder. Then a program is instituted that includes behavior modification, awareness and replacement of the habits with proper positive habits, which will help to motivate patients to succeed.

Joy L. Moeller, RDH, OMT
Academy of Orofacial Myofunctional Therapy (AOMT)

Email: joyleamoeller@aol.com

18.2 Brief history of myofunctional therapy

Myofunctional therapy is an area of specialization arising out of orthodontics, although there are some studies from Italy dating back to the 1400s, about training muscles of the orofacial complex. Many dentists during the 1800s and 1900s recognized that tongue rest position, mouth breathing and oral habits influenced dental occlusion.

Edward H. Angle, rightly termed by some as the one of the fathers of orthodontics, wrote "Malocclusion of the Teeth" appearing in Dental Cosmos in 1907, in which he recognized the influence of the facial muscles on dental occlusion. In his research Angle concluded that mouth breathing was the chief etiological factor in malocclusion.

The first program of MT in the USA began in 1918 with an article written by an orthodontist Dr. Alfred P. Rogers entitled "Living Orthodontic Appliances". He was one of the first doctors in the United States to suggest that corrective exercises would develop tonicity and proper muscle function, thereby influence proper occlusion, and that breathing was the chief etiological factor in malocclusion.

18.3 The mainstreaming of MT

The field of MT is gaining greater acceptance today because a greater number of peer-reviewed articles are published in well-regarded journals every year, and because MT is increasingly connected to the fields of sleep disorders [3], orthodontics and oral-facial pain. Evidence based science is focusing more on myofunctional disorders as the demand for services increases. Two meta-analyses were published in the last few years on applications of MT in snoring [4, 5] and sleep apnea [6, 7], which have lead the way for much interest in MT as an adjunctive treatment.

18.4 Etiology of myofunctional disorders and the role of nutrition

The etiology of myofunctional disorders relates to civilization and the desire of moms to become "modern" and efficient in child care. However, with the advent of processed baby foods, bottle feeding, pacifiers, spouted cups and baby furniture that amuses the infant during feeding, the growth and development of a baby is being led by industry instead of a mothers' intuition.

The suck, swallow, breathing mechanism of breastfeeding is being disrupted by a non-physiological rubber or silicone nipple on a bottle, which encourages the tongue to rest down on the floor of the mouth instead of up against the palate. The correct swallowing mechanism is being replaced by a tongue thrust swallow, in which the tongue pushes forward rather than upward against the palate as it would be the norm. Then with pacifiers, thumb or finger sucking, or spouted cups, the low rest posture of the tongue is reinforced, causing, over time, a high narrow palate, which also impacts the functionality of the nose and nasal breathing.

The molar teeth are the major grinding surface of the dentition. A toddler not used to gnaw and chew food over time develops aversion for tougher textures. Plus, unchecked tight or short lingual, labial and/or buccal frena may lead to the patient not having the ability to move the food efficiently into the molar area. The result is the desire for soft or refined foods in which minimal or no chewing is needed before swallowing the food. Therefore, the first oral stage of digestion is compromised, and the flow of enzymes contained in the saliva is limited, contributing to poor digestion [8]. The muscles of mastication do not develop correctly, which may lead to oral facial pain or the articular disk becoming displaced [9], which may also cause pain or discomfort.

Myofunctional therapy now includes frenum inspection and treatment with exercises and stretching both before and after frenum removal to restore normal function [10]. If the lingual, labial or buccal frenum are restricted, that may lead to not being able to move the food into a comfortable place on the molar teeth to chew properly or to be able to properly rest the tongue up against the palate, keep the lips together, and to swallow correctly.

For patients with restricted oral tissues, MT is mandatory and a key in obtaining a complete recovery of functionality [11]. This will reduce or possibly avoid relapse or surgical release revision in the future. For infants, it's necessary to implement stretching, stroking and massaging the tongue after surgery with a therapeutic salve such as coconut oil or vitamin E oil, combined with breastfeeding. The motion of breastfeeding then becomes easier, and it can be used as therapy tool for both parent and child.

If the patient is not chewing properly, the cranium and the head and neck muscles may not develop properly, affecting the underlining bones. Often there may not be enough space for the dentition to erupt properly. The width of the palate may be compromised and the anterior-posterior plane may be shortened causing an airway problem. Without attaining proper oral-rest posture, the palate and the maxilla may collapse into a narrow, ogival or gothic shape. The result of a high narrow palate may also lead to mouth breathing. The roof of the mouth is also the floor of the nose and to properly develop and maintain it, the nasal cavity requires proper postural support from the tongue.

Proper oral rest posture includes:

1) The entire dorsal surface of the tongue to be lightly suctioned to the palate comfortably
2) The lips comfortable sealed at rest, without "bracing" or tension during the swallow
3) The teeth slightly apart.

18.5 How does poor oral-rest posture effect proper nutrition?

The first stage of digestion starts in the mouth with chewing. If the patient does not take the time to chew [8], enzymes are not pre-digesting the food properly. Smelling food correctly increases appetite. When people do not breathe through their nose, they cannot smell, the desire to eat may decrease and hyposmia may develop. Moreover, those who habitually keep their mouth open struggle to breathe and chew at the same time, often become "picky" eaters and develop texture sensitivity problems.

Patients with habitual open lips or worse, mouth breathing, may experience dry mouth and dehydration, which in children, often becomes desire for sodas and sugary drinks. Open lips during chewing is unsightly and impolite, plus, because the swallowing sequence starts at the lips, if they are not in contact then a compensatory sequence occurs, usually defined as "tongue thrust swallow".

The patients may trap air when they swallow if the interaction tongue-palate is not adequate. This trapped air may cause stomach distress and bloating and lead to aerophagia and gastroenterological problems [12].

In general terms, the type of food eaten leads to the health of the patient. The patient may reach for soft, refined foods without the need for chewing which lead to consuming more calories than needed. This may lead to obesity and other eating and digestive disorders.

18.6 Treatment

Initially, in therapy, we will observe and bring to the awareness of the patient oral habits that have developed and explain how myofunctional therapists may help to eliminate them. Many therapists use behavior modification and rewards, but gaining awareness of the problems that may develop and how to stop it is usually a choice that the patient makes. A good therapist will guide the patients and support their success.

Depending on frequency, duration and intensity, these oral habits such as mouth breathing, thumb sucking, nail, lip, hair or object chewing, may interfere with proper growth and development of the mouth and face. The tongue and lips, once properly re-patterned to their optimal function, will replace the habit. If implemented early enough, the treatment may also help to prevent some orthodontic and periodontal problems.

The active retraining of the functions in myofunctional disorders thus include activating muscles in the face and neck, and re-patterning them to optimize proper functions. Myofunctional therapists generally work alongside a team of health care professionals: dentists, orthodontists, physicians, physical therapists, speech pathologists, occupational therapists and many others.

Myofunctional therapy is a therapeutic program by which even some problems of speech articulation are often improved because the patients have better control of their muscle functions and tongue placement. There are eight intrinsic and extrinsic muscles of the tongue, which need to work independently and interdependently to articulate sounds. These muscles are involved in breathing, chewing, swallowing, sleeping and rest posture, therefore their re-patterning may benefit more than one function at the time.

Therapy begins with training the tongue to rest up in the palate, to keep the lips closed and breathe nasally. One way this is accomplished is by having the patient to hold an orthodontic elastic to the roof of the mouth with the tongue, for a defined period of time, with the lips together [13]. During the same appointment, the patient may use different strings and buttons and chewing devices, in order to activate, coordinate or relax the muscles of mastication, the tongue muscles and the perioral muscles.

Proper symmetrical chewing, gathering the food in the middle of the tongue, and swallowing without the assistance of the perioral muscles is a very important part of myofunctional treatment, as monolateral chewing has been shown exacerbate TMD symptoms [9].

Myofunctional therapy is progressive, with sequential exercises that become more advanced over time. Certain exercises are repeated depending on the needs of the patient, focusing on the goals of therapy. The therapy program is usually done over a period of one year to attain long-term retention of the results. Many therapists will begin with an intensive eight-week program then follow ups every other week, then every three weeks and then slowly titrate the patients off of the exercises and encourage them to generalize and habituate the new pattern with an internal awareness of proper function. Therapists will also address proper table eating posture as an important part of success. If a patient is sitting with a forward head posture, it is much more difficult to swallow correctly. Many times, the collaboration with an osteopathic physician, a physical therapist or a chiropractor may be necessary in order to accomplish the best result on posture.

The reasons why people learn the abnormal habits and patterns may require more than what the myofunctional therapist is able to provide with behavior modification and awareness. Because so many learned behaviors and protective mechanisms may have a psychological component, sometimes a psychologist is also a professional whose collaboration may be needed.

18.7 Motivation

Since the success of myofunctional therapy relies on active patient participation, we must use several techniques that are based on the ten principles of neuroplasticity. Neuroplasticity refers to the ability of the brain to change, following physiologic or pathologic input, generating an adaptive response. Some techniques [14] used are:

- Use it or lose it: if the patient is given softer foods for a while, such as a holiday for the summer at a camp with a diet of processed soft foods, they will find it difficult to eat whole foods when they return home.
- Use it and improve it: when the patient returns home, the parents offer them raw vegetables, fruits and meats, and the muscle functions improve.
- Plasticity is experience specific: if the patient only eats soft foods, the muscles do not move much and atrophy or become plastic and stiff.
- Repetition matters: every day, at lunch, when they are very hungry, the patients are given a fresh, raw carrot and a whole delicious apple, so they develop a pattern of enjoying chewing harder foods.
- Intensity matters: if the patient is given harder foods and taught to chew very well before swallowing, the intensity for chewing may become enjoyable and the brain understands that foods must be masticated thoroughly before swallowing.
- Time matters: ever since the patients' teeth all erupted, they were allowed an hour to enjoy chewing their foods, even if they played in between swallows. Many times, children only have 5-10 minutes to dine and chewing is not possible.
- Salience matters: when the family, the therapist, and finally the patient understands the importance of proper chewing, the patient will remember to do it properly. We need to make sure the patient understands the benefits of chewing properly. For instance, discussing when food is chewed slowly and properly, stomachaches may disappear and the food may taste better.
- Age matters: a very young child may be in mixed dentition, and it may be uncomfortable to chew with loose teeth. An older patient may not have any teeth and their denture may not fit properly and it may be uncomfortable to chew. Then even if they are properly fitted with a new denture, the muscles may need to be strengthened in order to chew again.
- Transference: learning a new technique of eating will not transfer to a permanent behavior, unless the patient understands the value of the change and is willing to commit to the time and consistency of practicing. Practice makes permanent, not perfect, but the patient must understand the value and really want to make a change.

Quoting Abraham Maslow:

"Human life will never be understood unless its highest aspirations are taken into account. Growth, self-actualization, the striving toward health, the quest for identity and autonomy, the yearning for excellence (and other ways of phrasing the striving "upward") must by now be accepted beyond question as a widespread and perhaps universal human tendency..." (Maslow, 1954, Motivation and Personality, pp.xii-xiii)

Therapists may need to obtain a commitment from the patient to complete a minimum of one year of treatment, as it takes long time to establish new neuroplastic patterns. Moreover, they must look at what is the patient's perception of why they are pursuing the treatment and what they hope to accomplish by doing the therapy, with a clear understanding that the final goal is optimization of the basic functions of nasal breathing, chewing and swallowing. Therefore, eating meals becomes part of the therapeutic process, as eating different food textures and increasing chewing efficiency.

Use of videos for visual feedback has taken commitment to a whole new level of success. If the patient can see the dysfunction during the act of swallowing food or liquid, such a visual cue will encourage commitment. Photos can show occlusal relationships as well as posture, facial shape, asymmetry and other abnormalities. These visual aids may assist the patient in continuing the therapy because they are engaged in seeing the positive changes. Understanding the functional pattern allows the patients to self-monitor in their daily lives, thus facilitating generalization of the correct patterns over time.

Working in a team will help motivate the patient for better compliance because the reinforcement by the team allows the patient a greater sense of responsibility to do their exercises and to modify their eating habits and food choices. It helps the patient to know that other professionals see a value in MT and it is key to long-term stability.

18.8 Nutritional counseling

Part of a patient assessment should be a diet survey to look for the texture and quality of foods eaten. Therapists must encourage patients to eat "real" food, as whole as possible. Processed, blended foods will encourage the patient to eat soft food and stop chewing thereby inhibiting the muscle functions, while firm foods (such as raw carrots or apples) are encouraged. MT encourages chewing at least until the bolus or portion of chewed up food is smooth.

Nutritional counseling may begin with having the patients keep a diet diary of everything they eat or drink for one week and then circling in red the healthier whole foods to have the patient focus on eating more of those foods. Also, with liquids, water is preferable to sodas and juices because otherwise patients may satiate too soon and avoid solids.

Motivation is the key to creating change. Small children might like having small "parties" with their friends. Carrot sticks, celery, apples, cucumber wedges, pepper strips and other crunchy fruits and vegetables with different types of dips to try to make the food tasty and fun. When children see their friends trying the foods, they may be encouraged to try a little bit. Making the activity fun and making a game out of it, may start the ability to select better choices. Also, educating the parent to have these snacks available at home may be necessary to complete the behavior changes which will affect the entire family. Having easy-to-read articles and books available will also help to encourage changes.

18.9 Conclusion

Chewing, breathing and swallowing affects many aspects of health. Even oral facial pain [15], orthodontic instability and sleep disorders [5] may be improved by restoring basic functions. Myofunctional therapy must be included in a nutritional program to restore proper function in order to support the patient reaching a higher level of success in choosing proper nutritional choices. Even small decisions improve overall function and therapists will support the patient reaching better and more stable health.

REFERENCES

1. Guilleminault C, Sullivan SS. Towards restoration of continuous nasal breathing as the ultimate treatment goal in pediatric obstructive sleep apnea. Pediatr Neonatal Biol 2014; 1: 1-7.
2. Shahraki N, Yassaei S, Goldani Moghadam M. Abnormal oral habits: A review. Journal of Dentistry and Oral Hygiene 2012; 4(2): 12-5.
3. Guimarães KC, Drager LF, Genta PR, et al. Effects of oropharyngeal exercises on patients with moderate obstructive sleep apnea syndrome. Am J Respir Crit Care Med 2009; 179(10): 962-6.
4. Camacho M, Guilleminault C, Wei JM, Song SA, Noller MW, Reckley LK, Fernandez-Salvador C, Zaghi S. Oropharyngeal and Tongue Exercises (Myofunctional Therapy) for snoring: A Systemic Review and Meta-Analysis. Eur Arch Otorhinolaryngol 2018; 275(4): 849-55.
5. Camacho M, Certal V, Abdullatif J, Zaghi S, Ruoff CM, Capasso R, Kushida CA. Myofunctional Therapy to Treat Obstructive Sleep Apnea: A systemic review and Meta-Analysis: Sleep 2015; 38(5): 669-75.
6. Bandyopadhyay A, Kaneshiro K, CamachM. Effect of myofunctional therapy on Children with obstructive sleep apnea: a meta-analysis. Med 2020; 75: 210-7.
7. de Felício CM, da Silva Dias FV, Trawitzki LVV. Obstructive sleep apnea: focus on myofunctional therapy. Nat Sci Sleep 2018; 10: 271-86.
8. Coceani Paskay L. Chewing, Biting, Clenching, Bruxing, and Oral Health, Oral Health, March 2016.
9. Ferreira CL, Machado BC, Borges CG, Rodrigues Da Silva MA, Sforza C, De Felício CM. Impaired Orofacial Motor Functions on Chronic Temporomandibular Disorders. J Electromyogr Kinesiol 2014; 24(4): 565-71.
10. Marchesan IQ, Martinelli RL, Gusmão RJ. Lingual frenulum: changes after frenectomy. J Soc Bras Fonoaudiol 2012; 24(4): 409-12.
11. Zaghi S, Valcu-Pinkerton S, Jabara M, Norouz-Knutsen L, Govardhan C, Moeller J, Sinkus V, Thorsen RS, Downing V, Camacho M, Yoon A, Hang WM, Hockel B, Guilleminault C, Liu SY. Lingual frenuloplasty with myofunctional therapy: Exploring safety and efficacy in 348 cases. Laryngoscope Investig Otolaryngol 2019; 4(5): 489-96.
12. Morabito G, Romeo C, Romano C. Functional Aerophagia in Children: A Frequent, Atypical Disorder. Case Rep Gastroenterol 2014; 8(1): 123-8.
13. Cabrera Mde C, Cabrera CA, de Freitas KM, Janson G, de Freitas MR. Lateral open bite: treatment and stability. Am J Orthod Dentofacial Orthop 2010; 137(5): 701-11.
14. Robbins J, Butler SG, Daniels SK, et al. Swallowing and dysphagia rehabilitation: translating principles of neural plasticity into clinically oriented evidence. J Speech Lang Hear Res 2008; 51(1): S276-300.
15. de Felício CM, de Oliveira MM, da Silva MA. Effects of Orofacial Myofunctional Therapy on Temporomandibular Disorders. Cranio 2010; 28(4): 249-59.

19 Team building for the treatment of myofunctional disorders

Wes Leffingwell

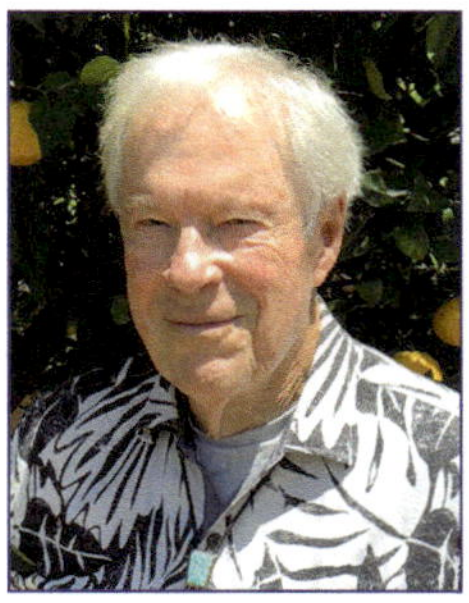

The rapid expansion of the number of disciplines needed to successfully treat this multifaceted disorder is impressive and demanding of practitioners to keep pace with this expansion. Modern medicine has divided itself into specialties and yet we treat one patient at a time for various maladies which occur within one individual body, often with too little success. Focus on symptom and not seeking cause is an invitation for poor outcome to complete failure to affect accurate treatment and long-term maintenance of health.

The human body is a group of systems all designed to work in cooperation to create a sense of well-being and vitality. If one or more of the systems is malfunctioning, associated systems will go into compensation. Crisis occurs when the ability to compensate is exhausted. That is the point at which things become expensive. It is highly improbable that one individual could perform all of the disciplines to successfully treat myofunctional disorder patients.

19.1 The Care Team

A team approach is a must for success in treatment. The qualities most important for teams are competence, open mindedness and excellent communication skills. All of your team members will need to willingly exchange information regarding patients undergoing treatment following HiPAA requirements.

For the G.P. dentist or specialist who is willing to expand their offices' proficiency in the diagnosis and treatment of MFT, it will no doubt take some experiential time to create a harmonious team.

1. The first member of the team is the Myofunctional Therapist. She or he is the best source of information for the entire office team. The Myofunctional Therapist is most likely to be up to date on all the newer inclusions in the discipline and have a list of potential referrals to round out the team.
2. Orthodontist: ideally, someone who is up to date on ALF and similar concept appliances with the goal of increasing palatal width and length (tongue space), splint types and their use, an appreciation of the cranio-sacral movement and the mechanics of the cranio-sacral dura mater relationship. It is vital that the orthodontist understands the processes involved in the treatment of MFT disorders.
3. Osteopath (D.O.): a practitioner who uses the "old school" manipulation for cranio-sacral balance and release.
4. Oral Surgeon or Periodontist: for surgeries and frenum releases and appropriate follow up. Must comprehend the frenum's part in myofunctional function and dysfunction for successful care and maintenance.

Wes Leffingwell, DDS Retired
Leucadia, CA, USA

Email: west@ad.com

5. Pediatrician: prevention, recognition and referral, also as co-educator of other M.D.s
6. Speech Therapist: may be helpful in reinforcing positive habit patterns. Must fully understand the principles and practice of MFT and work as a team player.
7-8. Allergist and ENT may be needed for evaluation of nasal structure and management of allergies, which can impact orofacial and nasal functions.
9. A psychologist or Psychiatrist: MFT patients often require counseling to aid in reducing resistances to the required disciplines of MFT. Please keep in mind, for children you are also treating the parents.
   It is critical the entire office staff is informed about MFT. The team is the theme.

19.2 TMD-Headaches-Allergies

As mentioned before, the body runs a compensation economy.

Most humans are operating at far less than optimum level. Television ads will point out which systems are usually decompensated: analgesics are used for headaches, back muscle aches, pain in any form. Digestives are used predominantly for acid reflux, followed by diarrhea, gas and constipation. All of these varied symptoms are signs of imbalances that are beyond the individuals' ability to compensate.

In lieu of using over the counter remedies to obscure symptoms, finding cause is the best method to activate long-term healing.

A health practitioner (chiropractor, osteopath or dentist) who is well trained in applied kinesiology can be of assistance to screen/scan symptoms for weakness [1, 2].

Once the imbalanced systems are located, evidence-based diagnostics and laboratory examination by a competent physiological chemist and a nutritional counselor can accurately direct treatment strategies. Musculoskeletal alignment is mandatory for comfort and ease of daily life. This alignment starts with the mothers' nutritional choices, well before, during and after pregnancy [3]. Preparation for the first breath begins with the initiation of labor. The natural unmedicated birth process is the ideal situation. Medicated cesarean is the most unfavorable. If the labor goes as desired, the first breath is normal. The infant initiated cross crawl and cranio-sacral movement. The C1 and C2 vertebrae are located properly in relation to the foramen magnum and the cranial bones have the desired space between them [3]. This data was compiled by W. G. Sutherland D.O. a truly original thinker.

Breastfeeding, if possible, is the sequel to a healthy birth, as the act of nursing continues to guide the desired development of the cranio-sacral complex and a competent airway.

The diet has a powerful impact on the cranial and dental arch development as described by Weston A. Price, D.D.S. [4]. The soft, greasy, carbo loaded western diet, of two chews and swallow is not serving our body's needs. The dental complex has receded posteriorly and narrowed, thus restricting the airway with resultant breathing difficulties including mouth breathing, tonsil/adenoid pathologies, sleep apnea, sleep deprivation snoring and more.

The MFT patient has an additional handicap in that the tongue's inappropriate movement patterns are devastating to the dental mechanism. The tongue becomes a destructive orthodontic appliance. Anterior thrusters most often occlude only on the rear molars. It is not possible for the patient to comminute food adequately, so a bolus of food is bolted down. The stomach will not be able to break down what it receives within the two-hour normal transit time and the pyloric valve won't open until the chyme content has a pH of two. The stomach contents being held too long allow fermentation, digestive distress, hiatal hernia and gas. Once the stomach finally releases its partially digested contents, the small intestine is handicapped to enzymatically perform its job. The large intestine now has to deal with an inappropriately composed mass. The lower intestine cannot do its functions, namely: to reabsorb water, provide substrates for the liver to build cholesterol factions, precursors for hormones, neurotransmitters, and immune cell production. Moreover, by virtue of its vast surface area, the lower intestine assists the body in maintaining appropriate cell wall pH, which is required for waste and nutrient transfer.

Proper nasal breathing is the result of appropriate dietary input, healthy orofacial development, necessary musculoskeletal alignment, positive health habits and posture.

A consequence of poor diet choices, misaligned bone muscle relationships, TMJ dysfunction, headaches, backaches, mouth breathing, negative habits ad nauseam is why most people operate well below optimum function level.

Allergies are reactions to irritants. Many are reactions of an already overburdened system loaded with the debris of digestive malfunction and environmental toxins. The immune system becomes overburdened, it becomes over reactive and hence requires more allergy medications and develops more sensitivities. An overburdened immune system, poor breathing habits, poor dietary choices, poor posture, contaminated environment, poor digestion and inappropriate mental/emotional posture, all contribute to the allergy profile. An allergist is helpful to sort out specifics. It is difficult to be sure of what specifically is an allergen to an individual. The answer is clearer when the appropriate diet is used, the breathing profile is corrected, the lower gut chemistry is balanced, and the mental emotional posture is healthy.

The TMJ and its muscular components play a major role in the protection of the dural membrane complex. The dura is a reciprocal tension organ that bends but doesn't stretch [3]. Thus, if there are any subluxations in the cranium, spinal structure, or extremities, all of the nervous system is informed and the muscular compensations are activated. Head, neck and spinal misalignments may demand the TMJ complex to be of assistance in easing dural membrane tensions. The TMJ complex and the associated external pterygoid muscles are the mediators. The TMJ often has local surrounding pathologies: damaging trauma, malocclusions, atypical swallow or dysphagia, tooth loss, restricted airway, negative genetics, habits and poor posture, and intense pain, just to name a few.

If inappropriate dural tension is sensed by the dura madre complex, then the external pterygoid's origin and insertion from the cranial base to the medial posterior inferior mandible, the mandible attachment from its inferior aspect to the hyoid area and the hyoid to the thorax via the neck musculature, all give the external pterygoid muscle (usually unilaterally) the ability to deform the cranial osseous structure to relieve tension in the dura mater complex.

If the cranial bones are misaligned, the TMJ socket is displaced as well as the TMJ disc. In most TMJ disorders the disc is bunched in front of or behind the condyle which can be perforated due to pathologic pressure. If the cranium, TMJ components and cervical vertebrae are misaligned, then the sacrum will rotate the ilium to aid in relieving dural tension. The average patient is expending significant vital energy just to remain functional. TMJ pain is often the result of trauma. Focusing on the joint itself is not enough, the cause of TMJ dysfunction could be from anywhere from the bottom of the feet to the top of the cranium and in between. For accurate treatment strategies the entire person needs scrutiny and experienced professionals to decipher the factors for a comprehensive diagnosis. Overlooking important factors often causes relapse.

19.3 Conclusion

The treatment of swallowing and breathing disorders is obviously complex and involved. To successfully treat this disorder, it takes commitment to learn, be observant, ask questions, seek answers and develop communication skills. At any point in dealing with patients, parents, and other professionals it is vital to sincerely convey "I CARE".

REFERENCES

1. Walther DS. Applied Kinesiology: Synopsis, 2nd ed.; Systems DC, Pueblo (CO), 2000.
2. Walther DS. Applied Kinesiology, Vol. 2, 1st ed.; Systems DC, Pueblo (CO), 1983.
3. Magoun HI. Osteopathy in the Cranial Field, 3rd ed.; Harold Ives Magoun, Sr., Denver (CO), 1976.
4. Price WA. Nutrition and Physical Degeneration, 8th ed.; Price-Pottenger Nutrition Foundation, Lemon Grove (CA), 2009.

SECTION 4 From the mouth to the entire organism

20 Alzheimer's, Parkinson's and Multiple Sclerosis: neuromuscular implication in eating and nutrition

Licia Coceani Paskay

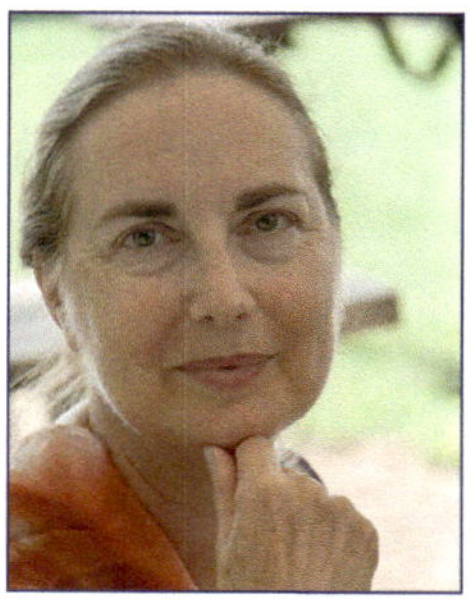

Neurological and neuromuscular disorders affect over a billion people worldwide, according to a WHO study published in 2007. The number has been increasing yearly as the world population increases and ages as well. The most common and well-known neurological disorders in adults are Alzheimer's and dementias in general, Parkinson's, Multiple Sclerosis (MS), strokes and traumatic brain injuries (TBIs). Each disorder implies various difficulties with the basic functions of self-feeding, eating, chewing and swallowing.

In this chapter we'll analyze some of the challenges posed by three disorders: Alzheimer's, Parkinson's and MS, as they have a chronic development, unlike a TBI which happens suddenly, and unlike strokes which usually affect one side of the body.

According to the National Institute of Environmental Health and Sciences, an estimated 5.4 million Americans were living with Alzheimer's disease in 2016 [1]. ParkinsonDisease.net estimates that about a million Americans are living with Parkinson's disease [2]. Similarly, a study funded by the National Multiple Sclerosis Society, finds that almost a million Americans have Multiple Sclerosis [3]. Given the chronic trajectory of these disorders, the cost to the people affected, their families, caregivers and society is staggering. Alzheimer's and Parkinson's in particular pose more challenges to those affected.

20.1 Alzheimer's disease (AD)

Alzheimer's disease is characterized by a progressive and currently incurable dementia, in which cognitive faculties deteriorate first, followed by motor skills and finally the deterioration of the basic physiological functions. Alzheimer's is caused by accumulation of proteins in the brain that stick together in clumps (plaques), killing neurons, and by the presence of filaments of protein (tangles) also contributing to the death of neurons. The neuronal destruction follows a specific pattern, affecting first higher functions like thinking, speaking, remembering and reasoning, then progressively losing some visual and motor skills. The basic vital functions are compromised only at the very end stage of the disease. Understanding the progression of Alzheimer's disease helps understand the progressive difficulties encountered by those affected and suggests compensative strategies that care partners can adopt in optimizing feeding and nutrition.

Licia Coceani Paskay, MS, CCC-SLP
Speech-Language Pathologist, Private Practice
Los Angeles, USA

Email: lcpaskay@gmail.com

20.1.1 Progression of the disease

Initially a person with Alzheimer's might encounter difficulties in shopping for food, buying the appropriate foods or realizing the need to buy food. Often the diet becomes over simplified and monotonous. People who live alone might repeatedly eat the same thing such as milk and cereals. A very restricted diet may cause malnutrition, which by itself affects the brain function. Coupled with this is the inability of people with Alzheimer's to be aware of the need for adequate hydration. Dehydration by itself causes cognitive impairment, fatigue and lethargy. Difficulties in remembering how to cook even a simple food, how to operate a stove, a microwave or a coffee maker are also among the signs of Alzheimer's in the middle to late stage. Sequence of movements well known for decades become increasingly difficult. Distractions and confusion lead to frustration, then refusal to eat anything that needs to be prepared unsupervised.

Often people with late stage Alzheimer's do not distinguish food from non-food, so the danger of ingesting foreign objects, unsafe foods or the drinking of cleaning products is a concern for care partners. Then people with Alzheimer's develop inability to "see" the food placed in front of them during a meal, requiring meals to be supervised and the person aided in eating. It's not that the person does not see the food visually, but they do not recognize it as food (visual agnosia). Quite often there is an inability to recognize when food in their mouth, causing some to spit the food, pocket the food in their cheeks, or chew it for a very long time, then eventually cough it out when the food spills prematurely into the pharynx. At this stage the food is either a soft texture (like boiled potatoes, soft meat, fish and bread) or even pureed, and there is a loss of chewing opportunity. Drinking liquids becomes difficult, causing choking and coughing episodes. At this point, it's not unusual, especially for institutionalized elderly with dementia, to receive a nasogastric or a gastric tube to supplement nutrition as oral feeding becomes more and more difficult, with a meal lasting for over an hour.

20.1.2 Managing some of the symptoms

Managing the disease eventually requires supervision and implementation of strategies to enable the person with Alzheimer's to be as independent as possible. Initially the supervision could be limited to helping with shopping and meal preparation, in which the care partner suggests steps to be taken during cooking, table set up and cleaning. At this time, safety in cooking and cleaning is also a concern that needs to be addressed, as gas or electric stoves, scalding water or cleaning products may pose serious health hazards. Safety hazards at this stage include small hard candies, pebbles, small toys, objects can be ingested or kept in the mouth for a long time.

Maintaining a routine for meals is very important, and so is creating the context for a meal in a quiet and calming room, free from distractions like a TV. Plate, drinking glass and silverware should be clearly visible and well contrasted from the place mat or tablecloth. Anti-skid mats and plates with a containing lip are useful, so is finger food (small sandwiches and cut-up fruit and veggies) and flexible eating hours with "food on the go" available for those who suffer from agitation and are in constant movement. Supervision with a care partner reminding to put available food on the plate and naming where it's located. Eating together stimulates imitation and inhibition of putting too much food in one's mouth are strategies to assist people with Alzheimer's.

The selection of appropriate foods requires some considerations due to the difficulty in processing visuo-motor and kinestetic impulses. If the person is still able to self-feed, the food should be "whole" as opposed to fragmented such as rice, peas or corn. Sauces such as gravy can create cohesion among fragmented foods that are otherwise difficult to manage. Using the spoon as opposed to the fork can be helpful in maintaining self-feeding skills as long as possible. Drinking fluids may be simplified by either offering water away from meals freely (according to the Frazier Water Protocol) or offering smoothies, thick juices or any liquid mixed with appropriate thickeners. The importance of keeping up with hydration cannot be overestimated.

Because swallowing disorders (dysphagia) may ensue at a later stage of the disease, often causing secondary aspiration pneumonia, protective mechanisms are encouraged, such as gentle coughing if the voice is "wet" and gurgly, clearance of the mouth from food debris and thorough oral hygiene. Moreover, Alzheimer's causes a diminished sense of smell, so people tend to "taste" only basic flavors such as sweet and salty and they tend to prefer foods that abound with them, often creating other health risks. Finally, preservation of the oral manipulation allowing self-feeding as long as possible takes advantage of the hand-to-mouth reflex that persists until late in life.

20.2 Parkinson's disease (PD)

This neurological disease is caused by death of the neurons in a specific area called *locus caeruleus* which regulates the smoothness of movements. Parkinson's manifests itself with a host of different symptoms ranging from lack of balance, cog-like movement of arms, hand tremor during intentional movement, tiny handwriting, mask-like face (one of the early symptoms), festination (fast, tiny steps) or bradykinesia (slow movements), sudden stops during walking and other movements, and attempts to "unglue" legs or feet from the floor to walk.

More localized symptoms affecting the face and mouth are compensatory exaggerated movement of the neck and jaw, slurred speech, low voice, reduced and ineffective airway protective mechanisms such as coughing or throat clearing due to difficult breathing coordination. Forty-one percent of people with PD experiences swallowing disorders such as difficulty chewing and dysphagia [4]. Dysphagia tends to be so significant that aspiration pneumonia is still a common occurrence, especially at a later stage of the disease.

20.2.1 Progression of the disease

The first symptoms may manifest as early as the 4th decade of life, with reduced facial expressivity that is interpreted as being uncaring or disinterested. Slurred speech and low voice are disturbing symptoms that often go unaddressed for years. Presence of balance problems, hand or lip tremor and unexplained falls may also require a differential diagnosis. During the initial and the middle phases of the disease, the person with PD might experience episodes of food or drinks "going down the wrong pipe". Difficult chewing, frequent coughing during and after meals, gurgly voice after eating are also characteristics of this stage.

As the disease progresses the symptoms become more frequent and intense and although people maintain a good appetite, they tend to lose weight. They might need assistance with feeding, due to tremors, bradykinesia (slow movements), dyskinesia (usually cog-wheel type movements) or inability to move that impede self-feeding, especially for soups or rice. The food may need to be modified to optimize chewing and facilitate intake of enough calories to maintain a healthy weight. To facilitate swallowing and proper nutrition, protein boosters and thickened liquids may need to be included in this stage.

At later stages, although the food is pureed to facilitate safe swallowing, the caloric intake by mouth is inadequate and a gastric tube may be necessary. Due to disordered movements and reduced protective mechanisms during swallowing, the patient is likely to experience aspiration pneumonia even in presence of a gastric tube (enteral nutrition).

20.2.2 Managing some of the symptoms

The best and most common approach to reduce some of the symptoms of PD is the Lee Silverman Voice Treatment (LSVT®), a behavioral approach focusing on increasing exaggeration of speech, voice and body movements, to counterbalance the tendency of this disease to manifest bradykinesia and small movements [5-8]. The LSVT®, both in its subsets LOUD and BIG, is a research-based, validated therapy that has been implemented and studied for over 20 years. It works on recalibrating the sensory system associated with movement, by exaggerating all the movements, therefore strengthening and coordinating the oro-pharingo-laryngeal muscles and their functions. Moreover, the LSVT® promotes breath support and protective mechanisms such as a proper closure of the vocal folds during swallowing and appropriate coughing to clear the airways of food liquids that spilled into the airways. The treatment protocol is standardized and intensive (16 one-hour sessions within one month), unlike traditional methods of dysphagia therapy, and it focuses on increasing the amplitude or intensity of movements, through effortful repetitions that maximizes learning and promotes neuroplasticity.

Apart from retraining the muscles, other symptoms requiring management are weak coughing, therefore requiring promotion of protective mechanisms such as a productive cough to clear the airways; the inability to chew, requiring changes in food texture; and dysphagia, requiring liquid thickening and food texture changes.

20.3 Multiple sclerosis (MS)

Multiple sclerosis is an inflammatory autoimmune disease that affects the axons of the neurons which transmit the neuro-electrical impulse from a neuron to its axon and onto another neuron. The axon is wrapped in a protective cover, called the myelin sheath which is made of lipids. This sheath is interrupted along the axon, in the Nodes of Ranvier, making it look like a string of sausages. The neuro-electrical impulse usually jumps from node to node thus speeding transmission. The myelin sheath acts like the insulating plastic surrounding copper electric wires. Due to a complex neuro-hormonal interaction, MS causes the myelin sheath to shrink, expanding the surface of the nodes which are then unable to continue transmitting the impulse downstream. Multiple Sclerosis has four different courses: Clinically Isolated Syndrome (CIS), relapsing-remitting MS (RRMS) affecting about 85% of cases, primary progressive MS (PPMS) and Secondary Progressive MS (SPMS) [9]. Each one presents different symptoms which become more severe as the disease progresses, especially in PPMS and SPMS, affect not only oral functions but movement, balance, cognition, vision, bowels and bladder control and much more. Regarding oral functions, about a third of people with MS experiences problems ranging from neck muscle weakness which affects head position during eating, reduced chewing efficiency, poor oral clearance, dysphagia and speech/voice problems [4].

20.3.1 Progression of the disease

Dysphagia is by itself one of the most common symptoms, affecting over one third of people with MS.

A study by Solaro et al. [10] indicated a correlation between severity of dysphagia and progress of the disease. According to Mische and Mowry [11], although many patients try to manage their symptoms through various diets and nutrition options, the current evidence to support any type of nutritional regimen to help with MS is inconclusive. Because various diets (such as the Mediterranean Diet) and supplements may be of help in other health aspects affecting the patients with MS, such as high blood pressure, cholesterol or diabetes, proper nutrition is still helpful.

20.3.2 Managing some of the symptoms

Depending on the type and severity of the MS symptoms drug therapy, exercise regimen and proper nutrition are still the cornerstones of MS management. Good nutrition starts also with good chewing, which may prevent episodes of dysphagia and even choking which often cause a drastic change in the texture of food consumed (soft or pureed vs. regular food). Many patients report reduced MS symptoms following a low sugar diet as sugar needs to be consumed in moderation for other health benefits. Patients who are wheelchair or scooter bound might experience constipation for which increased veggies and fruit consumption, raw, boiled or steamed, may be useful. Any medication that may affect muscle activity (such as spasms or stiffness) or medications for fatigue, depression and even bladder control may affect oral and digestive functions such as salivation (xerostomia), swallowing (dysphagia and oral dyskinesia), gastric (nausea or vomiting) and intestinal motility (constipation or sometimes diarrhea). Food choices need to be kept into account to address whichever issue arises and co-morbidities, with preference to plant-based food, fish and unsaturated fats, reduced gluten, dairy and eggs [11-13].

20.3.3 Conclusion

Given that alterations to the nervous system, being it central or peripheral, affect multiple functions of the oro-digestive system, proper nutrition is a basic rule. As Hirshbergh et al. note, a proper diet and nutrition affect the gut biome which itself is now linked to so many aspects of health and disease [14].

Therefore, although neurological diseases add complexity to the daily functions of eating and digesting, the same therapeutic principles apply, related to learn as early as possible in life the proper chewing mechanics, proper eating techniques and making healthy choices with food, along with daily physical activity and social relationships.

REFERENCES

1. Neurodegenerative Diseases. https://www.niehs.nih.gov/research/supported/health/neurodegenerative/index.cfm
2. How Common Is Parkinson's Disease? https://parkinsonsdisease.net/basics/statistics/
3. Preliminary Results of MS Prevalence Study Estimate Nearly 1 Million Living with MS in the U.S. https://www.nationalmssociety.org/About-the-Society/News/Preliminary-Results-of-MS-Prevalence-Study
4. Hartelius L, Svensson P. Speech and swallowing symptoms associated with Parkinson's disease and multiple sclerosis: a survey. Folia Phoniatr Logop 1994; 46(1): 9-17.
5. El Sharkawi A, Ramig L, Logemann JA, Pauloski BR, Rademaker AW, Smith CH, Pawlas A, Baum S, Werner C. Swallowing and voice effects of Lee Silverman Voice Treatment (LSVT): a pilot study. J Neurol Neurosurg Psychiatry 2002; 72(1): 31-6.
6. Miles A, Jardine M, Johnston F, de Lisle M, Friary P, Allen J. Effect of Lee Silverman Voice Treatment (LSVT LOUD®) on swallowing and cough in Parkinson's disease: A pilot study. J Neurol Sci 2017; 383: 180-7.
7. Fox CM, Ramig LO, Ciucci MR, Sapir S, McFarland DH, Farley BG. The science and practice of LSVT/LOUD: neural plasticity-principled approach to treating individuals with Parkinson disease and other neurological disorders. Semin Speech Lang 2006; 27(4): 283-99.
8. Fox C, Ebersbach G, Ramig L, Sapir S. LSVT LOUD and LSVT BIG: Behavioral Treatment Programs for Speech and Body Movement in Parkinson Disease. Parkinsons Dis 2012; 2012: 391946.
9. Lublin FD, Reingold SC, Cohen JA, Cutter GR, Sørensen PS, Thompson AJ, et al. Defining the clinical course of multiple sclerosis: the 2013 revisions. Neurology 2014; 83(3): 278-86.

10. Solaro C, Rezzani C, Trabucco E, Amato MP, Zipoli V, Portaccio E, et al. Prevalence of patient-reported dysphagia in multiple sclerosis patients: an Italian multicenter study (using the DYMUS questionnaire). J Neurol Sci 2013; 331(1-2): 94-7.
11. Mische LJ, Mowry EM. The Evidence for Dietary Interventions and Nutritional Supplements as Treatment Options in Multiple Sclerosis: a Review. Curr Treat Options Neurol 2018; 20(4): 8.
12. Fellows Maxwell K, Wahls T, Browne RW, Rubenstein L, Bisht B, Chenard CA, Snetselaar L, Weinstock-Guttman B, Ramanathan M. Lipid profile is associated with decreased fatigue in individuals with progressive multiple sclerosis following a diet-based intervention: Results from a pilot study. PLoS One 2019; 14(6): e0218075.
13. Yadav V, Marracci G, Kim E, Spain R, Cameron M, Overs S, Riddehough A, Li DK, McDougall J, Lovera J, Murchison C, Bourdette D. Low-fat, plant-based diet in multiple sclerosis: A randomized controlled trial. Mult Scler Relat Disord 2016; 9: 80-90.
14. Hirschberg S, Gisevius B, Duscha A, Haghikia A. Implications of Diet and The Gut Microbiome in Neuroinflammatory and Neurodegenerative Diseases. Int J Mol Sci 2019; 20(12): 3109.

21 Food and kidney disease

Domenico Santoro, Alfredo Laudani and Rossella Siligato

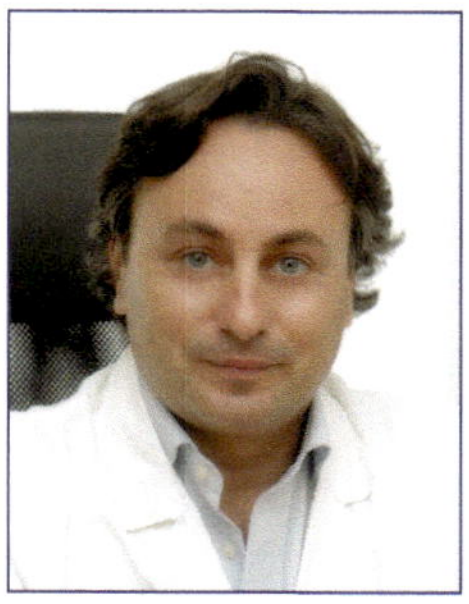

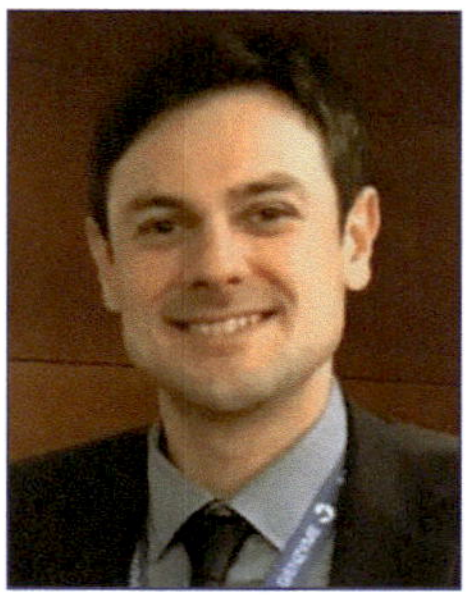

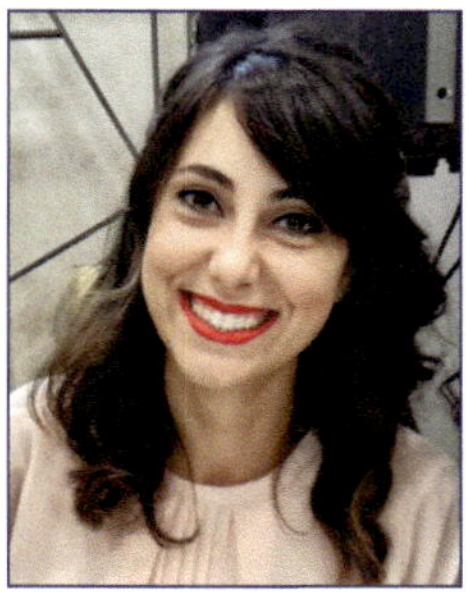

21.1 Introduction

Kidney disease is a substantial worldwide clinical and public health problem. Acute Kidney Injury (AKI) and Chronic Kidney Disease (CKD) are linked to high health care costs, a poor quality of life and serious adverse health outcomes (including the risk of CardioVascular Disease or CVD, infections, depression, the need for Renal Replacement Therapy or RRT, and elevated mortality) [1].

According to the National Health and Nutrition Examination Survey (NHANES) performed from 2011 to 2014, the overall CKD prevalence in the United States adult population was higher than that of the period between 1988 and 1994 [14.8%, 95% CI = 13.6-16.0% versus 10.0%, 95% CI = 9.2-10.9%], after which the overall prevalence of CKD raised significantly [2, 3].

The prevalence of End-Stage Renal Disease (ESRD) increased too. According to the United States Renal Data System (USRDS), a total of 124,114 ESRD patients beginning RRT in the USA in 2015, with an age-gender-race adjusted incidence rate of 357 patients per million/year [4].

CKD and ESRD are associated with higher mortality and morbidity than in the general population [5], as well as with an increased need for health care and hospitalizations. Mortality is related, in part, to the progression of kidney disease and its complications, such as CVD and protein-energy wasting.

Different degrees of albuminuria were demonstrated to correlate with a risk of mortality, progression of CKD and ESRD, independent of the estimated Glomerular Filtration Rate (eGFR), without an apparent threshold value. The increase in risk is significant for urine Albumin-to-Creatinine Ratio (ACR) values ≥ 30 mg/g, even when eGFR is > 60 mL/min/1.73 m^2 [6].

In addition, malnutrition is common in patients with advanced CKD because of a lower food intake (principally due to anorexia), decreased intestinal absorption and digestion, and metabolic acidosis [7]. Therefore, appropriate dietary interventions may have an effect on clinical outcomes, and it is important to monitor the nutritional status in the CKD population. The optimal diet varies

Domenico Santoro, MD
Full Professor, University of Messina, Italy
Director Postgraduate School of Nephrology
Director Unit of Nephrology and Dialysis, AOU G. Martino, Messina, Italy

Email: dsantoro@unime.it

Alfredo Laudani, MD
Unit of Nephrology and Dialysis, University of Messina, Italy

Rossella Siligato, MD
Unit of Nephrology and Dialysis, University of Messina, Italy

Table 21.1 Recommended dietary and nutrient intake in adults according to the Chronic Kidney Disease (CKD) stage*

Dietary constituent	*Moderate-to-advanced CKD*
Protein (g/kg/day)	0.6-0.8, including 50% high biological value proteins
Sodium (g/day)	< 4-3
Potassium (g/day)	< 3 if hyperkalemia occurs frequently during high-fiber intake
Phosphorus (mg/day)	< 800; minimize added inorganic phosphorus and encourage consumption of more plant-based foods
Calcium (mg/day)	< 1500
Fibers, alkali and plant-based foods (g/day)	38 for men and 25 for women, considering > 70% plant-based foods
Fats	Mostly monounsaturated and polyunsaturated lipids, including n-3 fatty acids; increase proportion with low-protein intake
Energy (kcal/kg/day)	30-35

* Modified from [12].

depending upon eGFR, specific kind of kidney disease (i.e., proteinuric or non-proteinuric) and the presence of other comorbidities such as CVD, diabetes or hypertension.

21.2 Overview and current recommendations

Large prospective epidemiologic studies of diet and chronic diseases have facilitated major advances in our understanding of the dietary contribution to the pathogenesis of diseases [8].

Uremic syndrome is due to a progressive reduction in renal function, leading to the impairment of several biochemical and physiological functions, with the accumulation of uremic toxins in extra- and intracellular compartments. These toxins mainly include protein-bound substances and free water-soluble molecules of low or medium molecular weight, most of which derive from protein breakdown [9].

Another possible source of amino acid/protein-derived toxic compounds is the set of intestinal microorganisms, defined as microbiota, which in CKD patients is typically altered. It may produce higher levels of indoxyl sulfate and p-cresyl sulfate, which have been associated with CKD progression and CKD-related complications and may contribute to an acceleration in the development of CVD and uremic bone disease [10, 11].

Uremic retention solutes accumulate in patients with CKD, including those described by the Kidney Disease Outcomes Quality Initiative (KDOQI) as affected by stage 5 disease or ESRD [9].

In medical literature there are evidence-based examples of the possible role of nutritional therapy in lowering serum urea nitrogen levels and managing uremia as well as other complications, such as electrolyte and acid-base imbalances, water and salt retention, blood pressure control, insulin resistance, mineral and bone disorders. Dietary interventions may also be intended as a therapeutic strategy for the conservative management of uremia in order to delay or avoid dialysis therapy [12].

It is important to understand that a renal diet does not only mean restriction, but a comprehensive nutritional approach of macro- and micronutrients in order to prevent protein catabolism, maintain a neutral nitrogen balance as well as an adequate nutritional status and body composition [13].

Macronutrients are the main chemical compounds assumed with diet and provide energy. The primary macronutrients include carbohydrates, proteins, fats and fiber. On the other hand, nutrients needed in very small amounts are called micronutrients and include several minerals (e.g., sodium, potassium, calcium, phosphorus) and vitamins (e.g., vitamin D) [14].

When nutritional therapy is implemented, each dietary component should be considered separately as protein waste products, sodium, fluids, potassium, phosphate, calcium and vitamin D, carbohydrates, fiber and fats (Table 21.1).

21.2.1 Benefits of protein restriction in patients with CKD on protein waste products, proteinuria and albuminuria, progression of CKD and metabolic control

Experimental evidence suggests that high dietary protein intake, usually defined as > 1.2 grams per kilogram of body weight per day (g/kg/day), induces significant alterations in renal function [15].

Higher protein intake modulates renal hemodynamic by increasing renal blood flow and elevating intraglomerular pressure. This mechanism is similar to the adaptive response that occurs to compensate for the loss of renal mass [16] and initially leads to a higher Glomerular Filtration Rate (GFR) and more efficient excretion of protein-derived nitrogenous waste products. However, in the long term, both glomerular hyperfiltration and the resultant increased urinary albumin excretion may have deleterious consequences on the kidney, as showed by experimental studies which correlated this condition to progressive glomerular damage and sclerosis [17, 18].

Conversely, dietary protein restriction demonstrated to be protective in patients with CKD because it reduces the amount of nitrogen waste products and decreases kidney workload by lowering intraglomerular pressure [17], thus limiting glomerular damage and preventing the loss of kidney function, even if this benefit is modest [16, 19, 20]. Protein restriction has been demonstrated to lower proteinuria by 20-50% in patients with CKD, with a linear relationship between reduction of protein intake and decrease in urinary excretion [16, 17]. The Kidney Disease Improving Global Outcomes (KDIGO) suggests restriction in protein intake for CKD patients [21], and 0.6-0.8 g/kg/day Low Protein Diet (LPD) is the most frequently recommended target for adults with moderate-to-advanced CKD (eGFR < 45 mL/min/1.73 m^2) to manage substantial proteinuria (urinary protein excretion > 0.3 g per day). It is essential that 50% of proteins has a high biological value (rich in essential amino acids), while the remaining half may be plant proteins [12]. However, nutritional studies suggest that protein intake can be safely lowered to 0.6 g/kg/day [22].

The so-called Very-Low Protein Diet (VLPD) at < 0.6 g of protein/kg/day, supplemented with calcium, folates, group B vitamins and mixtures of essential amino acids and ketoacids, is another therapeutic strategy [12] because more restricted protein intakes have been shown to further reduce amino acid oxidation and uremic toxicity [23]. Obviously, VLPD management requires significant expertise by nephrologists to ensure adequate daily energy intake (35 kcal/kg/day for patients aged < 60 years and 30 kcal/kg/day for those aged > 60 years) to prevent malnutrition, but it also needs a high degree of patient compliance to accept lifestyle changes, as well as social and family support and, above all, a high doctor-patient empathy [13].

Many studies suggest that protein restriction may slow the progression of CKD. The balance of evidence suggests a benefit of dietary protein restriction, even if more recent studies suggest that the benefit is modest [19, 20].

A restricted protein intake, as in LPD, proved to be effective by also improving metabolic acidosis in CKD. Acid is generated during metabolism of proteins including sulfur-containing amino acids, and pre-dialysis analysis of serum bicarbonate concentration demonstrated that it was lower in patients with higher protein intake [24].

A high dietary acid load invokes adaptive mechanisms to increase acid excretion despite a reduced nephron number, such as increased per nephron ammoniagenesis and augmented distal acid excretion mediated by the renin-angiotensin system and endothelin-1 and may contribute to the progression of renal damage. Additionally, high dietary acid loads produce low-grade, subclinical acidosis that may result in bone and muscle loss [25].

Another significant effect of acidosis is potassium shift from the intracellular to the extracellular fluid and the consequent hyperkalemia typical of severe CKD and ESRD.

Additionally, Insulin Resistance (IR) is a common report in CKD, as a consequence of kidney dysfunction. Mechanisms leading to IR are complex and multifactorial, but the role of inflammation, uremic toxicity, acidosis and vitamin D deficiency has been clearly recognized both in experimental studies and in humans [26].

Hence, metabolic acidosis represents a modifiable risk factor for the development of insulin resistance and an attainable therapeutic target in CKD. The use of sodium bicarbonate or alkali supplementation, a low protein or even vegetarian diet, suggests that serum bicarbonate can be maintained within the normal range [27].

A low protein diet, especially with plant protein, also helps control CKD-Mineral and Bone Disorder (MBD). Dietary control is essential in the management of hyperphosphatemia because dietary proteins, especially of animal origin, are the major source of phosphorus. This could result in slowing the progression of vascular calcification and improving cardiovascular outcome [17].

21.2.2 Sodium and fluids

A reduction of GFR determines the increase of the total body sodium pool and causes hypertension and edema. This is due to the activation of the sympathetic nervous system and the Renin-Angiotensin-Aldosterone System (RAAS). There is also an association between dietary sodium intake, reduction in

24-hour urinary sodium (a surrogate for sodium chloride intake) and blood pressure, especially in persons who consume a high-sodium diet.

A reduction in salt intake causes significant falls in blood pressure and, thereby, improves cardiovascular outcomes [28].

Therefore, a daily dietary sodium intake of less than 4 g (< 174 mmol/day – 6 g of salt) is recommended for the overall management of CKD and its associated risks, while a sodium intake of less than 3 g (< 131 mmol/day – 5 g of salt) is recommended for the specific management of symptomatic fluid retention or proteinuria [12].

Whereas adequate fluid intake may mitigate the risk of kidney disease, patients with CKD may have isosthenuria. This is the basis for recommending that patients with stage 3 CKD limit their fluid intake to less than 1.5 liters per day in order to avoid hyponatremia; adjustment of that limit for conditions associated with high insensible fluid losses is necessary. Finally, treatment with loop diuretics is often prescribed if the patients have symptomatic fluid retention or hypervolemic hyponatremia [12].

21.2.3 Potassium

Potassium levels outside of normal range have been associated with an increased risk of all-cause and cardiovascular mortality as well as cardiac arrhythmias and ESRD [29].

In general, potassium restriction is not required until the eGFR decreases to < 30 mL/min/1.73 m^2.

In patients with a tendency toward hyperkalemia (serum potassium levels > 5.5 mmol/L), a dietary potassium intake of less than 3 g per day (< 77 mmol/day) is recommended, without compromising a balanced intake of fresh fruits and vegetables (fiber rich foods) [12]. Fruits and vegetables that are low in potassium might be consumed in moderation.

However, dietary potassium recommendations need to be individually based on the patient's serum potassium levels.

21.2.4 Phosphorus

Patients with CKD may suffer from phosphate overload and hyperphosphatemia. Higher serum phosphorus concentrations have been associated with increased cardiovascular risk, both in the general and CKD populations [30, 31].

Excess of phosphate causes the increase of parathyroid hormone (PTH) and fibroblast growth factor-23 (FGF-23) levels, which promote urinary phosphorus excretion, inhibits the production of 1,25-dihydroxyvitamin D3 [1,25(OH)D3], promotes renal bone disease, left ventricular hypertrophy, vascular calcification with increased risk of coronary heart disease, heart failure and an accelerated progression of kidney disease from vascular and tubulointerstitial injury [12].

Phosphate is mainly found in foods with high protein content, such as meat and cheese. Restricting dietary phosphorus intake to less than 800 mg per day (26 mmol/day) is recommended for patients with moderate-to-advanced kidney disease and processed foods with a high phosphorus-to-protein ratio should be minimized [12].

Plant sources have the lowest bioavailability of phosphorus; in grains it is 50%, while bioavailability of phosphorus from casein is 100%. A low phosphate diet requires a moderate protein restriction and avoidance of preservatives used in processed and precooked meals [32].

21.2.5 Calcium and vitamin D

Renal insufficiency is associated with a decline in 1,25-dihydroxyvitamin D (1,25-D) and gastrointestinal absorption of calcium. In advanced stages (4 and/or 5) of CKD, serum calcium concentrations decrease, as circulating 1,25-D continues to decrease. A diet of 2000 mg/day of calcium in CKD patients might result in a positive calcium balance, with the extra calcium deposited in tissues [33].

For these reasons, in 2000, the KDOQI guideline suggests limiting total calcium intake (both dietary and medication sources) to 1500 mg/day [34]. Native vitamin D supplementation (cholecalciferol or ergocalciferol) may be offered to patients with CKD in whom circulating vitamin D levels are low [12] to prevent secondary hyperparathyroidism.

21.2.6 Carbohydrates, fiber and fats

Carbohydrates account for 45-65% of the usual daily energy intake, as recommended by the United States Dietary Guidelines [35].

Several prospective studies have associated diets high in glycemic index with a risk of developing type 2 diabetes mellitus, coronary heart disease and some cancers; therefore, it is important to replace high glycemic index carbohydrates (e.g., white rice) with low glycemic index carbohydrates (e.g., green vegetables, lentils), which are higher in fiber content. Fruits and vegetables are a rich source of fiber and essential vitamins and minerals, as well as carbohydrates with a low glycemic index. Added sugars should be limited and comprise no more than 10% of total calories consumed [12, 14].

Such a diet is thought to promote a more favorable microbiome with less constipation, with less risk for each renal outcome and cardiovascular disease [12, 36].

In fact, a lower ratio of dietary fiber to protein has been associated with higher blood levels of indoxyl sulfate and p-cresyl sulfate [37].

The US Department of Agriculture and US Department of Health and Human Services has recommended a daily intake of 14 g per 1000 calories or 38 g of fiber for men and 25 g for women [35].

Fat should make up 20% to 35% of total caloric intake, as recommended by the United States Dietary Guidelines [35]. The type of fat consumed appears to be important: unsaturated fat (n-3 and n-6 fatty acids) is the preferred lipid, while saturated fats should be limited because they contribute to coronary heart disease.

The United States Dietary Guidelines also recommend keeping consumption of saturated fat under 10% of calories per day [35]. There is currently no evidence that low-fat diets, recommended by some guidelines, improve kidney disease outcomes [12].

21.3 Dietary energy and protein energy wasting

Patients with advanced CKD (stage 3b-4-5) and ESRD requiring maintenance dialysis treatment may develop Protein-Energy Wasting (PEW) and low dietary energy and nutrient intakes are often associated. The PEW syndrome encompasses a number of nutritional and metabolic alterations, which result in a progressive loss of protein body mass and energy fuels (i.e., body muscle and fat mass) [38].

There are many important consequences with a negative impact on not only the patient's prognosis, complications, management and quality of life, but also on health economics [38].

The PEW prevalence in patients with CKD stage 3-5 ranges from 11% to 54% and in patients on maintenance dialysis from 28% to 54%, while a PEW prevalence of 60-82% was reported in AKI patients [38]. PEW is caused by malnutrition (specifically negative nitrogen balance and low energy intake), hypercatabolic status, uremic toxins, inflammation, metabolic acidosis, decreased physical activity, comorbidities, lifestyle and dialysis (Table 21.2) [39].

The criteria for the diagnosis of PEW, proposed in 2007 by the International Society of Renal Nutrition and Metabolism (ISRNM), are listed in the table 21.3 [40].

Table 21.2 Causes of PEW in CKD patients*

1. Decrease protein and energy intake
   a. Anorexia
      i. Dysregulation in circulating appetite mediators
      ii. Hypothalamic amino acid sensing
      iii. Nitrogen-based uremic toxins
   b. Dietary restrictions
   c. Alterations in organs involved in nutrient intake
   d. Depression
   e. Inability to obtain or prepare food
2. Hypermetabolism
   a. Increased energy expenditure
      i. Inflammation
      ii. Increased circulating proinflammatory cytokines
      iii. Insulin resistant secondary to obesity
      iv. Altered adiponectin and resistin metabolism
   b. Hormonal disorders
      i. Insulin resistance
      ii. Increased glucocorticoid activity
3. Metabolic acidosis
4. Decreased physical activity
5. Decreased anabolism
   a. Decreased nutrient intake
   b. Resistant to GH/IGF-1
   c. Testosterone deficiency
   d. Low thyroid hormone levels
6. Comorbidities and lifestyle
   a. Comorbidities (diabetes, CHF, depression, coronary artery disease, peripheral vascular disease)
7. Dialysis
   a. Nutrient losses into dialysate
   b. Dialysis-related inflammation
   c. Dialysis-related hypermetabolism
   d. Loss of residual renal function

* Adapted from [39].

Therefore, a crucial aspect of nutrient intake in CKD, to maintain a neutral or positive nitrogen balance and prevent loss of lean body mass, is the amount of energy supply, which should be at least 30 kcal/kg/day for those aged > 60 years and 35 kcal/kg/day for patients aged < 60 years [13, 39].

21.4 Cost-benefit analysis and delayed initiation of dialysis therapy

The increasing economic burden of CKD is attributable to the management of ESRD patients, mostly due to kidney transplants. For example, in Italy the management of ESRD patients represented 1.8% of health care expenditures in 2001, corresponding to an average cost of 36,000 € per patient per year [41].

Table 21.3 Criteria for the clinical diagnosis of PEW in CKD*

1. Serum chemistry
   a. Serum albumin < 3.8 g/dL
   b. Serum prealbumin (transthyretin) < 30 mg/dL (for maintenance dialysis patients only)
   c. Serum cholesterol < 100 mg/dL
2. Body mass
   a. Body mass index (edema free) < 23
   b. Unintentional weight loss over time: 5% over 3 months or 10% over 6 months
   c. Total body fat percentage < 10%
3. Muscle mass
   a. Reduced muscle mass 5% over 3 months or 10 over 6 months
   b. Reduced mid-arm muscle circumference (reduction > 10% in relation to 50th percentile of reference population)
   c. Creatinine appearance (influenced by both muscle mass and meat intake)

Dietary intake
a. Unintentional low DPI < 0.80 g/kg/day for at least 2 months for dialysis patients or < 0.6 g/kg/day for patients with CKD stages 2-5
b. Unintentional low DEI < 25 kcal/kg/day for at least 2 months

* Adapted from [39].
CKD, Chronic Kidney Disease; DEI, Dietary Energy Intake; DPI, Dietary Protein Intake; GFR, Glomerular Filtration Rate; PEW, Protein Energy Wasting.

Less accumulation of uremic toxins relieves clinical manifestations in the late stages of CKD. Consequently, a low protein diet can be used effectively to delay the initiation of dialysis therapy with clinical benefits and contemporaneous economic advantages for the health care system [42].

Delaying dialysis could also save time for maturation of arteriovenous fistula and avoid the insertion of central venous catheter [43].

21.5 Conclusion

Given the high incidence and prevalence of CKD (millions of people worldwide), high health care costs and serious adverse health outcomes, nutritional interventions represent an important additional strategy in the field of conservative treatment, in order to improve uremic symptoms and prolong the dialysis-free interval.

Patients with CKD who are on a protein-restricted diet should be carefully monitored to prevent PEW, in particular body mass as well as serum albumin, with follow-up on adequate caloric intake and ingested proteins (high biologic value).

REFERENCES

1. Bello A, Levinv A, Tonelli M, Okpechi IG, Feehally J, Harris D, Jindal K, Salako BL, Rateb A, Osman MA, Qarni B, Saad S, Lunney M, Wiebe N, Ye F, Johnson DW. Assessment of Global Kidney Health Care Status. JAMA 2017; 317(18): 1864-81.
2. Coresh J, Selvin E, Stevens LA, Manzi J, Kusek JW, Eggers P, Van Lente F, Levey AS. Prevalence of chronic kidney disease in the United States. JAMA 2007; 298(17): 2038-47.
3. Murphy D, McCulloch CE, Lin F, Banerjee T, Bragg-Gresham JL, Eberhardt MS, Morgenstern H, Pavkov ME, Saran R, Powe NR, Hsu CY; Centers for Disease Control and Prevention Chronic Kidney Disease Surveillance Team. Trends in Prevalence of Chronic Kidney Disease in the United States. Ann Intern Med 2016; 165(7): 473-81.
4. United States Renal Data System. 2017 USRDS Annual Data Report: Epidemiology of kidney disease in the United States. National Institutes of Health, National Institute of Diabetes and Digestive and Kidney Diseases, Bethesda, MD, 2017.
5. Keith DS, Nichols GA, Gullion CM, Brown JB, Smith DH. Longitudinal follow-up and outcomes among a population with chronic kidney disease in a large managed care organization. Arch Intern Med 2004; 164(6): 659-63.
6. Levey AS, de Jong PE, Coresh J, El Nahas M, Astor BC, Matsushita K, Gansevoort RT, Kasiske BL, Eckardt KU. The definition, classification, and prognosis of chronic kidney disease: a KDIGO Controversies Conference report. Kidney Int 2011; 80(1): 17-28.
7. Kopple JD, Greene T, Chumlea WC, Hollinger D, Maroni BJ, Merrill D, Scherch LK, Schulman G, Wang SR, Zimmer GS. Relationship between nutritional status and the glomerular filtration rate: results from the MDRD study. Kidney Int 2000; 57(4): 1688-703.
8. Willett WC. Nutritional Epidemiology. 2nd ed. New York: Oxford University Press; 1998.
9. Vanholder R. Uremic toxins. In: UpToDate 2019. https://www.uptodate.com/contents/uremic-toxins
10. Ellis RJ, Small DM, Vesey DA, Johnson DW, Francis R, Vitetta L, Gobe GC, Morais C. Indoxyl sulphate and kidney disease: causes, consequences and interventions. Nephrology (Carlton) 2016; 21(3): 170-7.
11. Barreto FC, Barreto DV, Liabeuf S, Meert N, Glorieux G, Temmar M, Choukroun G, Vanholder R, Massy ZA, European Uremic Toxin Work Group (EUTox). Serum indoxyl sulfate is associated with vascular disease and mortality in chronic kidney disease patients. Clin J Am Soc Nephrol 2009; 4(10): 1551-8.

12. Kalantar-Zadeh K, Fouque D. Nutritional Management of Chronic Kidney Disease. N Engl J Med 2017; 377(18): 1765-76.
13. Bellizzi V, Cupisti A, Locatelli F, Bolasco P, Brunori G, Cancarini G, Caria S, De Nicola L, Di Iorio BR, Di Micco L, Fiaccadori E, Garibotto G, Mandreoli M, Minutolo R, Oldrizzi L, Piccoli GB, Quintaliani G, Santoro D, Torraca S, Viola BF; "Conservative Treatment of CKD" study group of the Italian Society of Nephrology. Low-protein diets for chronic kidney disease patients: the Italian experience. BMC Nephrol 2016; 17(1): 77.
14. Colditz G. Healthy diet in adults. Up-to-date 2019. https://www.uptodate.com/contents/healthy-diet-in-adults
15. Kalantar-Zadeh K, Moore LW, Tortorici AR, Chou JA, St-Jules DE, Aoun A, Rojas-Bautista V, Tschida AK, Rhee CM, Shah AA, Crowley S, Vassalotti JA, Kovesdy CP. North American experience with Low protein diet for Non-dialysis-dependent chronic kidney disease. BMC Nephrol 2016; 17(1): 90.
16. Riccio E, Di Nuzzi A, Pisani A. Nutritional treatment in chronic kidney disease: the concept of nephroprotection. Clin Exp Nephrol 2015; 19(2): 161-7.
17. Ko GJ, Obi Y, Tortorici AR, Kalantar-Zadeh K. Dietary protein intake and chronic kidney disease. Curr Opin Clin Nutr Metab Care 2017; 20(1): 77-85.
18. Fouque D, Aparicio M. Eleven reasons to control the protein intake of patients with chronic kidney disease. Nat Clin Pract Nephrol 2007; 3(7): 383-92.
19. Levey AS, Adler S, Caggiula AW, England BK, Greene T, Hunsicker LG, Kusek JW, Rogers NL, Teschan PE. Effects of dietary protein restriction on the progression of advanced renal disease in the Modification of Diet in Renal Disease Study. Am J Kidney Dis 1996; 27(5):652-63.
20. Levey AS, Greene T, Beck GJ, Caggiula AW, Kusek JW, Hunsicker LG, Klahr S. Dietary protein restriction and the progression of chronic renal disease: what have all of the results of the MDRD study shown? Modification of Diet in Renal Disease Study group. J Am Soc Nephrol 1999; 10(11): 2426-39.
21. KDIGO 2012 Clinical Practice Guideline for the Evaluation and Management of Chronic Kidney Disease. Kidney Int Suppl 2013; 3(1): 5-14.
22. Fouque D, Laville M. Low protein diets for chronic kidney disease in non diabetic adults. Cochrane Database Syst Rev 2009; (3): CD001892.
23. Masud T, Young VR, Chapman T, Maroni BJ. Adaptive responses to very low protein diets: the first comparison of ketoacids to essential amino acids. Kidney Int 1994; 45(4): 1182-92.
24. Scialla JJ, Anderson CA. Dietary acid load: a novel nutritional target in chronic kidney disease? Adv Chronic Kidney Dis 2013; 20(2): 141-9.
25. Kalantar-Zadeh K. Moderator's view: Higher serum bicarbonate in dialysis patients is protective. Nephrol Dial Transplant 2016; 31(8): 1231-4.
26. Xu H, Carrero JJ. Insulin resistance in chronic kidney disease. Nephrology (Carlton) 2017; 22 Suppl 4: 31-4.
27. Bellasi A, Di Micco L, Santoro D, Marzocco S, De Simone E, Cozzolino M, Di Lullo L, Guastaferro P, Di Iorio B; UBI study investigators. Correction of metabolic acidosis improves insulin resistance in chronic kidney disease. BMC Nephrol 2016; 17(1): 158.
28. He FJ, Li J, Macgregor GA. Effect of longer-term modest salt reduction on blood pressure. Cochrane Database Syst Rev 2013; (4): CD004937.
29. Chen Y, Sang Y, Ballew SH, in A, Chang AR, Matsushita K, Coresh J, Kalantar-Zadeh K, Molnar MZ, Grams ME. Race, Serum Potassium, and Associations With ESRD and Mortality. Am J Kidney Dis 2017; 70(2): 244-51.
30. Dhingra R, Sullivan LM, Fox CS, Wang TJ, D'Agostino RB Sr, Gaziano JM, Vasan RS. Relations of serum phosphorus and calcium levels to the incidence of cardiovascular disease in the community. Arch Intern Med 2007; 167(9): 879-85.
31. Palmer SC, Hayen A, Macaskill P, Pellegrini F, Craig JC, Elder GJ, Strippoli GF. Serum levels of phosphorus, parathyroid hormone, and calcium and risks of death and cardiovascular disease in individuals with chronic kidney disease: a systematic review and meta-analysis. JAMA 2011; 305(11): 1119-27.
32. Gonzalez-Parra E, Tuñón J, Egido J, Ortiz A. Phosphate: a stealthier killer than previously thought? Cardiovasc Pathol 2012; 21(5): 372-81.
33. Spiegel DM, Brady K. Calcium balance in normal individuals and in patients with chronic kidney disease on low- and high-calcium diets. Kidney Int 2012; 81(11): 1116-22.
34. K/DOQI Nutrition in Chronic Renal Failure Guidelines, 2000. Dietary Energy Intake (DEI) for Nondialyzed Patients. https://www.kidney.org/sites/default/files/docs/kdoqi2000nutritiongl.pdf (Accessed on August 31, 2015).
35. U.S. Department of Health and Human Services and U.S. Department of Agriculture. 2015 – 2020 Dietary Guidelines for Americans. 8th Edition. December 2015. Available at http://health.gov/dietaryguidelines/2015/guidelines/
36. Sumida K, Molnar MZ, Potukuchi PK, Thomas F, Lu JL, Matsushita K, Yamagata K, Kalantar-Zadeh K, Kovesdy CP. Constipation and incident CKD. J Am Soc Nephrol 2017; 28(4): 1248-58.
37. Rossi M, Johnson DW, Xu H, Carrero JJ, Pascoe E, French C, Campbell KL. Dietary protein-fiber ratio associates with circulating levels of indoxyl sulfate and p-cresyl sulfate in chronic kidney disease patients. Nutr Metab Cardiovasc Dis 2015; 25(9): 860-5.
38. Carrero JJ, Thomas F, Nagy K, Arogundade F, Avesani CM, Chan M, Chmielewski M, Cordeiro AC, Espinosa-Cuevas A, Fiaccadori E, Guebre-Egziabher F, Hand RK, Hung AM, Ikizler TA, Johansson LR, Kalantar-Zadeh K, Karupaiah T, Lindholm B, Marckmann P, Mafra D, Parekh RS, Park J, Russo S, Saxena A, Sezer S, Teta D, Ter Wee PM, Verseput C, Wang AYM, Xu H, Lu Y, Molnar MZ, Kovesdy CP. Global Prevalence of Protein-Energy Wasting in Kidney Disease: A Meta-analysis of Contemporary Observational Studies From the International Society of Renal Nutrition and Metabolism. J Ren Nutr 2018; 28(6): 380-92.
39. Obi Y, Qader H, Kovesdy CP, Kalantar-Zadeh K. Latest consensus and update on protein-energy wasting in chronic kidney disease. Curr Opin Clin Nutr Metab Care 2015; 18(3): 254-62.
40. Fouque D, Kalantar-Zadeh K, Kopple J, Cano N, Chauveau P, Cuppari L, Franch H, Guarnieri G, Ikizler TA, Kaysen G, Lindholm B, Massy Z, Mitch W, Pineda E, Stenvinkel P, Treviño-Becerra A, Wanner C. A proposed nomenclature and diagnostic criteria for protein-energy wasting in acute and chronic kidney disease. Kidney Int 2008; 73(4): 391-8.
41. Pontoriero G, Pozzoni P, Del Vecchio L, Locatelli F. International study of Health Care Organization and Financing for renal replacement therapy in Italy: an evolving reality. Int J Health Care Finance Econ 2007; 7(2-3): 201-15.

42. Scalone L, Borghetti F, Brunori G, Viola BF, Brancati B, Sottini L, Mantovani LG, Cancarini G. Cost-benefit analysis of supplemented very low-protein diet versus dialysis in elderly CKD5 patients. Nephrol Dial Transplant 2010; 25(3): 907-13.

43. Duenhas M, Gonçalves E, Dias M, Leme G, Laranja S. Reduction of morbidity related to emergency access to dialysis with very low protein diet supplemented with ketoacids (VLPD+KA). Clin Nephrol 2013; 79(5): 387-93.

22 Food and osteoporosis

Francesco Bove, Daniela Prosperi and Gabriele Bove

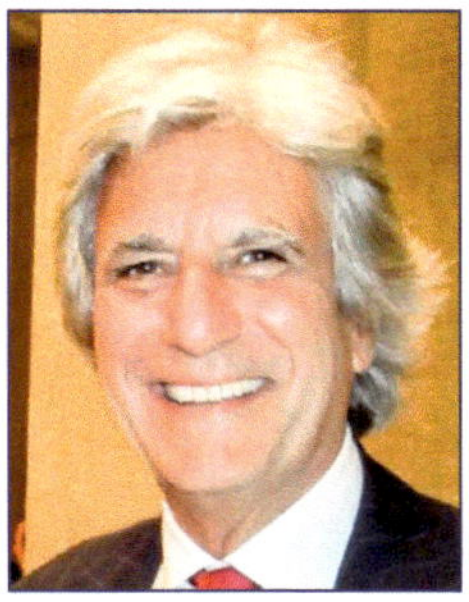

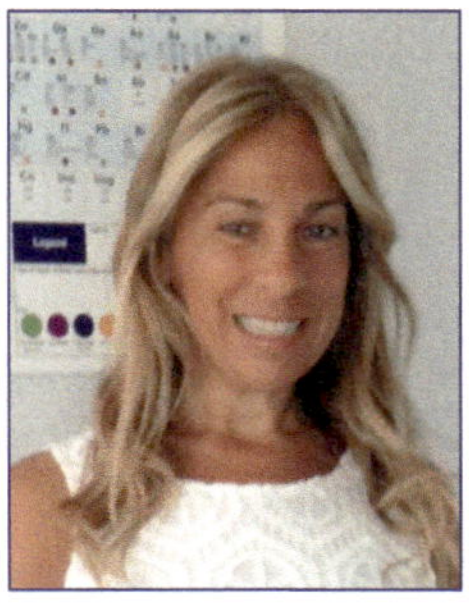

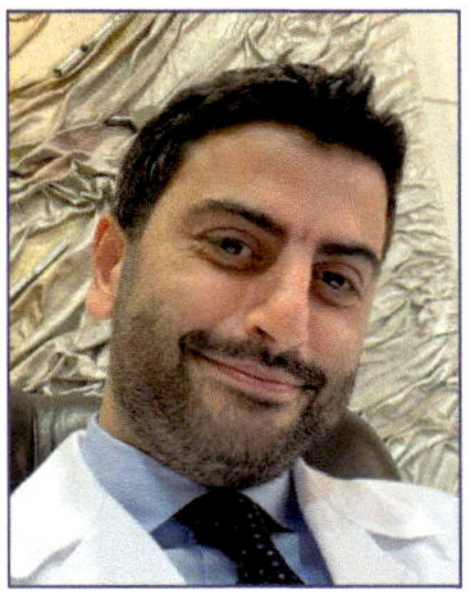

22.1 Introduction

The progressive aging of the population has focused attention on degenerative pathologies that occur in the skeletal system, and which are therefore increasing with age. Hence the interest of orthopedic specialists to prevent the progressive and physiological weakening of the bone structure; to analyze the regulatory mechanisms of bone turnover and possible improvements; to bridge the deficiencies easily corrected with adequate lifestyles and, in particular, with a correct diet.

Coping with skeletal degeneration, in particular osteoporosis, has become of fundamental importance to ensure optimal functionality of the locomotor system and to give autonomy to the individual in later age, with a primary goal of individual benefits and a secondary goal of social benefits that positively affect the economy of any family and, in general, public spending.

Osteoporosis is one condition that best can be fought with nutrition, adequate preventive measures and with awareness, through progressive measures that can ensure good stability of the bone apparatus, counteracting its weakening.

22.2 The importance of calcium

The fundamental constituent of bone is calcium, a mineral that is deposited in our skeletal system from birth to completion of growth. The value amount of the calcium thus accumulated constitutes the Peak of Bone Mass (PBM) which varies in the individual according to the constitution and dietary intake. This is nothing more than our heritage, which can be identified with the CBM (Computerized Bone Mineralometry) DEXA (Dual-Energy X-Ray Absorptiometry) which can detect the conditions of osteopenia and osteoporosis, with consequent risk of fracture, through the analysis of the neck of the femur and vertebrae.

During growth and development, a deficit in calcium intake can negatively affect the achievement of the peak bone mass and negatively expose the individual to osteoporosis.

The bone density remains constant in women until menopause then progressively begins to decrease, mainly due to the lack of estrogens that act on bone metabolism by increasing the activity of osteoclasts. This metabolic change exposes the bones, in the long years that follow, to the loss of mass which makes them naturally more brittle. Men are not exempt from this aging process, how-

Francesco Bove, MD; Gabriele Bove, MD, PhD
I.N.I. Italian Neurotraumatology Institute, Grottaferrata, Rome, Italy

Email: francesco.bove@studiomedicobove.com

Daniela Prosperi MD
Nuclear Medicine Unit; Sant'Andrea University Hospital, Rome, Italy

ever, which begins a little later around age 60/65.

Calcium intake is therefore essential during the various stages of life. In children it has been observed that minimal amounts of daily calcium are needed to achieve an adequate PBM. The Italian National Institute of Nutrition has identified the recommended nutrient intake levels, or LARN in Italian [1].

For children under the age of 10, the quantity of calcium between 70-150 mg/day is considered sufficient to reach adequate bone mass, but the accumulation of the mineral in the skeleton is proportional to the food intake, so the LARN propose an assumption 10 times higher than those indicated. The daily intake levels are therefore 800 mg daily for children up to 6 years, 1000 mg for those from 7 to 10 years of age, and 1200 mg for adolescents.

In addition to calcium, in these stages of life, even adequate protein intake, typical of a normal nutritional status, favors the achievement of an ideal bone stock identified by the PBM.

It is very understandable how the condition of malnutrition in the growing phase, as in anorexia for example, exposes a child to a depletion of the bone mass with negative repercussions after menopause and during aging, favoring the onset of osteoporosis and well-feared complications such as fractures [2].

During adulthood 800 mg of calcium are considered sufficient, whereas after menopause, 1000 mg (as in the case of elderly men) are needed, which increase to 1200 mg in the absence of replacement therapy during menopause.

Among the risk factors for fracture, in addition to the ones listed above, the risk factor of having hypovitaminosis D, found in the laboratory with the evaluation of 25OH-Vitamin D, was extensively evaluated. A reduced intake of vitamin D, an important factor for the absorption of calcium in the intestine, has been shown to influence the onset of osteoporosis [3].

When calcium intake is inadequate or cannot be absorbed in the intestine for whatever reason, plasma levels are reduced, leading to an increase in parathyroid hormone. Calcium is thus recalled from the bones to maintain the plasma levels of the mineral itself. Consequently, the bone mass decreases. Therefore, adequate dietary intake is one of the fundamental lifestyles, along with physical activity and reduced use of alcohol and caffeine to counteract bone loss and subsequent osteoporosis [4].

In the absence of pathologies, food is essential to reduce the attacks of what is considered the *silent worm*. In fact, osteoporosis is often underestimated and without adequate monitoring and knowledge of bone mass values, the *worm* attacks and manifests itself with fractures causing individual, family and society pain and discomfort.

Fractures without adequate preventive measures are in fact on the increase, also due to the aforementioned demographic factors. There are about 4.5 million women with osteoporosis in our country, Italy, and 200 million worldwide. Fractures of the femoral neck alone causes the expenditure of about 1 billion euros (source AIFA), similar to the expenditure for vertebral fractures. That translate to almost 2% of healthcare spending, amounting to around € 116 billion.

An adequate diet containing the principles of calcium and vitamin D and making the patient aware of the problem and being proactive can do so much. The calcium that we have to introduce daily, to reduce the losses we have described, plays a fundamental role and, in reality, many people do not take a sufficient amount of calcium, exposing the bone to a weakening that in the elderly can also cause a rarefaction of the alveolar bone with consequent loss of teeth.

Calcium is mainly contained in milk and milk derivatives and can be found in minimum quantity in other foods. Cheeses in general are in first place and alone can ensure the daily requirement. Milk and soft cheeses such as mozzarella and ricotta instead provide a reduced calcium quantity equal to 20-30% of the requirement. Another source is represented by waters in which the calcium content, both in tap water and in mineral water, varies from case to case.

In general, experts from the Nutrition Institute attribute 65% of the needs to dairy products, 12% to vegetables, 6.5% to fish and meat and 8.5% to cereals. By giving preference to milk and derivatives such as cheese in the daily diet, however, it is easy to run into collateral problems of which the subjects are aware, such as the increase in cholesterol and various intolerances.

Trying to reach the necessary levels of calcium with milk, mozzarella and parmesan is not possible every day, so the use of supplements is almost necessary. In the absence of a mathematical calculation, it is thought that integrating 500-600 mg of calcium a day with a healthy and varied diet, into the elderly population foreseeing however at least one element of the milk or its derivatives, the requirement can be satisfied.

22.3 The importance of vitamin D

The same applies to the vitamin D3 that we develop from sunlight. This physiological phenomenon is decreasing due to smog and reduced exposure to the sun, especially for the elderly population. Moreover, on the sun exposure for the development of vitamin D, the incidence of the solar rays that varies according to the latitude is decisive. This is greater when approaching the equator, less towards the poles. In fact, the Nordic populations are lacking in vitamin D more than those in the South.

A recent study of an elderly population admitted to hospitals showed insufficient vitamin D levels through mass screening [4]. Vitamin D is scarcely present in foods and therefore, if we do not produce it with ultraviolet rays, blood levels will be deficient, and calcium simply cannot be absorbed. Few foods, in fact, contain vitamin D. The greater quantity can be introduced with the diet rich in milk and cereals, commonly used in breakfast, with cod liver oil, with tuna, sardines, salmon and with egg yolk.

As mentioned, the primary function of vitamin D is to maintain the homeostasis of blood levels of calcium. Vitamin D activates the intestinal absorption of calcium and phosphates. In the kidney, vitamin D with PTH (parathyroid hormone) increases calcium reabsorption in the distal renal tubule. In the absence of vitamin D, the absorption of calcium and phosphates in the intestine is reduced to 50% and PTH increases to keep the calcium-phosphate ratio normal for the correct mineralization of the collagen matrix.

Many authors [5, 6] consider 30 mg/mL as the minimum limit necessary for a PTH response and optimal calcium absorption, as established in 2010 by the International Osteoporosis Foundation. When nutrition and exposure to sunlight do not exceed this level, supplements from 600 IU to 800-2000 IU per day are recommended for the elderly population.

Vitamin D is necessary for many other protective functions for the cardiovascular system and the immune system. Therefore, by knowing your own blood level of vitamin D you can correct the defi-

Table 22.1 Calcium content every 100 grams of food expressed in mg

Cereals		**Fresh meat**	
Rice	14	Beef	7
Corn flour	6	Chicken	9
Common bread	10	Veal	10
Fresh legumes		**Sausages**	
Green beas	54	Cooked ham	10
Beans	35	Cured ham/prosciutto	10
Peas	12		
Dried legumes		**Fresh fish**	
Beans	137	Anchovy	26
Lentils	56	Snapper	25
Peas	64	Cod	19
		Sole	15
Vegetables and greens		Tuna	34
Asparagus	8	Red mullet	23
Beet	20		
Broccoli rabe	177	**Conserved fish**	
Broccoli	91	Anchovies in oil	44
Artichokes	17	Stockfish	25
Carrots	27	Tuna in oil	44
Cauliflowers	18		
Cucumber	9		
Chicory	47	**Milk, cheese and dairy products**	
Fresh mushrooms	8		
Lettuce	14	Whole cow milk	119
Aubergines/eggplants	14	Skimmed cow milk	122
Peppers	5	Gruyere	1033
Tomatoes	8	Parmesan	1049
Spinach	73	Provolone	828
Courgettes	17	Soft cheese	162
		Mozzarella	162
Fresh fruit		Cheese (average)	274
Oranges	24		
Apples	5	**Egg**	
Pears	11	Hen egg (yolk)	147
Dried fruit		**Fats**	
Dried figs	182	Butter	15
Almond	102	Olive oil	0
Walnuts	29		

ciency by integrating it adequately through its monitoring for optimal function.

In the countries of northern Europe, vitamin D is now added to many packaged foods such as biscuits, yogurt, milk, contributing to the reduction of environmental solar deficiencies. However, although calcium and vitamin D introduced with food and supplements are essential for bone biochemistry, they are not always able to perform their function of contributing significantly to bone turnover [7].

22.4 Risk factors

Many factors negatively affect the absorption of calcium, such as alcohol, sodium and acidosis conditions that recall calcium from the bone to balance the body biochemistry. Other risk factors and causes of hypovitaminosis D are obesity (adipocytes sequester vitamin D), malabsorption, drugs for hypercholesterolemia, liver and kidney diseases, glucocorticoids and hyperthyroidism.

22.5 Conclusion

In conclusion, among the lifestyles necessary to fight osteoporosis, food plays a decisive role. A balance between calcium-containing foods, the control of vitamin D, and the possible use of supplements, are fundamental for the balance of bone quality necessary to sustain a population destined to live longer.

Table 22.1 presents the calcium content every 100 grams of dairy food.

REFERENCES

1. Livelli di Assunzione Raccomandati di Energia e Nutrienti per la Popolazione Italiana (LARN - ediz. 1996) -Società Italiana di Nutrizione Umana.
2. Consensus development conference: prophylaxis and treatment of osteoporosis. Am J Med 1991; 90(1): 107-10.
3. Bove G. Vitamina D e Osteoporosi. Il Patologo Clinico, Journal of Molecular and Clinical Pathology (Vol.48, N.2/2012, p. 10).
4. Burckhardt P. Calcium and Vitamin D in the treatment and prevention of osteoporosis: the actual dilemma. Ther Umsch 2012; 69(3): 153-61. [Article in German]
5. Del Toma E. Dietoterapia e Nutrizione Clinica. Il Pensiero Scientifico, Roma, 1995.
6. Grimston SK, Morrison K, Harder JA, et al. In Nutritional Aspects of Osteoporosis. Raven Press 1991; vol 85: 77-89.
7. Jackson RD, LaCroix AZ, Gass M, et al. Calcium plus vitamin D supplementation and the risk fractures. N Engl J Med 2006; 354(7): 669-83.

23 Food and cardiovascular risk

Emiliano Angeloni, Daniela Prosperi and Giovanni Melina

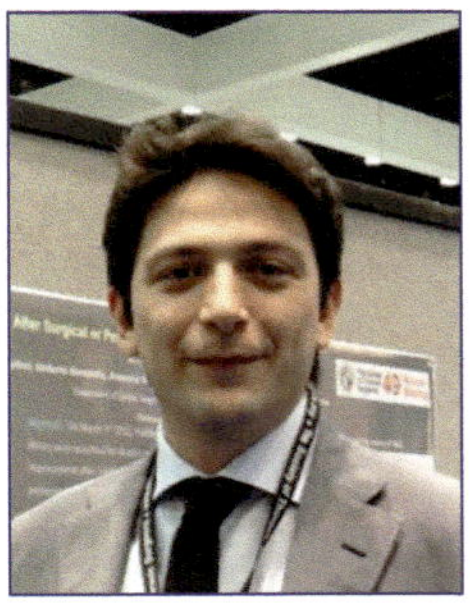

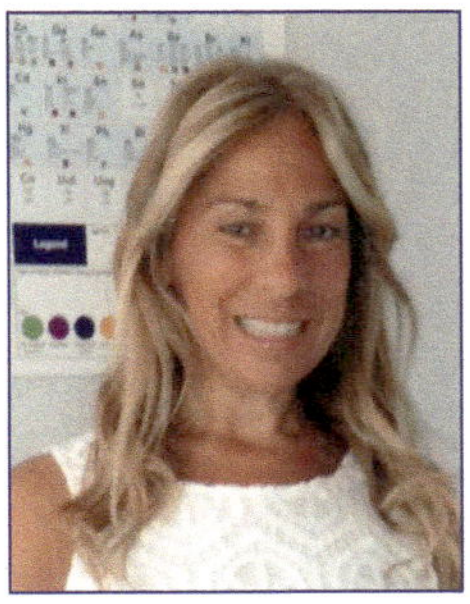

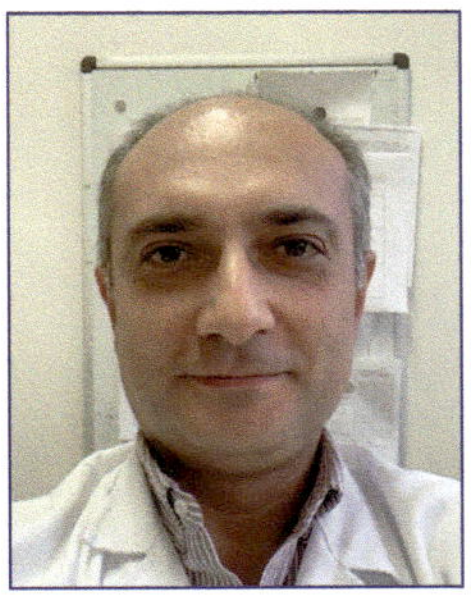

23.1 Clinical scenario

As already known in popular tradition and reiterated in the prevention guidelines of the European Society of Cardiology [1], diet is among the major modifiable cardiovascular risk factors. Indeed, modification of alimentary habits is a key issue in the first-line treatment and prevention of arterial hypertension [2] and dyslipidemias [3].

Consequently, the beneficial effects of a healthy diet, in terms of blood pressure, optimal levels of lipids and glycemia, and maintenance of a healthy weight, are a cornerstone to prevent hypertension, dyslipidemias and diabetes. These systemic disorders determine and/or accelerate atherosclerosis, thus resulting in major cardiovascular adverse events such as myocardial infarction or stroke.

The previous considerations become more compelling since major cardiovascular accidents are the most frequent causes of death and disability among adults in industrialized countries [1]. As a matter of fact, according to the 2018 American Heart Association (AHA) statistical report [4], in the USA, 45% of deaths due to myocardial infarction, stroke and/or diabetes was correlated with poor dietary habits, in particular due to elevated intake of sodium, red meats, sweetened beverages, and low consumption of fruits, vegetables and omega-3 rich fatty acids [4].

Thus, a balanced diet with maintenance of a healthy weight is recommended in all individuals, regardless of their specific risk profile [1]; although it is clear that healthiest diet patterns bear increased costs of about 1.50 USD per person per day, according to the AHA 2018 statistical report [4].

Nevertheless, the cost-effectiveness of a healthy diet is definitely clear: among different prevention strategies (statin therapy, smoking cessation, nurse assistance and counseling), a deep and stable improvement of the diet is the cheapest option (almost 20-900 USD per year of life gained) [4]. Conversely, each year more than 33 billion USD in medical costs and 9 billion USD in lost productivity due to heart disease, cancer, stroke, and diabetes are accountable to poor nutrition [4].

As a result, a healthy diet is not only cost-effective, bust cost-saving. For example, it has been calculated that, in the USA, a 1.2 g/day reduction in dietary sodium consumption would reduce the annual cases of coronary artery disease to 60,000 from 120,000, stroke to 32,000 from 66,000, and total mortality to 44,000 from 92,000 [4]. If accomplished through a regulatory intervention, estimated savings in healthcare costs would be between 10 and 24 billion USD annually [4]. Such an intervention, leading to halving the incidence of cardiovascular events,

Emiliano Angeloni, MD; Daniela Prosperi, MD; Giovanni Melina, MD
Sant'Andrea University Hospital, Rome, Italy

Email: emilianoangeloni@gmail.com

would be surely less expensive than using medications to lower blood pressure in all people with hypertension.

23.2 Current recommendations

From a nutritional point of view, a healthy diet is defined, in the cardiovascular prevention ESC guidelines [1], as that in which energy intake is limited to the amount of energy needed to maintain (or obtain) a healthy weight in the absence of dietary supplements, that is a Body Mass Index between 20 and 25 kg/sm.

According to the cited cardiovascular prevention guidelines [1], ten major points deserve attention (Table 23.1).

23.2.1 Fats

Moving from the evidence that the impact of dietary cholesterol on serum cholesterol levels is weak, compared to that of the fatty acid composition of the diet, European guidelines [1, 3] do not give specific recommendations regarding dietary cholesterol intake, but only regarding fatty acids consumption. Indeed, a lower saturated fat intake generally leads to a reduced dietary cholesterol intake, which ideally should be no greater than 300 mg/day [1].

Table 23.1 Healthy diet characteristics*

1.	Saturated fatty acids (dairy products, red meats, cured meats, eggs) to account for < 10% of total energy intake, through replacement by polyunsaturated fatty acids
2.	Trans unsaturated fatty acids (fries, cakes, cookies): as little as possible, referably no intake from processed food, and < 1% of total energy intake from natural origin
3.	< 5 g of salt per day
4.	30-45 g of fiber per day, preferably from wholegrain products (rice, cereals)
5.	≥ 200 g of fruit per day (2-3 servings)
6.	≥ 200 g of vegetables per day (2-3 servings)
7.	Fish 1-2 times per week, one of which to be oily
8.	30 g unsalted nuts (almonds, hazelnuts, walnuts, cashews) per day
9.	Consumption of alcoholic beverages should be limited to 2 glasses per day (20 g/day of alcohol) for men and 1 glass per day (10 g/day of alcohol) for women
10.	Sugar-sweetened soft drinks and alcoholic beverages consumption must be discouraged

* Adapted from [1].

Thus, the first two recommendations [1] focus on fatty acids consumption, as it is clearly demonstrated that, in the context of cardiovascular disease prevention, the types of fatty acids assumed are more important than the total fat content. The risk of coronary artery disease is lowered by 2-3% when 1% of daily energy intake from saturated fatty acids is replaced by polyunsaturated fatty acids, which are known to significantly lower LDL cholesterol [1]. Polyunsaturated fatty acids belong to two principal subsets: omega-6 fatty acids (mainly deriving from plant foods) and omega-3 fatty acids (mainly deriving from fish oils and fats). Within the subclass of the latter, eicosapentaenoic acid and docosahexaenoic acid are particularly important, but there is no consensus whether they exert a favorable effect on all-causes, coronary and stroke mortality [1, 3, 5].

In addition, mono-unsaturated fatty acids showed a beneficial effect on HDL cholesterol levels, although they were not found to be correlated with reduced cardiovascular risk [1].

On the other hand, trans fatty acids (a subclass of unsaturated fatty acids formed during the industrial processing of fats, which are present in, for example, margarine and baked goods), have been shown to be especially harmful due to their detrimental effect on both total/LDL cholesterol (increase) and HDL cholesterol (decrease).

There are strong evidences that a 2% increase in energy intake from trans fatty acids increases the risk of coronary artery disease by 23% [6]; thereby it is recommended to derive the least amount possible of total energy intake from trans fatty acids, in any case no more than 1% [1, 3].

23.2.2 Sodium

It is estimated that even a modest reduction in sodium intake of 1 g/day reduces systolic blood pressure by 3.1 mmHg in hypertensive patients and 1.6 mmHg in normotensive patients, with a clear dose-response relation between sodium and BP reductions [1, 2, 7].

Anyway, optimal daily salt intake should be around 3 g, with a maximum recommended of 5 g, whereas in most Western countries it ranges between 9-10 g/day [1].

On average, 80% of salt intake comes from processed foods, while only 20% is added later on. Salt reduction can be achieved by making different dietary choices (fewer processed foods, more basic foods) and the reformulation of foods (lowering salt content).

In addition, still remaining in the minerals' field, an inverse statistically significant association exists between potassium intake and the risk of incident stroke, mainly because potassium (mostly derived from fruits and vegetables) exerts favorable effects on blood pressure [1].

23.2.3 Other nutrients

Even if the mechanism is not clear yet, a high fiber intake reduces postprandial glucose responses after carbohydrate-rich meals and lowers total and LDL-cholesterol levels [1]. Indeed, recent studies showed that higher intakes of fiber are associated with a 9% lower risk of coronary artery disease, a 16% lower risk of stroke, and with a 6% lower risk of type 2 diabetes [1].

High-quality evidences identified a risk reduction for stroke by 11% for 3-5 daily servings of fruits and vegetables and by 26% for more than five servings, compared to less than three daily servings [8].

Cardiovascular beneficial effects of fish are attributed to its n-3 fatty acid content; in fact, scientific reports showed that eating fish at least once a week results in a 16% reduction of the risk of coronary artery disease, and in a 6% reduction of the risk of stroke [1]. Furthermore, the highly increased cardiovascular risk observed in the range of no/very low fish intake, determines that a small increase of fish consumption may bear a potentially large impact on public health.

Regarding fish oil, randomized trials have failed to demonstrate a significant reduction of cardiovascular events among patients with coronary artery disease who received omega-3 fatty acids supplementation of 400-1000 g/daily [1, 5].

Latest evidence suggests that daily consumption of 30 g of nuts is associated with a 30% reduction of cardiovascular risk [1].

Although daily drinking of 3 (or more) alcoholic beverages is strongly associated with elevated cardiovascular risk, lower risk has been observed among moderate alcohol consumption (1-2 units per day) in comparison with non-drinkers, even if the real beneficial effects of moderate drinking are still not conclusive.

Regular consumption of sugar-sweetened soft drinks is clearly correlated with excessive weight, diabetes and metabolic syndrome [1]. As recommended even in the World Health Organization's guidelines [9], those beverages should be avoided and maximum sugar intake (including added sugars as well as sugars present in fruits and fruit juices) should not exceed 10% total energy intake.

Although many observational investigations have indicated inverse associations between levels of vitamins A, B, C and E and the risk of cardiovascular disease, intervention trials have failed to confirm these findings [1]. Slightly more robust evidence is available for vitamin D, as in the bottom tertile of its serum levels, cardiovascular and total mortality appears higher, while an 11% risk reduction in all-cause mortality was observed for vitamin D3 supplementation [1].

Moreover, functional foods providing phytosterols, as plant sterols, and stanols were found to be effective in lowering LDL cholesterol levels by an average of 10% when consumed in the amount of 2 g/day [1, 3].

In addition, based on the apparent relationship of plasma homocysteine to cardiovascular disease risk and the estimated influence of folic acid on homocysteine levels, it has been suggested that a 350 mg increase in folic acid daily intake in men, and a 280 mg/d increase in women, could potentially prevent around 30,500 and 19,000 vascular deaths annually in men and women, respectively. However, in the absence of prospective, placebo-controlled intervention trials on the effects of diet- or vitamin-mediated homocysteine reductions on incidence of cardiovascular disease, the clinical benefits of such interventions are unknown [1].

In conclusion, with regards to dietary patterns, it has to be pointed out that the Mediterranean diet provides many of the nutrients discussed above, warranting a high intake of fruits, vegetables, legumes, wholegrain products, fish and unsaturated fatty acids (Fig. 23.1). The Mediterranean diet, indeed, has been correlated with a 10% reduction in cardiovascular mortality and morbidity, with a 8% reduction in all-cause mortality, and with a 29% reduction at 5 year of cardiovascular risk among high-risk individuals [1, 10].

23.2.4 Specific populations

Individuals with high blood pressure

A healthy diet is the first-line treatment for arterial hypertension: in fact, salt restriction, moderation of alcohol consumption, high consumption of vegetables and fruits, weight reduction and maintaining an ideal body weight are the main lifestyle measures recommended in order to lower blood pressure [2], although the effect of reduced dietary sodium on cardiovascular adverse events remains unclear [11-13].

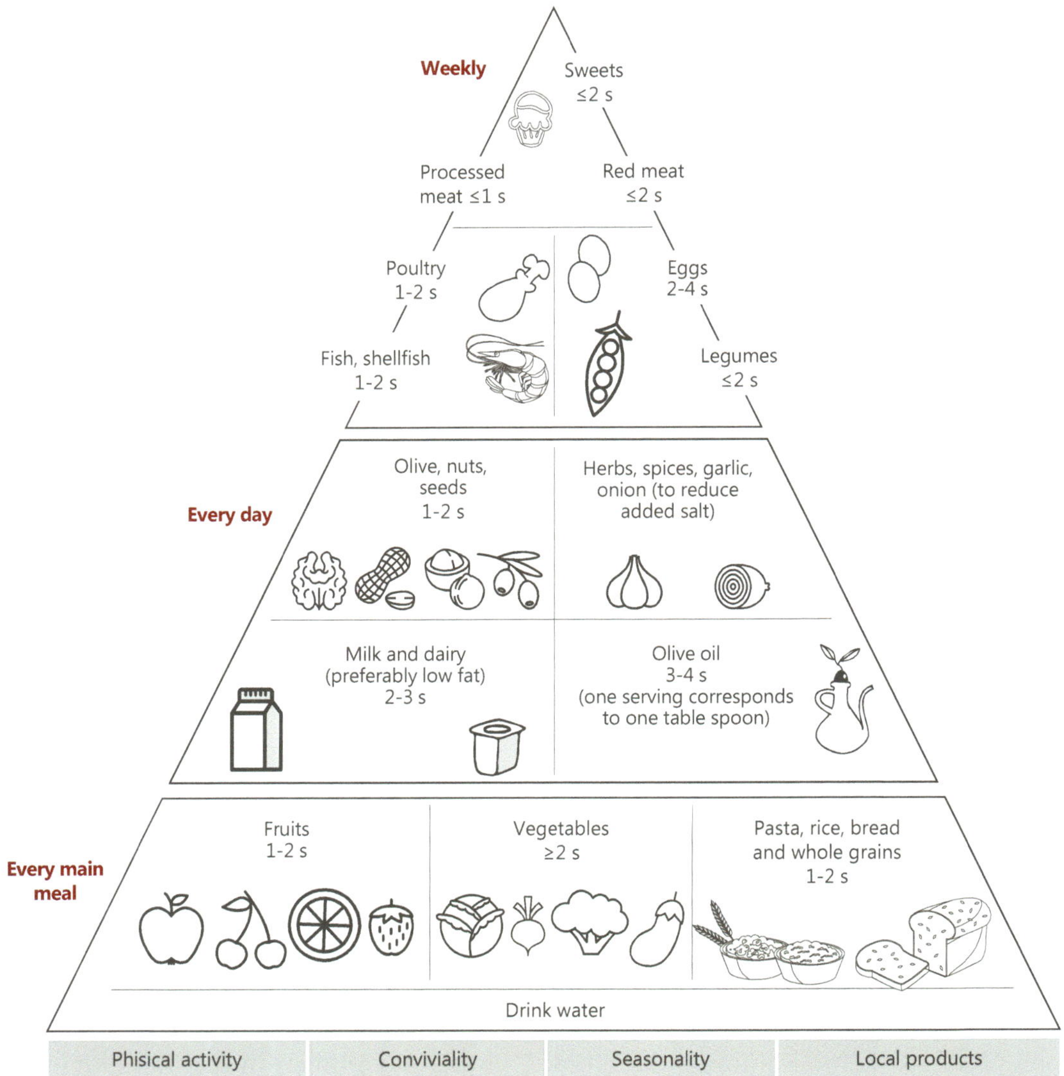

Fig. 23.1 Mediterranean diet pyramid (from Fondazione Umberto Veronesi).

Current evidence has reported an overall increased risk of mortality and cardiovascular events linked to high sodium intake, but, on the other hand, some studies also reported that reducing sodium intake below 3 g/daily further reduced blood pressure. However, paradoxically, that was also associated with an increased risk of all-cause and cardiovascular mortalities in both the general and the hypertensive population, suggesting a J-curve phenomenon [14], for which the underlying mechanisms are still not clear.

In summary, hypertensive patients should be advised to eat a healthy balanced diet containing vegetables, legumes, fresh fruits, low-fat dairy products, whole grains, fish and unsaturated fatty acids (especially olive oil), and to have a low consumption of red meat and saturated fatty acids. Of note, the Mediterranean diet includes many of these nutrients and foods, with a moderate consumption of alcohol (mostly wine with meals).

Several different studies and meta-analyses have shown that the Mediterranean diet significantly lowers blood pressure, blood glucose and lipid levels, and is associated with a reduction in cardiovascular events and all-cause mortality [1, 2].

Individuals with elevated lipids levels

The role of nutrition in the prevention of cardiovascular diseases has been extensively reviewed and there is strong evidence showing that dietary factors may influence atherogenesis directly or through effects by traditional risk factors, such as plasma lipids, blood pressure or glucose levels [1, 3, 15].

As outlined in the guidelines on prevention and treatment of dyslipidemias [3], in most cases several strategies are available in order to control lipids levels before recurring to medical therapy. Among them, the reduction of trans and saturated fats is the cornerstone, and could be aided by increasing consumption of fiber, daily physical activity and functional foods providing phytosterols (Table 23.2). The latter lifestyle modifications had shown much more efficacy than any other one in reducing LDL cholesterol and triglycerides, and in increasing HDL cholesterol [3].

It must be noted anyway that there are several dysfunctional patterns of HDL, which may be not beneficial on cardiovascular outcomes [3, 16], therefore the main goal of lipid control should be LDL lowering to a threshold that should be identified through individual risk-stratification [3]. According to the Heart Score stratification [3], the target LDL level is 130, 115, 100 or 70 mg/dL for those with low, moderate, high or very high cardiovascular risk, respectively. In addition, lifestyle intervention is strongly recommended for low-risk individuals with LDL cholesterol ≥ 190 mg/dL, and for moderate-risk individuals with LDL cholesterol ≥ 100 mg/dL [3]. Conversely, drug therapy is strongly recommended for those high-risk individuals with LDL cholesterol ≥ 100 mg/dL, and for the very high-risk ones with LDL cholesterol ≥ 70 mg/dL [3].

Regarding further lifestyle interventions, beside smoking cessation and physical activity, a healthy diet is of main importance. Cited guidelines provide a detailed description of what is allowed and what should be preferred or avoided in a daily diet (Table 23.3). At a glance, wholegrain cereals, vegetables, fruits, legumes, nuts and low-fat products should be preferred; while saturated and trans fats, especially those deriving from food processing and/or frying, should be completely avoided [3].

Table 23.2 Impact of specific lifestyle changes on lipid levels*

Strategies	*Magnitude*	*LoE*
To reduce TC and LDL-C		
Reduce dietary trans fat	+++	A
Reduce dietary saturated fat	+++	A
Increase dietary fiber	++	A
Use functional foods with phytosterols	++	A
Use red yet rice supplements	++	A
Reduce excessive body weight	++	A
Reduce dietary cholesterol	+	B
Increase habitual physical activity	+	B
Use of soy protein products	+/–	B
To reduce TG-rich lipoproteins		
Reduce excessive body weight	+++	A
Reduce alcohol intake	+++	A
Increase habitual physical activity	++	A
Reduce total amount of dietary carbohydrate	++	A
Use supplement of n-3 polyunsaturated fat	++	A
Reduce intake of mono- and disaccharides	++	B
Replace saturated fat with mono- or polyunsaturated fat	+	B
To increase HDL-C		
Reduce dietary trans fat	+++	A
Increase habitual physical activity	+++	A
Reduce excessive body weight	++	A
Reduce dietary carbohydrates and replace with unsaturated fat	++	A
Modest alcohol consumption	++	B
Quit smoking	+	B
Prefer carbohydrates with low glycemic index and high fiber content	+/–	C
Reduce intake of mono- and disaccharides	+/–	C

* Adapted from [3].
LoE, level of evidence; TC, total cholesterol; LDL-C, low-density lipoprotein-cholesterol; HDL-C, high-density lipoprotein-cholesterol

23.3 Controversies

The recent Prospective Urban Rural Epidemiology (PURE) trial [17] added a new level of understanding of some key environmental components of health. The main findings of the PURE investigators were:

- High carbohydrate intake was associated with higher risk of total mortality, whereas total fat and individual types of fat were related to lower total mortality. Total fat and types of fat were not associated with cardiovascular disease, myocardial infarction, or cardiovascular disease mortality, whereas saturated fat had an inverse association with stroke [17].
- Dairy consumption was associated with lower risk of mortality and major cardiovascular disease events in a diverse multinational cohort [18].

Such conclusions obviously raised many concerns among the scientific community and gained consent through mass media diffusion. Therefore, those reports need to be deeply analyzed in order to properly understand the real message learnable from them.

Table 23.3 Dietary recommendations to lower low-density lipoprotein-cholesterol and improve the overall lipoprotein profile*

Nutrients	*Preferred*	*Moderation*	*Limited*
Cereals	Whole grains	Refined bread, rice and pasta, biscuits, corn flakes	Pastries, muffins, pies, croissants
Vegetables	Raw and cooked vegetables	Potatoes	Vegetables cooked with butter or cream
Legumes	Lentils, beans, fava beans, peas, chickpeas, soybean		
Fruit	Fresh or frozen fruit	Dried fruit, jelly, jam, canned fruit, sorbets, popsicles, fruit juice	
Sweets	Non-caloric sweeteners	Sucrose, honey, chocolate, candies	Cakes, ice creams, fructose, soft drinks
Meat and fish	Lean and oily fish poultry without skin	Lean cuts of beef, lamb, pork or veal, seafood, shellfish	Sausages, salami, bacon, spare ribs, hot dogs, organ meats
Dairies and eggs	Skim milk and yogurt	Low-fat milk, low-fat cheese and other milk products, eggs	Regular cheese, cream, whole milk and yogurt
Fats and dressing	Vinegar, mustard, fat-free dressings	Olive oil, non-tropical vegetable oils, soft margarines, salad dressing, mayonnaise, ketchup	Trans fats and hard margarines (AVOID), palm and coconut oils, butter, lard, bacon fat
Nuts and seeds		All (except coconut) unsalted	Coconut
Cooking procedures	Grilling, boiling, steaming	Stir-frying, roasting	Frying

* Adapted from [3].
Preferred: to be preferred in daily consumption; Moderation: not to be assumed daily; Limited: to be avoided or only occasionally consumed.

This large epidemiological multi-center study is based on food frequency questionnaires compiled between 2003 and 2013 by more than 135,000 individuals (age 35-70 years), from 18 different countries, that were clinically followed-up for nearly 10 years (median 7.4 years, IQR 5.3-9.3 years).

By the way, food questionnaires are historically known for under-reporting food intake, and, notably, fat intake, thus altering dietary data sets [19]. In addition, the questionnaires were administered only at baseline, thus assuming that the dietary habits of each participant did not change over that long follow-up.

Much more important, the macronutrient analysis did not discern the type of dietary carbohydrates as either simple or complex, nor in function of their glycemic index.

Indeed, it has to be pointed out that in many of those low-income countries showing high carbohydrates consumption, the latter were coming from refined products, such as white rice and white bread, which appear to correlate with the obesity epidemic and the rapid increase of diabetes in such populations [19]. Moreover, consumption of foods with a high glycemic index is also associated with a linear increase in the risk of coronary heart disease, cardiovascular events and total mortality [19]. Consistently, it has been demonstrated that plant-based diets composed of healthful complex carbohydrates were associated with decreased incidence of cardiovascular disease, whereas the opposite happens with plant-based diets but with refined foods [20]. However, dietary modifications towards whole grains, vegetables, fruit, and fish or other omega-3 fatty acids were associated with decreased mortality [21], hence emphasizing the value and clinical impact of complex carbohydrates, fruits and vegetables as the fundamental components of the optimal diet.

Consequently, according to the PURE trial findings, as superficially interpreted, we should conclude that saturated fats do not have a negative impact on population health. However, this would mean ignoring much of the earlier data showing a correlation between saturated fats and increased cardiovascular disease, including the guidelines [1, 3] and the powerful data on animal protein that comes coupled with saturated fat, linking the downstream products (trimethylamine N-oxide) to the development of atherosclerosis [22].

Another significant limitation of the PURE study is that most of the subjects eating refined carbohydrates were poor, thus confounding variables associated with being poor cannot fully be ruled out. In addition, access to medical care was not specifically examined, although it would be expected that it would be closely tied to income and urban vs. rural location, which were controlled for.

However, the findings of the PURE trial were an "eye-opener" with respect to the nutritional concerns that are likely different in economically depressed areas. This is of even greater concern at a time when low and middle-income countries such as Brazil and India are incorporating Westernized, highly processed, inexpensive food into their diet, leading to significant increases in obesity, diabetes, and heart disease on top of the health concerns of poverty and famine. This type of poor-quality carbohydrate as the bulk of the diet is certainly an unfair comparator to saturated fat.

In addition, the oversimplification of macronutrients in fats, carbohydrates and proteins as *good* or *bad*, set the stage that maybe triggered the epidemic of obesity and diabetes observed in the past decades. As recommended by international guidelines [1-3], largely plant-based dietary patterns are associated with excellent health and longevity, as supported by the largest and better designed studies to date.

Therefore, consistent with several recent publications indicating higher mortality with refined grains and sugar, the PURE study demonstrated that consuming highly refined carbohydrates exceeds the mortality rate associated with eating fats. That should not be interpreted as a call to increase fat consumption, but to decrease low-fiber, low-quality, and high-sugar items, which so many people consume daily, and which provide sustenance for people in countries with lower economic status.

23.4 Conclusion

Dietary patterns are clearly correlated with cardiovascular health and outcomes. Specifically, reduced consumption of salt, fats and high glycemic index carbohydrates is effective in both reducing the prevalence of cardiovascular diseases and the incidence of adverse cardiovascular events. In particular, trans fats and processed foods should be completely avoided.

A balanced diet rich of vegetables and mono-unsaturated fats, typical of the Mediterranean diet, has been shown to be the best dietary pattern in the context of cardiovascular prevention.

Finally, in patients with previous adverse events, although dietary patterns are always of cornerstone importance, they cannot replace pharmacological therapy as recommended by the current guidelines [1-3].

REFERENCES

1. The Sixth Joint Task Force of the European Society of Cardiology and Other Societies on Cardiovascular Disease Prevention in Clinical Practice. 2016 European Guidelines on cardiovascular disease prevention in clinical practice. Eur Heart J 2016; 37: 2315-81.
2. The Task Force for the management of arterial hypertension of the European Society of Cardiology (ESC) and the European Society of Hypertension (ESH). 2018 ESC/ESH Guidelines for the management of arterial hypertension. Eur Heart J 2018; 39: 3021-104.
3. The Task Force for the Management of Dyslipidaemias of the European Society of Cardiology (ESC) and European Atherosclerosis Society (EAS). 2016 ESC/EAS Guidelines for the Management of Dyslipidaemias. Eur Heart J 2016; 37: 2999-3058.
4. A Report From the American Heart Association. Heart Disease and Stroke Statistics - 2018 Update. Circulation 2018; 137: e67-e492.
5. Rizos EC, Ntzani EE, Bika E, Kostapanos MS, Elisaf MS. Association between omega-3 fatty acid supplementation and risk of major cardiovascular disease events: a systematic review and meta-analysis. JAMA 2012; 308: 1024-33.
6. Mozaffarian D, Katan MB, Ascherio A, Stampfer MJ, Willett WC. Trans fatty acids and cardiovascular disease. N Engl J Med 2006; 354: 1601-13.
7. Sacks FM, Svetkey LP, Vollmer WM, et al. Effects on blood pressure of reduced dietary sodium: the Dietary Approaches to Stop Hypertension (DASH) diet. DASH-Sodium Collaborative Research Group. N Engl J Med 2001; 344: 3-10.
8. He FJ, Nowson CA, MacGregor GA. Fruit and vegetable consumption and stroke: meta-analysis of cohort studies. Lancet 2006; 367: 320-6.
9. World Health Organization. Guideline: Sugars Intake for Adults and Children. Geneva: World Health Organization, 2015.
10. Estruch R, Ros E, Salas-Salvado J, et al. Primary prevention of cardiovascular disease with a Mediterranean diet. N Engl J Med 2013; 368: 1279-90.
11. Bibbins-Domingo K, Chertow GM, Coxson PG, Moran A, Lightwood JM, Pletcher MJ, Goldman L. Projected effect of dietary salt reductions on future cardiovascular disease. N Engl J Med 2010; 362: 590-9.
12. He FJ, Burnier M, Macgregor GA. Nutrition in cardiovascular disease: salt in hypertension and heart failure. Eur Heart J 2011; 32: 3073-80.
13. He FJ, MacGregor GA. Salt reduction lowers cardiovascular risk: meta-analysis of outcome trials. Lancet 2011; 378: 380-2.
14. Mente A, O'Donnell M, Rangarajan S, et al. Associations of urinary sodium excretion with cardiovascular events in individuals with and without hypertension: a pooled analysis of data from four studies. Lancet 2016; 388: 465-75.

15. Eckel RH, Jakicic JM, Ard JD, et al. 2013 AHA/ACC guideline on lifestyle management to reduce cardiovascular risk: a report of the American College of Cardiology/ American Heart Association Task Force on Practice Guidelines. Circulation 2014; 129: S76-S99.
16. Angeloni E, Paneni F, Landmesser U, et al. Lack of protective role of HDL-C in patients with coronary artery disease undergoing elective coronary artery bypass grafting. Eur Heart J 2013; 34: 3557-62.
17. Dehghan M, Mente A, Zhang X, et al. Associations of fats and carbohydrate intake with cardiovascular disease and mortality in 18 countries from five continents (PURE): a prospective cohort study. Lancet 2017; 390: 2050-62.
18. Dehghan M, Mente A, Rangarajan S, et al. Association of dairy intake with cardiovascular disease and mortality in 21 countries from five continents (PURE): a prospective cohort study. Lancet 2018; 392: 2288-97.
19. Gianos E, William KA, Freeman AM, Kris-Etherton P, Aggarwal M. How Pure is PURE? Dietary Lessons Learned and Not Learned From the PURE Trials. Am J Med 2018; 131: 457-8.
20. Satija A, Bhupathiraju SN, Spiegelman D, et al. Healthful and Unhealthful Plant-Based Diets and the Risk of Coronary Heart Disease in U.S. Adults. J Am Coll Cardiol 2017; 70: 411-22.
21. Soto-Prieto M, Bhupathiraju SN, Mattei J, et al. Association of Changes in Diet Quality with Total and Cause-Specific Mortality. N Eng J Med 2017; 377: 143-53.
22. Tang WH, Wang Z, Levison BS, et al. Intestinal microbial metabolism of phosphatidylcholine and cardiovascular risk. N Engl J Med 2013; 368: 1575-84.

24 Diabetes and nutrition

Francesca De Leva, Linda Tartaglione, Mauro Di Leo,
Federica Costantini and Dario Pitocco

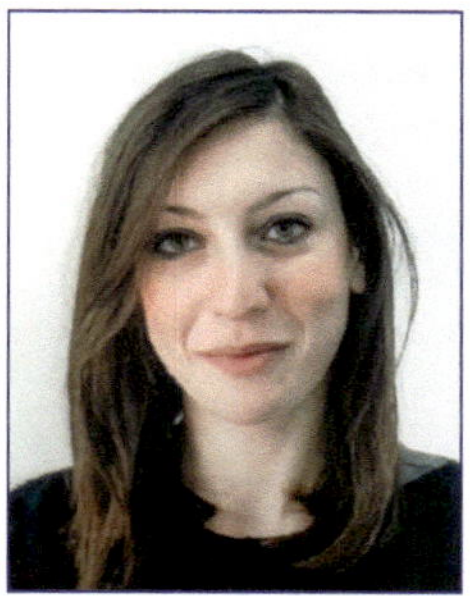

Federica Costantini

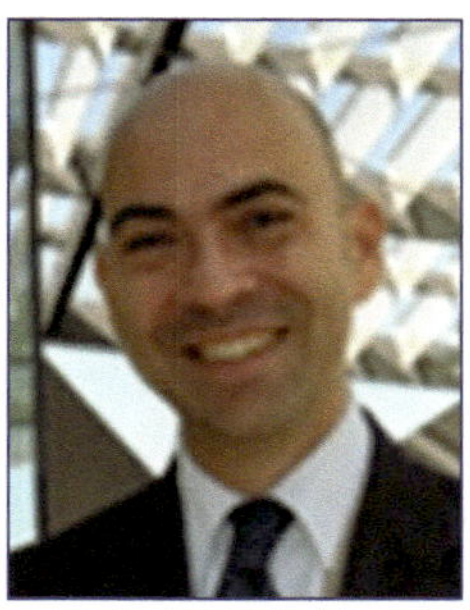

Dario Pitocco

24.1 Diabetes mellitus

Diabetes Mellitus (DM) is certainly among the diseases of the metabolism that has the greatest impact in public health, in relation to the frequency and related burden of the disease itself, with its complications and disabilities. According to current estimates, there are around 415 million people with diabetes mellitus in the world and this number is predicted to increase to 642 million in 2040. The occurrence of this disease, affecting all age groups, and the severity of its associated complications, make diabetes one of the major health problems on a global scale [1].

24.1.1 Diagnosis and classification

In the presence of symptoms typical of the disease (polyuria, polydipsia, weight loss), the diagnosis of diabetes is made after finding, even with a single occasion of random blood testing, a glucose level of > 200 mg/dL (regardless of food intake).

In the absence of the typical symptoms of the disease, the diagnosis of diabetes must rely on the confirmation of positive results on at least two different factors [2]:

- Fasting blood glucose ≥ 126 mg/dL (where fasting means at least 8 hours of food withdrawal)
- Glycemia ≥ 200 mg/dL 2 hours after oral glucose load (75 g)
- HbA1c ≥ 48 mmol/mol (6.5%)

In addition to diabetes, other dysglycemias are known, which identify individuals at risk of diabetes and cardiovascular disease, in particular [2]:

- "Altered fasting glycemia" or impaired fasting glucose (IFG), if fasting blood sugar is 100-125 mg/dL;
- "Reduced glucose tolerance" or impaired glucose tolerance (IGT), if, after 2 hours, the blood sugar oral glucose load is 140-199 mg/dL
- Glycated hemoglobins (HbA1c) is equal to 42-48 mmol/mol (6.0-6.49%)

In these subjects the presence of other risk factors for diabetes (obesity, familiarity for diabetes, etc.) or cardiovascular diseases (dyslipidemia, hyperten-

Dario Pitocco, MD
UOSA Director of Diabetology University Policlinico Foundation A. Gemelli,
Università Cattolica del Sacro Cuore, Rome, Italy

Email: dario.pitocco@policlinicogemelli.it

sion, etc.) must be investigated in order to implement the correct intervention to reduce the risk of onset of the disease and to establish appropriate therapeutic interventions based on the global cardiovascular risk.

A correct differential diagnosis between type 2 diabetes mellitus and other forms of diabetes (late-onset type 1 diabetes, LADA, MODY) is important in order to prescribe the best therapy for that particular type of diabetes.

Type 1 diabetes mellitus (DMT1) is caused by β-cell destruction, triggered by an autoimmune or idiopathic cause, and is characterized by an absolute insulin deficiency (the LADA variant, Latent Autoimmune Diabetes in Adults, has a slow course and appears only in adults).

Type 2 diabetes mellitus (DMT2) is caused by a partial deficiency of insulin secretion, which generally progresses over time but never leads to an absolute lack of the hormone, and which often occurs because of a condition of insulin resistance or a multifactorial condition.

Gestational diabetes appears in the second or third trimester of pregnancy and is caused by functional defects similar to those of DMT2. The first time it is diagnosed is during pregnancy and then it generally regresses after delivery. But can recur, often later, usually with the characteristics of DMT2 [2].

24.1.2 Notes of epidemiology

While DMT1 predominantly affects young people, the much more widespread DMT2 has the highest incidence in adulthood and is related to both socio-economic and individual behavioral factors: its onset can therefore be prevented with an appropriate lifestyle [3].

The diagnosis of diabetes is preceded by an asymptomatic phase in which a marked phenotypic variability of the manifestations associated with the alteration of glucose homeostasis can be observed. The presence of fasting hyperglycemia (IFG), reduced glucose tolerance (IGT) or the combination of both of these conditions should be considered not only as risk factors for the development of diabetes, but also factors associated with the development of both macrovascular and microvascular complications.

According to data recently published by the IDF (International Diabetes Federation) [1], the world prevalence of IGT stands at 6.7%. Approximately 318 million people, aged between 20 and 79, are at risk for diabetes and cardiovascular disease. After 10 years, the conversion rate to diabetes is 7.6%, with an 11 times higher risk among subjects with IFG, 3.9 times among the IGT subjects and 20.5 times higher among those presenting the IFG/IGT combination [4].

Until a few years ago, DMT2 was considered a pathology exclusively for adults, but the spread of obesity has triggered its appearance even in the current younger population. Insulin resistance and β-cell defects are the factors that correlate obesity to DMT2, while genetic and environmental factors are involved in their genesis.

The incidence of DMT2 has been strongly increasing in children, along with obesity [5, 6]. It mainly affects obese adolescents, with familiarity for DMT2, preceded by a history of glucose intolerance. Its onset is insidious because it often presents the same characteristics of DMT1, including ketoacidosis.

In Western Europe over 80% of diabetes cases are attributable to obesity, according to the IDF estimates. It is easy to understand how the fight against obesity and the one against diabetes go hand in hand, and how another fight is needed that focuses efforts on social and health policies to stem a growing debilitating phenomenon.

Diabetes still remains one of the main causes of death due to its widespread occurrence [7]. Its high prevalence and high mortality make it a disease with a significant social impact. The appearance of both microvascular and macrovascular complications is a determining factor in reducing the life expectancy in patients with diabetes mellitus. Therefore, there is an evident need for better maintenance of good glycemic control, especially in the earliest stages of the disease, combined with careful prevention and correction of the coexisting cardiovascular risk factors and renal damage [8].

24.2 Nutritional medical therapy

Nutritional Medical Therapy (NMT) is essential in both the prevention and in the treatment of DM which, among the most widespread chronic diseases, is surely the one that benefits most from a correct diet.

Numerous studies, and in particular the American study *Diabetes Control and Complication Trial* (DCCT) [9], have shown that, in addition to pharmacological and educational therapy, an adequate diet assumes the value of "real therapy". A proper diet represents a tool essential to obtaining and maintaining an optimal metabolic compensation, to reduce the cardiovascular risk, to prevent and best treat the microvascular and macrovascular complications of the diabetic patient.

24.2.1 Nutritional medical therapy: prevention and care of diabetes mellitus

The conditions of dysglycemia (IFG and IGT), besides involving a high risk of developing type 2 diabetes and cardiovascular disease, are associated with obesity, dyslipidemia and arterial hypertension.

The treatment of obesity is of great importance in the whole population and especially in diabetic patients or those at risk of developing diabetes. There is a direct correlation between Body Mass Index (BMI) and diseases related to obesity, including DMT2. The risk of diabetes is greatly increased by being overweight (BMI > 25 kg/m^2). In fact, in overweight or obese individuals, insulin sensitivity is reduced and there is an overall deterioration in diabetes control. In particular, the distribution of visceral fat and an increase in abdominal circumference, are associated with an increase in insulin resistance [10].

To date, no drug has been specifically approved for use in pre-diabetes and/or the prevention of type 2 diabetes.

According to the Italian Standards of Care 2018 [2] for diabetes mellitus, achieving and maintaining a 7% weight loss and performing regular physical activity are the most appropriate means to reduce the risk of developing DMT2 in individuals with IGT (level of test I, strength of recommendation A).

For patients with normal weight, it is not important to change the daily energy intake. Conversely, in overweight or obese patients, and particularly in patients with visceral fat distribution, it is important to reduce the daily calorie intake. Dietary restriction should be assessed based on the patient's energy expenditure. Generally, we recommend a reduction of the energy intake of 500-1000 kcal compared to the calculated daily energy expenditure, decreasing in particular the contribution of high energy density foods, rich in fats and/or carbohydrates, and increasing the intake of plant-based fibers. Indeed, most observational epidemiological studies suggest that a diet rich in fibers and foods with a low glycemic index is protective against the risk of type 2 diabetes [11, 12].

In subjects who have an elevated daily consumption of high energy density foods (rich in fats and/or carbohydrates such as sweets, cookies, sugary drinks, seasoning fats, cheeses, sausages), the reduction of these foods alone can lead to weight loss. Most of the available evidence indicates that, more than the total quantity, the quality of dietary fatty acids is important; in particular, saturated fatty acids increase the risk of DMT2, while the partial replacement of these with unsaturated fatty acids reduces it [13].

The reduction of caloric intake must therefore be associated with the increase in physical activity, which is important not only to facilitate weight loss but also in the maintenance period to prevent recovery of lost weight. It has been shown that interventions to improve lifestyle, which include moderate-intensity aerobic physical activity lasting at least 20-30 minutes a day, or 150 minutes-a-week, and a weight loss of 5-10% reduce the incidence of DMT2 by about 60%, and therefore represent particularly effective preventive tools for halting or slowing the diabetes epidemic [14].

These patients should therefore be encouraged to change their eating habits by:

- reducing the total fat intake (< 30% of the daily intake) and particularly the intake of fatty acids (less than 10% of the daily calorie intake)
- increasing the intake of vegetable fibers (at least 15 g/1000 kcal).

The diet in diabetic patients, both in DMT1 and in DMT2, must be calibrated and individualized based on some needs such as: glycemic goals, the degree of glycometabolic compensation, lipid values, renal function, hypoglycemic drug therapy, and last but not least, the social context in which patients find themselves.

It should also be remembered that even patients with type 1 diabetes, who are overweight, can become insulin-resistant and weight loss can reduce insulin requirements and improves glycemic control.

24.2.2 Nutritional medical therapy in the patient with type 2 diabetes mellitus

Most patients with DMT2 are overweight or obese, therefore, in these patients, weight loss is the most important aspect of diet therapy. Several studies have shown that even a modest weight loss induces a reduction in blood glucose levels, thanks to the decrease in peripheral insulin resistance and hepatic glucose production. The reduction in body weight also leads to an improvement in all the cardiovascular risk factors present in diabetic patients, in particular hyperlipidemia and arterial hypertension along with a significant reduction in the need for hypoglycemic drugs [3, 15, 16].

Weight loss is recommended for all overweight adults (BMI 25-29.9 kg/m^2) or obese adults (BMI ≥ 30 kg/m^2). The main approach to achieving and maintaining weight loss is lifestyle modification, which includes a reduction in caloric intake and an increase in physical activity. A moderate reduction in caloric intake (300-500 kcal/day) and a modest increase in energy expenditure (200-300 kcal/day) allow a slow but progressive weight loss.

Weight loss can be achieved by a low fat and low calories diet, a low carbohydrate diet, and a Mediterranean diet, naturally rich in vegetable fibers, which can be effective in the short term (up to 2 years).

A pharmacological treatment for obesity should be implemented only after the efficacy of diet, exercise and, where indicated, cognitive-behavioral therapy has been considered, and these therapeutic approaches were proven to be ineffective in inducing weight loss or in maintaining the lost weight.

Carbohydrates

The amount and type of carbohydrates (CHO) ingested are the main determinants of a post-meal blood glucose level. The amount of carbohydrates can vary according to individual and local habits and may complement the consumption of fats and proteins in the range between 45-60% of the total food energy intake, but never be less than 130 g/day [10, 17]. The 60% share of the total energy intake can be recommended as long as the consumption of carbohydrates derives mainly from foods rich in water-soluble fibers (fruit, vegetables, legumes) and/or foods with low glycemic index (pasta, legumes, parboiled rice).

The intake of carbohydrates should be reduced in patients with non-optimal glycemic control and/or with hypertriglyceridemia. When that is not possible, it's advisable to use, in significant quantities, foods rich in water-soluble fibers with a low glycemic index. Moreover, in these cases it is advisable to reduce the intake of carbohydrates to up to 45% of the total daily energy needs while isoenergetically increasing the intake of cis-monounsaturated fats. However, particular attention should be paid when increasing the total fat content to over 35% of the total energy needs, as a diet that is too rich in fat has a high energy density and can therefore facilitate the onset of obesity.

Glycemic Index

The glycemic response to foods is influenced both by the quantity and quality of carbohydrates. In fact, it is known that, with the same CHO content, different foods can produce very different effects on post-meal blood glucose levels. The "Glycemic Index" (GI) is defined as "the incremental level of glycemia after ingestion of 50 g of available carbohydrates, expressed as a percentage of the corresponding level obtained after intake". To assess the glycemic response of a given food, glucose or white bread is introduced as reference items: a food with a glycemic index of 50% determines a rise in blood sugar equal to half that induced by glucose or white bread.

Among the most common foods with a high carbohydrate content and a low glycemic index (less than 55) we should mention: pasta, legumes, fruit, milk. Foods with a high glycemic index (greater than 75) are bread, rice and potatoes.

For example, 50 g of carbohydrates contained in a portion of 100 g of dried beans have a lower impact on blood sugar than the same amount of carbohydrates contained in a slice of bread of 90 g.

The GI takes into account only the quality of carbohydrates while the glycemic response to a food is also influenced by the quantity of carbohydrates. For this reason, another index, called "Glycemic Load" (GL), was introduced that best expresses the impact of carbohydrates on blood sugar. The GL is calculated as: "quantity of carbohydrates contained in a portion of the food, multiplied by the GI of the food itself and divided by 100" (GL = GI x g of CHO content/100), and allows comparing the effect on the glycemic response of equivalent portions of different foods: the lower the glycemic load the lower the effect on the blood sugar of that portion of food.

The GI and GL are very useful for predicting the effect on blood sugar of a mixed meal, such as a meal that is composed of very different GI foods. To obtain the GL of the entire meal, the percentage of carbohydrates contained in each food is multiplied by its glycemic index and the results obtained for each component of the meal are summed up.

The GI can be influenced by a series of factors that cause a certain variability, such as the fat and protein content of the meal, the fiber content, the technological process used for the production of food, the type and duration of cooking.

Fats

The main objective for recommendations on the intake of fat, in the diet for people with diabetes, is to limit the intake of saturated fatty acids (< 10%, to be reduced to < 8% in the presence of high LDL) and drastically reduce trans fatty acids which are the main determinants of plasma LDL cholesterol and cholesterol intake [2].

In fact, numerous studies document that reducing the intake of saturated fats within a diet is effective in reducing the cardiovascular risk of the general population. If we consider that diabetics have a high cardiovascular risk, the recommendation to reduce dietary fat intake is even more important in the diabetic population. A reduction in plasma cholesterol levels in diabetics also achieves a reduction of cardiovascular events higher than that obtained in the general population.

In general, it is recommended that dietary fat intake should not exceed 20-35% of the total daily calories, with a quantity of cholesterol not exceeding 300 mg/day, to be reduced to 200 mg/day when plasma level values are high [2]. In obese subjects, a further 30% reduction in fat intake is recommended to promote weight loss [18]. Furthermore, it is recommended to introduce at least 2 portions per week of fish, preferably blue, as it supplies polyunsaturated fatty acids N-3 [2].

Protein

Current nutritional recommendations regarding the protein content in the diet of people with diabetes without overt nephropathy are similar to those of the general population, according to major national and international scientific societies. In patients without evident nephropathy, proteins should provide 10-20% of the total daily energy.

In people with any degree of chronic kidney disease, to reduce the risk of progression towards terminal renal failure, the protein intake should be limited to the recommended dietary ration of 0.8 g per day of good quality protein per kg of body weight.

In people with DMT2, the introduction of proteins can affect the increase in post-meal insulin levels, without increasing the concentration of glucose; for this reason, proteins should not be used to treat an acute hypoglycemic episode or prevent nocturnal hypoglycemia [2].

Dietary proteins must include all 8 essential amino acids (or 9, including histidine, which is not strictly an essential amino acid for adult humans and adolescents, while it is essential for early childhood). High quality proteins are present in meat, poultry, eggs, dairy products, fish and soy. Proteins of lower quality are contained in cereals, grains, nuts and vegetables.

Fibers

A diet rich in fiber is recommended to people with diabetes in order to improve glycemic control and reduce cholesterol (total and LDL), thus helping to reduce cardiovascular risk and contribute to weight management [10].

Alcohol

A moderate introduction of alcohol, up to 10 g/day in women (one portion) and 20 g/day in men (two servings), has no effect on blood glucose and is acceptable if the patient wishes to drink alcohol. However, the carbohydrates contained in alcoholic beverages can have an important negative impact [2].

Alcohol intake should be limited in obese or subjects with hypertriglyceridemia and it is not recommended in pregnant women and patients with a history of pancreatitis.

It is advisable for any intake of alcohol, in patients who are treated with insulin, to take place during meals that include carbohydrate-containing foods, to prevent, especially at night, the risk of prolonged hypoglycemia.

24.2.3 Nutritional medical therapy in the patient with type 1 diabetes mellitus

Although general dietary recommendations for people with DMT1 do not differ from those in the general population, specific nutritional intervention is an essential component of the treatment of DMT1 [2].

The nutritional medical therapy of DMT1 is necessary to adapt insulin therapy to the supply of nutrients, guaranteeing the achievement of satisfactory glycemic control [19]. The adoption of specific nutritional education programs leads to an improvement in blood glucose control and a reduction in the risk of hospitalization in people with DMT1 [20].

Insulin therapy must be integrated into an individual's nutritional and physical activity program. Patients on basal-bolus insulin therapy should modify the preprandial insulin boluses based on the carbohydrates contained in the meals. Therefore, carbohydrate counting represents an essential component in the context of Nutritional Medical Treatment and identifies the most effective strategy for glycemic control in patients with diabetes in intensive insulin treatment, both in multi-injective therapy and with insulin pumps [21, 22].

In patients treated with constant insulin doses, the introduction of carbohydrates with meals must be kept constant as well, in terms of quantity and schedule [23].

During scheduled exercise, adjustment of insulin therapy is recommended. On the other hand, if physical exercise is not planned, it is advisable to suggest taking glucose supplements.

Counting carbohydrates

It is a method that allows adjusting the dose of insulin to the carbohydrate content of a particular meal. To learn the carbohydrate count it is necessary to learn how to recognize which foods contain them and, above all, to be able to count the contents in grams [24].

Below are the food groups that contain carbohydrates:

- cereals and derivatives: flour, pasta, rice, polenta (grits), bread, crackers, etc.
- legumes and potatoes
- fruit
- confectionery products: cakes, pies, snacks, chocolate, ice cream, etc.
- milk and yogurt
- sugary drinks

And others that do not contain CHO, or contain them in negligible quantities:

- meat and fish
- vegetables (excluding legumes and potatoes)
- eggs
- cheeses
- water and unsweetened drinks.

Carbohydrates are essentially divided into 2 groups:

- "Simple" carbohydrates, which are rapidly absorbed: sugar, fruit juice, sweetened drinks, candies, honey.
- "Complex" carbohydrates, whose absorption is slower: cereals and derivatives, legumes and potatoes.

This distinction is very important, especially when CHO are taken as a treatment for hypoglycemia (in these cases, simple ones are preferred).

Different foods have different percentages of CHO. To accurately calculate the content of carbohydrates in foods, special tables must be available that supply the CHO content per 100 g of food.

If the portion of food to be consumed does not correspond to 100 g it will be necessary to apply a proportion. For example, if the common bread has 65 g of carbohydrates in 100 g, and if they take 50 g, applying a proportion, the content in grams of carbohydrates (X) of the portion:

$$X/50 = 65/100 \text{ then } X = 65 \times 50/100 = 32.5$$

which corresponds to the grams of carbohydrates contained in 50 g of bread.

The same is true for other foods, but for pasta and cereals such as rice and spelt, it is important to note that the carbohydrate contents shown in the tables refer to the raw weight; therefore, if they are weighed after cooking the value must be adjusted (usually half for pasta and a third for rice, barley and polenta or grits).

At the beginning it is necessary to weigh all the foods containing carbohydrates, but with time and practice people usually learn to "eyeball" the weight of food [25].

Commercial foods have a variable carbohydrate content, depending on the preparation process and the brand, therefore when possible, it is always better to consult the label of the product being consumed (among other things, it is also very convenient, as it provides values per portion or per piece). The carbohydrate tables are basically correct, but they remain a simplification nevertheless.

REFERENCES

1. http://www.diabetesatlas.org/resources/2015-atlas.html.
2. Associazione Medici Diabetologi (AMD) - Società Italiana di Diabetologia (SID) - Standard italiani per la cure del diabete mellito. 2018.
3. Tuomilehto J, Lindström J, Eriksson JG, et al; Finnish Diabetes Prevention Study Groups. Prevention of type 2 diabetes mellitus by changes in lifestyle among subjects with impaired glucose tolerance. N Engl J Med 2001; 344(18): 1343-50.
4. Lazzeri C, Dei S, Mennuti N, Papini D, Salvadori P, Caciagli L, Coletta D. Progetto "prediabete". Valutazione della tolleranza glucidica neri soggetti a rischio di diabete mellito tipo 2 nell'ASL 11 di Empoli. G It Diabetol Metab 2008; 28: 168-72.
5. Brufani C, Tozzi A, Fintini D, Ciampalini P, Grossi A, Fiori R, Kiepe D, Manco M, Schiaffini R, Porzio O, Cappa M, Barbetti F. Sexual dimorphism of body composition and insulin sensitivity across pubertal development in obese Caucasian subjects. Eur J Endocrinol 2009; 160(5): 769-75.
6. ISPAD Clinical Practice Consensus Guidelines 2009 Compendium. Type 2 diabetes in children and adolescent. Pediatr Diabetes 2009: 10 Suppl 12: 17-32.
7. Waugh NR, Dallas JH, Jung RT, Newton RW. Mortality in a cohort of diabetic patients: Causes and relative risks. Diabetologia 1989, 32: 103-4.
8. Tancredi M, Rosengren A, Svensson AM, Kosiborod M, Pivodic A, Gudbjörnsdottir S, Wedel H, Clements M, Dahlqvist S, Lind M. Excess Mortality among Persons with Type 2 Diabetes. N Engl J Med 2015; 373: 1720-32.
9. Nathan DM; DCCT/EDIC Research Group. The Diabetes Control and Complications Trial/Epidemiology of Diabetes Interventions and Complications Study at 30 Years: Overview. Diabetes Care 2014; 37(1): 9-16.
10. ADI - AMD - SID. Raccomandazioni 2013-2014 - La terapia medica nutrizionale nel Diabete Mellito.
11. Shai I, Schwarzfuchs D, Henkin Y, et al.; Dietary Intervention Randomized Controlled Trial (DIRECT) Group. Weight loss with a low-carbohydrate, Mediterranean, or low-fat diet. N Engl J Med 2008; 359(3): 229-41.

12. Thomas D, Elliott EJ, Baur L. Low glycaemic index or low glycaemic load diets for overweight and obesity. Cochrane Database of Systematic Rev 2007; 2007(3): CD005105.
13. Raccomandazioni nutrizionali basate sull'evidenza per la terapia e la prevenzione del diabete mellito. Il diabete 2005; 164: 947-54.
14. Knowler WC, Barrett-Connor E, Fowler SE, Hamman RF, Lachin JM, Walker EA, Nathan DM; Diabetes Prevention Program Research Group. Reduction in the incidence of type 2 diabetes with lifestyle intervention or metformin. N Engl J Med 2002; 346(6): 393-403.
15. SIO- ADI. Standard Italiani per la Cura dell'Obesità.
16. Look AHEAD Research Group, Wing RR. Long-term effects of a lifestyle intervention on weight and cardiovascular risk factors in individuals with type 2 diabetes mellitus: four-year results of the Look AHEAD trial. Arch Intern Med 2010; 170 (17): 1566-75.
17. Sheard NF, Clarck NG, Brand-Miller JC, Franz MJ, Pi-Sunyer FX, Mayer-Davus E, Kulkarni K, Geil P. Dietary carbohydrate (amount and type) in the prevention and management of diabetes: a statement of the American Diabetes Association. Diabetes Care 2004; 27: 2266-71.
18. Astrup A, Ryan L, Grunwald GK, et al. The role of dietary fat in body fatness: evidence from a preliminary meta-analysis of ad libitum low-fat dietary intervention studies. Br Nutr 2000; 83 (Suppl. 1): S25-S32.
19. American Diabetes Association. Standard of medical care in diabetes, 2019. Diabetes care.
20. Kulkarni K, Castle G, Gregory R, et al. Nutrition Practice Guidelines for Type 1 Diabetes Mellitus positively affect dietitian practices and patient outcomes. The Diabetes Care and Education Dietetic Practice Group. J Am Diet Assoc 1998; 98(1): 62-70; quiz 71-2.
21. Bell KJ, Barclay AW, Petocz P, Colagiuri S, Brand-Miller JC. Efficacy of carbohydrate counting in type 1 diabetes: a systematic review and meta-analysis. Lancet Diabetes Endocrinol 2014; 2(2): 133-40.
22. Bozzetto L, Giorgini M, Alderisio A, et al. Glycaemic load versus carbohydrate counting for insulin bolus calculation in patients with type 1 diabetes on insulin pump. Acta Diabetol 2015; 52(5): 865-71.
23. Bonora E, Kiechl S, Willeit J, et al.; Bruneck study. Population-Based Incidence Rates and Risk Factors for Type 2 Diabetes in White Individuals. The Bruneck Study. Diabetes 2004, 53(7): 1782-9.
24. Brocco S, Visentin C, Fedeli U, et al. Monitoring the occurrence of diabetes mellitus and its major complications: the combined use of different administrative databases. Cardiovasc Diabetol 2007; 6: 5.
25. Lindström J, Ilanne-Parikka P, Peltonen M, et al.; Finnish Diabetes Prevention Study Group. Sustained reduction in the incidence of type 2 diabetes by lifestyle intervention: follow-up of the Finnish Diabetes Prevention Study. Lancet 2006; 368(9548): 1673-9.

25 Food and skin

Steven Paul Nisticò, Martina Silvestri,
Luigi Bennardo and Federica Tamburi

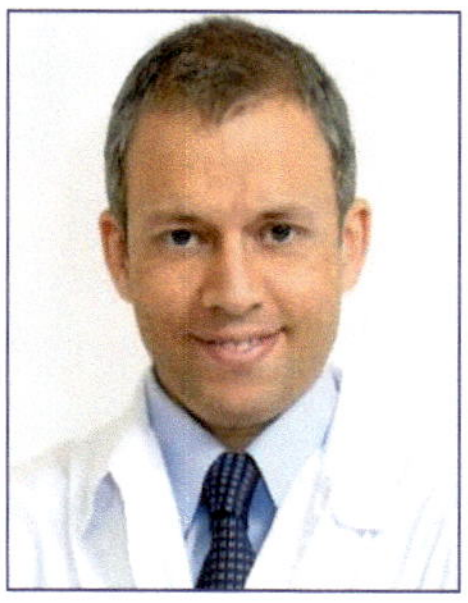

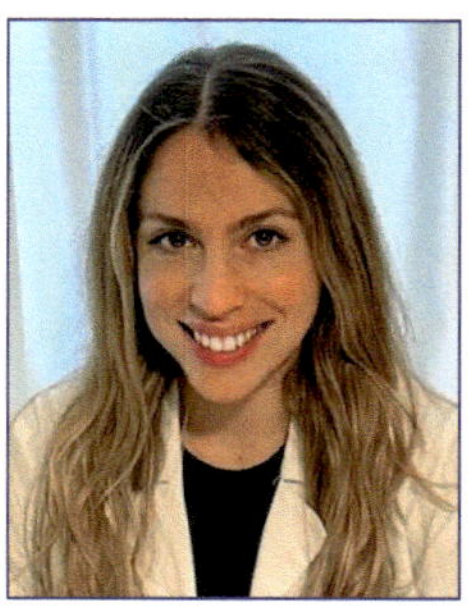

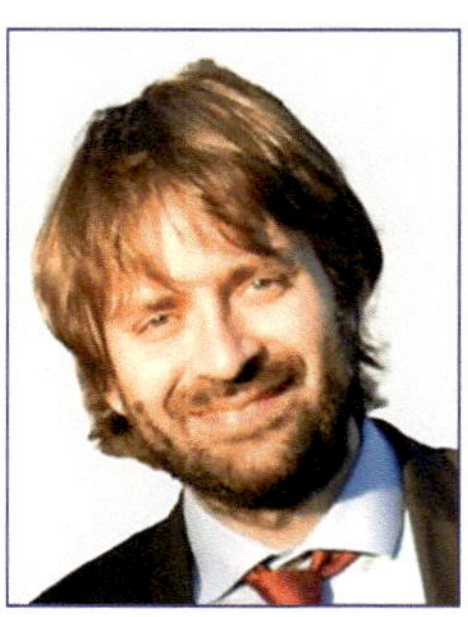

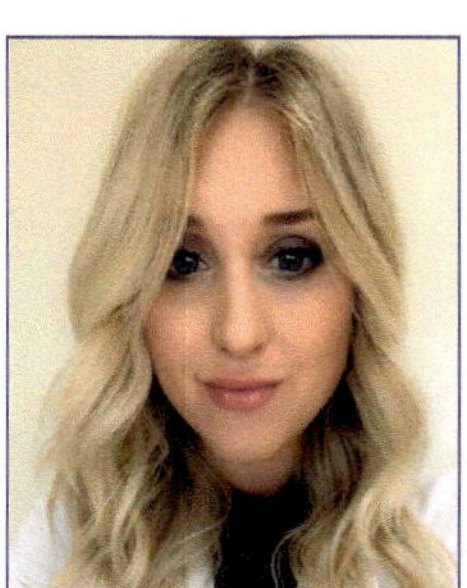

25.1 Introduction

Since ancient times, the intake of particular foods or specific diets has been considered one of the fundamental cornerstones for the treatment of skin diseases and blemishes. To date, the number of research studies indicating the modification of eating behavior as a fundamental step in the treatment of dermatological diseases is increasing. In this chapter we will focus on the most frequent and common skin diseases, for which dietary change can be recommended as one of the main components of the treatment of the skin pathology in question.

The Internet is full of "tips" and "scams" regarding dietary regimes to be adopted which, while on one hand are totally ineffective, on the other hand can even be harmful, such as the use of untested dietary supplements or specific item elimination diets that are severely restrictive. By analyzing specific nutrients, foods or dietary patterns, it is possible to highlight both the triggering factors of the disease and substances that can be useful in therapy.

Studies published in recent years have clarified, if ever there was a need, that diet can influence the outcome of many common dermatological conditions. In some cases, dermatological diseases can be linked to a systemic disease, and dietary changes can affect its severity. In other cases, the intake of particular foods and substances can be useful in prevention, such as in skin cancer and skin aging. Not the least of which, the systemic therapies used for dermatological diseases, such as steroid therapies, that are known to increase the risk of other related diseases. However, even in this case, the diet regimen plays a key role, and it is crucial in trying to reduce these related risks.

25.2 Food and the aging skin

Different behaviors are commonly accepted by people as negative factors affecting skin aging, such as smoking and sun exposure. Like these, however, dietary factors should also be taken into consideration.

In people with diabetes, it is known that higher blood sugar values can accelerate skin aging. In this regard, sugar promotes the cross-linking of collagen

Martina Silvestri, MD; Luigi Bennardo, MD
Università Magna Graecia, Catanzaro, Italy

Steven Paul Nisticò, MD;
Sapienza Università di Roma, Italy

Email: steven.nistico@uniroma1.it

Federica Tamburi, MD
Università Cattolica del Sacro Cuore, Rome, Italy

fibers which occurs through a process known as glycation. This process leads to the production of Advanced Glycation End-products (AGEs) and cross-linking of collagen fibers. These changes, in turn, results in a loss of elasticity and sagging skin due to changes in collagen and elastic fibers. In this process, a covalent bond is established between the amino acids present in the collagen and the elastin present in the dermis. These amino acids are linked together by glucose and fructose, resulting in increased rigidity and a reduction in elasticity. This glycation process develops much faster during adulthood and is significantly influenced by the dietary regime a person follows. Also, the intake of preformed AGEs, which develop during some cooking processes, such as frying, can be harmful. Once these structural changes have occurred in the skin, the body is no longer able to repair the cytoarchitectural cutaneous damage, and it is for these reasons that food prevention becomes important. Recently, research has focused on the study of foods that are able to inhibit the production of AGEs, including herbs and spices, such as oregano, cinnamon, cloves, ginger and garlic, as well as substances that are naturally found in some fruits and vegetables, such as lipoic acid.

Several studies conducted both *in vitro* and *in vivo* have shown that various foods (fruits, vegetables, tea leaves and seeds) containing Anti-Oxidant (AO) substances act to limit the harmful skin effects of Ultra-Violet (UV) radiation. It is important to note that research indicates AOs consumed through food sources seem to work differently than those found in isolated supplements. Just like the daily consumption of tomato paste for 12 weeks, in one study, showed a reduction in UV-induced erythema (redness of the skin), and the presence of lower levels of metalloproteinases in the skin matrix.

It has been reported that a greater intake of vegetables, legumes and olive oil serves to protect the skin from actinic damage. Similarly, a diet with a high content of potassium and vitamins A and C has been related to fewer wrinkles. From this it can be inferred that a diet rich in phytonutrients can limit photo-damage and delay skin aging.

25.3 Food and acne

During the 1960s, several research groups focused on a possible relationship between chocolate and acne. The largest study of the time, involving 65 acne patients compared the effects of chocolate consumption with that of a placebo over a four-week period, and did not find substantial differences in the severity of acne in the patient groups involved. However, while recently reviewing the study, it was noted that it presented methodological flaws.

In fact, more recent research studies carried out in the USA have provided strong support for the theory that sees diet as a contributing cause of acne, demonstrating a primary role of some types of food, such as dairy products, as well as in high glycemic index diets, typical of Western diets. To confirm this theory, it has been observed that acne is absent in non-westernized native populations, as in Papua New Guinea and in Paraguay. Similar results were noted by researchers in Italy and Malaysia. The strongest evidence regarding the acne pathology has been highlighted on high glycemic dietary patterns.

In several Randomized Controlled Trials (RCTs), it was shown that patients who followed a low-glycemic load dietary pattern for 10/12 weeks had a significant improvement in the clinical manifestations of the disease. This type of diet produced less bioavailability of androgens and an altered production of cutaneous sebum, confirmed by histopathological examination, with a decrease in skin inflammation and sebaceous glands.

At the base of this mechanism there is the glycemic load which does not only consider the quantity of carbohydrates consumed, but also the rate of carbohydrates that are absorbed. There are foods that have a high glycemic index such as sugar, white bread or white rice and which are rapidly absorbed, thus rapidly raising glucose levels and causing high levels of insulin as a result.

In terms of dairy products, various RCTs suggest a mechanism that focuses instead on the high carbohydrate content, with relative effects on serum insulin and insulin-like growth factor-1 (IGF-1). Recent RCTs have shown that insulin as well as IGF-1 are able to increase sebum production, stimulate androgen synthesis and at the same time increase their bioavailability, considering their fundamental role in the pathogenesis of acne.

Supplements containing probiotics, omega-3 fatty acids, zinc, antioxidants or fiber and vitamin A, have shown promising results *in vitro* and on animal testing, but given the scarcity of human studies, a level of high recommendation cannot be reached at this time.

Several studies in this regard have concluded that both omega-3 fatty acids and gamma linolenic acid supplements and minocycline-integrated probiotics, for a treatment period of about 10 weeks, have led to a decrease in both the number of total acne lesions, and a clinical and histopathological improvement of the same lesions.

It should be noted that further scientific studies are necessary because of the contrasting results in terms of both efficacy and negative results obtained in various RTCs that tested zinc at different doses and in various formulations (gluconate, sulfate). That is also true for zinc linked to methionine or in combination with antioxidants and lactoferrin.

25.4 Food and atopic dermatitis

Atopic dermatitis (AD) is a chronic-recurrent dermatitis that presents clinical manifestations with characteristic topographical destruction that varies in different age groups. Food allergies are highly correlated with AD. Foods can trigger an exacerbation of AD through three main mechanisms. Immediate type 1 or hypersensitivity reactions mediated by immunoglobulins E (IgE) can trigger an exacerbation over a period of time ranging from a few minutes to a few hours. The six trigger foods are *wheat, soy, milk, eggs, nuts* and *seafood*. Tests for the diagnosis of food allergies, prick tests or specific blood chemistry tests can be used as a screening, but given the high rate of false positive results, confirmation requires the execution of a double-blind placebo-controlled oral challenge test. Late eczematous reactions, due to trigger foods, can cause an exacerbation of atopic dermatitis up to 48 hours later. The trophoallergens can act as histamine-liberating agents, causing itching or cutaneous inflammation, or they can cause an IgE-mediated urticarial reaction, capable of causing eczematous dermatological lesions. Some experimental studies have shown the worsening of AD, following ingestion of cow's milk, is probably due to activation of T lymphocytes stimulated by casein contained in milk. It has also been shown that in Peru's balsam allergy, some people allergic to fragrance additives may experience a skin flare following the ingestion of certain foods, including tomatoes, citrus fruits and cinnamon. The correlation between AD and food allergies is strongly supported by the benefit patients derive from restrictive dietary measures.

25.5 Food and psoriasis

Psoriasis is a chronic inflammatory disease characterized by erythematous desquamative patches. It is an established fact that psoriasis represents an important risk factor for cardiovascular diseases. In the last decade, this association has been studied more closely and numerous reports have presented substantial evidence that patients with psoriasis are at a higher risk of cardiovascular disease (acute coronary syndromes, stroke). The evidence is such that psoriasis patients should be informed about this association and, above all, how to reduce their risk. It is therefore important to evaluate cardiovascular risk factors, including those that can be modified through lifestyle changes (diet, physical activity). Patients with psoriasis have been shown to have a higher prevalence of comorbidities that increase the risk of cardiovascular disease (CVD). These include obesity, diabetes, hypertension and dyslipidemia. A meta-analysis of 27 observational studies found that psoriasis is associated with an increased prevalence and incidence of diabetes. A review of 25 observational studies, with more than 265,000 patients with psoriasis, found that psoriasis was significantly associated with greater chances of dyslipidemia. Furthermore, the mere presence of psoriasis may represent an independent risk factor for Myocardial Infarction (MI). In a study of women, psoriasis was found to be an independent predictor for non-fatal CVD. In patients undergoing coronary angiography, patients with psoriasis were more likely to have an angiographically confirmed CVD than in controls. In a study that specifically targeted patients with severe psoriasis, these patients had an increased risk of cardiovascular mortality, regardless of traditional CV risk factors. Recent theories on the pathogenesis of CVD have focused on the key role of vascular inflammation. In numerous studies, the increased severity of psoriasis or the duration of the disease, and therefore a greater and prolonged skin inflammation, has been associated with a higher risk of CVD. In examining the link between psoriasis and CVD, several studies have found similar pathogenic features, including an activation of inflammatory cells and increased circulating levels of proinflammatory cytokines. A murine model showed that prolonged skin inflammation favored both inflammation of the aortic root and thrombosis, with significant increases in serum levels of proinflammatory cytokines. A better delineation of the mechanisms underlying the link between psoriasis and CVD can provide an important basis for the choice of psoriasis therapies in the future. In particular, some therapies may improve psoriasis while reducing the risk of CVD. While the research focused on specific therapies, the studies to date have not provided definitive answers. However, it is possible to reduce this risk in the current time, without the use of expensive systemic therapies that have the potential for significant side effects. Dietary intervention should be recommended to patients with psoriasis as a fundamental therapy for reducing cardiovascular risk. The initial goal should be to improve the conditions known as important cardiac risk factors. Dietary intervention is the basis of therapy for diabetes, hypertension and hypercholesterolemia. However, even in patients without these associated cardiac risk factors, a change in diet can help reduce the risk of CVD. Numerous studies have shown that some dietary approaches can be considered "anti-inflammatory". In a randomized trial, the intervention group was treated with a Mediterranean-type diet. This was associated with improved endothelial function scores as well as a reduction in serum levels of C-reactive protein and interleukin-18. As some dietary patterns have been shown to improve markers of vascular inflammation, many doctors now recommend a diet rich in fruits and vegetables, which favors whole grains over processed grains and omega-3 fatty acids compared to omega-6 fatty acids. In the literature it has been observed that the degree of severity of the disease is directly related to BMI (body mass index): obese psoriatic patients must be encouraged to lose weight through an appropriate hypocaloric diet and adequate physical activity.

25.6 Food and rosacea

Rosacea is a cutaneous dermatosis characterized by persistent erythema, papules, pustules and telangiectasias located in the central region of the face. In a survey of patients from the National Rosacea Society, 78% presented an unbalanced diet. Some foods have been indicated as triggers of the disease, in particular: *pepper, cinnamon, chili pepper, tea, coffee, chocolate* and *alcohol* seem to be directly responsible for the typical erythema of rosacea. The underlying pathophysiological mechanism is unknown, but it appears that transient receptor potential ion channels may play a role. These are expressed throughout the body, including neuronal tissues, and can be activated by cold or hot temperatures, as well as by certain foods; in particular, capsaicin and cinnamaldehyde act on some of these channels to stimulate an increase in cutaneous blood flow through neuro-genetic vasodilation. Capsaicin is found in some spices, while cinnamaldehyde is found in cinnamon, tomatoes, citrus fruits and chocolate. It is therefore appropriate for patients suffering from rosacea to limit the consumption of certain foods.

All things considered, the correct food intake plays a crucial role in various chronic skin conditions. Furthermore, a balanced diet will help to achieve optimal outcomes for pharmacological treatments.

REFERENCES

1. Michaelsson G, Juhlin L, Ljunghall K. A double-blind study of the effect of zinc and oxytetracycline in acne vulgaris. Br J Dermatol 1977; 97(5): 561-6.
2. Hambidge KM, Miller LV, Westcott JE, et al. Zinc bioavailability and homeostasis. Am J Clin Nutr 2010; 91(5): 1478S-83S.
3. Danby F. Nutrition and aging skin: sugar and glycation. Clin Dermatol 2010; 28(4): 409-11.
4. Dreno B, Moyse D, Alirezai M, et al. Multicenter randomized comparative double-blind controlled clinical trial of the safety and efficacy of zinc gluconate versus minocycline hydrochloride in the treatment of inflammatory acne vulgaris. Dermatology 2001; 203(2): 135-40.
5. Duffey K, Popkin B. High-fructose corn syrup: is that what's for dinner? Am J Clin Nutr 2008; 88: 1722S-32S.
6. Kowalczyk MC, Kowalczyk P, Tolstykh O, et al. Synergistic effects of combined phytochemicals and skin cancer prevention in SENCAR mice. Cancer Prev Res 2010; 3(2): 170-8.
7. O'Brien J, Morrissey P. Nutritional and toxicological aspects of the Maillard browning reaction in foods. Crit Rev Food Sci Nutr 1989; 28(3): 211-48.
8. Dearlove R, Greenspan P, Hartle D, et al. Inhibition of protein glycation by extracts of culinary herbs and spices. J Med Food 2008; 11(2): 275-81.
9. Sardana K, Garg VK. An observational study of methionine-bound zinc with antioxidants for mild to moderate acne vulgaris. Dermatol Ther 2010; 23(4): 411-8.
10. Nguyen HP, Katta R. Sugar Sag: Glycation and the role of diet in aging skin. Skin Therapy Lett 2015; 20(6): 1-5.
11. Chan H, Chan G, Santos J, et al. A randomized, double-blind, placebo-controlled trial to determine the efficacy and safety of lactoferrin with vitamin E and zinc as an oral therapy for mild to moderate acne vulgaris. Int J Dermatol 2017; 56(6): 686-90.
12. Noordam R, Gunn DA, Tomlin CC, et al. High serum glucose levels are associated with a higher perceived age. Age (Dordr) 2013; 35(1): 189-95.
13. Fulton J, Plewig G, Kligman A. Effect of chocolate on acne vulgaris. JAMA 1969; 210(11): 2071-4.
14. Goh W, Kallianpur K, Chow DA, et al. Chocolate and acne: how valid was the original study? Clin Dermatol 2011; 29(4): 459-60.
15. Adebamowo C, Spiegelman D, Danby F, et al. High school dietary dairy intake and teenage acne. J Am Acad Dermatol 2005; 52(2): 207-14.
16. Adebamowo C, Spiegelman D, Berkey C, et al. Milk consumption and acne in teenaged boys. J Am Acad Dermatol 2008; 58(5): 787-93.
17. Adebamowo C, Spiegelman D, Berkey C, et al. Milk consumption and acne in adolescent girls. Dermatol Online J 2006; 12(4): 1.
18. Bowe W, Joshi S, Shalita A. Diet and acne. J Am Acad Dermatol 2010; 63(1): 124-41.
19. Cordain L, Lindeberg S, Hurtado M, et al. Acne vulgaris: a disease of Western civilization. Arch Dermatol 2002; 138(12): 1584-90.
20. Di Landro A, Cazzaniga S, Parazzini F, et al. GISED Acne study group. Family history, body mass index, selected dietary factors, menstrual history, and risk of moderate to severe acne in adolescents and young adults. J Am Acad Dermatol 2012; 67(6): 1129-35.

21. Ismail NH, Manaf ZA, Azizan NZ. High glycemic load diet, milk and ice cream consumption are related to acne vulgaris in Malaysian young adults: a case control study. BMC Dermatol 2012; 12: 13.
22. Kendall SN. Remission of rosacea induced by reduction of gut transit time. Clin Exp Dermatol 2004; 29(3): 297-9.
23. Egeberg A, Gislason GH, Hansen PR. Risk of major adverse cardiovascular events and all-cause mortality in patients with hidradenitis suppurativa. JAMA Dermatol 2016; 152(4): 429-34.
24. Zeevi D, Korem T, Zmora N, et al. Personalized nutrition by prediction of glycemic responses. Cell 2015; 163(5): 1079-94.
25. Sofi F. The Mediterranean diet revisited: evidence of its effectiveness grows. Curr Opin Cardiol 2009; 24(5): 442-6.
26. Smith RN, Mann NJ, Braue A, et al. The effect of a high-protein, low glycemic-load diet versus a conventional, high glycemic-load diet on biochemical parameters associated with acne vulgaris: a randomized, investigator-masked, controlled trial. J Am Acad Dermatol 2007; 57(2): 247-56.
27. Kwon HH, Yoon JY, Hong JS, et al. Clinical and histological effect of a low glycaemic load diet in treatment of acne vulgaris in Korean patients: a randomized, controlled trial. Acta Derm Venereol 2012; 92(3): 241-6.
28. Adebamowo CA, Spiegelman D, Danby FW, et al. High school dietary dairy intake and teenage acne. J Am Acad Dermatol 2005; 52(2): 207-14.
29. Silverberg NB. Whey protein precipitating moderate to severe acne flares in 5 teenaged athletes. Cutis 2012; 90(2): 70-2.
30. Bowe WP, Joshi SS, Shalita AR. Diet and acne. J Am Acad Dermatol 2010; 63(1): 124-41.
31. Jung JY, Kwon HH, Hong JS, et al. Effect of dietary supplementation with omega-3 fatty acid and gamma-linolenic acid on acne vulgaris: a randomised, double-blind, controlled trial. Acta Derm Venereol 2014; 94(5): 521-5.
32. Jung GW, Tse JE, Guiha I, et al. Prospective, randomized, open-label trial comparing the safety, efficacy, and tolerability of an acne treatment regimen with and without a probiotic supplement and minocycline in subjects with mild to moderate acne. J Cutan Med Surg 2013; 17(2): 114-22.
33. Werfel T, Breuer K. Role of food allergy in atopic dermatitis. Curr Opin Allergy Clin Immunol 2004; 4(5): 379-85.
34. Katta R, Schlichte M. Diet and dermatitis: food triggers. J Clin Aesthet Dermatol 2014; 7(3): 30-6.
35. Sampson HA, McCaskill CC. Food hypersensitivity and atopic dermatitis: evaluation of 113 patients. J Pediatr 1985; 107(5): 669-75.
36. Salam TN, Fowler JF Jr. Balsam-related systemic contact dermatitis. J Am Acad Dermatol 2001; 45(3): 377-81.
37. Brenaut E, Horreau C, Pouplard C, et al. Alcohol consumption and psoriasis: a systematic literature review. J Eur Acad Dermatol Venereol 2013; 27 Suppl 3: 30-5.
38. Fleming P, Kraft J, Gulliver WP, et al. The relationship of obesity with the severity of psoriasis: a systematic review. J Cutan Med Surg 2015; 19(5): 450-6.
39. Barrea L, Nappi F, Di Somma C, et al. Environmental risk factors in psoriasis: the point of view of the nutritionist. Int J Environ Res Public Health 2016; 13(5): 743.
40. Debbaneh M, Millsop JW, Bhatia BK, et al. Diet and psoriasis, part I: impact of weight loss interventions. J Am Acad Dermatol 2014; 71(1): 133-40.
41. Barrea L, Balato N, Di Somma C, et al. Nutrition and psoriasis: is there any association between the severity of the disease and adherence to the Mediterranean diet? J Transl Med 2015; 13: 18.
42. Egeberg A, Weinstock LB, Thyssen EP, et al. Rosacea and gastrointestinal disorders: a population-based cohort study. Br J Dermatol 2017; 176(1): 100-6.

26 Food and eye

Ciro Tamburrelli and AnnaClara Tamburrelli

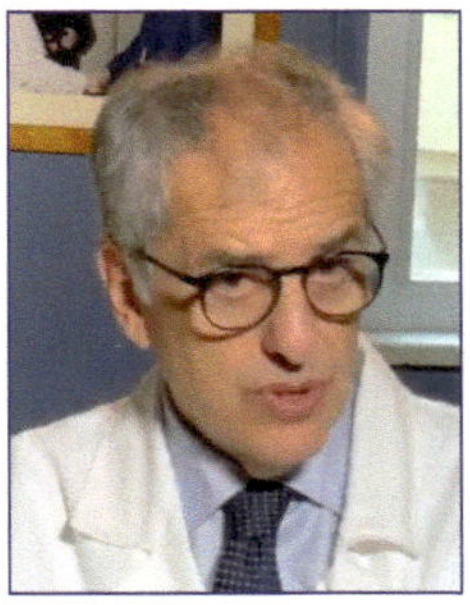

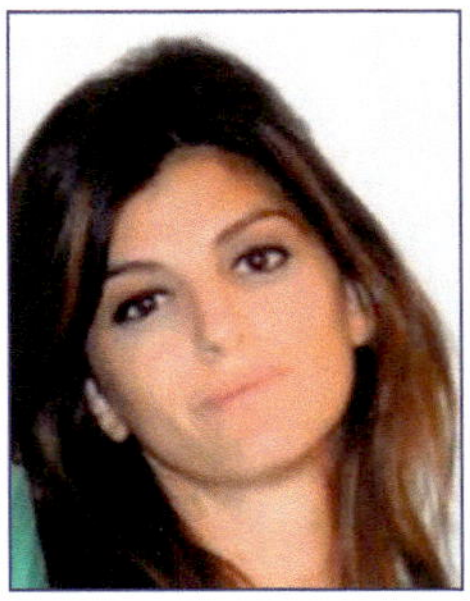

26.1 Vitamin A and eye disorders

Vitamin A is a fat-soluble vitamin absorbed in the small intestine in the form of retinol. Retinol is crucial in maintaining conjunctival and corneal epithelial integrity, while in the retina it plays a major role in phototransduction in rod and cone cells. Anything compromising absorption in the small intestine will therefore affect vitamin A absorption.

While one of the leading causes of preventable blindness in the low-income/middle-income countries [1], vitamin A deficiency (VAD) is uncommon in developed countries. It has however been reported in severely malnourished patients [2] and following intestinal or bariatric surgery [3-5] due to the resultant malabsorption [6, 7].

VAD can lead to significant dysfunction of the ocular epithelial lining, resulting in a range of ocular manifestations, from xerosis (dry eye) to corneal ulceration and keratomalacia (necrosis and softening of the cornea leading to its perforation), and if left untreated, blindness.

Due to retinol's role in phototransduction, night blindness is classically an early symptom of xerophthalmia. Cone function appears to be preserved in the early stages [8]. Clinical findings suggestive of VAD include conjunctival and corneal xerosis and the presence of Bitot's spots. Bitot's spots are non-specific white plaques that develop on the conjunctiva due to collection of corneal substances. The clinical features of xerophthalmia have been classified by the WHO [9] as follows: *XN*, night blindness; *X1A*, conjunctival xerosis; *X1B*, Bitot's spots; *X2*, corneal xerosis; *X3A*, corneal ulceration/keratomalacia < 1/3 corneal surface; *X3B*, corneal ulceration/keratomalacia ≥ 1/3 corneal surface; *XS*, corneal scar; and *XF*, xerophthalmic fundus.

We had the chance to examine two patients with undiagnosed deficit of vitamin A, both consecutive to major surgery on the small intestine consecutive to bariatric surgery, that were hospitalized at our institution (Ospedale Oftalmico di Roma) as secondary treatment center after previous treatment in a primary care hospital.

They presented with a 8-10 week history of progressive loss of vision in one eye due to a perforated corneal ulcer and a 1-week history of progressive loss of vision in the second eye, due to incipient corneal ulcer and night blindness.

Their medical history included bariatric surgery for marked obesity.

Ciro Tamburrelli, MD
Professor, Ospedale Oftalmico di Roma, Rome, Italy

Email: citam@tiscali.it

AnnaClara Tamburrelli, MD
Sapienza University, Istituto di Oftalmologia, Rome, Italy

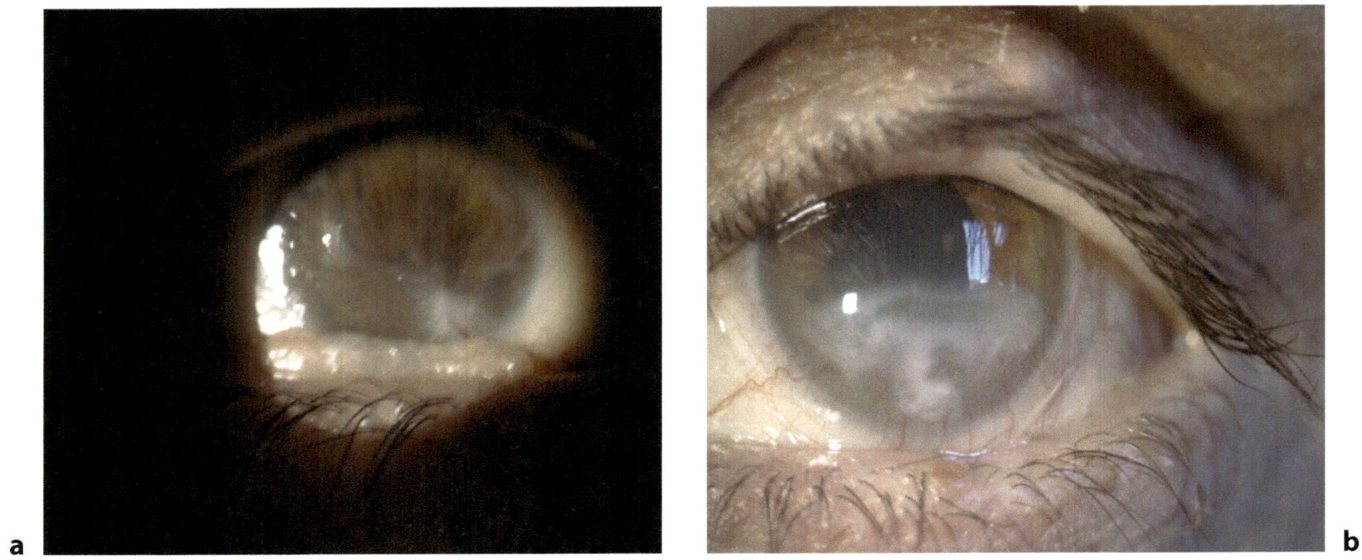

Fig. 26.1 **a**, OD: perforated ulcer anterior synechia. **b**, OS: inferior corneal ulcer and xerophthalmia.

26.1.1 Differential diagnosis

A diagnosis of xerophthalmia due to VAD can usually be made clinically. A history of night blindness and the presence of Bitot's spots and corneal ulceration are pathognomonic of VAD.

Xerophthalmia, the pathological drying of the conjunctiva and cornea, can also occur in autoimmune conditions such as rheumatoid arthritis, scleroderma and systemic lupus erythematosus, and so could be considered in the list of differentials; however, none were relevant in both of them.

They presented with a perforated corneal ulcer in one eye and prephtisical condition and a corneal ulcer in the lower portion of the cornea considered secondary to marked dry eye syndrome.

The clinical picture and the anamnestic data of a previous bariatric surgery, prompted our diagnosis of xerophthalmia in avitaminosis (Fig. 26.1).

26.1.2 Treatment

Initial oral vitamin A supplementation with 200,000 IU failed to correct either the patient's serum vitamin A levels or symptoms, so they were switched to intravenous supplementation.

26.1.3 Outcome and follow-up

A month after diagnosis, serum vitamin A levels had returned to within normal limits (1.9 μmol/L). The epithelial defects and the corneal ulcers progressive-

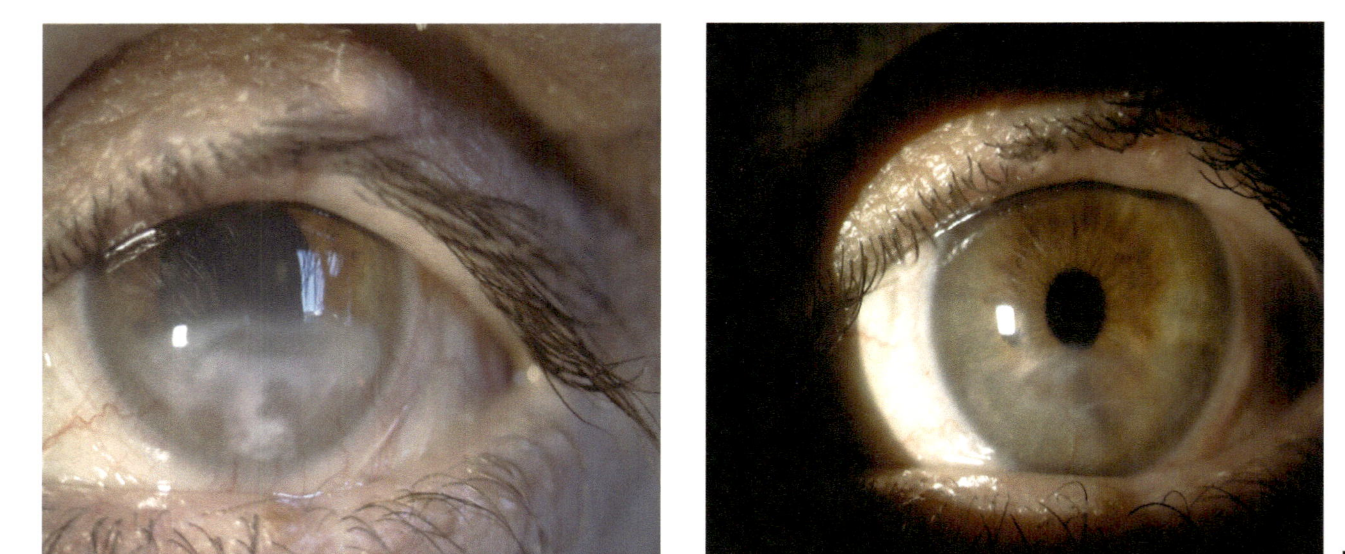

Fig. 26.2 **a**, Pre-vitamin A supplementation. **b**, Post-vitamin A supplementation.

ly healed with a permanent inferior scar functionally not relevant (Fig. 26.2).

While the diagnosis of VAD is mainly clinical, serum vitamin A levels can be requested to confirm the diagnosis but should not delay treatment.

The WHO recommends an oral dose of 200,000 IU of vitamin A for 2 days followed by another dose 1-4 weeks later [10, 11]. Typically, in cases of malabsorption, the WHO recommends treatment of VAD via the intramuscular route rather than the oral route.

26.2 Zeaxanthin: metabolism, properties, and antioxidant protection of eyes

26.2.1 Introduction

Zeaxanthin (β,β-carotene-3,3′-diol), with a molecular weight of 568.8 Daltons and 11 conjugated double bonds, is a carotenoid that belongs to the xanthophyll family. These conjugated bonds are distributed between the polyene chain and the ionone rings. The ionone rings contain a hydroxyl group that can attach to fatty acids during esterification [12].

Lutein is the stereoisomer of zeaxanthin, and both of these carotenoids are generally found together in plant sources including green leafy vegetables, where the content can be as high as 40 mg per 100 g, while in the yellow-orange fruit and vegetables such as carrots, papaya, orange and peaches, the concentration is less than 1 mg per 100 g.

These xanthophylls can also be found in animal products, where they are more bioavailable because they are incorporated into the lipid matrix of the food, as is the case of egg yolks and cheese. Wheat can also be considered a source of zeaxanthin and lutein, mainly because wheat products are a common staple in some parts of the world [13]. Neither of these xanthophylls possess provitamin A activity.

Zeaxanthin has three stereoisomeric forms (i.e., (3R,3′R)-zeaxanthin, (3R,3′S)-zeaxanthin, and (3S,3′S)-zeaxanthin). The main form of zeaxanthin in nature is (3R,3′R)-zeaxanthin, while (3R,3′S)-zeaxanthin, also called meso-zeaxanthin, is absent from dietary sources, the liver, or in circulation, but it can be found in ocular tissues [14]. It is important to mention that humans are unable to synthesize zeaxanthin and therefore it needs to be obtained from dietary sources [15].

It is recognized that both lutein and zeaxanthin predominantly accumulate in the retina, and the concentrations increase gradually towards the center of the macula, where it can be approximately 1000-fold higher than in other tissues [16]. Their presence in eyes is relevant as they have been shown to protect against age-related macular degeneration (AMD) [17] and cataracts. In addition, zeaxanthin has been shown to protect against oxidative stress in different tissues as well as systemic inflammation.

26.2.2 Factors affecting zeaxanthin bioavailability

Carotenoids are normally very poorly absorbed. Absorption varies widely depending on other dietary components present in the meal and can fluctuate from 5-50%. Several factors have been identified as having important effects on zeaxanthin availability, including thermal processing, esterification, and some dietary components such as lipids, polysaccharides and minerals.

Thermal processing

Thermal processing can have both beneficial and deleterious effects on zeaxanthin bioavailability during food preparation. For example, it can damage the content of zeaxanthin in raw food, while it can also facilitate the release and solubilization of zeaxanthin for greater bioavailability [18]. During food processing, a high temperature may substantially reduce the concentrations of zeaxanthin, as has been reported in sweet corn, where canning at 121 °C decreased zeaxanthin content by 29% [18]. The loss of zeaxanthin can also vary due to the temperatures used for cooking [19]. For example, in comparison with raw egg yolk, zeaxanthin decreased by 11.6%, 5.9% and 6% in boiled, microwaved and fried eggs, respectively [19].

Thermal treatments, however, can also increase the release and bioavailability of zeaxanthin. For example, pasteurization at 98 °C for 21 s of an orange-carrot juice mixture increased the concentration of zeaxanthin by 45%, which may be associated with a disruption in the food matrix, promoting a better extraction of the carotenoid [20]. It has also been shown that wolfberries homogenized into hot skimmed milk are much more bioavailable compared with those in warm skimmed milk, with a three-fold increase of zeaxanthin with the hot milk [21], indicating that the higher temperature facilitates the incorporation of zeaxanthin into mixed micelles, thus increasing zeaxanthin bioavailability.

Bioavailability of carotenoids appears to be higher in the trans-isomers compared with the cis-counterparts [22]. Although some studies suggest that conversion of cis to trans form occurs in zeaxanthin, the impact of this conversion on bioavailability is still not clear [23].

26.2.3 Esterification

Most zeaxanthin in foods exists esterified as zeaxanthin di-palmitate [22], which needs to be hydrolyzed before incorporation into chylomicrons [24]. Yet, esterified zeaxanthin has been shown to have higher bioavailability than the free form. To evaluate which form was more bioavailable, 12 healthy subjects were administered 5 mg of free or zeaxanthin di-palmitate dissolved in palm oil and blended into yogurt, in a crossover design [25]. Supplementation with the esterified zeaxanthin resulted in two-fold greater mean area under the curve values compared with supplementation with the free form [25].

26.2.4 Dietary polysaccharides

The bioavailability of zeaxanthin is affected by the type of polysaccharides in meals. For instance, a recent report indicated that zeaxanthin exhibits different bioavailability whether consumed in a starch-based or an alginate-based matrix [26]. These results suggested that zeaxanthin in a starch-based matrix has a higher bioavailability than the one in an alginate-based matrix.

26.2.5 Dietary lipids

As a carotenoid, zeaxanthin is also a lipophilic compound. Its absorption partially depends on bile acid solubilization and micelle incorporation. Dietary fats are considered to be essential for stimulating bile production in the intestine and subsequent micelle formation [27]. Although no study has specifically looked into the impact of fat amount on zeaxanthin bioavailability, it has been reported that dietary fat increased lutein bioavailability in human subjects [28].

26.2.6 Absorption and metabolism of zeaxanthin

Zeaxanthin is a lipophilic compound and therefore is insoluble in aqueous media. However, zeaxanthin possesses two hydroxyl groups with a higher polarity compared with other carotenoids, suggesting that zeaxanthin might be absorbed and transported differently. Zeaxanthin needs first to be released from the food matrix, a process that starts in the stomach by the action of acid and digestive enzymes. Other carotenoids have been shown to be partially released from the food matrix in the stomach [29]. Similarly, zeaxanthin will solubilize into lipid droplets that convert to lipid emulsion particles smaller in size [12]. The distribution of carotenoids in emulsion particles is based on their polarity, thus those with lower polarity would migrate to the lipid core of the particles, while those with higher polarity (e.g., zeaxanthin) will locate in the surface where proteins and phospholipids are found [28].

26.2.7 Digestion in the intestinal lumen

Lipid emulsion particles containing zeaxanthin and other carotenoids move from the stomach to the duodenum. Dietary fat present in the emulsion stimulates the gallbladder to secrete bile acids and triggers the release of lipases from the pancreas. All enzymes produced by the pancreas hydrolyze the food matrix and promote the release of zeaxanthin. Pancreatic lipases also help in the transfer of zeaxanthin from the emulsion particles to the lipid phase of the micelles [25].

Zeaxanthin is present in plants in the esterified form [30]; however, this xanthophyll is found in the free form in chylomicrons and other lipoproteins [31], indicating that the esterified zeaxanthin needs to be hydrolyzed before it is transported into the lymph or blood. Carboxyl ester lipase, one of the dietary fat-induced pancreatic lipases, has been found to hydrolyze esterified carotenoids [30].

26.2.8 Absorption by enterocytes

The concentration gradient of zeaxanthin between the enterocyte and the cell membrane will control the rate of passive diffusion, which is the most accepted approach by which carotenoids are absorbed into the small intestine [32, 33].

The mixed micelles directly contact and diffuse into the membrane of enterocytes, releasing carotenoids including zeaxanthin into the cytoplasm of enterocytes [32].

However, there is more recent evidence showing that xanthophylls can also be transported into enterocytes by receptors

26.2.9 Efflux from enterocytes

There are two different pathways by which zeaxanthin may efflux from the enterocytes, one of which is the assembly into chylomicrons and release into the lymph [34], or it can be secreted into the lymph or the portal vein from the enterocytes within the small intestine-derived high-density lipoprotein (HDL) [35].

26.2.10 Transport in blood

Following efflux, chylomicrons travel through the lymphatic system and reach systemic circulation at the thoracic duct, where they transport zeaxanthin along with other carotenoids and dietary lipids to the extrahepatic tissues. Chylomicrons in circulation are rapidly hydrolyzed by lipoprotein lipase bound to the capillary endothelium, converting them into chylomicron remnants that are later removed by the liver.

After uptake by the liver, zeaxanthin can be stored, eliminated in the bile, or re-distributed to extrahepatic tissues via VLDL secretion [36]. Zeaxanthin and other carotenoids in VLDL are distributed into intermediate density lipoprotein (IDL) and LDL following the delipidation cascade. Zeaxanthin in LDL is taken up by the LDL receptor or LDL receptor-related protein (LRP).

26.2.11 Tissue distribution

The major sites of carotenoid storage are the liver and the adipose tissue, but they can also be found in kidney, adrenals and testes [37]. Few studies, if any, have specifically looked into the distribution of zeaxanthin among different tissues.

Since lutein and zeaxanthin are absorbed and transported similarly, accumulation of lutein and zeaxanthin in different tissues might follow a similar pattern. Recently, the distribution of lutein in tissues was studied [38]. The highest accumulation was observed in eyes, followed by adrenal gland and liver.

26.2.12 Effects of zeaxanthin in human health

Carotenoids play essential roles in protecting cellular membranes and lipoproteins against reactive oxygen species (ROS)-induced oxidative stress [39]. Results from *in vitro* and *in vivo* studies involving animal models and human have demonstrated that lutein and zeaxanthin potentially protect against chronic eye and cardiovascular diseases, such AMD, cataract, coronary heart disease and stroke [40]. Further, the hydrophilic properties of zeaxanthin may enhance its antioxidant properties in aqueous media, such as in the blood circulation. In human plasma, loss of zeaxanthin upon photo-irradiation in the presence of photo-oxidation sensitizer methylene blue was faster than that of β-carotene and lycopene [41]. The data from this *in vitro* study indicate that zeaxanthin reacts with singlet oxygen more efficiently than nonpolar carotenoids in the water phase, probably due to its higher polarity [41]. Oxidative stress is involved in the initiation and progression of these chronic diseases [42, 43]. Therefore, it is necessary to study the antioxidant effects of these two xanthophylls and the underlying mechanisms.

In comparison with lutein, zeaxanthin has only one additional conjugated double bond [44]. However, this small difference in the molecular structure still leads to a difference in their antioxidant activities. Evidence shows zeaxanthin is a more potent antioxidant than lutein.

26.2.13 Lutein and eye health

Lutein and zeaxanthin are found along with long-chain PUFA in human rod outer segment membranes, in which oxidative stress is the highest [45]. The identification of β,β-carotene-3,3′-dione, 3′-Hydroxy-βββ-carotene-3-one and 3-Hydroxy-ββ-carotene-3′-one as oxidation products of lutein and zeaxanthin in human retina also supports that these xanthophylls function as antioxidants in human eyes [46]. Age-related macular degeneration is the major cause of visual impairment and irreversible blindness among the senior population in the USA [47]. In 2010, the estimated number of AMD patients was 2.07 million, which is anticipated to increase by more than two-fold in the following forty years [47]. AMD may lead to vision blurry or loss of vision in patients' central visual field, which can cause difficulty in reading, writing, driving, or other daily activities [47]. About two decades ago, antivascular endothelial growth factor (VEGF) treatment was introduced as an effective therapy, which can recover the vision of AMD patients [48]. Nevertheless, this treatment requires frequent intravitreal injections along with a high cost. Therefore, an alternative treatment that does not come with a steep price and is less invasive would be a better choice.

Several studies have investigated the relationship between AMD and retinal lutein and zeaxanthin levels in human subjects. For example, Bone et al. measured lutein and zeaxanthin concentrations in donated retinas from healthy controls and AMD patients (n = 56 for each group) [49]. They reported that compared with healthy subjects, the combined concentrations of lutein and zeaxanthin in three concentric regions of the macula were decreased in AMD patients.

A recently published article evaluated relationships among macular pigment optical density (MPOD), which represents macular pigment levels within the retina, and age among Irish subjects [50]. This study indicates that aging may lead to AMD onset by depleting retinal xanthophylls. In addition to retinal xanthophyll contents, plasma xanthophyll concentrations are also negatively associated with AMD risk in humans. However, in the case of lutein, the association was not statistically significant. Therefore, plasma xanthophyll levels can be an indicator of AMD risk, with plasma zeaxanthin level probably serving as a better indicator than plasma lutein level.

Supplementation of lutein and zeaxanthin has shown improvement in visual performance of patients with early age-related macular degeneration. Forty-seven patients with early AMD were supplemented with a combination of lutein and zeaxanthin (20 mg and 0.86 mg per day, respectively) or meso-zeaxanthin, lutein and zeaxanthin (17 mg, 3 mg and 2 mg per day, respectively) for 36 months [51]. Both dosages were equivalent to 22 mg of total macular carotenoids. Both supplementations significantly increased MPOD in patients compared with the basal level, along with a significant improvement in letter contrast sensitivity [51].

Another study by Seddon et al. suggested AMD risk reduced with increased dietary intake of lutein and zeaxanthin. In this case-control study, 356 patients diagnosed with the advanced stage of AMD and 520 control subjects aged 55 to 80 years were recruited [52]. The lesion in the retinal pigment epithelium initiates development of AMD due to RPE cells death and degeneration [53].

During the development of AMD, cellular oxidative stress plays a vital role in RPE cell death [53]. The previous section demonstrated that zeaxanthin exhibits a strong antioxidant property by quenching ROS and inducing GSH production *in vitro* and thereby inhibiting oxidative stress-induced RPE cell apoptosis. Moreover, zeaxanthin can protect RPE cells by inhibiting lipofuscin production. Excessive oxidation also induces the formation of lipofuscin in the RPE, which is an undegradable complex of intracellular protein aggregation [54]. The accumulation of lipofuscin can lead to cellular toxicity and functional impairment of RPE cells, which may be involved in AMD development [55].

Zeaxanthin treatment has also been shown to decrease the accumulation of lipofuscin formed in cultured RPE cells and *in vivo*. Treatment of lutein or zeaxanthin for two weeks significantly reduced lipofuscin accumulation induced by normobaric hyperoxia in rabbit or calf RPE cells compared with the control group [56].

Light exposure, especially blue light (wavelength ranged between 400 and 500 nm), has been hypothesized as a risk factor for AMD. An age-matched control study among 838 watermen revealed patients with advanced AMD had significantly higher exposure to blue light over the past 20 years [57]. Similar to other carotenoids, the presence of a conjugated polyene chain in the zeaxanthin molecule allows it to absorb light [58]. The maximum light absorbance of zeaxanthin is between 445 and 472 nm in dichloromethane and 451 nm in ethanol, which falls in the blue light wavelength range [59]. Therefore, zeaxanthin can function as a blue light filter and reduce the intensity of blue light that reaches the retina and thus protect against AMD development [49]. Supplementation with pure zeaxanthin (2.2 mg/kg/day) for 22 weeks significantly reduced the area of lesion induced by acute blue light exposure in the fovea of monkeys, which supports this hypothesis [60].

26.2.14 Conclusion

There is sufficient evidence documenting the importance of zeaxanthin as an antioxidant, especially in the eyes. There are also accumulated data demonstrating that zeaxanthin intake from supplement or dietary sources may protect against AMD development via its antioxidant and blue-filtering properties. However, it is still necessary to provide evidence to support that zeaxanthin reduces the risk of AMD onset or slows the progression of AMD in the long-term. Current zeaxanthin supplementation studies only showed the effect of zeaxanthin in years, instead of in decades [50, 61]. Further, to have a better interpretation of the protective functions of zeaxanthin against AMD development, a complete understanding of the AMD pathophysiology is necessary. For instance, although this review highlights that zeaxanthin treatment inhibits lipofuscin accumulation, the potential role of lipofuscin in the development of AMD is not clearly elucidated.

Zeaxanthin has also been found in organs other than eyes, such as skin and brain [62, 63], which strongly suggests that zeaxanthin supplementation may protect skin against UV light damage and may have a beneficial role on cognitive function in seniors [63]. However, the delivery of zeaxanthin to these two organs and subsequent intra-organ metabolism has not been reported. Future studies should address all these pending questions.

26.3 Sugar intake and eye disorders

The "western" lifestyle is spreading across the globe. Associated with this lifestyle is less activity and increased consumption of processed foods. A majority of processed foods contain added sugars or polysaccharides that are broken down rapidly to sugars which raise blood sugar levels [64].

In order to optimize dietary practices, promote healthy aging, and develop policies that improve dietary practices, it is useful to evaluate and review the scientific literature regarding sugar intake and its effects on health. A growing number of reports indicate that chronic exposure to high glycemia diets contributes to increased risk for multiple human disorders including type II diabetes, cerebrovascular, cardiovascular and eye-related diseases.

The latter include cataract, diabetic retinopathy and macular degeneration [65-69]. Although these diseases may have multiple and different etiologies, all of them have been linked to a common pathogenic factor that accelerates under hyperglycemic conditions: the formation of toxic advanced glycation end products (AGEs) [68, 69].

AGEs are a heterogeneous array of compounds that accumulate in multiple human tissues during normal aging and, especially, under conditions of hyperglycemia [65-67]. AGEs accumulate particularly rapidly in tissues with a low capacity of regeneration [67-69].

AGEs are deposited intracellularly or in the extracellular environments thus participating in the onset of the ocular damage in different ways (Fig. 26.2).

Retinal pigmented epithelia cells have the highest proteolytic burden in the body because each RPE cell must digest the outer tips of 30 photoreceptor cells that are shed each morning. Usually, RPE cells do not proliferate. The vast majority of lens cells also do not proliferate. Thus, in these cells, opportunities for dilution of AGEs by replication, or repair of AGEs-associated damage, are limited, making hyperglycemic conditions a major risk factor for eye diseases. Or for example, AGEs in circulation may bind at the plasma membrane to cell surface receptors, including scavenger receptors. The best-studied AGE-receptor is called receptor for advanced glycation end-products (RAGE or also AGER), a transmembrane receptor of the immunoglobulin superfamily [70]. When AGEs are bound to RAGE, several signaling pathways are activated, including Ras/MAPK/NF-κB, JAK/STAT, and Rac1/Cdc42 leading to oxidative stress and NF-κB activation [71-73]. Other receptors capable of binding AGEs are AGE-R1/OST-48/p60, AGE-R2/80K-H/p90, AGE-R3/galectin-3, SR-A (I/II), SR-B/CD36, SR-BI, SR-E/LOX-1, FEEL-1/FEEL-2 [74-81].

26.3.1 Cornea

Advanced glycation end products (AGEs) accumulate in the corneal stroma and lamina during normal aging. A specific example is glycation and crosslinking of corneal collagen [82]. Some AGEs fluoresce. Higher values of corneal AGE fluorescence are found in patients with proliferative diabetic retinopathy compared to control subjects [83]. Furthermore, enhanced levels of AGEs are detected in diabetic cornea with a more prominent reactivity in stroma, basal laminae and Bowman's membrane. Importantly, collagen crosslinking appears to be involved in the central corneal thickening, which alters corneal biomechanics properties [84-86]. *In vitro* data showed that AGEs can delay corneal epithelial wound healing and also induce apoptosis in human corneal epithelial cells through increased generation of intracellular ROS via NADPH oxidase activation and upregulation of JNK and p38 MAPK pathways [87, 88]. Glycation in the stromal matrix is thought to increase aggregation of collagen fibrils in the cornea contributing to diabetic keratopathy [89, 90]. High concentrations of AGEs are also found *in vivo* in the corneal epithelium, basement membrane and stromal keratocytes of long-term diabetic monkeys and in streptozotocin-injected Sprague-Dawley rats [89, 90].

26.3.2 Lens

The lens is probably the eye tissue in which the pathogenic role of AGEs has been best characterized at the molecular level both in normal aging and in a diabetic context [91-101]. The role of sugar in diabetic cataract has been extensively studied and several reports established a plasma glycemic threshold above which incidence of diabetic cataract increases exponentially [102, 103]. High levels of AGEs are found in diabetic patients [98, 104].

As might be expected, protein glycation increases dramatically with age [100, 105]. Associated with this glycation are covalent crosslinking of crystallins, resulting in altered tertiary structure, and aggregation. Chaperone activity is also lost and lens fiber cell integrity is compromised [93, 106]. For example, αA-crystallin and γB-crystallin have been shown to be thus modified, resulting in aggregation, insolubility, and lens opacity [107-111].

The lens capsule is also a target for glycation. Recently, different AGEs were found accumulated in human lens capsules in an age-dependent manner, with higher levels observed in cataractous lens capsules compared to normal lens capsules. It was suggested that AGEs in the lens capsule could promote the TGFβ2-mediated fibrosis of lens epithelial cells during posterior capsule opacification [105].

In addition, *in vitro* and *in vivo* data support a cytotoxic effect of AGEs on the vitality of lens epithelial cells through the induction of apoptosis in a NF-κB-dependent manner, suggesting that AGEs accumulation might be a causative factor of injury to the lens epithelium [104, 112]. We also demonstrated that lens proteolytic potential is compromised upon aging [113-117]. This would have the effect of accelerating accumulation of AGEs, and associated pathology.

Both carbohydrate restriction and calorie restriction, and compounds inhibiting the accumulation of AGEs have shown efficacy to delay cataract progress in humans and mice [118-121]. Several other studies report anti-cataract activity of dietary flavonoids through the reduction of glycation-induced protein aggregation [122-124]. Interestingly, treatment with an AGE cross-link breaker has been shown to be sufficient in disrupting aggregates from diabetic human lenses [125].

26.3.3 Vitreous humor

Structural changes in the vitreous humor are associated with normal aging, but are detected earlier in diabetic conditions. These include posterior vitreous detachment and liquefaction [126-128]. Glycation seems to play a pathologic role in vitreous degeneration in diabetic vitreopathy, and is associated with aberrant crosslinks in collagenous fibrils [129]. Glycated collagen dissociates from hyaluronan, a hydrophilic glycosaminoglycan, destabilizing the vitreous gel structure and causing morphological changes within the cortical gel, leading to vitreous dysfunction [127, 129]. From a chemical perspective, it is likely that the hyaluronan is also subject to glycative modification, but this remains to be fully investigated. Vitreous AGE-associated fluorescence increases in a glucose-concentration dependent manner in streptozotocin-induced diabetic rats [130]. Data from ex vivo porcine vitreous show that AGEs accumulation compromises the vitreous permeability, thus impeding the diffusion of molecules [131]. Changes in vitreous permeability might increase the retention of cytokines or drugs, with implications in the pathogenesis of ocular diseases such as diabetic retinopathy. High glucose concentrations in bovine vitreous recapitulates the phenotype of crosslinked-collagen fibers and, interestingly, the process is inhibited by aminoguanidine, an inhibitor of AGE formation [127].

26.3.4 Retina

Similar to cornea, lens and vitreous, retinal AGEs increase with age and diabetes, especially in the outer retina. This insult has been proposed as a major pathological factor in age-related macular degeneration (AMD) [97, 132-134]. Modification due to glycation is thought to lead to thickening and changes in the physical properties of Bruch's membrane and extracellular matrix, causing a dysfunctional outer retina. Extracellular deposits, called drusen, and changes in biomechanical properties of Bruch's membrane are two of the major early features of AMD. Interestingly, Bruch's membrane and drusen deposits display high AGE-immunoreactivity in an age-dependent manner [135-137]. Additionally, higher AGEs levels are found in AMD-patients compared to control subjects as well as in AMD-mouse models [69, 135, 137-140]. In addition, thickening of Bruch's membrane and breakdown of the blood retinal barrier takes place even in non-diabetic animals when infused with pre-formed AGEs [141, 142].

Another complication is that high concentrations of AGEs result in aberrant levels of platelet derived growth factor B (PDGF-B) and vascular endothelial growth factor (VEGF). This is thought to contribute to the early vascular damage in diabetic retinopathy [136, 143-145]. In addition, exposure to glycative stress compromises the vitality of cells within the retinal pigment epithelium [146-149]. As indicated above, these cells are ultimately responsible for the maintenance of the functionality of photoreceptors and the integrity of choriocapillaris.

Hyperglycemia is also associated with compromises to inner vasculature, particularly in diabetic patients. This is associated with accumulation of AGEs in Müller glia [150-154]. High levels of diet-induced AGEs have been associated with Müller glial malfunction in diabetic retinopathy [151, 155].

As with lens and cataract, compounds that inhibit AGEs formation delay the onset of diabetic retinopathy, at least in animal models [152, 156-158]. Also, consistent with a role for AGEs in the initiation of diabetic retinopathy, the overexpression of glyoxalase 1, the limiting enzyme in the methylglyoxal-detoxifying glyoxalase system, reduces retinal AGEs in diabetic rats [159].

Recently it has been shown that specific loss of autophagy, one of the proteolytic activities involved in the clearance of AGEs, in the retinal pigment epithelium also induces AMD-features in an age-dependent manner with a concomitant accumulation of AGEs [160]. Compromised redox status of glycatively/oxidatively stressed RPE can also lead to cytotoxicity due to limited UPS activity [161].

REFERENCES

1. Sherwin JC, Reacher MH, Dean WH, Ngondi J. Epidemiology of vitamin A deficiency and xerophthalmia in at-risk populations. Trans R Soc Trop Med Hyg 2012; 106(4): 205-14.
2. Velasco Cruz AA, Attié-Castro FA, Fernandes SL, et al. Adult blindness secondary to vitamin A deficiency associated with an eating disorder. Nutrition 2005; 21(5): 630-3.
3. De Salvo G, Maguire JI, Lotery AJ. Vitamin A deficiency-related retinopathy after bariatric surgery. Graefes Arch Clin Exp Ophthalmol 2012; 250(6): 941-3.
4. Lee WB, Hamilton SM, Harris JP, Schwab IR. Ocular complications of hypovitaminosis a after bariatric surgery. Ophthalmology 2005; 112(6): 1031-4.
5. Danesh-Meyer HV, Savino P, Sergott R. The correlation of phenylephrine 1% with hydroxyamphetamine 1% in Horner's syndrome. Br J Ophthalmol 2004; 88(4): 592-3.
6. Clifford LJ, Turnbull AMJ, Denning AM. Reversible night blindness – A reminder of the increasing importance of vitamin A deficiency in the developed world. J Optom 2013; 6(3): 173-4.
7. Chae T, Foroozan R. Vitamin A deficiency in patients with a remote history of intestinal surgery. Br J Ophthalmol 2006; 90(8): 955-6.
8. Kemp CM, Jacobson SG, Faulkner DJ, et al. Visual function and rhodopsin levels in humans with vitamin A deficiency. Exp Eye Res 1988; 46(2): 185-97.
9. World Health Organization, UNICEF, United Sates Agency for International Development, Helen Keller International, Group IVAC. Control of vitamin A deficiency and xerophthalmia: report of a Joint WHO/UNICEF/USAID/Helen Keller International/IVACG meeting. Geneva, 1982.
10. Sommer A. Vitamin A deficiency and its consequences: a field guide to detection and control. 3rd ed Geneva: World Health Organization, 1995.
11. Ross DA. Recommendations for vitamin A supplementation. J Nutr 2002; 132(9 Suppl): 2902S-2906S.
12. Sajilata MG, Singhal RS, Kamat MY. The Carotenoid Pigment Zeaxanthin – A Review. Compr Rev Food Sci Food Saf 2008; 7(1): 29-49.
13. Sparrow JR, Kim SR. The carotenoids of macular pigment and bisretinoid lipofuscin precursors in photoreceptor outer segments. In Carotenoids: Physical, Chemical and Biological Functions and Properties; CRC Press: Boca Raton, FL, USA, 2009; pp. 355-63.
14. Nwachukwu ID, Udenigwe CC, Aluko RE. Lutein and zeaxanthin: Production technology, bioavailability, mechanisms of action, visual function, and health claim status. Trends Food Sci Technol 2016, 49: 74-84.
15. Delgado-Pelayo R, Hornero-Méndez D. Identification and Quantitative Analysis of Carotenoids and Their Esters from Sarsaparilla (Smilax aspera L.) Berries. J Agric Food Chem 2012; 60(33): 8225-32.
16. Billsten HH, Bhosale P, Yemelyanov A, Bernstein PS, Polivka T. Photophysical properties of xanthophylls in carotenoproteins from human retinas. Photochem Photobiol 2003; 78(2): 138-45.
17. Mozaffarieh M, Sacu S, Wedrich A. The role of the carotenoids, lutein and zeaxanthin, in protecting against age-related macular degeneration: a review based on controversial evidence. Nutr J 2003; 2: 20.
18. Maiani G, Castón MJP, Catasta G, et al. Carotenoids: actual knowledge on food sources, intakes, stability and bioavailability and their protective role in humans. Mol Nutr Food Res 2009; 53 Suppl 2: S194-S218.
19. Nimalaratne C, Lopes-Lutz D, Schieber A, Wu J. Effect of domestic cooking methods on egg yolk xanthophylls. J Agric Food Chem 2012, 60(51): 12547-52.
20. Torregrosa F, Cortés C, Esteve MJ, Frigola A. Effect of high-intensity pulsed electric fields processing and conventional heat treatment on orange-carrot juice carotenoids. J Agric Food Chem 2005, 53(24): 9519-25.
21. Benzie IF, Chung WY, Wang J, Richelle M, Bucheli P. Enhanced bioavailability of zeaxanthin in a milk-based formulation of wolfberry (Gou Qi Zi; Fructus barbarum L.). Br J Nutr 2006; 96: 154-60.
22. Khoo HE, Prasad KN, Kong KW, Jiang Y, Ismail A. Carotenoids and their isomers: color pigments in fruits and vegetables. Molecules 2011; 16(2): 1710-38.
23. Schieber, A.; Carle, R. Occurrence of carotenoid cis-isomers in food: Technological, analytical, and nutritional implications. Trends Food Sci Technol 2005; 16(9): 416-22.
24. Pérez-Gálvez A, Martin HD, Sies H, Stahl W. Incorporation of carotenoids from paprika oleoresin into human chylomicrons. Br J Nutr 2003; 89(6): 787-93.
25. Breithaupt DE, Weller P, Wolters M, Hahn A. Comparison of plasma responses in human subjects after the ingestion of 3R,3R'-zeaxanthin dipalmitate from wolfberry (Lycium barbarum) and non-esterified 3R,3R'-zeaxanthin using chiral high-performance liquid chromatography. Br J Nutr 2004; 91(5): 707-13.
26. Evans M, Beck M, Elliott J, Etheve S, Roberts R, Schalch W. Effects of formulation on the bioavailability of lutein and zeaxanthin: a randomized, double-blind, cross-over, comparative, single-dose study in healthy subjects. Eur J Nutr 2013; 52(4): 1381-91.
27. Furr, H.C.; Clark, R.M. Intestinal absorption and tissue distribution of carotenoids. J Nutr Biochem 1997; 8: 364-77.
28. Borel P, Grolier P, Armand M, Partier A, Lafont H, Lairon D, Azais-Braesco V. Carotenoids in biological emulsions: solubility, surface-to-core distribution, and release from lipid droplets. J Lipid Res 1996; 37(2): 250-61.
29. Tyssandier V, Reboul E, Dumas JF, Bouteloup-Demange C, Armand M, Marcand J, Sallas M, Borel P. Processing of vegetable-borne carotenoids in the human stomach and duodenum. Am J Physiol Gastrointest Liver Physiol 2003; 284(6): G913-23.
30. Chitchumroonchokchai C, Failla ML. Hydrolysis of zeaxanthin esters by carboxyl ester lipase during digestion facilitates micellarization and uptake of the xanthophyll by Caco-2 human intestinal cells. J Nutr 2006; 136(3): 588-94.
31. Wingerath T, Sies H, Stahl W. Xanthophyll esters in human skin. Arch Biochem Biophys 1998; 355(2): 271-4.
32. Deming DM, Erdman JW. Mammalian carotenoid absorption and metabolism. Pure Appl Chem 1999; 71(12): 2213-23.
33. Parker RS. Absorption, metabolism, and transport of carotenoids. FASEB J 1996; 10(5): 542-51.
34. Borel P. Genetic variations involved in interindividual variability in carotenoid status. Mol Nutr Food Res 2012; 56(2): 228-40.
35. Niesor EJ, Chaput E, Mary JL, Staempfli A, Topp A, Stauffer A, Wang H, Durrwell A. Effect of compounds affecting ABCA1 expression and CETP activity on the HDL

pathway involved in intestinal absorption of lutein and zeaxanthin. Lipids 2014; 49(12): 1233-43.
36. Desmarchelier C, Borel P. Overview of carotenoid bioavailability determinants: From dietary factors to host genetic variations. Trends Food Sci Technol 2017; 69: 270-80.
37. Kiokias S, Proestos C, Varzakas T. A review of the structure, biosynthesis, absorption of carotenoids-analysis and properties of their common natural extracts. Curr Res Nutr Food Sci J 2016; 4: 25-37.
38. Jeon S, Li Q, Rubakhin SS, Sweedler JV, Smith JW, Neuringer M, Kuchan M, Erdman JW Jr. 13C-lutein is differentially distributed in tissues of an adult female rhesus macaque following a single oral administration: a pilot study. Nutr Res 2019; 61: 102-8.
39. Sies H, Stahl W. Vitamins E and C, beta-carotene, and other carotenoids as antioxidants. Am J Clin Nutr 1995; 62(6 Suppl): 1315S-1321S.
40. Ribaya-Mercado JD, Blumberg JB. Lutein and zeaxanthin and their potential roles in disease prevention. J Am Coll Nutr 2004; 23(6 Suppl): 567S-587S.
41. Ojima F, Sakamoto H, Ishiguro Y, Terao J. Consumption of carotenoids in photosensitized oxidation of human plasma and plasma low-density lipoprotein. Free Radic Biol Med 1993; 15(4): 377-84.
42. Dhalla NS, Temsah RM, Netticadan T. Role of oxidative stress in cardiovascular diseases. J Hypertens 2000; 18(6): 655-73.
43. Vinson JA. Oxidative stress in cataracts. Pathophysiology 2006; 13(3): 151-62.
44. Lee SH, Min DB. Effects, quenching mechanisms, and kinetics of carotenoids in chlorophyll-sensitized photooxidation of soybean oil. J Agric Food Chem 1990; 38: 1630-4.
45. Rapp LM, Maple SS, Choi JH. Lutein and zeaxanthin concentrations in rod outer segment membranes from perifoveal and peripheral human retina. Invest Ophthalmol Vis Sci 2000; 41(5): 1200-9.
46. Khachik F, Bernstein PS, Garland DL. Identification of lutein and zeaxanthin oxidation products in human and monkey retinas. Invest Ophthalmol Vis Sci 1997; 38(9): 1802-11.
47. National Eye Institute. Age-Related Macular Degeneration (AMD). Available online: https://nei.nih.gov/eyedata/amd (accessed on 15 June 2019).
48. Kovach JL, Schwartz SG, Flynn HW Jr, Scott IU. Anti-VEGF Treatment Strategies for Wet AMD. J Ophthalmol 2012; 2012: 786870.
49. Bone RA, Landrum JT, Mayne ST, Gomez CM, Tibor SE, Twaroska EE. Macular pigment in donor eyes with and without AMD: a case-control study. Invest Ophthalmol Vis Sci 2001; 42(1): 235-40.
50. Nolan JM, Kenny R, O'Regan C, Cronin H, Loughman J, Connolly EE, Kearney P, Loane E, Beatty S. Macular pigment optical density in an ageing Irish population: The Irish Longitudinal Study on Ageing. Ophthalmic Res 2010; 44(2): 131-9.
51. Akuffo KO, Nolan JM, Howard AN, Moran R, Stack J, Klein R, Klein BE, Meuer SM, Sabour-Pickett S, Thurnham DI, Beatty S. Sustained supplementation and monitored response with differing carotenoid formulations in early age-related macular degeneration. Eye (Lond) 2015; 29(7): 902-12.
52. Seddon JM, Ajani UA, Sperduto RD, Hiller R, Blair N, Burton TC, Farber MD, Gragoudas ES, Haller J, Miller DT, et al. Dietary carotenoids, vitamins A, C, and E, and advanced age-related macular degeneration. Eye Disease Case-Control Study Group. JAMA 1994; 272(18): 1413-20.
53. Young RW. Pathophysiology of age-related macular degeneration. Surv Ophthalmol 1987; 31(5): 291-306.
54. Keller JN, Dimayuga E, Chen Q, Thorpe J, Gee J, Ding Q. Autophagy, proteasomes, lipofuscin, and oxidative stress in the aging brain. Int J Biochem Cell Biol 2004; 36(12): 2376-91.
55. Nociari MM, Kiss S, Rodriguez-Boulan E. Lipofuscin Accumulation into and Clearance from Retinal Pigment Epithelium Lysosomes: Physiopathology and Emerging Therapeutics. In Lysosomes-Associated Diseases and Methods to Study Their Function; IntechOpen: London, UK, 2017.
56. Sundelin SP, Nilsson SE. Lipofuscin-formation in retinal pigment epithelial cells is reduced by antioxidants. Free Radic Biol Med 2001; 31(2): 217-25.
57. Taylor HR, West S, Muñoz B, Rosenthal FS, Bressler SB, Bressler NM. The long-term effects of visible light on the eye. Arch Ophthalmol 1992; 110(1): 99-104.
58. Krinsky NI, Landrum JT, Bone RA. Biologic mechanisms of the protective role of lutein and zeaxanthin in the eye. Annu Rev Nutr 2003; 23: 171-201.
59. Junghans A, Sies H, Stahl W. Macular pigments lutein and zeaxanthin as blue light filters studied in liposomes. Arch Biochem Biophys 2001; 391(2): 160-4.
60. Barker FM 2nd, Snodderly DM, Johnson EJ, Schalch W, Koepcke W, Gerss J, Neuringer M. Nutritional manipulation of primate retinas, V: effects of lutein, zeaxanthin, and n-3 fatty acids on retinal sensitivity to blue-light-induced damage. Invest Ophthalmol Vis Sci 2011; 52(7): 3934-42.
61. Gale CR, Hall NF, Phillips DI, Martyn CN. Lutein and zeaxanthin status and risk of age-related macular degeneration. Invest Ophthalmol Vis Sci 2003; 44(6): 2461-5.
62. Roberts RL, Green J, Lewis B. Lutein and zeaxanthin in eye and skin health. Clin Dermatol 2009; 27(2): 195-201.
63. Johnson EJ. A possible role for lutein and zeaxanthin in cognitive function in the elderly. Am J Clin Nutr 2012; 96(5): 1161S-5S.
64. Popkin BM, Hawkes C. Sweetening of the global diet, particularly beverages: patterns, trends, and policy responses. Lancet Diabetes Endocrinol 2016; 4(2): 174-86.
65. Aragno M, Mastrocola R. Dietary Sugars and Endogenous Formation of Advanced Glycation Endproducts: Emerging Mechanisms of Disease. Nutrients 2017; 9(4): 385.
66. Chiu CJ, Taylor A. Dietary hyperglycemia, glycemic index and metabolic retinal diseases. Prog Retin Eye Res 2011; 30(1): 18-53.
67. Semba RD, Nicklett EJ, Ferrucci L. Does accumulation of advanced glycation end products contribute to the aging phenotype? J Gerontol A Biol Sci Med Sci 2010; 65(9): 963-75.
68. Weikel KA, Chiu CJ, Taylor A. Nutritional modulation of age-related macular degeneration. Mol Aspects Med 2012; 33(4): 318-75.
69. Weikel KA, Fitzgerald P, Shang F, Caceres MA, Bian Q, Handa JT, Stitt AW, Taylor A. Natural history of age-related retinal lesions that precede AMD in mice fed high or low glycemic index diets. Invest Ophthalmol Vis Sci 2012; 53(2): 622-32.
70. Neeper M, Schmidt AM, Brett J, Yan SD, Wang F, Pan YC, Elliston K, Stern D, Shaw A. Cloning and expression of a

cell surface receptor for advanced glycosylation end products of proteins. J Biol Chem 1992; 267(21): 14998-5004.
71. Huang RF, Hsu YC, Lin HL, Yang FL. Folate depletion and elevated plasma homocysteine promote oxidative stress in rat livers. J Nutr 2001; 131(1): 33-8.
72. Hudson MB, Hosick PA, McCaulley GO, Schrieber L, Wrieden J, McAnulty SR, Triplett NT, McBride JM, Quindry JC. The effect of resistance exercise on humoral markers of oxidative stress. Med Sci Sports Exerc 2008; 40(3): 542-8.
73. Lander HM, Tauras JM, Ogiste JS, Hori O, Moss RA, Schmidt AM. Activation of the receptor for advanced glycation end products triggers a p21(ras)-dependent mitogen-activated protein kinase pathway regulated by oxidant stress. J Biol Chem 1997; 272(28): 17810-4.
74. Araki N, Higashi T, Mori T, Shibayama R, Kawabe Y, Kodama T, Takahashi K, Shichiri M, Horiuchi S. Macrophage scavenger receptor mediates the endocytic uptake and degradation of advanced glycation end products of the Maillard reaction. Eur J Biochem 1995; 230(2): 408-15.
75. Jono T, Miyazaki A, Nagai R, Sawamura T, Kitamura T, Horiuchi S. Lectin-like oxidized low density lipoprotein receptor-1 (LOX-1) serves as an endothelial receptor for advanced glycation end products (AGE). FEBS Lett 2002; 511(1-3): 170-4.
76. Li D, Devaraj S, Fuller C, Bucala R, Jialal I. Effect of alpha-tocopherol on LDL oxidation and glycation: in vitro and in vivo studies. J Lipid Res 1996; 37(9): 1978-86.
77. Ohgami N, Nagai R, Ikemoto M, Arai H, Kuniyasu A, Horiuchi S, Nakayama H. CD36, a member of class B scavenger receptor family, is a receptor for advanced glycation end products. Ann N Y Acad Sci 2001; 947:350-5.
78. Ohgami N, Nagai R, Ikemoto M, Arai H, Kuniyasu A, Horiuchi S, Nakayama H. Cd36, a member of the class b scavenger receptor family, as a receptor for advanced glycation end products. J Biol Chem 2001; 276(5): 3195-202.
79. Ohgami N, Nagai R, Ikemoto M, Arai H, Miyazaki A, Hakamata H, Horiuchi S, Nakayama H. CD36, serves as a receptor for advanced glycation endproducts (AGE). J Diabetes Complications 2002; 16(1): 56-9.
80. Tamura Y, Adachi H, Osuga J, Ohashi K, Yahagi N, Sekiya M, Okazaki H, Tomita S, Iizuka Y, Shimano H, Nagai R, Kimura S, Tsujimoto M, Ishibashi S. FEEL-1 and FEEL-2 are endocytic receptors for advanced glycation end products. J Biol Chem 2003; 278(15): 12613-7.
81. Vlassara H, Li YM, Imani F, Wojciechowicz D, Yang Z, Liu FT, Cerami A. Identification of galectin-3 as a high-affinity binding protein for advanced glycation end products (AGE): a new member of the AGE-receptor complex. Mol Med 1995; 1(6): 634-46.
82. Malik NS, Moss SJ, Ahmed N, Furth AJ, Wall RS, Meek KM. Ageing of the human corneal stroma: structural and biochemical changes. Biochim Biophys Acta 1992; 1138(3): 222-8.
83. Sato E, Mori F, Igarashi S, Abiko T, Takeda M, Ishiko S, Yoshida A. Corneal advanced glycation end products increase in patients with proliferative diabetic retinopathy. Diabetes Care 2001; 24(3): 479-82.
84. Brummer G, Littlechild S, McCall S, Zhang Y, Conrad GW. The role of nonenzymatic glycation and carbonyls in collagen cross-linking for the treatment of keratoconus. Invest Ophthalmol Vis Sci 2011; 52(9): 6363-9.
85. Kaji Y, Usui T, Oshika T, Matsubara M, Yamashita H, Araie M, Murata T, Ishibashi T, Nagai R, Horiuchi S, Amano S. Advanced glycation end products in diabetic corneas. Invest Ophthalmol Vis Sci 2000; 41(2): 362-8.
86. Sady C, Khosrof S, Nagaraj R. Advanced Maillard reaction and crosslinking of corneal collagen in diabetes. Biochem Biophys Res Commun 1995; 214(3): 793-7.
87. Shi L, Chen H, Yu X, Wu X. Advanced glycation end products delay corneal epithelial wound healing through reactive oxygen species generation. Mol Cell Biochem 2013; 383(1-2): 253-9.
88. Shi L, Yu X, Yang H, Wu X. Advanced glycation end products induce human corneal epithelial cells apoptosis through generation of reactive oxygen species and activation of JNK and p38 MAPK pathways. PLoS One 2013; 8(6): e66781.
89. Kim J, Kim CS, Sohn E, Jeong IH, Kim H, Kim JS. Involvement of advanced glycation end products, oxidative stress and nuclear factor-kappaB in the development of diabetic keratopathy. Graefes Arch Clin Exp Ophthalmol 2011; 249(4): 529-36.
90. Zou C, Wang S, Huang F, Zhang YA. Advanced glycation end products and ultrastructural changes in corneas of long-term streptozotocin-induced diabetic monkeys. Cornea 2012; 31(12): 1455-9.
91. Abiko T, Abiko A, Ishiko S, Takeda M, Horiuchi S, Yoshida A. Relationship between autofluorescence and advanced glycation end products in diabetic lenses. Exp Eye Res 1999; 68(3): 361-6.
92. Ahmed MU, Brinkmann Frye E, Degenhardt TP, Thorpe SR, Baynes JW. N-epsilon-(carboxyethyl)lysine, a product of the chemical modification of proteins by methylglyoxal, increases with age in human lens proteins. Biochem J 1997; 324(2): 565-70.
93. Chellan P, Nagaraj RH. Protein crosslinking by the Maillard reaction: dicarbonyl-derived imidazolium crosslinks in aging and diabetes. Arch Biochem Biophys 1999; 368(1): 98-104.
94. Frye EB, Degenhardt TP, Thorpe SR, Baynes JW. Role of the Maillard reaction in aging of tissue proteins. Advanced glycation end product-dependent increase in imidazolium cross-links in human lens proteins. J Biol Chem 1998; 273(30): 18714-9.
95. Lyons TJ, Silvestri G, Dunn JA, Dyer DG, Baynes JW. Role of glycation in modification of lens crystallins in diabetic and nondiabetic senile cataracts. Diabetes 1991; 40(8): 1010-5.
96. Matsumoto K, Ikeda K, Horiuchi S, Zhao H, Abraham EC. Immunochemical evidence for increased formation of advanced glycation end products and inhibition by aminoguanidine in diabetic rat lenses. Biochem Biophys Res Commun 1997; 241(2): 352-4.
97. Nagaraj RH, Linetsky M, Stitt AW. The pathogenic role of Maillard reaction in the aging eye. Amino Acids 2012; 42(4): 1205-20.
98. Pokupec R, Kalauz M, Turk N, Turk Z. Advanced glycation endproducts in human diabetic and non-diabetic cataractous lenses. Graefes Arch Clin Exp Ophthalmol 2003; 241(5): 378-84.
99. Stevens VJ, Rouzer CA, Monnier VM, Cerami A. Diabetic cataract formation: potential role of glycosylation of lens crystallins. Proc Natl Acad Sci USA 1978; 75(6): 2918-22.
100. Tessier F, Obrenovich M, Monnier VM. Structure and mechanism of formation of human lens fluorophore LM-1. Relationship to vesperlysine A and the advanced Maillard reaction in aging, diabetes, and cataractogenesis. J Biol Chem 1999; 274(30): 20796-804.
101. Zarina S, Zhao HR, Abraham EC. Advanced glycation end

products in human senile and diabetic cataractous lenses. Mol Cell Biochem 2000; 210(1-2): 29-34.
102. Nagaraj RH, Kern TS, Sell DR, Fogarty J, Engerman RL, Monnier VM. Evidence of a glycemic threshold for the formation of pentosidine in diabetic dog lenses but not in collagen. Diabetes 1996; 45(5): 587-94.
103. Swamy-Mruthinti S, Shaw SM, Zhao HR, Green K, Abraham EC. Evidence of a glycemic threshold for the development of cataracts in diabetic rats. Curr Eye Res 1999; 18(6): 423-9.
104. Hashim Z, Zarina S. Advanced glycation end products in diabetic and non-diabetic human subjects suffering from cataract. Age (Dordr) 2011; 33(3): 377-84.
105. Raghavan CT, Smuda M, Smith AJ, Howell S, Smith DG, Singh A, Gupta P, Glomb MA, Wormstone IM, Nagaraj RH. AGEs in human lens capsule promote the TGFβ2-mediated EMT of lens epithelial cells: implications for age-associated fibrosis. Aging Cell 2016; 15(3): 465-76.
106. Shamsi FA, Sharkey E, Creighton D, Nagaraj RH. Maillard reactions in lens proteins: methylglyoxal-mediated modifications in the rat lens. Exp Eye Res 2000; 70(3): 369-80.
107. Beswick HT, Harding JJ. Conformational changes induced in lens alpha- and gamma-crystallins by modification with glucose 6-phosphate. Implications for cataract. Biochem J 1987; 246(3): 761-9.
108. Casey EB, Zhao HR, Abraham EC. Role of glycine 1 and lysine 2 in the glycation of bovine gamma B-crystallin. Site-directed mutagenesis of lysine to threonine. J Biol Chem 1995; 270(35): 20781-6.
109. Kumar PA, Kumar MS, Reddy GB. Effect of glycation on alpha-crystallin structure and chaperone-like function. Biochem J 2007; 408(2): 251-8.
110. Nahomi RB, Wang B, Raghavan CT, Voss O, Doseff AI, Santhoshkumar P, Nagaraj RH. Chaperone peptides of α-crystallin inhibit epithelial cell apoptosis, protein insolubilization, and opacification in experimental cataracts. J Biol Chem 2013; 288(18): 13022-35.
111. Perry RE, Swamy MS, Abraham EC. Progressive changes in lens crystallin glycation and high-molecular-weight aggregate formation leading to cataract development in streptozotocin-diabetic rats. Exp Eye Res 1987; 44(2): 269-82.
112. Kim MJ, Kim JH, Kim SJ, Yu YS. Long-term follow-up of changes in corneal endothelium after primary and secondary intraocular lens implantations in children. Graefes Arch Clin Exp Ophthalmol 2012; 250(6): 925-30.
113. Jahngen-Hodge J, Cyr D, Laxman E, Taylor A. Ubiquitin and ubiquitin conjugates in human lens. Exp Eye Res 1992; 55(6): 897-902.
114. Jahngen JH, Haas AL, Ciechanover A, Blondin J, Eisenhauer D, Taylor A. The eye lens has an active ubiquitin-protein conjugation system. J Biol Chem 1986; 261(29): 13760-7.
115. Jahngen JJ, Eisenhauer D, Taylor A. Lens proteins are substrates for the reticulocyte ubiquitin conjugation system. Curr Eye Res 1986; 5(10): 725-33.
116. Jahngen JH, Lipman RD, Eisenhauer DA, Jahngen EG Jr, Taylor A. Aging and cellular maturation cause changes in ubiquitin-eye lens protein conjugates. Arch Biochem Biophys 1990; 276(1): 32-7.
117. Shang F, Taylor A. Oxidative stress and recovery from oxidative stress are associated with altered ubiquitin conjugating and proteolytic activities in bovine lens epithelial cells. Biochem J 1995; 307 (1): 297-303.
118. Chiu CJ, Robman L, McCarty CA, et al. Dietary carbohydrate in relation to cortical and nuclear lens opacities in the melbourne visual impairment project. Invest Ophthalmol Vis Sci 2010; 51(6): 2897-2905.
119. Nagaraj RH, Sarkar P, Mally A, Biemel KM, Lederer MO, Padayatti PS. Effect of pyridoxamine on chemical modification of proteins by carbonyls in diabetic rats: characterization of a major product from the reaction of pyridoxamine and methylglyoxal. Arch Biochem Biophys 2002; 402(1): 110-9.
120. Swamy-Mruthinti S, Green K, Abraham EC. Inhibition of cataracts in moderately diabetic rats by aminoguanidine. Exp Eye Res 1996; 62(5): 505-510.
121. Taylor A, Jacques PF, Epstein EM. Relations among aging, antioxidant status, and cataract. Am J Clin Nutr 1995; 62(6 Suppl): 1439S-1447S.
122. Du L, Hao M, Li C, Wu W, Wang W, Ma Z, Yang T, Zhang N, Isaac AT, Zhu X, Sun Y, Lu Q, Yin X. Quercetin inhibited epithelial mesenchymal transition in diabetic rats, high-glucose-cultured lens, and SRA01/04 cells through transforming growth factor-β2/phosphoinositide 3-kinase/Akt pathway. Mol Cell Endocrinol 2017; 452: 44-56.
123. Muthenna P, Akileshwari C, Saraswat M, Bhanuprakash Reddy G. Inhibition of advanced glycation end-product formation on eye lens protein by rutin. Br J Nutr 2012; 107(7): 941-9.
124. Patil KK, Meshram RJ, Gacche RN. Effect of monohydroxylated flavonoids on glycation-induced lens opacity and protein aggregation. J Enzyme Inhib Med Chem 2016; 31(sup1): 148-56.
125. Hollenbach S, Thampi P, Viswanathan T, Abraham EC. Cleavage of in vitro and in vivo formed lens protein cross-links by a novel cross-link breaker. Mol Cell Biochem 2003; 243(1-2): 73-80.
126. Géhl Z, Bakondi E, Resch MD, et al. Diabetes-induced oxidative stress in the vitreous humor. Redox Biol 2016; 9: 100-3.
127. Stitt AW, Moore JE, Sharkey JA, et al. Advanced glycation end products in vitreous: Structural and functional implications for diabetic vitreopathy. Invest Ophthalmol Vis Sci 1998; 39(13): 2517-23.
128. van Deemter M, Pas HH, Kuijer R, van der Worp RJ, Hooymans JM, Los LI. Enzymatic breakdown of type II collagen in the human vitreous. Invest Ophthalmol Vis Sci 2009; 50(10): 4552-60.
129. Sebag J, Buckingham B, Charles MA, Reiser K. Biochemical abnormalities in vitreous of humans with proliferative diabetic retinopathy. Arch Ophthalmol 1992; 110(10): 1472-6.
130. Villa M, Parravano M, Micheli A, et al. A quick, simple method for detecting circulating fluorescent advanced glycation end-products: Correlation with in vitro and in vivo non-enzymatic glycation. Metabolism 2017; 71: 64-9.
131. Lee OT, Good SD, Lamy R, Kudisch M, Stewart JM. Advanced glycation end-product accumulation reduces vitreous permeability. Invest Ophthalmol Vis Sci 2015; 56(5): 2892-7.
132. Glenn JV, Stitt AW. The role of advanced glycation end products in retinal ageing and disease. Biochim Biophys Acta 2009; 1790(10): 1109-16.
133. Karachalias N, Babaei-Jadidi R, Ahmed N, Thornalley PJ. Accumulation of fructosyl-lysine and advanced glycation end products in the kidney, retina and peripheral nerve of streptozotocin-induced diabetic rats. Biochem Soc Trans 2003; 31(Pt 6): 1423-5.
134. Uchiki T, Weikel KA, Jiao W, et al. Glycation-altered prote-

olysis as a pathobiologic mechanism that links dietary glycemic index, aging, and age-related disease (in non-diabetics). Aging Cell 2012; 11(1): 1-13.
135. Farboud B, Aotaki-Keen A, Miyata T, Hjelmeland LM, Handa JT. Development of a polyclonal antibody with broad epitope specificity for advanced glycation end-products and localization of these epitopes in Bruch's membrane of the aging eye. Mol Vis 1999; 5: 11.
136. Handa JT, Reiser KM, Matsunaga H, Hjelmeland LM. The advanced glycation endproduct pentosidine induces the expression of PDGF-B in human retinal pigment epithelial cells. Exp Eye Res 1998; 66(4): 411-9.
137. Handa JT, Verzijl N, Matsunaga H, et al. Increase in the advanced glycation end product pentosidine in Bruch's membrane with age. Invest Ophthalmol Vis Sci 1999; 40(3): 775-9.
138. Hammes HP, Hoerauf H, Alt A, et al. N(epsilon)(carboxymethyl)lysin and the AGE receptor RAGE colocalize in age-related macular degeneration. Invest Ophthalmol Vis Sci 1999; 40(8): 1855-9.
139. Rowan S, Weikel K, Chang ML, et al. Cfh genotype interacts with dietary glycemic index to modulate age-related macular degeneration-like features in mice. Invest Ophthalmol Vis Sci 2014; 55(1): 492-501.
140. Rowan S, Jiang S, Korem T, et al. Involvement of a gut-retina axis in protection against dietary glycemia-induced age-related macular degeneration. Proc Natl Acad Sci USA 2017; 114(22): E4472-E4481.
141. Clements RS Jr, Robison WG Jr, Cohen MP. Anti-glycated albumin therapy ameliorates early retinal microvascular pathology in db/db mice. J Diabetes Complications 1998; 12(1): 28-33.
142. Stitt AW, Bhaduri T, McMullen CB, Gardiner TA, Archer DB. Advanced glycation end products induce blood-retinal barrier dysfunction in normoglycemic rats. Mol Cell Biol Res Commun 2000; 3(6): 380-8.
143. Kandarakis SA, Piperi C, Moschonas DP, Korkolopoulou P, Papalois A, Papavassiliou AG. Dietary glycotoxins induce RAGE and VEGF up-regulation in the retina of normal rats. Exp Eye Res 2015; 137: 1-10.
144. Lu M, Kuroki M, Amano S, et al. Advanced glycation end products increase retinal vascular endothelial growth factor expression. J Clin Invest 1998; 101(6): 1219-24.
145. Murata T, Nagai R, Ishibashi T, Inomuta H, Ikeda K, Horiuchi S. The relationship between accumulation of advanced glycation end products and expression of vascular endothelial growth factor in human diabetic retinas. Diabetologia 1997; 40(7): 764-9.
146. Reber F, Kasper M, Siegner A, Kniep E, Seigel G, Funk RH. Alteration of the intracellular pH and apoptosis induction in a retinal cell line by the AGE-inducing agent glyoxal. Graefes Arch Clin Exp Ophthalmol 2002; 240(12): 1022-32.
147. Roehlecke C, Valtink M, Frenzel A, et al. Stress responses of human retinal pigment epithelial cells to glyoxal. Graefes Arch Clin Exp Ophthalmol 2016; 254(12): 2361-72.
148. Wang Y, Hanus JW, Abu-Asab MS, et al. NLRP3 Upregulation in Retinal Pigment Epithelium in Age-Related Macular Degeneration. Int J Mol Sci 2016; 17(1): 73.
149. Yamagishi S, Inagaki Y, Amano S, Okamoto T, Takeuchi M, Makita Z. Pigment epithelium-derived factor protects cultured retinal pericytes from advanced glycation end product-induced injury through its antioxidative properties. Biochem Biophys Res Commun 2002; 296(4): 877-82.
150. Chiarelli F, de Martino M, Mezzetti A, et al. Advanced glycation end products in children and adolescents with diabetes: relation to glycemic control and early microvascular complications. J Pediatr 1999; 134(4): 486-91.
151. Curtis TM, Hamilton R, Yong PH, et al. Müller glial dysfunction during diabetic retinopathy in rats is linked to accumulation of advanced glycation end-products and advanced lipoxidation end-products. Diabetologia 2011; 54(3): 690-8.
152. Gardiner TA, Anderson HR, Stitt AW. Inhibition of advanced glycation end-products protects against retinal capillary basement membrane expansion during long-term diabetes. J Pathol 2003; 201(2): 328-33.
153. Hammes HP, Wellensiek B, Klöting I, Sickel E, Bretzel RG, Brownlee M. The relationship of glycaemic level to advanced glycation end-product (AGE) accumulation and retinal pathology in the spontaneous diabetic hamster. Diabetologia 1998; 41(2): 165-70.
154. Stitt AW, He C, Friedman S, et al. Elevated AGE-modified ApoB in sera of euglycemic, normolipidemic patients with atherosclerosis: relationship to tissue AGEs. Mol Med 1997; 3(9): 617-27.
155. Zong H, Ward M, Madden A, et al. Hyperglycaemia-induced pro-inflammatory responses by retinal Müller glia are regulated by the receptor for advanced glycation end-products (RAGE). Diabetologia 2010; 53(12): 2656-66.
156. Hammes HP, Martin S, Federlin K, Geisen K, Brownlee M. Aminoguanidine treatment inhibits the development of experimental diabetic retinopathy. Proc Natl Acad Sci USA 1991; 88(24): 11555-8.
157. Hammes HP, Brownlee M, Edelstein D, Saleck M, Martin S, Federlin K. Aminoguanidine inhibits the development of accelerated diabetic retinopathy in the spontaneous hypertensive rat. Diabetologia 1994; 37(1): 32-5.
158. Hammes HP, Federoff HJ, Brownlee M. Nerve growth factor prevents both neuroretinal programmed cell death and capillary pathology in experimental diabetes. Mol Med 1995; 1(5): 527-34.
159. Berner AK, Brouwers O, Pringle R, et al. Protection against methylglyoxal-derived AGEs by regulation of glyoxalase 1 prevents retinal neuroglial and vasodegenerative pathology. Diabetologia 2012; 55(3): 845-54.
160. Zhang Y, Cross SD, Stanton JB, Marmorstein AD, Le YZ, Marmorstein LY. Early AMD-like defects in the RPE and retinal degeneration in aged mice with RPE-specific deletion of Atg5 or Atg7. Mol Vis 2017; 23: 228-41.
161. Jahngen-Hodge J, Obin MS, Gong X, et al. Regulation of ubiquitin-conjugating enzymes by glutathione following oxidative stress. J Biol Chem 1997; 272(45): 28218-26.

27 Food, allergies and intolerances

Gabriele Rumi

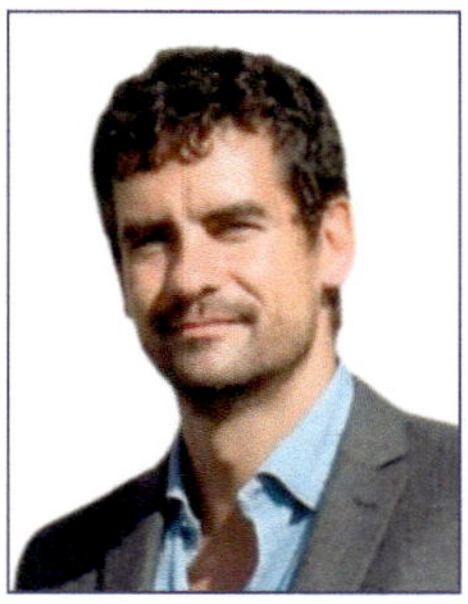

In 2014, the European Academy of Allergy and Clinical Immunology (EAACI) clarified that an adverse reaction to food should be called food *hypersensitivity*. Once immunologic mechanisms have been demonstrated, the appropriate term is food *allergy*, and, if the role of IgE is highlighted, the term is *IgE-mediated food allergy*. All other reactions, previously sometimes referred to as "food intolerance", should be referred to as *non-allergic food hypersensitivity* [1]. Severe, generalized allergic reactions to food can be classified as *anaphylaxis*. Food allergy has been defined as adverse reactions to food in which "immunologic mechanisms have been demonstrated"; this term therefore encompasses both Immunoglobulin E (IgE)-mediated and non-IgE-mediated food allergies [2].

27.1 Clinical scenario

27.1.1 IgE-mediated food allergy

Food allergy (FA), oral allergy syndrome and food-dependent exercise-induced anaphylaxis are adverse immune responses to food protein(s). Gastrointestinal (GI) symptoms associated with food allergic reactions may affect all the GI tract and the patient might suffer from a local reaction to a systemic and fatal one. Oral itching (pruritus), oral swelling or angioedema (lips, tongue or palate) and pharyngeal itching/tightness may represent a local reaction or a prelude of a systemic reaction involving other GI aspects as colicky abdominal pain, nausea, vomiting and diarrhea; or involving other organs such as the skin (urticaria and/or angioedema); the upper and lower respiratory airways (rhinitis, cough, bronchial hyperactivity and asthma) and the cardiovascular system (hypotension and shock). In the healthy GI tract, the epithelial lumen and GI immunity develop active immune tolerance to dietary antigens, combat invading microbes, and limit their persistence in the mucosa. It is unclear why some individuals fail to establish oral tolerance toward innocuous food allergens and develop allergic reactions to food allergens at the mucosal sites of the GI tract. Particularly, it is perplexing as to why only some of the individuals with a FA, who have high levels of dietary allergen-specific serum IgE, acquire susceptibility thus developing life threatening anaphylactic reactions. FA is thought to develop because of a failed induction of tolerance upon initial exposure to a food antigen or a break-

Gabriele Rumi, MD
Area Gastroenterologia ed Oncologia Medica
UOC di Allergologia
Fondazione Policlinico Universitario A. Gemelli IRCCS
Università Cattolica del Sacro Cuore, Rome, Italy

Email: gabriele.rumi@policlinicogemelli.it

down of an established tolerance to food antigen. Clinically, individuals with atopy (elevated immune response to common allergens) and skin sensitization in infancy often develop an allergic response to ingested food in the GI tract later in life. Although this observation has led to the "dual-allergen exposure" hypothesis, the molecular and cellular mechanisms that support this plausible hypothesis remain to be established [3].

After exposure to common allergens, IgE-mediated type I hypersensitivity reactions present different manifestations, such as hives, wheezing or vomiting. The most allergenic foods in the USA are milk, eggs, peanuts, tree nuts, soy, wheat, fish and shellfish. This class of FA is associated with the risk of severe or even fatal reactions. Whereas IgE-mediated allergies to cow's milk, egg, wheat and soy tend to be outgrown, atopic responses to peanuts, tree nuts and shellfish usually persist into adulthood. Estimating the prevalence of FA is challenging because the gold standard for confirming the diagnosis of FA is the Double-Blind, Placebo-Controlled Food Challenge (DBPCFC), a time-consuming and expensive process that can trigger adverse reactions. Thus, most FA prevalence estimates rely on self-reporting and vary in FA definitions and study methodology. FA is increasing in prevalence for reasons that are not yet clear. A rigorous population-based study utilizing food challenges to demonstrate FA showed that approximately one in 10 Australian children had a FA at one year of age. Estimates in the USA and Canada indicate a prevalence rate of one in 15 to one in 20. Regardless of the rate there is a need to differentiate prevalence of self-reported FA from the established oral food challenge (OFC). While the incidence of FA appeared stable over time, there was some evidence that the prevalence – alleged or real – may be increasing [4]. Roughly 70-80% of children allergic to egg, milk, wheat and soy will outgrow these allergies by adolescence. Approximately 50% of children outgrow egg and cow's milk allergy by age 6. In contrast, only about 20% of children with peanut allergy and 10% with tree nut allergy will outgrow these allergies [5]. A recent report notes that both the public and health providers often misinterpret a FA and its symptoms; they are having trouble in differentiating a FA from other immune and GI diseases, such as lactose intolerance and gluten sensitivity; and they don't know which management and prevention approaches are best. FA is both common and costly. In a recently published epidemiological study defining a retrospective cross-sectional cohort of 333,200 children in the United States, the results in costs to the USA healthcare system was approximately $24.8 billion. In addition, the global prevalence of all FA seems to be increasing [6].

27.1.2 Oral allergy syndrome

Another immunological condition that may affect GI organs, and especially the oral and throat mucosa, is the Oral Allergy Syndrome (OAS). The patient often displays itching after ingestion of fresh or raw fruits and vegetables or other allergens. Signs and symptoms of OAS include immediate oral itching, mucosal swelling (angioedema) and/or abdominal pain. Under the term OAS, if fact, we have to ascribe different situations that are defined as pollen-food syndromes and associations, such as birch-apple, cypress-peach and celery-mugwort (also called Artemisia) spice syndromes, mugwort-peach, mugwort-chamomile, mugwort-mustard, ragweed-melon-banana, goosefoot (also called pigweed or wild spinach)-melon. OAS may be of fungal origin, such as *Alternaria* mould-spinach syndrome, or may be of invertebrate, mammalian or avian origin, such as mite-shrimp, cat-pork and bird-egg syndromes. In these patients we may observe IgE sensitization via the respiratory route to aeroallergens and the establishment of FA due to cross-reactivities between some allergen components. This phenomenon should be distinguished from the common FA without sensitization to cross-reactive aeroallergens, in which heat and enzyme-resistant class 1 food allergens induce allergic sensitization via the digestive tract, typically being responsible for systemic allergic reactions. Class 2 food allergens are more heat-labile and susceptible to digestion and therefore do not cause GI sensitization, but instead lead to allergic reactions in patients already sensitized to cross-reactive aeroallergens through the respiratory route. Typically, pollen-food syndromes are produced by class 2 food allergens. In contrast to class 1 FA, which mainly affects young children, class 2 FA is observed especially in adults, as a consequence of sensitization to cross-reactive aeroallergens. Patients with allergic rhinitis produce IgE molecules specific for pollen-derived epitopes (which are the part of an antigen that is recognized by the immune system) that are cross reactive with fruit- or vegetable-protein epitopes. Several molecules with different characteristics act as food allergens. Some of them are stable, enduring heating, cooking, storage and digestion (linear epitopes), while others are less stable (conformational epitopes) losing their allergenicity in cooking and preservation. The patient with FA can be sensitized to both labile and stable components. The stability/lability to physical agents (heat, gastric pH, enzymes like protease, pepsin and so on) is a requisite for an allergen to interact with the IgE antibody. Thus, a component sensitive to heat will be virtually absent in a cooked food, while a determinant resistant to heat, pH and peptidase (for example,

Lipid Transfer Protein or LTP) will reach the bowel practically intact despite cooking and passage through the gastric and pancreatic digestion. As the cross-reactive IgE antibodies may be specific for a heat-labile food epitope, uncooked fruits or vegetables should be used in diagnostic testing for OAS. In recent years, Component Resolved Diagnosis (CRD) helps clinician and patient in treating OAS. Regarding peanut allergy, testing for IgE antibodies specific for particular components of peanut protein (IgE recombinant component testing) can be used to distinguish OAS from standard IgE-mediated allergy. For instance, in individuals with birch-pollen allergy, IgE antibodies specific for the pollen antigen Bet v 1 may cross react with the peanut component Ara h 8 to cause OAS, but reactivity against Ara h 8 is also associated with a decreased risk of clinically relevant IgE-mediated peanut allergy. By contrast, reactivity against the peanut components Ara h 1 or Ara h 2 is more likely to be associated with clinically relevant IgE-mediated peanut allergy. IgE- and T cell-mediated cross reactivities have also been observed between Bet v 1 and the hazelnut allergen Cor a 1. Finally, oral mite anaphylaxis is a new syndrome characterized by severe allergic symptoms occurring immediately after eating mite-contaminated foods, in patients with a previous history of house dust mite-allergic rhinitis and/or asthma [7].

27.1.3 Food dependent exercise-induced anaphylaxis

Exercise-Induced Anaphylaxis (EIAn) is defined as the occurrence of anaphylactic symptoms (skin, respiratory, GI, and cardiovascular symptoms) after physical activity. When the associated cofactor is food ingestion, the correct diagnosis is Food-Dependent EIAn (FDEIAn). Some of these patients present a characteristic pattern of IgE-mediated sensitization. The literature describes numerous reports of FDEIAn after intake of very different foods, from vegetables and nuts to meats and seafood. One of the best-characterized types of FDEIAn is that due to ω5-gliadin of wheat, though cases of FDEIAn after wheat ingestion by sensitization to wheat LTP are described. Some other conditions are strictly correlated with this syndrome, in fact, in about a third of cases, cofactors, such as food intake, temperature (warm or cold), alcohol consumption and drugs (especially nonsteroidal anti-inflammatory drugs) can be identified. Each of these cofactors may contribute to improving intestinal blood perfusion as this process may improve food allergen and GI mucosa contact causing allergy symptoms [8].

27.1.4 Alpha-gal mammalian meat allergy

A novel unusual IgE-mediated allergy has been described in the last ten years. In contrast to conventional food allergies which require IgE antibodies specific to a food protein, for the first time a pattern was detected of IgE antibodies against a sugar moiety galactose-alpha-1,3-galactose (also known as alpha-gal) that lines the surface of non-primate mammalian tissue. That kind of antibodies were well known in acute organ rejection, and then were associated with anaphylactic reactions to cetuximab, a chimeric mouse-human IgG1 monoclonal antibody that has the oligosaccharide galactose-alpha-1,3-galactose on the Fab portion of the cetuximab heavy chain. Unlike other IgE-mediated food allergies, IgE-mediated allergic reactions to alpha-gal in ingested mammalian meat are typically delayed in onset, frequently developing 3-6 hours after ingestion, although alcohol and exercise may decrease time frame to reaction. Reactions to alpha-gal are intermittent and may not occur with every allergen exposure. Variability in adverse reactions to alpha-gal depends on how much allergen is ingested which may depend on fat content of the cut of mammalian meat consumed. Additional factors include how much alpha-gal is digested, processed, packaged and presented to the immune system. Therefore, the anamnestic history (i.e., alcohol consumption and/or exercise) of chronic infection, autoimmune disease, malignancy, etc. may be investigated to better understand time frame to reaction and induced symptoms [9].

27.1.5 Allergic and immunologic reactions to food additives

Food additives are potential hidden allergens, and every human being is inevitably exposed to them every day. They should be considered and classified into eight groups: (1) antioxidants; (2) colors; (3) emulsifiers and stabilizers; (4) solvents; (5) glazing agents; (6) preservatives; (7) sweetening agents; (8) thickeners. Although it is mentioned that the calculation of FA prevalence is so hard, a prediction of FA is indicated between 3% and 35% in literature. Among sensitive subjects, potential of allergic reaction to food additives is reported as 0.03-0.23% As a result, allergic reactions to food additives can be considered triggers or aggravating factors in sensitive individuals, rather than etiological factors. Clinicians and consumers, especially sensitive individuals, must take into consideration allergic features of food additives [9]. Even a pseudoallergen-rich challenging diet (see below), that includes natural foods in addition to additives as triggers, elicits symptoms only in a portion of those who respond to diet. This observation suggests that healing may be initiated by a diet that avoids known triggers for a limited period of time. The justification for a low-pseudoallergenic diet is supported by observations in patients with chronic urticaria (an intensely itching rash with welts and swelling): especially those patients whose gastroduodenal permeability profits from diet. The permeability of the gastric mucosa normalizes in patients who profit from the diet over 3-4 weeks [9]. Food-additive intolerance occurs less often than supposed by patients, and, contrary to the lay and news media perception, food-additive intolerance occurs more often in children and adults with pre-existing disease such as atopic dermatitis or asthma. In such patients, atopic dermatitis, chronic urticaria, rhinitis and asthma may be aggravated. They rarely induce GI symptoms, headache, or mood change, but occasionally they cause life-threatening anaphylactic reactions. In the latter situation, an IgE-mediated mechanism is at work. Some foods and food additives can precipitate an attack of a vascular headache, particularly pharmacologic agents present in foods, such as tyramine, phenylethylamine, histamine, ethyl alcohol, nitrates and monosodium glutamate.

27.2 Current recommendations

Medical history is essential in every field of medicine because it allows us to obtain all the information and data that can help to move towards the diagnosis of a certain disease. It comprises the physiological, family (investigating all possible genetic risk factors or any family predisposition) and the past and current medical history. The latter investigates the disorder for which the patient consulted a doctor. In suspected FA, repeated clinical manifestations related to the ingestion of given meals are highly indicative. Medical history should be addressed to establish: (a) the presence or absence of similar symptoms in other people when they consumed the same food(s); (b) the ingested food(s) in the 2-4 hours before the onset of symptoms; (c) the allergens that may contaminate food preparation (for example, casein, latex, ovomucoid); (d) the cooking and storage of food; (e) the presence of triggering factors; (f) the existence of other allergies (such as respiratory or skin allergy) or other diseases.

Skin prick test (SPT) is a well-standardized, simple, cheap and low-risk diagnostic test. It should be the first step performed and both inhalant and food allergens should be tested. *Prick + prick* (P + P) is performed with fresh food, in particular vegetables, when the commercial extract is negative (or unavailable) but the clinical history is suggestive. When the food is solid, the technique involves firstly puncturing the fresh food (some allergens are located just under the skin of the fruit) and then the patient's skin with a lancet according to the SPT standard procedure. The assay of specific IgE (sIgE) for food extracts is a second-level test in the view of costs. Thus, it should be requested only after SPT. However, it may still be exceptionally considered as a first-level test in those conditions in which a SPT cannot be performed (e.g., very young pediatric patients, concomitant antihistamine therapy or skin alterations, risk of systemic reactions). Diagnostics based on allergenic extracts allow the identification of the allergen source (e.g., fish, egg, milk, etc.) but not the molecular component to which a patient is sensitized, which can be studied instead through *in vitro* allergenic molecules (Molecular-Based Diagnosis, MBD) and therefore used to improve the result of a sIgE test. *In vitro* MBD uses molecular allergens isolated from a given allergen source (purified or native allergens) or produced by recombinant DNA technology (recombinant allergens) (Tables 27.1 and 27.2). This approach improves the description of the IgE repertoire against food allergens or their molecular components and explains cross-reactions and their role in FA [10]. Oral food challenges are usually required to confirm the diagnosis of a FA, to monitor a FA, or to prove oral tolerance to a given food. Oral food challenges can be performed in an open or blind manner. Blinded challenges can be single or double-blind. In many cases, an open OFC with an objective and unequivocal reaction is sufficient for the diagnosis of FA. The DBPCFC is considered the gold standard diagnostic test for the diagnosis of a FA. Immediate reactions usually appear within 2 hours after the last food intake, atopic eczema may worsen several hours or days following an oral challenge. Urticaria and angioedema are the most common objective signs, and GI, respiratory or cardiovascular system involvement is also common. To optimize safety, vital signs should be closely monitored during OFC, while equipment and appropriately trained staff should be in place to deal with allergic reactions – including anaphylaxis. For patients with non-IgE-mediated reactions, challenges tailored to the individual modalities of reactions should be designed [1].

Recently the Italian Society of Allergy, Asthma and Clinical Immunology (SIAAIC) supported the "Doing more does not mean doing better" campaign and made a list of the 5 allergological procedures with the highest evidence of inappropriateness. In order to improve a clinical algorithm for the diagnosis and treatment of FA, the SIAAIC suggest not to perform aller-

Table 27.1 Major food allergens and components available for molecular diagnostics using ImmunoCAP (or ImmunoCAP ISAC)*

Allergens (or allergen source)	*Protein family*
Cupin superfamily	
Vicilins	Ara h 1 (peanut)
Legumins	Ara h 3 (peanut), Cor 9 (hazelnut)
Prolamin superfamily	
2S albumin	Ber e 1 (Brazil nut), Ara h 2 (peanut), Gly m 6
Lipid transfer protein (LTP) 3	Pru p 3 (peach), Cor 8 (hazelnut), Art v 3 (Composite) Jug r (walnut)
Cereal prolamines	Tri 19 (wheat) Tri a 14
Pathogenesis-related (PR) proteins	
PR10: intracellular proteins	Pru p 1 (peach), Api g 1 (celery), Gly m 4 (soy)
PR3: chitinase Class 1	Hev b 11, Hev b 2.6 (latex, banana, avocado)
Profilins	Pru p 4 (peach) (Bet v 2, Phl p 12, Hev b 8), MUXF3 (celery, tomato)
Cross-reactive carbohydrate determinants	
Tropomyosins	Pen a 1 (shrimp)
Calcium binding proteins	
Parvalbumin	Gad c 1 (codfish)
Milk proteins	Bos d 4 (α-albumin), Bos d 5 (β-lactoglobulin), Bos d 8 (casein), Bos d lactoferrin (lactoferrin)
Egg protein	Gal d 1 (ovomucoid) Gal d 2 (ovalbumin) Gal d 3 (conalbumin) Gal d 4 (lysozyme)

* Adapted from [10].

Table 27.2 Families of protein carbohydrate molecules mainly involved in food allergy*

Molecules associated with allergy to food source (or source allergen)
PR-10 proteins (homologous to Bet v 1)
Non-specific lipid transfer proteins (nsLTP)
Profilins
Storage proteins
Thaumatin-like-proteins (TLP)
Cross-reactive carbohydrate determinants (CCD)
Molecules associated with allergy to food of animal origin
Tropomyosins
Parvalbumins
Caseins
Lipocalin, family of lysozyme, transferrin family, ovomucoids

* Adapted from [10].

gy tests for drugs (including anesthetics) and/or foods when neither clinical history nor symptoms suggestive of hypersensitivity reactions are present.

Performing the so-called "food intolerance tests" is also not appropriate, apart from those which are validated for suspect celiac disease and lactose enzymatic intolerance. Several assays and techniques are constantly proposed to many patients to identify supposed food intolerance. These methods include, for example, VEGA-test, Cytotoxic test, serum specific

IgG4 dosage, chemical analysis of hair, applied kinesiology, iridology and "bioresonance" analysis. None of these methods have reached sufficient evidence of efficacy, accuracy and repeatability in diagnosing food allergy/intolerance. The third recommendation by the SIAAIC was not to perform serological allergy tests (i.e., total IgE, specific IgE, component-resolved diagnosis) as first-line tests or as "screening" of inhalants and food immediate hypersensitivity assays. Cutaneous allergometric tests, if possible, should be considered as the first diagnostic tests in cases of consistent clinical history and symptoms with a suspect allergic reaction, as they provide faster results, are less invasive and are cheaper than serological tests. Moreover, there is moderate evidence that, at least for food allergies, those skin tests have at least the same diagnostic accuracy of serological tests [11]. Due to the lack of standardized test substances and the lack of studies showing advantages of an atopy patch test (APT) over SPT or sIgE, APTs are not recommended for FA routine diagnosis [1]. Moreover, regarding FA, given the limitation of cutaneous and serological tests, oral food challenges (ideally DBPCFC) are still the gold standard in IgE and non-IgE-mediated FA in order to establish a firm diagnosis, to determine threshold reactivity, and to assess tolerance and response to immuno-modulation [11].

27.3 Gastrointestinal non-IgE-mediated symptoms

Infants in the first year of life may present GI food-related clinical manifestations such as Food Protein Induced Enterocolitis Syndrome (FPIES), proctocolitis and enteropathy. Usually, patients have negative food sIgE testing. The diagnosis is based on symptoms, clinical history, an elimination diet for up to 3 weeks, and specifically designed OFCs. Endoscopy with biopsies might be helpful confirming bowel inflammation. Currently, there is scarce evidence that APT is helpful in diagnosing a FA in such types of patients. Eosinophilic esophagitis is defined as a chronic, immune/antigen-mediated esophageal disease, clinically characterized by symptomatic esophageal disfunction and histologically by eosinophil-predominant inflammation. All age groups can be affected, and the current estimated prevalence is around one in 24,000 adults. Adult patients mostly present dysphagia, less frequently retrosternal pain and food bolus impaction, whereas the symptom presentation in children is much more variable and includes failure to thrive, vomiting, regurgitation, thoracic and abdominal pain. Eosinophilic esophagitis is diagnosed by an upper endoscopy and biopsies. Biopsies should be performed when the patient has been treated for at least 6 weeks with double the standard dose proton-pump inhibitors to rule out esophageal eosinophilia caused by GastroEsophageal Reflux Disease (GERD) and to exclude proton-pump inhibitor-responsive [1].

27.3.1 Lactose intolerance

Lactose intolerance is common, as most of the world population is lactase deficient. Treatment involves limiting the intake of fresh milk to an individually tolerated level. Cheese and fermented milk products, e.g., yogurt, are usually well tolerated. Lactase is commercially available and can be used by lactase-deficient individuals who wish to drink milk.

27.4 Pregnancy and breastfeeding

The development of allergic disease is shaped by genetics and the environment, including diet. Many studies suggest a role for maternal diet during pregnancy. The combination of in utero exposures and genetic predisposition may contribute to the development of allergic disease by altering immune and organ development. Inflammation predominates in the first and third trimesters, whereas the second trimester is characterized by anti-inflammatory and Th2 immune responses. Maternal dietary exposures during pregnancy may interact with inherited genetic risk factors that may influence the immune system development. Epidemiological studies have reported that high maternal dietary vitamin D intake during pregnancy is associated with a reduced risk of asthma and recurrent wheeze in children. Similarly, a meta-analysis showed that higher maternal vitamin E intake was associated with reduced childhood wheeze and the antioxidant properties of vitamin C are also thought to underline its main effects. An Australian cohort study found that higher maternal vitamin C intake was associated with a reduced risk of infant wheeze. Because supplemental folic acid during pregnancy reduces the risk of fetal neural tube defects, the US Department of Health recommends that pregnant women consume 400 µg of folic acid daily. Many found no significant association between maternal intake of folic acid and childhood wheeze, allergic rhinitis and eczema. In one prospective study of 2,640 pregnant mothers, maternal folic acid supplementation was not associated with an increased risk of wheeze, lung function, asthma or related atopic outcomes in children, but there was a dose-dependent trend towards decreased asthma risk at age 6 to 7 years with higher intracellular folic acid levels in pregnancy. Omega-3 PolyUnsaturated Fatty Acids (PUFAs) are thought to exert anti-inflammatory effects, with several studies reporting that they decrease Th2 cell responses and increase Th1 cell and Treg cell responses. More recent randomized controlled trials, though, support that omega-3 supplementation during the second and/or third trimester may decrease child risk of atopic disease and allergic disease/respiratory symptoms. Although some studies have reported no association between an inclusion of allergenic food in prenatal maternal diets and the development of atopic disease, other studies provide contrasting results. In some studies, maternal intake of specific foods was found to be associated with an increased risk of allergic sensitization and FA in children [12]. Finally, in a robust meta-analysis based on studies and extracted data, the assessed risk of bias and Grading of Recommendations Assessment, Development and Evaluation (GRADE) was used to assess certainty of the findings. Publication studies were searched across Medical Literature Analysis and Retrieval System Online (MEDLINE), Excerpta Medica dataBASE (EMBASE), Web of Science, Central Register of Controlled Trials (CENTRAL), and Literatura Latino-Americana e do Caribe em Ciências da Saúde (LILACS) between January 1946 and July 2013. The authors reported a mother's diet during pregnancy and lactation may influence the risk that her child develops an allergic disease, and this has implications for future research in this field. There are two specific implications for pregnant women. First, a daily probiotic supplement such as Lactobacillus rhamnosus, taken from around 36 to 38 weeks gestation through the first 3 to 6 months of lactation, may reduce the risk of eczema in the child. Although probiotics are generally considered safe, their pro-inflammatory effects may have potential adverse consequences when used earlier in pregnancy, and serious adverse effects in people with intestinal disorders or immune deficiency have been documented. Second, a fish oil supplement, taken from around 20 weeks gestation through the first 3 to 4 months of lactation, may reduce the risk of allergic sensitization to egg or peanut in the child [13]. Given the heterogeneous results, from studies of prenatal diet and childhood allergic disease thus far, current guidelines and practice parameters do not advise avoidance diets or the additional supplementation of specific nutrients during the prenatal period for the prevention of atopic disease. This is due to the lack of conclusive and consistent evidence on whether such interventions are effective. Thus, an important role of clinical allergists is to help expectant parents be informed about the available evidence and their limitations [12].

27.5 Weaning: present evidence

Of the many possible hypotheses that explain the recent increase in childhood FA, the dual-allergen exposure hypothesis has been the most extensively investigated. This chapter serves as a review and an update on the prevention of FA and focuses on recently published Randomized Controlled Trials (RCTs) exploring the efficacy of oral tolerance induction in infancy for the prevention of FA. As a result of these RCTs, the US National Institute of Health recommendations now actively encourage the early introduction of peanuts for the prevention of a peanut allergy, and other countries/settings recommend the inclusion of potential common food allergens, including peanuts and eggs, in complementary feeding regimens starting at approximately 6 months but not before 4 months of age. Further studies are required that explore the efficacy of oral tolerance induction to other common food allergens and that focus on optimal timing, duration and adherence [12].

A recent meta-analysis found that early feeding with egg and peanut, but not other potentially allergenic foods, led to a significant reduction in egg and peanut allergy. A careful review of the egg prevention RCTs suggests that cooked egg products might be safer and better tolerated than raw egg products, although more definitive evidence would be helpful. Based on this data, allergy societies outside of North America have endorsed early feeding of cooked eggs. There is concern that medicalizing infant feeding practices is unnecessary and that no data exists to support the delayed introduction of certain foods. Perhaps the best recommendation might be the common-sense approach suggested by the Australasian Society of Clinical Immunology and Allergy (ASCIA): which states, "When your infant is ready, introduce foods according to what the family eats, regardless of whether the food is considered to be a common food allergen" [13].

REFERENCES

1. Muraro A, Werfel T, Hoffmann-Sommergruber K, Roberts G, Beyer K, Bindslev-Jensen C, Cardona V, Dubois A, duToit G, Eigenmann P, Fernandez Rivas M, Halken S, Hickstein L, Høst A, Knol E, Lack G, Marchisotto MJ, Niggemann B, Nwaru BI, Papadopoulos NG, Poulsen LK, Santos AF, Skypala I, Schoepfer A, Van Ree R, Venter C, Worm M, Vlieg-Boerstra B, Panesar S, de Silva D, Soares-Weiser K, Sheikh A, Ballmer-Weber BK, Nilsson C, de Jong NW, Akdis CA; EAACI Food Allergy and Anaphylaxis Guidelines Group. EAACI food allergy and anaphylaxis guidelines: diagnosis and management of food allergy. Allergy 2014; 69(8): 1008-25.
2. Waserman S, Watson W. Food allergy. Allergy Asthma Clin Immunol 2011; 7 Suppl 1(Suppl 1): S7.
3. Wang YH. Developing food allergy: a potential immunologic pathway linking skin barrier to gut. F1000Res 2016; 5.
4. Food Allergy and Anaphylaxis Guidelines. EAACI 2014.
5. Iweala OI, Burks AW. Food Allergy: Our Evolving Understanding of Its Pathogenesis, Prevention, and Treatment. Curr Allergy Asthma Rep 2016; 16(5): 37.
6. Finding a Path to Safety in Food Allergy: Assessment of the Global Burden, Causes, Prevention, Management, and Public Policy (2016).
7. Popescu FD. Cross-reactivity between aeroallergens and food allergens. World J Methodol 2015; 5(2): 31-50.
8. Pravettoni V, Incorvaia C. Diagnosis of exercise-induced anaphylaxis: current insights. J Asthma Allergy 2016; 9: 191-8.
9. Reese I, Zuberbier T, Bunselmeyer B, Erdmann S, Henzgen M, Fuchs T, Jäger L, Kleine-Tebbe J, Lepp U, Niggemann B, Raithel M, Saloga J, Vieths S, Werfel T. Diagnostic approach for suspected pseudoallergic reaction to food ingredients. J Dtsch Dermatol Ges 2009; 7(1): 70-7.
10. Macchia D, Melioli G, Pravettoni V, Nucera E, Piantanida M, Caminati M, Campochiaro C, Yacoub MR, Schiavino D, Paganelli R, Di Gioacchino M; Food Allergy Study Group (ATI) of the Italian Society of Allergy, Asthma and Clinical Immunology (SIAAIC). Guidelines for the use and interpretation of diagnostic methods in adult food allergy. Clin Mol Allergy 2015; 13: 27.
11. Heffler E, Landi M, Quadrino S, Incorvaia C, Pizzimenti S, Vernero S, Crimi N, Rolla G, Canonica GW. Choosing wisely in Allergology: a Slow Medicine approach to the discipline promoted by the Italian Society of Allergy, Asthma and Clinical Immunology (SIAAIC). Clin Mol Allergy 2015; 13: 28.
12. Du Toit G, Sampson HA, Plaut M, Burks AW, Akdis CA, Lack G. Food allergy: Update on prevention and tolerance. J Allergy Clin Immunol 2018; 141(1): 30-40.
13. Bird JA, Parrish C, Patel K, Shih JA, Vickery BP. Prevention of food allergy: Beyond peanut. J Allergy Clin Immunol 2019; 143(2): 545-7.

28

Food and veins

Luca Revelli, Carmen Gravina and Angelo Santoliquido

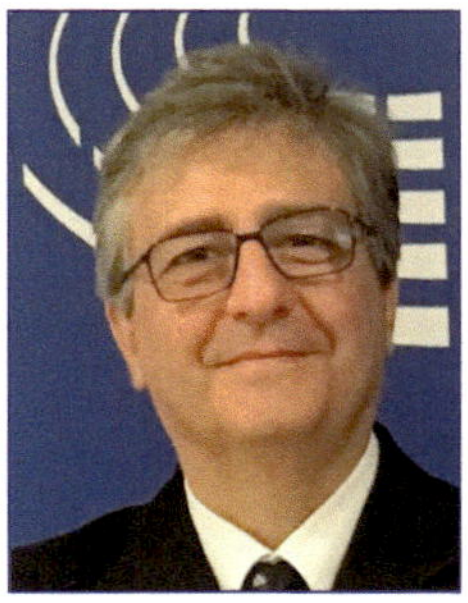

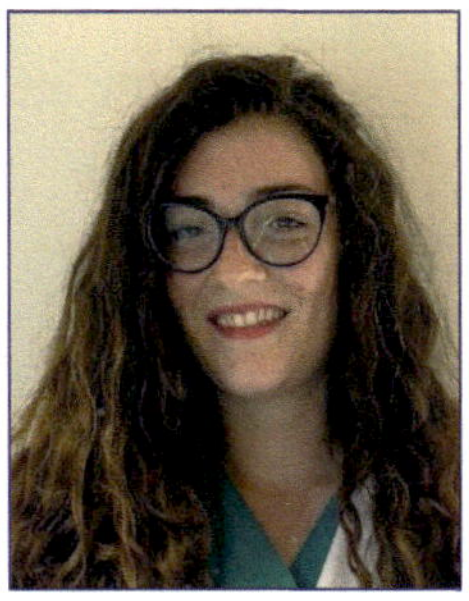

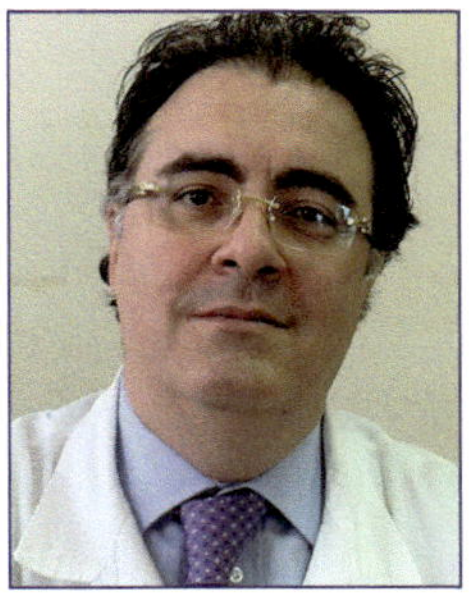

Lifestyle and **dietary habits** can improve venous tone and capillary permeability, especially in the lower limbs. Substances contained in some fruits and plants – through more sophisticated mechanisms – act on leukocytes and endothelium to modify the degree of venous inflammation, reducing edema and other symptoms related to **Chronic Venous Insufficiency (CVI)** such as heaviness, swelling, tingling and pain.

Good nutrition can help reduce the chances of developing varicose veins due to the protective effect of various substances contained in fruit and vegetables (molecules of the large family of **bioflavonoids**), **medicinal herb** (Centella Asiatica), **officinal plants** (Gingko Biloba), **micronutrients** such as **vitamins** (vitamin C, E, B6, and B12) and **minerals** (copper, magnesium and sodium), **proteins** of some type of meat and **fibers** [1].

An important role is played by the control of the **body weight** and an **adequate hydration** of the organism [2].

A CVI of the lower limb refers to a wide spectrum of disorders caused by damage to valves and vein walls. This leads to venous dilatation and the formation of twisted and swollen veins, visible under the surface of the skin [3].

The **mechanism of varicose vein formation** is complex. It is, however, based on blood stasis, hypoxia, inflammation, Reactive Oxygen Species (ROS) generation and oxidative stress. Damages to the capillary endothelium lead to the accumulation of fluids, proteins and red blood cells into the interstitial space, forming capillary edema and inflammation.

The importance of CVI is related to the number of people affected and the **socioeconomic impact** of its more severe manifestations. It represents one of the biggest strains on the national health services of European and North American countries and CVI is a major and worldwide socioeconomic burden. In Western Europe, 2% of the annual healthcare budget is spent on chronic venous conditions [4]. Moreover, CVI is a common problem, affecting up to 50% of the population in industrialized countries.

The incidence and prevalence of deep and superficial venous disease depend on the age and gender of the population, but – at any age – such disease is more common in women than in men. In younger men, the incidence is lower than 10%,

Luca Revelli, MD
Professor, Fondazione Policlinico Universitario A. Gemelli IRCCS,
Università Cattolica del Sacro Cuore, Rome, Italy

Email: luca.revelli@unicatt.it

Carmen Gravina, MD
Fondazione Policlinico Universitario A. Gemelli IRCCS,
Università Cattolica del Sacro Cuore, Rome, Italy

Angelo Santoliquido, MD
Professor, Fondazione Policlinico Universitario A. Gemelli IRCCS,
Università Cattolica del Sacro Cuore, Rome, Italy

Table 28.1 Risk factors for chronic venous insufficiency (CVI)

Non-modifiable risk factors
- advanced age
- family history of venous disease
- hereditary conditions
- female sex
- prior venous thrombosis
- pregnancies
- high estrogenic states
- ligamentous laxity

Modifiable risk factors
- smoking
- sedentary life
- low antioxidant food diet
- prolonged standing or sitting
- increased Body Mass Index (BMI)

compared with 30% in similarly aged women. In men older than 50 years, the incidence is 20%, compared with 50% in similarly aged women [5]. Peak incidence occurs in women aged 40-49 years and in men aged 70-79 years. This condition can be asymptomatic. Reticular veins usually appear or are first noticed in adolescence and young adulthood, with only a small number of new cases developing after a pregnancy.

More working hours are lost as a result of venous disorders than arterial disease. Varicose veins are a common condition found in "**standing workers**", people who stand for prolonged periods. It can be considered a work-related illness in various occupations such as: **cooks** (working in a warm and humid environment); ironers (also called pressers), barbers and hairdressers (warm and dry); surgeons, nurses in operating theater (cold and dry) and also salesmen, assembly line workers, waiters, room attendants and housewives [7]. It is also commonly found in pregnant women due to hormone influences.

Table 28.1 shows the risk factors for developing CVI classified into non-modifiable and modifiable risk factors.

Chronic Venous Insufficiency is a common disease with different **clinical signs** from spider veins, through varicose veins, to venous ulceration [5]. In particular, when the valves become incompetent, they allow retrograde blood flow with high hydrostatic pressure which progressively leads to reflux and chronic hypertension in the veins. This can lead to remodeling of the venous walls, the appearance of varicose veins and further complications linked to the progression of venous disease. Venous hypertension and changes in the hemodynamics of the superficial veins are internally transmitted into the microcirculation causing an increase of the venous pressure and capillary permeability [8].

Truncal varicosities and telangiectasias, on the other hand, are relatively less common in youth and can appear throughout life. Patients affected by CVI can also suffers with leg heaviness, aching or tingling, ankle swelling, dry skin, tightness, skin irritation, heaviness, muscle cramps (usually overnight), itching, lipodermatosclerosis, telangiectasias up to varicose veins and venous ulcerations. Disease progression and increasing severity of symptoms appear to be related to the extent of venous valvular incompetence [8].

The manifestations of CVI can be viewed in terms of a **clinical classification** scheme. The Clinical, Etiology, Anatomic, Pathophysiology (**CEAP**) classification was developed by an International Consensus Conference to provide a basis of uniformity in reporting, diagnosing and treating CVI. The CEAP clinical classification has 7 categories (0-6) and is further categorized by the presence or absence of symptoms [9].

The **diagnosis** of CVI is suggested by the presence of typical symptoms (leg pain, fatigue, heaviness) and confirmed by the presence of venous reflux, which is diagnosed on a duplex ultrasound by the duration of retrograde or reversed flow (> 500 m/s for superficial or perforating veins, > 1000 m/s for deep veins). However, visibly dilated superficial veins, in conjunction with typical symptoms, suggest CVI.

Treatment of CVI aims to both improve venous function and improve signs and symptoms of CVI. Management should also address the progressive nature of CVI and act as a prophylaxis against aggravation and progression [7]. Treatment comprises both conservative and invasive therapeutic options. Conservative treatments include an increase of physical activity or sports, compression treatment and pharmacological therapy. Invasive treatments include surgery of superficial and deep veins, such as percutaneous phlebectomy with hooks and stripping techniques. New less-invasive treatment options include foam sclerotherapy, endovenous thermal ablation and radiofrequency ablation techniques.

28.1 Lifestyle, nutrition and weight control

An important role in the management of CVI is played by **lifestyle** and **nutrition**. Many pieces of evidence show how some bioactive compounds – present in many foods and beverages – have a **veno-active action** and may help reduce venous wall inflammation, edema, development of skin changes and help with the healing of ulcers. A healthy lifestyle such as maintaining an ideal **body weight** (or weight reduction if overweight) may improve manifestations of CVI.

Obesity is a well-established risk factor for the development of CVI and its complications. Weight reduction after bariatric surgery has been shown to improve manifestations of CVI, including edema and ulcers. It may be extrapolated that weight reduction – by other means – might also assist in the treatment of CVI.

Flavonoids are a group of natural substances, with variable phenolic structures, that are found – among others – in fruits, vegetables, buckwheat, legumes, tea, wine, beer, young pepper, chocolate, cocoa and olive oil [10].

They act as dyes, antioxidants and natural fungicides. Flavonoids are plant pigments responsible for color in the flowers' petals designed to attract pollinating animals. In higher plants, flavonoids are involved in ultraviolet (UV) absorption and act as chemical messengers, physiological regulators and cell cycle inhibitors.

These natural products are considered an indispensable component in a variety of nutraceutical, pharmaceutical, medicinal and cosmetic applications. The beneficial effect of flavonoids is connected with their absorption and bioavailability; antioxidant properties (free radical scavenging, and reaction with other reactive oxygen species); support of cellular antioxidants and antioxidant enzymes; transition metals chelation; ability of distribution in cells, tissues and extracellular fluids; effects on gene expression, DNA repair activity, tissue repair and regeneration.

Flavonoids are mainly water-soluble and usually are present as glycosides in plants. They are also known to be inhibitors for several enzymes, such as Xanthine Oxidase (XO), Cyclo-Oxygenase (COX), lipoxygenase and phosphoinositide 3-kinase.

More than 4,000 flavonoids are currently known. The term is completely interchangeable with **bioflavonoids** (the name by which these nutrients are commonly known). Sometimes they are grouped under the name **vitamin P**. Flavonoids, and in particular **Rutin** and **Quercetin**, which are mostly associated with venous benefits, are found in green tea, grape seeds, red pepper, apples, citrus fruits, berries and peaches.

Rutin assumption for management of symptoms associated to CVI is strongly recommended based on a grade A evidence. Many properties can be attributed to this compound. The most important is the capability to allow the physiological permeability of capillaries, thus avoiding edema formation. This is why it is also called "Vitamin P". Rutin can also stimulate vessel wall trophism and elasticity, improving circulation. It can be useful in reducing bad circulation symptoms, like edema and itching. Many studies have shown Rutin's antioxidant properties, being able to protect cells from oxidative stress. It also has antiplatelet and antithrombotic properties. **Quercetin** has very important antioxidant properties that allow it to prevent radical free damages, lipoproteins oxidation and tissue inflammation and aging. It can be used to prevent leg swelling and pain. Its use is based on a grade B evidence [11].

Aescin is the major active principle from the horse chestnut tree seed (*Aesculus hippocastanum*). It has shown satisfactory evidence for clinically significant activity in CVI. The therapeutic benefit is well supported by a number of experimental studies, indicative of anti-edematous, anti-inflammatory and venotonic properties, mainly related to the molecular mechanism of the agent, allowing improved entry of ions into channels, thus raising venous tension *in vitro* and *in vivo* conditions. Venotonic properties may be also attributable to decreased vascular permeability. Other mechanisms, like the release of PGF2 from veins, antagonism to 5-HT (serotonin) and histamine, reduced catabolism of tissue mucopolysaccharides, further underline the wide-ranging mechanisms of the therapeutic activity of aescin [12].

Anthocyanins (ACs) are a group of flavonoids, which are present in various fruits, vegetables and beverages, and are commonly consumed in the human diet. Anthocyanins are water-soluble vacuolar pigments: red, purple or blue, with the color depending on the pH value. The largest quantity of anthocyanins can be found in red cabbage, aronia berries, aubergine, black raspberry and wild blueberry. They are present also in bilberry, chokeberry, raspberry, black rice, cranberry, elderberry, black soybean, strawberry and other plants. Anthocyanin are a group of flavonoids with antioxidants properties and have antithrombotic action by inhibiting platelet activation and thrombus growth. They are vital in the control of angiogenesis, inflammation, platelet aggregation and vascular remodeling [13].

Pro-anthocyanidins (also called **tannins**) are the grape constituents, responsible for part of the organoleptic properties of grapes and wines. They can also be found in many plants such as green and black tea, cocoa beans, cinnamon, aronia berries, grape seed, grape skin (pro-cyanidins and pro-delphinidins), bilberry, cranberry and black currant. Pro-anthocyanidins are oligomeric flavonoids containing catechin and epicatechin and their gallic acid esters (dimer and trimer polymerizations of catechins). These compounds have a broad spectrum of therapeutic properties and can be used in the treatment of many diseases such as atherosclerosis, cataracts, diabetes, gingivitis (periodontal disease), macular degeneration, night blindness, retinopathy and varicose veins.

28.2 Medicinal herbs

Centella Asiatica (or *Hydrocotyle asiatica*) is a herb that has received substantial attention for improving signs and symptoms of CVI. It is a perennial herb plant native to India and Madagascar that grows in wet and shady places, typically along the waterways. It has purple flowers, and its active compounds are found in the leaves.

It is also known as the "tiger herb" because tigers are said to use it to heal wounds. Centella leaves are rich in triterpene saponins (asiaticoside, asiatic acid and madecassoside) which improve venous circulation by stimulating fibroblasts. These cells synthesize collagen, essential for the health of different tissues, such as the dermis, the connective tissue and the walls of the vessels. Several clinical trials have shown significantly greater improvement while using centella, compared to the control group, in treating the signs and symptoms of CVI (especially leg heaviness, pain and edema).

Centella is useful for preventing and treating venous insufficiency and therefore swelling and heaviness in the legs and ankles that derive from it, but also pain in the veins, night cramps and hemorrhoids. It is also useful in case of highlighted capillaries. After a first treatment it is possible to carry out maintenance cycles that help prevent a new weakening of the blood vessels. In addition, the centella extract is also able to accelerate the healing of sores, skin lesions and first and second degree burns.

28.3 Officinal plants

Ginkgo biloba, also known as the "maidenhair tree", is the only living species in the division Ginkgophyta: all others being extinct. It is found in fossils dating back 270 million years. Native to China, the tree is widely cultivated. It has various uses in traditional medicine and as a source of food. Ginkgo biloba leaves contain terpenes, (ginkgolide B) which block the lipid peroxidation, implicated in platelet aggregation. These active ingredients, in fact, inhibit the platelet activation factor (PAF), preventing the formation of thrombi in the blood vessels and decreasing capillary permeability, improving tissue spraying.

Polyphenols and flavonoids (ginketol, isiginketol, bilabetol, ginkolide) act on cell membranes, stabilizing them and contrasting the formation of free radicals. Particularly known for its activity on venous, arterial and capillary circulation, the plant is also widely used as a blood thinner, because it decreases its viscosity, in the prevention of thrombo-embolic diseases.

Because of its ability to promote correct distribution of oxygen and glucose to the brain, ginkgo biloba increases mental acuity, concentration, short-term memory, and cognitive faculties. For these reasons it is particularly suitable for students. Numerous research studies have also shown that the use of ginkgo counteracts the phenomena of atherosclerosis in the elderly and slows the progression of Alzheimer's disease.

Its active principles also make it a powerful remedy for allergies: it is a vasodilator of the arteries, while it has a vasoconstrictor action in the veins; therefore, it is recommended in asthma attacks. Furthermore, favoring more efficient peripheral circulation, it is recommended in the treatment of chilblains at the extremities due to the cold; and it is also used in cases of tinnitus, dizziness, intermittent pain in legs and headache.

The vasoprotective property of ginkgo biloba is given by the ability to improve the tone and elasticity of the walls of veins, arteries and capillaries, and therefore it is recommended for the treatment of neuropathies caused by diabetes, in macular degeneration of the retina and other circulatory problems, such as hemorrhoids, varices and capillary fragility. Finally, ginkgo biloba is considered a free radical scavenger. This feature makes it an excellent antioxidant, because it activates cellular metabolism and above all protects the nervous system from damage caused by free radicals (anti-aging effect).

28.4 Micronutrients and veins

28.4.1 Vitamins

Vitamin C helps the body make the connective tissues collagen and elastin, which the body uses to repair and maintain veins, keeping them flexible and strong. Top sources of vitamin C are oranges, guava, kiwi, sweet red and green peppers, grapefruit and vegetable juice, strawberries, cantaloupe and Brussels sprouts.

Vitamin E keeps platelets from sticking together and adhering to the sides of blood vessel walls. This prevents blood from clotting. Load up on vitamin E by adding to the diet: wheat germ, corn, nuts, seeds, olives, asparagus, and spinach or other green leafy vegetables.

Vitamins B6 and B12 help clear the blood of homocysteine, which has been linked to recurring blood clots.

B6 sources are primarily meats, poultry and fish (including tuna and cod), calf liver, beef, chicken, turkey, venison and halibut. B6 is also found in potatoes and sunflower seeds.

B12-rich foods are mostly meat, fish and dairy products. Top choices are clams, oysters, crabs, salmon, rainbow trout, herring, beef, chicken, turkey and fortified cereals.

28.4.2 Minerals

Copper is an oligoelement essential in building, repairing and maintaining endothelial cells. It helps the organism knit together collagen and elastin and is believed to help protect blood vessels against microscopic tears and rough spots that can lead to blood clots and plaque-filled veins. It is found in all body tissues and plays a role in making red blood cells and maintaining nerve and immune system cells. It also helps absorb iron and plays a role in energy production. It has venotonic properties. Copper is found in shellfish, lean red meat, calf liver, sesame seeds, cashews, sunflower seeds, barley, tempeh, soybeans, garbanzo beans, lentils and lima beans.

28.5 Fibers

Fibers help to prevent constipation which is a risk factor for increased abdominal pressure which reduces the flow of blood back from legs, weakening vein walls over time. The strain of moving the bowels can put pressure on the veins, particularly veins located in the lower legs. Since these veins already have to work against the forces of gravity to pump blood back up to the heart, the additional pressure may be enough to create varicosities in some of the lower leg veins.

Fiber-rich foods include beans, whole grains, brown rice, popcorn, nuts, baked potatoes (leaving the skin on), bran cereal, oatmeal, berries and crisp vegetables. Large population studies have confirmed this link between varicose veins and fiber-rich diets. Cultures that tend to eat less fiber (Western countries) also have a higher prevalence of varicose veins. However, further studies are needed to determine if additional fiber alone is effective in preventing varicose veins. At this time, it appears appropriate to recommend a high-fiber diet as one component in lowering the risk for CVI.

28.6 Meat proteins

Meat proteins may have a protective role on the blood vessel wall. According to a recent observational study by the University of Chang Mai (Thailand) patients who had regularly consumed chicken, but not other meat (beef, pork, fish and egg), had a lower risk of venous disease than those patients who sometimes or never consumed chicken [12]. The part it plays is probably due to vitamin B6 and B12 contained in chicken which can help to treat (and prevent) venous disease by strengthening blood vessel walls. This data is controversial: other studies have shown that chicken intake may cause varicose veins.

28.7 Hydration

It is strongly recommended to drink enough water to stay well hydrated and to have a healthy and varied diet that includes high-fiber foods (fruits and vegetables) to avoid constipation. Constipation is proven to promote hemorrhoidal outbreak, increasing intra-abdominal pressure (during bowel evacuation) and lower limb venous pressure.

Drinking plenty of water helps to improve vein health in two ways: improving the overall circulation of the blood by thinning it and strengthening the muscles that support veins. Both poor blood circulation and blood clots can cause a number of painful problems such as varicose veins or deep vein thrombosis (DVT).

Avoiding dehydration by staying properly hydrated will also improve the strength of the muscles that support lower limb veins. These vessels rely upon strong muscles to provide additional support when they encounter high pressure from the blood that circulates throughout the body. If the muscles are not strong enough to provide support to the veins when faced with high pressure, the veins will start to weaken and collapse. If left weakened and collapsed, it is possible to experience vein disease.

The amount of water to drink on a daily basis varies from person-to-person (including individual variables such as BMI, environment and type of activity). In order to stay properly hydrated, it is recommended that everyone aim to try and drink at least 8 ounces (250 mL) of water every two hours. This recommendation is given because it is easy to remember and it keeps almost everyone properly hydrated. Since 350 mL of metabolic water is produced daily in the body, it is necessary to introduce 2400 mL of water per day: 1200-1500 mL through food; the rest with drinks between meals. Drinking during meals means diluting the active compounds of foods and reducing their effectiveness; but it also means diluting the gastric juices, making them less effective in the digestive process.

Many foods contain important quantities of water. Vegetables contain amounts of water from 78% in potatoes to 96.5% in cucumbers. Fruit contain from 80% water in grapes to 95.3% in watermelon. Even bananas contain 76% of water. Fish and shellfish contain from 61.5% of water in tuna and river eel to 85.7% in oysters. The water contained in fresh fruit and vegetables is a very pure, biological water, free from impurities, filtered by the metabolic processes of the plant. A water that no aqueduct – and that perhaps not even the purest of sources – could guarantee [14].

REFERENCES

1. Melet JJ. The importance of nutrition among the risk factors in varicose veins. Phlebologie 1981; 34(3): 469-88. [Article in French]
2. Kulprachakarn K, Abkom P, Pongtam O, Ounjaijean S, Thongkham P, Saengyo S, Rerkasem K. Higher Level of Chicken Consumption Associated With Less Severe Venous Disease. Int J Low Extrem Wounds 2017; 16(4): 251-4.
3. Revelli L, Santoliquido A, Tinelli G. Anatomia delle vene degli arti inferiori. In Mandolesi S: Flebologia Emodinamica, SEU, Roma 2010.
4. Bozkurt K, Rabe E, Sharkawy MI. Chronic venous insufficiency: management and treatment. Eur Med J 2017; 5[Suppl 2]: 2-13.
5. Robertson L, Evans C, Fowkes FG. Epidemiology of chronic venous disease. Phlebology 2008; 23(3): 103-11.
6. Revelli L, Mandolesi D, Stammegna I, Flore R, Mandolesi S, Lombardi CP, Santoliquido A. Lifestyle, environment and risk factors for varicose veins in Italian chef de cuisine. G Ital Med Lav Erg 2017: 39: 4, suppl.
7. Lichota A, Gwozdzinski L, Gwozdzinski K. Therapeutic potential of natural compounds in inflammation and chronic venous insufficiency. Eur J Med Chem 2019; 176: 68-91.
8. Eberhardt RT, Raffetto JD. Chronic venous insufficiency. Circulation 2014; 130(4): 333-46.
9. Porter JM, Moneta GL. Reporting standards in venous disease: an update. International Consensus Committee on Chronic Venous Disease. J Vasc Surg 1995; 21(4): 635-45.
10. Ding EL, Hutfless SM, Ding X. Chocolate and prevention of cardiovascular disease: a systematic review. Nutr Metab (Lond) 2006; 3: 2.
11. Panche AN, Diwan AD, Chandra SR. Flavonoids: an overview. J Nutr Sci 2016; 5: e47.
12. Rabe E, Guex JJ, Morrison N, Ramelet AA, Schuller-Petrovic S, Scuderi A, Staelens I, Pannier F. Treatment of chronic venous disease with flavonoids: recommendations for treatment and further studies. Phlebology 2013; 28(6): 308-19.
13. Millar CL, Duclos Q, Blesso CN. Effects of Dietary Flavonoids on Reverse Cholesterol Transport, HDL Metabolism, and HDL Function. Adv Nutr 2017; 8(2): 226-39.
14. Valerio N. L'alimentazione naturale, Oscar Mondadori (1980).

29 Food and oncology

Alessio Filippone, Maria Maddalena Rossi,
Cristina Rossi and Donatella Guarino

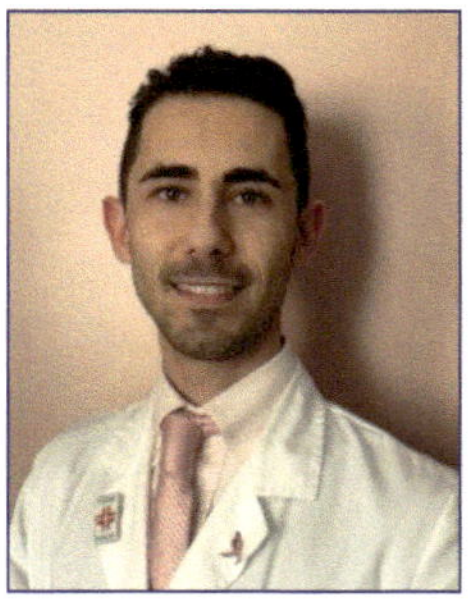

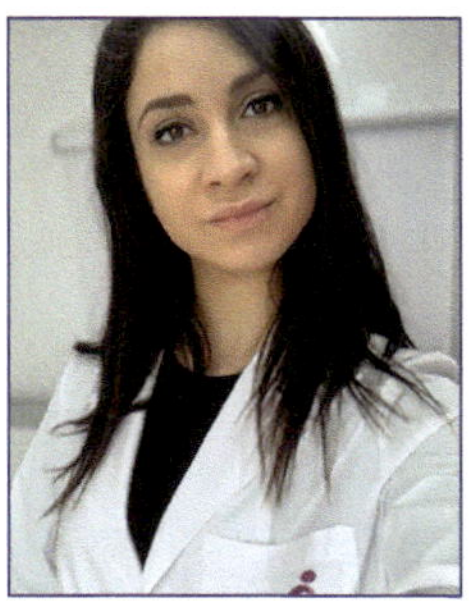

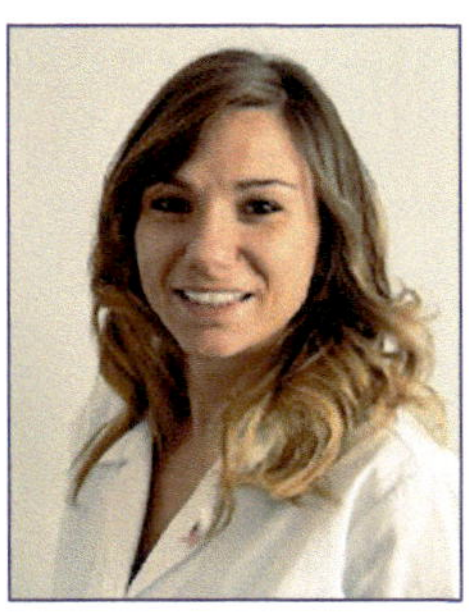

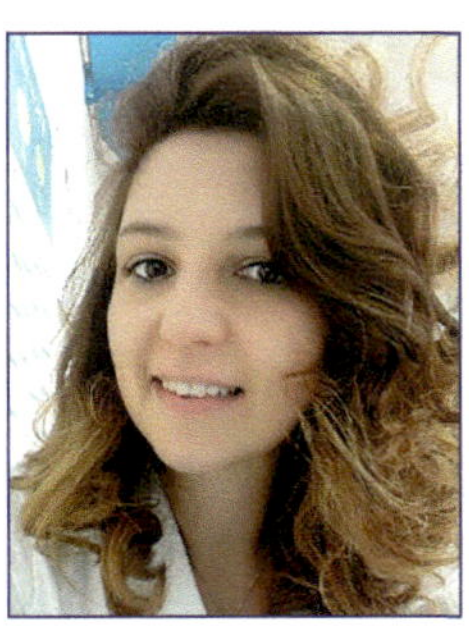

29.1 Introduction

It is widely known that lifestyles including diet, nutrition and physical activity play a key role in cancer prevention, and that about 30-50% of cancers worldwide could be avoided by following healthy behaviors. The relationship between foods, diet and cancer is very complex and needs a multidisciplinary team of scientists, oncologists, epidemiologists and nutritionists to achieve a global vision in this field. A recent and updated systematic review conducted by the World Cancer Research Fund (WCRF) and the American Institute for Cancer Research (AICR) on "Diet, Nutrition, Physical Activity and Cancer: a Global Perspective" highlighted the correlation between body composition including body mass index (BMI), waist-hip ratio and body fat, physical activity, food and the risk of developing at least 13 types of cancer [1]. This huge compendium contains the current knowledge about the oncological impact of food, body composition and physical activity, paving the way for cancer's primary prevention and risk of recurrences.

Before getting deeper into the role of every single most interesting food in cancer prevention, initiation and progression, it is useful to remark that a single "super food" that could prevent or cure cancer does not exist, but there is solid and increasing evidence on the role of a general pattern diet. In this scenario, one of the most accredited is the Mediterranean Diet that is rich in vegetables, whole grains, legumes, fish and unsaturated fats like extra virgin olive oil, thus repre-

Alessio Filippone, PhD
Center for Integrative Oncology
Fondazione Policlinico Universitario Agostino Gemelli IRCCS, Rome, Italy

Email: alessiofilippone@hotmail.it

Maria Maddalena Rossi, MSc
Center for Integrative Oncology
Fondazione Policlinico Universitario Agostino Gemelli IRCCS, Rome, Italy

Email: mmaddalena.rossi@virgilio.it

Cristina Rossi, PhD
Center for Integrative Oncology
Fondazione Policlinico Universitario Agostino Gemelli IRCCS, Rome, Italy

Email: cristina.rossi13@yahoo.it

Donatella Guarino
Center for Integrative Oncology
Fondazione Policlinico Universitario Agostino Gemelli IRCCS, Rome, Italy

Email: donatella.guarino@gmail.com

senting one of the healthiest models worldwide, recognized in 2010 as Intangible Cultural Heritage of Humanity by UNESCO. On the other side, the so called "Western Diet", rich in processed and sugary foods, meat and saturated fats is related to major risks of weight gain all the way to obesity and related pathologies.

From this background, the aim of this chapter is to summarize the most updated evidence on foods as they relate to the risk of cancer, and its prevention and management.

29.2 Alcohol

Alcoholic drinks include beers, wines and spirits. Other alcoholic drinks that may be locally important include fermented milks, mead (fermented honey-water) and cider (fermented apples). Ethanol is the active ingredient in alcoholic drinks; the concentration varies, depending on the type of drink. The main alcoholic drinks consumed, in ascending order of ethanol content, are beers and ciders; wines; wines 'fortified' with spirits; and spirits and liqueurs. The consumption of alcoholic drinks is graded by the International Agency for Research on Cancer (IARC) as carcinogenic to humans (Group 1) [2].

The consumption of alcohol is correlated with many types of cancer: a meta-analysis on mouth, pharynx and larynx showed a statistically significant 15% increased risk of oral cavity cancer per 10 grams increase in alcohol (as ethanol) consumed per day (RR 1.15 [95% CI 1.09-1.22]; n = 5,617) [3-8].

Also, the esophagus (squamous cell carcinoma) is correlated with high alcohol consumption. A large meta-analysis showed a statistically significant 25% increased risk per 10 grams increase in alcohol (as ethanol) consumed per day (RR 1.25 [95% CI 1.12-1.41]; n = 1,079) [9-14].

A meta-analysis conducted on liver cancer showed a statistically significant 4% increased risk of liver cancer per 10 grams increase in alcohol (as ethanol) consumed per day (RR 1.04 [95% CI 1.02-1.06]; n = 5,650) [10, 15-27].

A meta-analysis on colorectal cancer showed a statistically significant 7% increased risk of colorectal cancer per 10 grams increase in alcohol (as ethanol) consumed per day (RR 1.07 [95% CI 1.05-1.08]; n = 15,896) [28-38].

Twenty-two of 34 identified studies were included in the dose-response meta-analysis, which showed a statistically significant 9% increased risk of postmenopausal breast cancer per 10 grams increase in alcohol (as ethanol) consumed per day (RR 1.09 [95% CI 1.07-1.12]; n = 35,221) [39-60].

Ten of 16 identified studies were included in the dose-response meta-analysis, which showed a statistically significant 5% increased risk of premenopausal breast cancer per 10 grams increase in alcohol (as ethanol) consumed per day (RR 1.05 [95% CI 1.02-1.08]; n = 4,227) [39, 42, 46-48, 51, 54, 55, 58, 61].

The precise mechanisms underlying the relationship between alcohol consumption and cancers are not completely understood for all of them. Probably the acetaldehyde disrupts DNA synthesis and repair and thus may contribute to a carcinogenic cascade [62, 63]. Higher ethanol consumption also induces oxidative stress through an increased production of reactive oxygen species, which are potentially genotoxic [64]. Reactive oxygen species (ROS) commonly identify chemical compounds that include oxygen such as: superoxide, hydrogen peroxide and other oxygen radicals. It is hypothesized that alcohol may also function as a solvent for cellular penetration of dietary or environmental (for example, tobacco) carcinogens or interfere with DNA repair mechanisms [65]. Heavy drinkers of alcohol may also have diets that are lacking in essential nutrients, such as folate, rendering target tissues more susceptible to the carcinogenic effects of alcohol.

Moreover, alcohol consumption can induce the expression of cytochrome P450 2E1 (CYP2E1) in the human esophagus in a dose-dependent manner, and CYP2E1 activity yields substantial quantities of reactive oxygen species that may cause carcinogenic DNA lesions through oxidative stress inflammation and lipid peroxidation [66].

More recent research has focused on the impact of chronic high alcohol intake on dysbiosis of the gut microbiome and weakened gut barrier function [67, 68]. Higher exposure to bacterial products leaked from the gut lumen has been observed to be associated with a higher risk of liver cancer development [69], presumably by inducing chronic inflammation in the liver, and with a higher risk of developing colorectal cancer [70].

For breast cancer, the mechanisms through which alcohol may increase the risk remain uncertain. Alcohol is metabolized by the liver, whose functional state and ability to metabolize other nutrients, non-nutritive dietary factors and hormones can be impaired by the alcohol itself. Thus, the potential mechanisms affecting breast carcinogenesis are probably multifactorial. Alcohol can also be metabolized in breast tissue into acetaldehyde, producing reactive oxygen species associated with DNA damage [2]. Alcohol may increase circulating levels of estrogen, which is an established risk factor for breast cancer [71]. Alcohol may also act as a solvent, potentially enhancing the penetration of carcinogens into

Table 29.1 Summary of principal evidence on food consumption and its role in the increase or decrease of cancer risk

Food	*Increases risk*	*Decreases risk*
Alcohol	Mouth, pharynx, larynx, esophagus (squamous cell carcinoma), stomach, liver, colon-rectum, breast premenopause, breast postmenopause	Kidney
Sugar sweetened drinks	Weight gain, overweight and obesity	
Whole grains		Colon-rectum
Food containig dietary fiber		Colon-rectum Weight gain, overweight and obesity
Non-starchy vegetables and fruits		Respiratory and digestive systems (aggregated)
Red and processed meat	Colon-rectum	
Food preserved in salt	Stomach	
Dairy products		Colon-rectum, breast premenopause
Coffee and mate	Esophagus (squamous cell carcinoma)	Liver, endometrium
Arsenic in drinking water	Lung, bladder, skin.	
Fish		Liver, colon-rectum

cells, which may be particularly relevant to tissues exposed to alcohol.

Therefore, according to these meta-analyses, the consumption of alcoholic drinks is a convincing cause of cancers of the mouth, pharynx and larynx, esophageal squamous cell carcinoma, liver, colorectal, postmenopausal breast cancer and a probable cause of premenopausal breast cancer.

29.3 Sugar sweetened drinks

As defined in the WCRF report, sugar sweetened drinks are liquids that are sweetened by adding free sugars, such as sucrose, high fructose corn syrup and sugars naturally present in honey, syrups, fruit juices and fruit juice concentrate. This includes, among others, sodas, sports drinks, energy drinks, sweetened waters, cordials, barley water, and coffee- and tea-based beverages with sugars or syrups added.

An interesting meta-analysis based on 3,869 women showed a relation between glycemic load and the risk of endometrial cancer (1.15; 95% CI 1.06-1.25) [72-77], and another dose-response meta-analysis based on 2,831 men shows that the consumption of foods and drinks containing fructose (25 g/day) increases the risk of pancreatic cancer (1.22; 95% CI 1.08-1.37) [78].

Moreover, consumption of sugar sweetened drinks is a convincing cause of weight gain and obesity that lead to an increasing risk of several cancers affecting the esophagus (squamous cell carcinoma), stomach, liver, colon-rectum, liver, breast (postmenopause) and kidney [79], as summarized in Table 29.1.

29.4 Whole grains

A whole grain is a grain of any cereal and pseudocereal that contains all three original parts: endosperm germ and bran, in contrast to refined grains, which retain only the endosperm while the germ and bran are removed during the milling process. The germ is the embryonic part of cereal plants and contains oils, proteins and fibers. The outer parts of the grain contain non-starch polysaccharides, a type of carbohydrate that is the major component of dietary fibers. Whole grains are good sources of fiber, B vitamins, and some trace minerals such as iron, magnesium and zinc [80-82]. These nutrients are found in the outer layer of the grains or the bran that function as a protective shell for the germ and endosperm inside. The germ is nourishment for the seed and contains antioxidants, vitamin E and some B vitamins, while the endosperm provides carbohydrates, protein and energy. Refining of whole grains usually removes the germ and outer layers of the grain, thereby reducing the presence of fibers and micronutrients.

Whole grain sources include wheat (spelt, emmer, farro, einkorn, Kamut®, durum), rice (black, red and other colored rice varieties), maize/corn, millet, sorghum, barley, oats and rye.

All the identified studies were included in the dose-response meta-analysis, which showed a statistically significant 17% decreased risk of colorectal cancer per 90 grams increase in whole grains consumed per day (RR 0.83 [95% CI 0.78-0.89]; n = 8,320 cases) [83-87].

Based on the Third Expert report from WCRF, there is strong evidence that consuming whole grains decrease the risk of colorectal cancer.

The possible mechanism is that whole grains provide various nutrients and bioactive non-nutrient compounds including vitamin E, selenium, copper, zinc, lignans (polyphenols found in plants), phytoestrogens and phenolic compounds as well as dietary fiber. Many of these compounds, which are largely found within the bran and germ of the grain, have plausible anti-carcinogenic properties [88-89]. Whole grains may also protect against colorectal cancer by binding carcinogens and regulating the glycemic response.

Particular biomarkers (alkylresorcinols), that are part of the whole grain wheat and rye intake, were shown to be inversely related to colorectal cancer risk in the European Prospective Investigation into Cancer and Nutrition (EPIC) [90].

29.5 Food containing fiber

Dietary fiber, or fiber, is sometimes referred to as "roughage". It is a type of carbohydrate found in plant foods and is made up of many sugar molecules linked together. But unlike other carbohydrates (such as starch), dietary fiber is bound together in such a way that it cannot be readily digested in the small intestine.

There are two types of dietary fiber, and most plant foods contain some of each kind:

- soluble fiber is dissolved in water to form a thick gel-like substance in the stomach that it is broken down by bacteria in the large intestine and provides some calories. It is found in beans, peas, fruits, oats, nuts, seeds and vegetables. Soluble fiber can interfere with the absorption of dietary fat and cholesterol. This, in turn, can help lower low-density lipoprotein (LDL or «bad») cholesterol levels in the blood. Soluble fiber also can help control the level of blood glucose by preventing rapid rises in blood glucose following a meal;
- insoluble fiber does not dissolve in water and passes through the gastrointestinal tract relatively intact and, therefore, is not a source of calories. It is found in a variety of foods, including fruits, nuts and seeds, vegetables and whole grain foods (such as brown rice and whole grain breads, cereals and pasta). Insoluble fiber provides "bulk" for stool formation and speeds up the movement of food and waste through the digestive system, which can help prevent constipation.

Fifteen studies were included in a dose-response meta-analysis, which showed a statistically significant 9% decreased risk of colorectal cancer per 10 grams increase in dietary fiber consumed per day (RR 0.91 [95% CI 0.88-0.94]; n = 14,876 cases) [85, 86, 91-102].

In humans, different types of fiber can, to varying degrees, be fermented or metabolized by the colonic microflora, and this ability can influence the types and patterns of bacterial populations found in the colon. Microbial fermentation within the large bowel forms short-chain fatty acids, such as butyrate, that have been shown in experimental studies to have anti-proliferative effects for colon cancer cells [88, 103]. Other mechanisms by which greater dietary fiber intake may lower colorectal cancer risk include the reduction of intestinal transit time, increased fecal bulk, which would lessen the potential for fecal mutagens to interact with the colon mucosa, and a reduction of secondary bile acid production [88, 103]. High-fiber diets may also reduce insulin resistance, which is a risk factor for colorectal cancer [104]. Overall, there is moderate mechanistic evidence linking dietary fiber intake with a reduced risk of colorectal cancer.

29.6 Non-starchy vegetables and fruits

The culinary term "vegetables" refers to the edible parts of plants (for example, edible leaves, roots, tubers, bulbs, stems and stalks, flowers and grains that are used as vegetables (such as sweet corn) and usually includes fungi (mushrooms, truffles) and algae (seaweed) [105].

Vegetables can be separated into groups according to their individual starch content: starchy vegetables, such as potatoes, sweet potatoes (yams), cassava (manioc), sago yams and taro, contain higher levels of carbohydrates than non-starchy vegetables. Levels of other nutrients also vary between the two groups.

The composition of fruit and vegetables depends on both species and subtype, as well as on the environmental, farming, production and storage conditions. In addition to dietary fiber, vegetables and fruit are sources of a wide variety of vitamins, minerals and other bioactive compounds.

Fruit and non-starchy vegetables contain many potential anti-tumorigenic agents, such as dietary fiber, carotenoids, vitamins C and E, selenium, dithiolthiones, glucosinolates and indoles, isothiocyanates, flavonoids, phenols, protease inhibitors, plant sterols, allium compounds and limonene [106].

It is likely that a combination of these nutrients is responsible for the lower risk of nasopharyngeal cancer that has been observed among high consumers of fruit and non-starchy vegetables.

A dose-response meta-analysis on vegetables and cancers of the mouth, pharynx and larynx could not be conducted. One of three identified published studies reported a statistically significant decreased risk of oral cavity cancer (RR 0.84 [95% CI 0.73-0.95], per serving/1,000 kcal, n = 319), and of head and neck cancer (RR 0.89 [95% CI 0.82-0.97], per serving/1,000 kcal, n = 787), with increased consumption of vegetables in dose-response meta-analyses [107].

Moreover, two published meta-analyses of case-control studies on vegetable intake and nasopharyngeal cancer were identified, and both of them showed a statistically significant decreased risk of nasopharyngeal cancer when comparing the highest with the lowest level of vegetables consumed (RR 0.60 [95% CI 0.47-0.76] and RR 0.64 [95% CI 0.48-0.85]) [108, 109].

There is limited evidence suggesting that the greater consumption of non-starchy vegetables decreases the risk of esophageal squamous cell carcinoma, and evidence is also limited on the greater consumption of non-starchy vegetables decreasing the risk of lung cancer, in people who smoke and people who used to smoke tobacco [110].

All three identified studies included in the dose-response meta-analysis, showed a statistically significant 21% decreased risk of estrogen receptor ER-negative/progesterone receptor-negative (PR-negative or PR–) breast cancer per 200 grams increase in vegetables consumed per day (RR 0.79 [95% CI 0.63-0.98]; n =1,346 cases) [111-113]. Moreover, a statistically significant decreased risk of ER-negative breast cancer was observed when comparing the highest with the lowest levels of vegetables consumed, while a statistically significant decreased risk of ER-negative breast cancer was also observed per 300 grams increase in vegetables consumed per day (approximately three servings per day) [114].

The impact of vegetables consumption on the risk of colorectal cancer was examined in 11 out of 23 identified studies. One of them showed a statistically significant 2% decreased risk of colorectal cancer per 100 grams increase in vegetables consumed per day (RR 0.98 [95% CI 0.96-0.99)]; n = 14,136 cases).

In summary, there is strong evidence that the consumption of non-starchy vegetables and fruit (aggregated) decreases the risk of cancers of the respiratory and digestive systems, but there is still limited evidence in bladder cancer. The consumption of non-starchy vegetables only, but not in association with fruit, has been shown to decrease the risk of the following cancers: mouth, pharynx and larynx; nasopharynx; esophagus (specifically adenocarcinoma and squamous cell carcinoma); lung (in people who smoke or used to smoke tobacco); but the evidence for breast cancer (ER-negative) is limited [115-120]. Moreover, there is limited evidence suggesting that the greater consumption of fruit decreases the risk of esophageal cancer (squamous cell carcinoma) [121-123] and lung cancer (for people who smoke or used to smoke tobacco); there is limited evidence suggesting that the greater consumption of citrus fruit decreases the risk of stomach cancer (cardia) [121, 124, 125]. There is also limited evidence that a low consumption of fruit increases the risk of colorectal and stomach cancer.

29.7 Fish

Fish contains functional components that are not present in terrestrial organisms. In the edible part (e.g., filet, abdominal muscle), fish provide many nutritional components beneficial for the human diet, like n-3 long chain polyunsaturated fatty acids (PUFAs), namely eicosapentaenoic acid (EPA) and docosahexaenoic acid (DHA), essential elements such as selenium and iodine, high potassium and low sodium concentrations, and vitamins D, A, E, and B12, as well as taurine (2-aminoethanesulfonic acid) among others [126, 127]. The Recommended Intake (RI) for EPA+DHA is associated with a healthier lifestyle [128].

Like meat, fish is also often processed, before consumption, by drying, salting and smoking it or by adding preservatives. These methods of processing and preparation may affect the chemical composition as well as the nutritional value. In fact, evidence from case-control studies showed an increased risk of nasopharyngeal cancer with the increased consumption of salted fish (including Cantonese-style salted fish) [129].

Fish contains about 6 to 25% protein by weight, B vitamins and minerals including potassium and selenium. It has a fat content between 0.7% by weight in low-fat fish, such as cod or skate, and 19% in oily fish such as Atlantic salmon [130]. As part of a healthy eating pattern, eating fish may also lower the risk of heart disease-related deaths and obesity, but research is less clear on the role that fish may play in cancer protection.

The AICR new report on liver cancer reveals that eating fish may protect against this cancer, although the evidence was not strong enough to draw a conclusion, while grilled (broiled) or barbecued (charbroiled) meat and fish increase the risk for stomach cancer [130].

For human hepatocellular carcinoma, increasing evidence from animal and *in vitro* studies indicates that n-3 fatty acids, especially the long-chain polyunsaturad fatty acids DHA and EPA inhibit carcinogenesis [131]. Most of the more recent data indicates a protective effects of a variety of fish oils, especially with regard to the formation of preneoplastic stages including foci and nodules [132, 133].

Some population studies have also linked higher fish consumption with a reduced risk of other cancers, including colon and breast [134]. In lab studies, the omega-3-fats of fish are well researched. Those studies have suggested the omega-3-fats from fish alter colon cell function and may cut down on inflammation, in particular when it comes to fish itself. Although fish oil is a popular dietary supplement, for people with no heart disease, the American Heart Association (AHA) recommends getting omega-3 fatty acids only through foods. For cancer prevention, AICR recommends not to use all doses and formulations of supplements, unless they have been advised by a qualified health professional who can assess potential risks and benefits [135].

However, evidence of the protective action of fish rich in omega-3 fatty acid was too limited to draw a conclusion for cancers of the following types: mouth, pharynx and larynx, nasopharynx, esophagus (adenocarcinoma and squamous cell carcinoma), lung, stomach, pancreas, gallbladder, breast (pre- and postmenopause), ovary, endometrium, prostate, kidney, bladder and skin.

Research shows that people eating diets with a moderate amount of fish have a lower risk of cancer and other chronic diseases and longer lives. This could be due to other parts of the diet. For example, if you're eating more fish for dinner, you may be eating less red and processed meats, which increase colorectal cancer risk. Fish is a staple of several dietary patterns also linked to lower cancer risk, such as the Mediterranean diet. People eating a Mediterranean diet are also eating plenty of beans, whole grains, vegetables and other plant foods, which all play a role in reducing cancer risk. Taken together, these diets high in plant foods, moderate in fish and seafood and low in sugar can help people stay within a healthy weight. Overweight and obesity is now linked to increased risk of 10 cancers, including postmenopausal breast, liver and colorectal cancers [135].

29.8 Red and processed meat

Meat contains about 11 to 23% protein by weight. The fat content by weight ranges from 1% in lean poultry to 47% in pork carcass [136]. Meat can be a valuable source of nutrients, in particular, protein, iron, zinc and vitamin B12.

Globally, about 43 kilograms per capita per year of meat (beef, lamb, mutton and goat, pork, poultry and other meat) are available for consumption [137].

Meat consumption generally increases with economic development. Worldwide, between 1961 and 2013, the quantity of meat available for consumption per person has nearly doubled from 23 kilograms to 43 kilograms per year [137]. Consumption of meat and other animal foods from undomesticated animals is low on a global basis, but these foods are a usual part of diets in many middle- and low-income countries, as well as being delicacies in high-income countries.

A large meta-analysis showed no statistically significant association between the risk of colorectal cancer and consumption of red meat (RR 1.12 [95% CI 1.00-1.25], per 100 grams increase per day; n = 6,662 cases) [101, 138-144]. But stratified by cancer type, a significant increased risk was observed for colon cancer (RR 1.22 [95% CI 1.06-1.39]), but not rectal cancer.

The evidence for red meat intake was generally consistent and showed an increased risk in the dose-response meta-analyses. The result was statistically significant for colon cancer but not for colorectal and rectal cancers.

Cooking meats at high temperatures, prolonged exposure to heat and cooking by various types of grilling results in the formation of heterocyclic amines and polycyclic aromatic hydrocarbons, both of which have been linked to colorectal cancer development in experimental studies [145]. In addition, heme iron, which is present at high levels in red meat, has been shown to promote colorectal tumorigenesis by stimulating the endogenous formation of carcinogenic N-nitroso compounds [146]. There is moderate mechanistic evidence to support a relationship between high consumption of red meat and colorectal cancer.

Polycyclic aromatic hydrocarbons, which are formed when organic substances like meat are burned incompletely, may also have carcinogenic potential [147]. Grilling (broiling) and barbecuing (charbroiling) meat, fish or other foods with intense heat over a direct flame result in fat dropping on the hot fire, causing flames; these flames contain polycyclic aromatic hydrocarbons that stick to the surface of food [145]. So, the consumption of red meat is probably a cause of colorectal cancer.

There is no generally agreed definition of "processed meat". The term is used inconsistently in epidemiological studies. In general, it refers to meat that has been transformed through salting, curing, fermentation, smoking or other processes to enhance flavor or improve preservation. Depending on food preparation practices, processed meat can include ham, salami, bacon and pastrami and some sausages.

There are a lot of studies about many types of cancer, but they are too limited to draw a conclusion regarding: mouth, pharynx and larynx [148]; esophagus (adenocarcinoma) [149]; stomach (cardia) [150]; liver [151]; breast (pre- and postmenopause) [152]; ovary [153]; endometrium [154]; prostate [155]; kidney [156]; bladder [157]; and skin [158].

For colorectal cancer, a meta-analysis showed a statistically significant 16% increased risk per 50 grams increase in processed meat consumed per day (RR 1.16 [95% CI 1.08-1.26]; n= 10,738 cases) [138, 139, 141, 142, 159-164].

Similar to red meat, processed meat is rich in fat, protein and heme iron, which can promote carcinogenesis [145]. Processed meats, such as sausages, are often cooked at high temperatures, which can lead to an increased exposure to heterocyclic amines and polycyclic aromatic hydrocarbons. Processed meat is invariably higher in fat content than red meat, which may promote carcinogenesis through synthesis of secondary bile acids; however, human data supporting this hypothesis are weak. Processed meat is also a source of exogenously derived N-nitroso compounds, which may have carcinogenic potential [165].

29.9 Food preserved by salting

Foods can be preserved and processed in several ways prior to consumption. These different methods affect the chemical composition of foods as well as their nutritional value and carcinogenic potential.

Apart from preserving meat and enhancing its flavor, salting is also a traditional method of preserving raw fish throughout much of the world. Depending on the precise conditions, salt-preserved fish may also undergo fermentation. Cantonese-style salted fish is characterized by using less salt and a higher degree of fermentation during the drying process compared with fish preserved (or salted) by other means, because of the relatively high outdoor temperature and moisture levels.

Although the use of salt as a preservative has generally decreased as industrial and domestic use of refrigeration has increased, some traditional diets still include substantial amounts of salt-preserved foods, including salted meat, fish, vegetables and sometimes also fruit [166].

The requirement for salt for human health has been estimated to be much lower than amounts currently consumed. The World Health Organization (WHO) pragmatically recommends restricting average salt consumption for populations to less than 5 grams per day (equivalent to less than 2 grams of sodium per day) [167].

Many types of cancer are correlated with a high salt consuming exposure: esophageal cancer (adenocarcinoma and squamous cell carcinoma) [168]; and lung cancer [169].

A meta-analysis showed a statistically significant 9% increased risk of stomach cancer per 20 grams increase in salt-preserved vegetables consumed per day (RR 1.09 [95% CI 1.05-1.13]; n = 3,932 cases) [170-178].

Animal models have shown that high salt levels alter the viscosity of the mucus protecting the stomach and enhance the formation of N-nitroso compounds [179]. In addition, high salt intake may stimulate the colonization of *H. pylori*, the strongest known risk factor for stomach cancer [180]. Finally, in animal models, high salt levels have been shown to be responsible for the primary cellular damage that results in the promotion of stomach cancer development [181].

29.10 Dairy products

Dairy products are foods derived from milk, produced by all mammalian species to feed their young. The principal source of milk used for human consumption derive from ruminants such as cows, sheep and goats, but a small percentage could come from other species. Fresh milk can be consumed raw or, as is common in many high-income countries, pasteurized. Milk is also commonly processed into a wide variety of foods including cream, concentrated milks, cheese, fats (such as butter and ghee), and fermented foods (such as yogurt, Greek yogurt, kefir and skyr). Currently, scientific evidence is available regarding dairy products consumption and risk of several kind of cancers including colon-rectum, breast (postmenopause) and prostate.

A meta-analysis on the consumption of dairy products and colon-rectum cancer, including a total of 56 studies and over of 43,000 cases, has shown that dairy products including milk and cheese are probably decreasing the risk of this tumor.

In particular, in a study based on 14,859 cases, the consumption of 400 g/day of dairy products shows a reduction of risk on colorectal cancer (RR 0.87; 95% CI 0.83-0.90). Another analysis on 10,783 cases shows that the consumption of 200 g/day of milk reduced the risk on colorectal cancer (RR 0.94; 95% CI 0.92-0.96). Another interesting study on postmenopause breast cancer, based on 2,862 women, shows that the consumption of 200 g of milk a day decreases the risk of colorectal cancer (RR 0.95; 95% CI 0.92-0.99).

Conversely, a study of 38,107 patients with a daily consumption of 400 g of cheese suggests an increased risk on prostate cancer (RR 1.07; 95% CI 1.02-1.12) [182].

29.11 Coffee and mate

Mate, a type of herbal tea, is an aqueous infusion prepared from the dried leaves of the plant Ilex paraguariensis [183, 184]. Regular consumption of mate, drank scalding hot above 65 °C, is the traditional style in South America.

Mate is consumed mainly and regularly in South America, specifically Argentina, Bolivia, Brazil, Chile, Ecuador, Paraguay and Uruguay. These countries correspond to areas of a higher incidence of esophageal squamous cell carcinoma within South America probably caused by drinking scalding hot mate over time [185-192].

Any carcinogenic effects of mate are believed to be due to the consumption at very hot temperatures (over 65 °C), increasing the incidence of nitrosamine-induced tumors [183, 193].

In 2016, an IARC Working Group declared that drinking very hot beverages, including mate, above 65 °C is probably carcinogenic to humans (Group 2A) [183]. Mate can also be consumed warm or cold [183]. In 2016, the IARC Working Group concluded that drinking mate that is not very hot is unclassifiable in terms of its carcinogenicity in humans (Group 3) [183].

Coffee is a beverage consisting of a decoction or infusion of the roasted ground or crushed seeds (coffee beans) of the two-seeded fruit (coffee berry) of certain coffee trees. Consumption of coffee probably protects against liver cancer and endometrial cancer.

Six of eight identified studies were included in the dose-response meta-analysis, which showed a statistically significant 14% decreased risk of liver cancer per cup increase in coffee consumed per day [171, 194-199].

The mechanism involved in the protection by coffee in liver cancer could be explained by the composition of coffee that is rich in bioactive compounds including caffeine, chlorogenic acids and other phenolic compounds. Recent studies suggest that these antioxidant and anti-inflammatory compounds may have beneficial effects on the liver, but the main underlying mechanisms of the role of coffee in liver cancer development are not fully elucidated [200]. Another mechanism that could be implicated in the protection from liver cancer is that the coffee is associated with improved insulin sensitivity [201], decreased incidence of metabolic syndrome [202] and a reduced level of liver injury [203].

Seven of eight identified studies were included in the dose-response meta-analysis, which showed a statistically significant 7% decreased risk of endometrial cancer per cup increase in coffee consumed per day (RR 0.93 [95% CI 0.91-0.96]; n = 3,571 cases) [204-210].

The mechanisms linking coffee consumption to a decrease in endometrial cancer risk remain unclear but, based on the evidence, a hormonal mechanism could be involved. Coffee drinking is correlated with higher levels of sex hormone-binding globulin (SHBG), which may decrease exposure to bioavailable estradiol levels [211-213]. Coffee drinking is also associated with reduced insulin levels, particularly among overweight women [214], and it has been hypothesized that coffee may reduce the risk of endometrial cancer through an insulin-mediated mechanism [215].

Coffee has also been shown to alter adipokines and inflammatory pathways and lead to an increase in adiponectin levels [216, 217], an adipokine that is down-regulated in obesity and has been linked to endometrial cancer development [218, 219].

The evidence is limited suggesting that consumption of coffee decreases the risk of cancers of the mouth, pharynx and larynx and skin cancer (basal cell carcinoma, and malignant melanoma in women). There are some inconsistencies, but the individual dose response analyses in some cohort-studies show a significant decreased risk with the increase of coffee consumed. The biological mechanism is unclear but probably drinking coffee provides exposure to bioactive compounds, such as phenolic phytochemicals and antioxidant compounds, that inhibit DNA methylation *in vitro* [220, 221]. Coffee is also a source of diterpenes such as cafestol and kahweol, which have been shown to induce apoptosis and have antioxidant and anti-inflammatory effects [222, 223].

29.12 Arsenic in drinking water

Access to clean drinking water is essential to health. However, drinking water can be contaminated by harmful substances, including arsenic. Agricultural, mining and industrial practices can contaminate water. Arsenic can also occur naturally in water due to natural geological deposits or volcanic activity. The IARC has judged drinking water contaminated with arsenic to be carcinogenic to humans (Group 1) [224]. The primary regions, where high concentrations of arsenic have been measured in drinking water, include large areas of Bangladesh, China and West Bengal (India).

There is no global recommendation for arsenic in

drinking water, as individuals do not have the power to control whether their local water supply is contaminated. However, contamination of water supplies with arsenic is a public health issue.

For lung cancer, studies showed a statistically significant increased risk with increasing levels of cumulative exposure to arsenic from drinking water. These studies were conducted in populations with a high exposure to arsenic [225-227] and one study was performed in an area with a low exposure to arsenic [228]. Measurements of people's level of exposure to arsenic in drinking water were based on arsenic levels in well water. Cumulative exposure was calculated from the amount of water consumed and the years of residence in the area. The mechanisms linking arsenic in drinking water with cancer development are poorly understood. Experimental studies suggest that exposure to arsenic and its metabolites induces the production of reactive oxygen species inducing DNA damage, altering transcription factor function and modulating the expression of genes involved in cell growth, survival and cancer risk [229, 230]. It is currently uncertain, however, whether these mechanisms are relevant specifically for lung cancer. For these reasons, consumption of arsenic in drinking water is a convincing cause of lung cancer.

Seven studies were conducted on consumption of arsenic in drinking water and the risk of bladder cancer, three studies conducted in populations with high exposure to arsenic [225, 226, 231], and the others in an area with low exposure to arsenic [228, 232-234]. Two of the three studies [226, 231] from areas with high exposure to arsenic showed a statistically significant increased risk of bladder cancer with increasing levels of cumulative exposure to arsenic from drinking water. No statistically significant increase or decrease in risk was observed in the studies from areas with low exposure to arsenic [228, 232-234]. For these reasons, consumption of arsenic in drinking water is probably a cause of bladder cancer.

Consumption of arsenic in drinking water is probably a cause of skin cancer as well. In fact, one study reported a statistically significant increased risk of skin cancer when comparing the highest with the lowest arsenic concentration in drinking water [235]. No statistically significant increase or decrease in risk was observed in two other studies from populations with low levels of exposure to arsenic in drinking water [228, 234].

29.13 Conclusion

There is strong evidence that dietary patterns influence the risk of several primary cancers and their recurrences. Specific foods have been shown to increase or decrease the risk of several types of cancer, depending on the exposure and frequency of consumption. Based on this evidence, specific recommendations are currently available on daily or weekly consumption for each kind of food groups, to minimize the cancer risk in the healthy population and help clinical management of cancer patients.

REFERENCES

1. World Cancer Research Fund/American Institute for Cancer Research. Diet, Nutrition, Physical Activity and Cancer: a Global Perspective. Continuous Update Project Expert Report 2018. Available at dietandcancerreport.org
2. International Agency for Research on Cancer (IARC). IARC Monographs on the Evaluation of Carcinogenic Risks to Humans. Volume 100 Part E: Personal Habits and Indoor Combustions. 2012: 373-472.
3. Hippisley-Cox J, Coupland C. Development and validation of risk prediction algorithms to estimate future risk of common cancers in men and women: prospective cohort study. BMJ Open 2015; 5: e007825.
4. Hsu WL, Chien YC, Chiang CJ, et al. Lifetime risk of distinct upper aerodigestive tract cancers and consumption of alcohol, betel and cigarette. Int J Cancer 2014; 135: 1480-6.
5. Maasland DH, van den Brandt PA, Kremer B, et al. Alcohol consumption, cigarette smoking and the risk of subtypes of head-neck cancer: results from the Netherlands Cohort Study. BMC Cancer 2014; 14: 187.
6. Shanmugham JR, Zavras AI, Rosner BA, et al. Alcohol-folate interactions in the risk of oral cancer in women: a prospective cohort study. Cancer Epidemiol Biomarkers Prev 2010; 19: 2516-24.
7. Freedman ND, Abnet CC, Leitzmann MF, et al. Prospective investigation of the cigarette smoking-head and neck cancer association by sex. Cancer 2007; 110: 1593-601.
8. Boffetta P, Garfinkel L. Alcohol drinking and mortality among men enrolled in an American Cancer Society prospective study. Epidemiology 1990; 1: 342-8.
9. Steevens J, Schouten LJ, Goldbohm RA, et al. Alcohol consumption, cigarette smoking and risk of subtypes of oesophageal and gastric cancer: a prospective cohort study. Gut 2010; 59: 39-48.
10. Allen NE, Beral V, Casabonne D, et al. Moderate alcohol intake and cancer incidence in women. J Natl Cancer Inst 2009; 101: 296-305.
11. Ishiguro S, Sasazuki S, Inoue M, et al. Effect of alcohol consumption, cigarette smoking and flushing response on esophageal cancer risk: a population-based cohort study (JPHC study). Cancer Lett 2009; 275: 240-6.
12. Weikert C, Dietrich T, Boeing H, et al. Lifetime and base-

line alcohol intake and risk of cancer of the upper aerodigestive tract in the European Prospective Investigation into Cancer and Nutrition (EPIC) study. Int J Cancer 2009; 125: 406-12.
13. Freedman ND, Abnet CC, Leitzmann MF, et al. A prospective study of tobacco, alco-hol, and the risk of esophageal and gastric cancer subtypes. Am J Epidemiol 2007; 165: 1424-33.
14. Lindblad M, Rodriguez LA, Lagergren J. Body mass, tobacco and alcohol and risk of esophageal, gastric cardia, and gastric non-cardia adenocarcinoma among men and women in a nested case-control study. Cancer Causes Control 2005; 16: 285-94.
15. Persson EC, Schwartz LM, Park Y, et al. Alcohol consumption, folate intake, hepatocellular carcinoma and liver disease mortality. Cancer Epidemiol Biomarkers Prev 2013; 22: 415-21.
16. Jung EJ, Shin A, Park SK, et al. Alcohol consumption and mortality in the Korean Multi-Center Cancer Cohort Study. J Prev Med Public Health 2012; 45: 301-8.
17. Yang L, Zhou M, Sherliker P, et al. Alcohol drinking and overall and cause-specific mortality in China: nationally representative prospective study of 220,000 men with 15 years of follow-up. Int J Epidemiol 2012; 41: 1101-13.
18. Koh WP, Robien K, Wang R, et al. Smoking as an independent risk factor for hepa-tocellular carcinoma: the Singapore Chinese Health Study. Br J Cancer 2011; 105: 1430-5.
19. Schutze M, Boeing H, Pischon T, et al. Alcohol attributable burden of incidence of cancer in eight European countries based on results from prospective cohort study. BMJ 2011; 342: d1584.
20. Kim MK, Ko MJ, Han JT. Alcohol consumption and mortality from all-cause and cancers among 1.34 million Koreans: the results from the Korea National Health Insurance Corporation's health examinee cohort in 2000. Cancer Causes Control 2010; 21: 2295-302.
21. Yi SW, Sull JW, Linton JA, et al. Alcohol consumption and digestive cancer mortality in Koreans: the Kangwha Cohort Study. J Epidemiol 2010; 20: 204-11.
22. Joshi S, Song YM, Kim TH, et al. Socio-economic status and the risk of liver cancer mortality: a prospective study in Korean men. Public Health 2008; 122: 1144-51.
23. Ohishi W, Fujiwara S, Cologne JB, et al. Risk factors for hepatocellular carcinoma in a Japanese population: a nested case-control study. Cancer Epidemiol Biomarkers Prev 2008; 17: 846-54.
24. Yuan JM, Gao YT, Ong CN, et al. Prediagnostic level of serum retinol in relation to reduced risk of hepatocellular carcinoma. J Natl Cancer Inst 2006; 98: 482-90.
25. Nakaya N, Tsubono Y, Kuriyama S, et al. Alcohol consumption and the risk of can-cer in Japanese men: the Miyagi Cohort Study. Eur J Cancer Prev 2005; 14: 169-74.
26. Goodman MT, Moriwaki H, Vaeth M, et al. Prospective cohort study of risk factors for primary liver cancer in Hiroshima and Nagasaki, Japan. Epidemiology 1995; 6: 36-41.
27. Ross RK, Yuan JM, Yu MC, et al. Urinary aflatoxin biomarkers and risk of hepatocellular carcinoma. Lancet 1992; 339: 943-6.
28. Shin A, Joo J, Yang HR, et al. Risk prediction model for colorectal cancer: National Health Insurance Corporation Study, Korea. PLoS One 2014; 9: e88079.
29. Bamia C, Lagiou P, Buckland G, et al. Mediterranean diet and colorectal cancer risk: results from a European cohort. Eur J Epidemiol 2013; 28: 317-28.
30. Everatt R, Tamosiunas A, Virviciute D, et al. Consumption of alcohol and risk of can-cer among men: a 30 year cohort study in Lithuania. Eur J Epidemiol 2013; 28: 383-92.
31. Nan H, Lee JE, Rimm EB, et al. Prospective study of alcohol consumption and the risk of colorectal cancer before and after folic acid fortification in the United States. Annals of Epidemiology 2013; 23: 558-63.
32. Razzak A, Oxentenko A, Vierkant RA, et al. Alcohol intake and colorectal cancer risk by molecularly defined subtypes in a prospective study of older women. Cancer Prev Res (Phila) 2011; 4: 2035-43.
33. Bongaerts BW, van den Brandt PA, Goldbohm RA, et al. Alcohol consumption, type of alcoholic beverage and risk of colorectal cancer at specific subsites. Int J Cancer 2008; 123: 2411-7.
34. Mizoue T, Inoue M, Wakai K, et al. Alcohol drinking and colorectal cancer in Japa-nese: a pooled analysis of results from five cohort studies. Am J Epidemiol 2008; 167: 1397-406.
35. Toriola AT, Kurl S, Laukanen JA, et al. Alcohol consumption and risk of colorectal cancer: the Findrink study. Eur J Epidemiol 2008; 23: 395-401.
36. Akhter M, Kuriyama S, Nakaya N, et al. Alcohol consumption is associated with an increased risk of distal colon and rectal cancer in Japanese men: the Miyagi Cohort Study. Eur J Cancer 2007; 43: 383-90.
37. Glynn SA, Albanes D, Pietinen P, et al. Alcohol consumption and risk of colorectal cancer in a cohort of Finnish men. Cancer Causes Control 1996; 7: 214-23.
38. Wu AH, Paganini Hill A, Ross RK, et al. Alcohol, physical activity and other risk fac-tors for colorectal cancer: a prospective study. Br J Cancer 1987; 55: 687-94.
39. Fagherazzi G, Vilier A, Boutron-Ruault MC, et al. Alcohol consumption and breast cancer risk subtypes in the E3N-EPIC cohort. Eur J Cancer Prev 2015; 24: 209-14.
40. Brinton LA, Smith L, Gierach GL, et al. Breast cancer risk in older women: results from the NIH-AARP Diet and Health Study. Cancer Causes Control 2014; 25: 843-57.
41. Falk RT, Maas P, Schairer C, et al. Alcohol and risk of breast cancer in postmeno-pausal women: an analysis of etiological heterogeneity by multiple tumor characteristics. Am J Epidemiol 2014; 180: 705-17.
42. Park SY, Kolonel LN, Lim U, et al. Alcohol consumption and breast cancer risk among women from five ethnic groups with light to moderate intakes: the Multiethnic Co-hort Study. Int J Cancer 2014; 134: 1504-10.
43. Couto E, Sandin S, Lof M, et al. Mediterranean dietary pattern and risk of breast cancer. PLoS One 2013; 8: e55374.
44. Hartz AJ, He T. Cohort study of risk factors for breast cancer in post menopausal women. Epidemiol Health 2013; 35: e2013003.
45. Sczaniecka AK, Brasky TM, Lampe JW, et al. Dietary intake of specific fatty acids and breast cancer risk among postmenopausal women in the VITAL cohort. Nutr Cancer 2012; 64: 1131-42.
46. Chen WY, Rosner B, Hankinson SE, et al. Moderate alcohol consumption during adult life, drinking patterns and breast cancer risk. JAMA 2011; 306: 1884-90.
47. Suzuki R, Iwasaki M, Inoue M, et al. Alcohol consumption-associated breast cancer incidence and potential effect modifiers: the Japan Public Health Center-based Prospective Study. Int J Cancer 2010; 127: 685-95.
48. Trichopoulou A, Bamia C, Lagiou P, et al. Conformity to traditional Mediterranean di-et and breast cancer risk in

the Greek EPIC (European Prospective Investigation into Cancer and Nutrition) cohort. Am J Clin Nutr 2010; 92: 620-5.
49. Ericson U, Sonestedt E, Ivarsson MI, et al. Folate intake, methylenetetrahydrofolate reductase polymorphisms and breast cancer risk in women from the Malmo Diet and Cancer cohort. Cancer Epidemiol Biomarkers Prev 2009; 18: 1101-10.
50. Nielsen NR, Gronbaek M. Interactions between intakes of alcohol and postmen-opausal hormones on risk of breast cancer. Int J Cancer 2008; 122: 1109-13.
51. Zhang SM, Lee IM, Manson JE, et al. Alcohol consumption and breast cancer risk in the Women's Health Study. Am J Epidemiol 2007; 165: 667-76.
52. Mellemkjaer L, Bigaard J, Tjonneland A, et al. Body composition and breast cancer in postmenopausal women: a Danish prospective cohort study. Obesity (Silver Spring) 2006; 14: 1854-62.
53. Suzuki R, Ye W, Rylander-Rudqvist T, et al. Alcohol and postmenopausal breast cancer risk defined by estrogen and progesterone receptor status: a prospective cohort study. J Natl Cancer Inst 2005; 97: 1601-8.
54. Horn-Ross PL, Canchola AJ, West DW, et al. Patterns of alcohol consumption and breast cancer risk in the California Teachers Study cohort. Cancer Epidemiol Biomarkers Prev 2004; 13: 405-11.
55. Petri AL, Tjonneland A, Gamborg M, et al. Alcohol intake, type of beverage and risk of breast cancer in pre- and postmenopausal women. Alcohol Clin Exp Res 2004; 28: 1084-90.
56. Sellers TA, Grabrick DM, Vierkant RA, et al. Does folate intake decrease risk of post-menopausal breast cancer among women with a family history? Cancer Causes Control 2004; 15: 113-20.
57. Feigelson HS, Jonas CR, Robertson AS, et al. Alcohol, folate, methionine and risk of incident breast cancer in the American Cancer Society Cancer Prevention Study II Nutrition Cohort. Cancer Epidemiol Biomarkers Prev 2003; 12: 161-4.
58. Rohan TE, Jain M, Howe GR, et al. Alcohol consumption and risk of breast cancer: a cohort study. Cancer Causes Control 2000; 11: 239-47.
59. Van den Brandt PA, Goldbohm RA, van't Veer P. Alcohol and breast cancer: re-sults from The Netherlands Cohort Study. Am J Epidemiol 1995; 141: 907-15.
60. Barrett-Connor E, Friedlander NJ. Dietary fat, calories, and the risk of breast cancer in postmenopausal women: a prospective population-based study. J Am Coll Nutr 1993; 12: 390-9.
61. Garland M, Hunter DJ, Colditz GA, et al. Alcohol consumption in relation to breast cancer risk in a cohort of United States women 25-42 years of age. Cancer Epidemiol Biomarkers Prev 1999; 8: 1017-21
62. Seitz HK, Stickel F. Molecular mechanisms of alcohol-mediated carcinogenesis. Nat Rev Cancer 2007; 7: 599-612.
63. International Agency for Research on Cancer (IARC). IARC Monographs on the Evaluation of Carcinogenic Risks to Humans. Volume 71, Part 2: Re-evaluation of Some Organic Chemicals, Hydrazine and Hydrogen Peroxide. 1999.
64. Albano E. Alcohol, oxidative stress and free radical damage. Proc Nutr Soc 2006; 65: 278-90.
65. Boffetta P, Hashibe M. Alcohol and cancer. Lancet Oncol 2006; 7: 149-56.
66. Linhart K, Bartsch H, Seitz HK. The role of reactive oxygen species (ROS) and cytochrome P-450 2E1 in the generation of carcinogenic etheno-DNA adducts. Redox Biol 2014; 3: 56-62.
67. Acharya C, Bajaj JS. Gut microbiota and complications of liver disease. Gastro-enterol Clin North Am 2017; 46: 155-69.
68. Engen PA, Green SJ, Voigt RM, et al. The gastrointestinal microbiome: alcohol ef-fects on the composition of intestinal microbiota. Alcohol Res 2015; 37: 223-36.
69. Fedirko V, Tran HQ, Gewirtz AT, et al. Exposure to bacterial products lipopolysaccha-ride and flagellin and hepatocellular carcinoma: a nested case-control study. BMC Med 2017; 15: 72.
70. Kong SY, Tran HQ, Gewirtz AT, et al. Serum endotoxins and flagellin and risk of col-orectal cancer in the European Prospective Investigation into Cancer and Nutrition (EP-IC) cohort. Cancer Epidemiol Biomarkers Prev 2016; 25: 291-301.
71. Singletary KW, Gapstur SM. Alcohol and breast cancer: review of epidemiologic and experimental evidence and potential mechanisms. JAMA 2001; 286: 2143-51.
72. Cui X, Rosner B, Willett WC, et al. Dietary fat, fiber, and carbohydrate intake in relation to risk of endometrial cancer. Cancer Epidemiol Biomarkers Prev 2011; 20: 978-89.
73. George SM, Mayne ST, Leitzmann MF, et al. Dietary glycemic index, glycemic load and risk of cancer: a prospective cohort study. Am J Epidemiol 2009; 169: 462-72.
74. Cust AE, Slimani N, Kaaks R, et al. Dietary carbohydrates, glycemic index, glycemic load and endometrial cancer risk within the European Prospective Investigation into Cancer and Nutrition cohort. Am J Epidemiol 2007; 166: 912-23.
75. Larsson SC, Friberg E, Wolk A. Carbohydrate intake, glycemic index and glycemic load in relation to risk of endometrial cancer: a prospective study of Swedish women. Int J Cancer 2007; 120: 1103-7.
76. Silvera SA, Rohan TE, Jain M, et al. Glycaemic index, glycaemic load and risk of endometrial cancer: a prospective cohort study. Public Health Nutr 2005; 8: 912-9.
77. Folsom AR, Demissie Z, Harnack L. Glycemic index, glycemic load and incidence of endometrial cancer: the Iowa women's health study. Nutr Cancer 2003; 46: 119-24.
78. World Cancer Research Fund/American Institute for Cancer Research. Continuous Update Project Expert Report 2018. Diet, Nutrition, physical activity and pancreatic cancer
79. World Cancer Research Fund/American Institute for Cancer Research. Continuous Update Project Expert Report 2018. Body fatness and weight gain and the risk of cancer.Available at dietandcancerreport.org
80. Slavin JL, Jacobs D, Marquart L, Wiemer K. The role of whole grains in disease prevention. J Am Diet Assoc. 2001 Jul; 101(7): 780-5.
81. US Department of Health and Human Services and US Department of Agriculture. Glossary: Dietary guidelines for Americans, 2015-2020, Eighth edition. 2015.
82. Frølich W, Åman P, Tetens I. Whole grain foods and health – a Scandinavian perspective. Food Nutr Res 2013; 57.
83. Kyro C, Skeie G, Loft S, et al. Intake of whole grains from different cereal and food sources and incidence of colorectal cancer in the Scandinavian HELGA cohort. Cancer Causes Control 2013; 24: 1363-74.
84. Fung TT, Hu FB, Wu K, et al. The Mediterranean and Di-

etary Approaches to Stop Hypertension (DASH) diets and colorectal cancer. Am J Clin Nutr 2010; 92: 1429-35.
85. Schatzkin A, Mouw T, Park Y, et al. Dietary fiber and whole-grain consumption in relation to colorectal cancer in the NIH-AARP Diet and Health Study. Am J Clin Nutr 2007; 85: 1353-60.
86. McCarl M, Harnack L, Limburg PJ, et al. Incidence of colorectal cancer in relation to glycemic index and load in a cohort of women. Cancer Epidemiol Biomarkers Prev 2006; 15: 8.
87. Larsson SC, Giovannucci E, Bergkvist L, et al. Whole grain consumption and risk of colorectal cancer: a population-based cohort of 60,000 women. Br J Cancer 2005; 92: 1803-7.
88. Slavin JL. Mechanisms for the impact of whole grain foods on cancer risk. J Am Coll Nutr 2000; 19: 300s-7s.
89. Kim K-H, Tsao R, Yang R, et al. Phenolic acid profiles and antioxidant activities of wheat bran extracts and the effect of hydrolysis conditions. Food Chemistry 2006; 95: 466-73.
90. Biskup I, Kyro C, Marklund M, et al. Plasma alkylresorcinols, biomarkers of whole-grain wheat and rye intake, and risk of type 2 diabetes in Scandinavian men and women. Am J Clin Nutr 2016; 104: 88-96.
91. Murphy N, Norat T, Ferrari P, et al. Dietary fibre intake and risks of cancers of the colon and rectum in the European Prospective Investigation into Cancer and Nutrition (EPIC). PLoS One 2012; 7: e39361.
92. Kabat GC, Shikany JM, Beresford SA, et al. Dietary carbohydrate, glycemic index and glycemic load in relation to colorectal cancer risk in the Women's Health Initiative. Cancer Causes Control 2008; 19: 1291-8.
93. Nomura AM, Hankin JH, Henderson BE, et al. Dietary fiber and colorectal cancer risk: the multiethnic cohort study. Cancer Causes Control 2007; 18: 753-64.
94. Otani T, Iwasaki M, Ishihara J, et al. Dietary fiber intake and subsequent risk of colorectal cancer: the Japan Public Health Center-based prospective study. Int J Cancer 2006; 119: 1475-80.
95. Shin A, Li H, Shu XO, et al. Dietary intake of calcium, fiber and other micronutrients in relation to colorectal cancer risk: results from the Shanghai Women's Health Study. Int J Cancer 2006; 119: 2938-42.
96. Sanjoaquin MA, Appleby PN, Thorogood M, et al. Nutrition, lifestyle and colorectal cancer incidence: a prospective investigation of 10998 vegetarians and non-vegetarians in the United Kingdom. Br J Cancer 2004; 90: 118-21.
97. Lin J, Zhang SM, Cook NR, et al. Dietary intakes of fruit, vegetables and fiber, and risk of colorectal cancer in a prospective cohort of women (United States). Cancer Causes Control 2005; 16: 225-33.
98. Michels KB, Fuchs CS, Giovannucci E, et al. Fiber intake and incidence of colorectal cancer among 76,947 women and 47,279 men. Cancer Epidemiol Biomarkers Prev 2005; 14: 842-9.
99. Mai V, Flood A, Peters U, et al. Dietary fibre and risk of colorectal cancer in the Breast Cancer Detection Demonstration Project (BCDDP) follow-up cohort. Int J Epidemiol 2003; 32: 234-9.
100. Terry P, Giovannucci E, Michels KB, et al. Fruit, vegetables, dietary fiber and risk of colorectal cancer. J Natl Cancer Inst 2001; 93: 525-33.
101. Pietinen P, Malila N, Virtanen M, et al. Diet and risk of colorectal cancer in a cohort of Finnish men. Cancer Causes Control 1999; 10: 387-96.
102. Wakai K, Date C, Fukui M, et al. Dietary fiber and risk of colorectal cancer in the Japan collaborative cohort study. Cancer Epidemiol Biomarkers Prev 2007; 16: 668-75.
103. Bingham SA. Mechanisms and experimental and epidemiological evidence relating dietary fibre (non-starch polysaccharides) and starch to protection against large bowel cancer. Proc Nutr Soc 1990; 49: 153-71.
104. Pi-Sunyer X. Do glycemic index, glycemic load and fiber play a role in insulin sensitivity, disposition index and type 2 diabetes? Diabetes Care 2005; 28: 2978-9.
105. International Agency for Research on Cancer (IARC). IARC Handbooks of Cancer Prevention. Volume 8: Fruit and Vegetables. Chapter 1, Definitions and classifications for fruit and vegetables. 2003.
106. Steinmetz KA, Potter JD. Vegetables, fruit and cancer. II. Mechanisms. Cancer Causes Control 1991; 2: 427-42.
107. Freedman ND, Park Y, Subar AF, et al. Fruit and vegetable intake, and head and neck cancer risk in a large United States prospective cohort study. Int J Cancer 2008; 122: 2330-6.
108. Jin J, Ouyang Z, Wang Z. Association of fruit and vegetables with the risk of nasopharyngeal cancer: evidence from a meta-analysis. Sci Rep 2014; 4: 5229.
109. Gallicchio L, Matanoski G, Tao XG, et al. Adulthood consumption of preserved and nonpreserved vegetables and the risk of nasopharyngeal carcinoma: a systematic review. Int J Cancer 2006; 119: 1125-35.
110. Smith-Warner SA, Spiegelman D, Yaun SS, et al. Fruits, vegetables and lung cancer: a pooled analysis of cohort studies. Int J Cancer 2003; 107: 1001-11.
111. Emaus MJ, Peeters PH, Bakker MF, et al. Vegetable and fruit consumption and the risk of hormone receptor- defined breast cancer in the EPIC cohort. Am J Clin Nutr 2016; 103: 168-77.
112. Suzuki R, Iwasaki M, Hara A, et al. Fruit and vegetable intake and breast cancer risk defined by estrogen and progesterone receptor status: the Japan Public Health Center-based Prospective Study. Cancer Causes Control 2013; 24: 2117-28.
113. Boggs DA, Palmer JR, Wise LA, et al. Fruit and vegetable intake in relation to risk of breast cancer in the Black Women's Health Study. Am J Epidemiol 2010; 172: 1268-79.
114. Jung S, Spiegelman D, Baglietto L, et al. Fruit and vegetable intake and risk of breast cancer by hormone receptor status. J Natl Cancer Inst 2013; 105: 219-36.
115. Buchner FL, Bueno-de-Mesquita HB, Linseisen J, et al. Fruits and vegetables consumption and the risk of histological subtypes of lung cancer in the European Prospective Investigation into Cancer and Nutrition (EPIC). Cancer Causes Control 2010; 21: 357-71.
116. Wright ME, Park Y, Subar AF, et al. Intakes of fruit, vegetables and specific botanical groups in relation to lung cancer risk in the NIH-AARP Diet and Health Study. Am J Epidemiol 2008; 168: 1024-34.
117. Liu Y, Sobue T, Otani T, et al. Vegetables, fruit consumption and risk of lung cancer among middle-aged Japanese men and women: JPHC study. Cancer Causes Control 2004; 15: 349-57.
118. Holick CN, Michaud DS, Stolzenberg-Solomon R, et al. Dietary carotenoids, serum beta-carotene, and retinol and risk of lung cancer in the alpha-tocopherol, beta-carotene cohort study. Am J Epidemiol 2002; 156: 536-47.
119. Voorrips LE, Goldbohm RA, Verhoeven DT, et al. Vegetable and fruit consumption and lung cancer risk in the

Netherlands Cohort Study on diet and cancer. Cancer Causes Control 2000; 11: 101-15.
120. Steinmetz KA, Potter JD, Folsom AR. Vegetables, fruit and lung cancer in the Iowa Women's Health Study.Cancer Res 1993; 53: 536-43.
121. Steevens J, Schouten LJ, Goldbohm RA, et al. Vegetables and fruits consumption and risk of esophageal and gastric cancer subtypes in the Netherlands Cohort Study. Int J Cancer 2011; 129: 2681-93.
122. Freedman ND, Park Y, Subar AF, et al. Fruit and vegetable intake and esophageal cancer in a large prospective cohort study. Int J Cancer 2007; 121: 2753-60.
123. Yamaji T, Inoue M, Sasazuki S, et al. Fruit and vegetable consumption and squamous cell carcinoma of the esophagus in Japan: the JPHC study. Int J Cancer 2008; 123: 1935-40.
124. Gonzalez CA, Lujan-Barroso L, Bueno-de-Mesquita HB, et al. Fruit and vegetable intake and the risk of gastric adenocarcinoma: a reanalysis of the European Prospective Investigation into Cancer and Nutrition (EPIC- EURGAST) study after a longer follow-up. Int J Cancer 2012; 131: 2910-9.
125. Freedman ND, Subar AF, Hollenbeck AR, et al. Fruit and vegetable intake and gastric cancer risk in a large United States prospective cohort study. Cancer Causes Control 2008; 19: 459-67.
126. Hosomi R, Yoshida M, Fukunaga K. Seafood consumption and components for health. Glob J Health Sci 2012; 4(3): 72-86.
127. Oehlenschläger J. Seafood: nutritional benefits and risk aspects. Int J Vitam Nutr Res 2012; 82(3): 168-76.
128. Marushka L, Batal M, Sadik T, Schwartz H, Ing A, et al. Seafood consumption patterns, their nutritional benefits and associated sociodemographic and lifestyle factors among First Nations in British Columbia, Canada. Public Health Nutr 2018; 21(17): 3223-36.
129. World Cancer Research Fund/American Institute for Cancer Research. Continuous Update Project Expert Report 2018. Meat, fish and dairy products and the risk of cancer. Available at dietandcancerreport.org
130. WCFR. FAO/INFOODS. Global Food Composition Database for Fish and Shellfish – Version 1.0 (uFiSh1.0). 2016. Food and Agriculture Organization of the United Nations. Accessed 12/05/2017; available from http://www.fao.org/ infoods/infoods/tables-and-databases/faoinfoods-databases/en/
131. Rose DP, Connolly JM. Omega-3 fatty acid sas cancer chemopreventive agents. Pharmacol Ther 1999; 83: 217-44.
132. Ko YJ, Lii CK, Ou CC, et al. Comparison of the effect of fish oil and corno oil on chemical-induced hepatic enzyme-altered foci in rats. J Agric food Chem 2000; 48: 4144-50.
133. Lee SO, Liu H, Cinnick JE, et al. Menhden oil-inhibitedgamma-glutamyltransferase-poitive altered hepatic foci in female Sprague-Dawley rats. Nutr Cancer 2002; 44: 71-9.
134. Kaizer L, Boyd NF, Kriukov V, Tritchler D. Fish consumption and breast cancer risk: an ecological study. Nutr Cancer 1989; 12(1): 61-8.
135. World Cancer research Fund/American Institute for Cancer Research. Continuous Update Project Expert Report 2018. Recommendations and public health and policy implications.
136. FAO. Animal Production and Health – Meat and Meats Products; Meat Consumption. 2014. Food and Agriculture Organization of the United Nations. Accessed 12/05/2017; available from http://www.fao.org/ag/againfo/themes/en/meat/background.html
137. FAO. FAOSTAT Food Balance Sheets. 2017. Food and Agriculture Organization of the United Nations. Accessed 12/05/2017; available from http://www.fao.org/faostat/en/#data/FBS
138. Norat T, Bingham S, Ferrari P, et al. Meat, fish, and colorectal cancer risk: the European Prospective Investigation into cancer and nutrition. J Natl Cancer Inst 2005; 97: 906-16.
139. Ollberding NJ, Wilkens LR, Henderson BE, et al. Meat consumption, heterocyclic amines and colorectal cancer risk: The Multiethnic Cohort Study. Int J Cancer 2012; 131: 1125-33.
140. Lee SA, Shu XO, Yang G, et al. Animal origin foods and colorectal cancer risk: a report from the Shanghai Women's Health Study. Nutr Cancer 2009; 61: 194-205.
141. Larsson SC, Rafter J, Holmberg L, et al. Red meat consumption and risk of cancers of the proximal colon, distal colon and rectum: the Swedish Mammography Cohort. Int J Cancer 2005; 113: 829-34.
142. English DR, MacInnis RJ, Hodge AM, et al. Red meat, chicken, and fish consumption and risk of colorectal cancer. Cancer Epidemiol Biomarkers Prev 2004; 13: 1509-14.
143. Tiemersma EW, Kampman E, Bueno de Mesquita HB, et al. Meat consumption, cigarette smoking, and genetic susceptibility in the etiology of colorectal cancer: results from a Dutch prospective study. Cancer Causes Control 2002; 13: 383-93.
144. Jarvinen R, Knekt P, Hakulinen T, et al. Dietary fat, cholesterol and colorectal cancer in a prospective study. Br J Cancer 2001; 85: 357-61.
145. Cross AJ and Sinha R. Meat-related mutagens/carcinogens in the etiology of colorectal cancer. Environ Mol Mutagen 2004; 44: 44-55.
146. Cross AJ, Pollock JR, Bingham SA. Haem, not protein or inorganic iron, is responsible for endogenous intestinal N-nitrosation arising from red meat. Cancer Research 2003; 63: 2358-60.
147. Bouvard V, Loomis D, Guyton KZ, et al. Carcinogenicity of consumption of red and processed meat. Lancet Oncol 2015; 16: 1599-600.
148. World Cancer Research Fund/American Institute for Cancer Research. Continuous Update Project Expert Report 2018. Diet, nutrition, physical activity and cancers of the mouth, pharynx and larynx.
149. World Cancer Research Fund/American Institute for Cancer Research. Continuous Update Project Expert Report 2018. Diet, nutrition, physical activity and oesophageal cancer.
150. World Cancer Research Fund/American Institute for Cancer Research. Continuous Update Project Expert Report 2018. Diet, nutrition, physical activity and stomach cancer.
151. World Cancer Research Fund/American Institute for Cancer Research. Continuous Update Project Expert Report 2018. Diet, nutrition, physical activity and liver cancer.
152. World Cancer Research Fund/American Institute for Cancer Research. Continuous Update Project Expert Report 2018. Diet, nutrition, physical activity and breast cancer.
153. World Cancer Research Fund/American Institute for Cancer Research. Continuous Update Project Expert Report 2018. Diet, nutrition, physical activity and ovarian cancer.
154. World Cancer Research Fund/American Institute for Cancer Research. Continuous Update Project Expert Report 2018. Diet, nutrition, physical activity and endometrial cancer.

155. World Cancer Research Fund/American Institute for Cancer Research. Continuous Update Project Expert Report 2018. Diet, nutrition, physical activity and prostate cancer.
156. World Cancer Research Fund/American Institute for Cancer Research. Continuous Update Project Expert Report 2018. Diet, nutrition, physical activity and kidney cancer.
157. World Cancer Research Fund/American Institute for Cancer Research. Continuous Update Project Expert Report 2018. Diet, nutrition, physical activity and bladder cancer.
158. World Cancer Research Fund/American Institute for Cancer Research. Continuous Update Project 2017. The Associations between Food, Nutrition and Physical Activity and the Risk of Skin Cancer. https://www.wcrf.org/sites/default/files/Skin-cancer-slr.pdf
159. Cross AJ, Ferrucci LM, Risch A, et al. A large prospective study of meat consumption and colorectal cancer risk: an investigation of potential mechanisms underlying this association. Cancer Research 2010; 70: 2406-14.
160. Balder HF, Vogel J, Jansen MC, et al. Heme and chlorophyll intake and risk of colorectal cancer in the Netherlands cohort study. Cancer Epidemiol Biomarkers Prev 2006; 15: 717-25.
161. Sato Y, Nakaya N, Kuriyama S, et al. Meat consumption and risk of colorectal cancer in Japan: the Miyagi Cohort Study. Eur J Cancer Prev 2006; 15: 211-8.
162. Lin J, Zhang SM, Cook NR, et al. Dietary fat and fatty acids and risk of colorectal cancer in women. Am J Epidemiol 2004; 160: 1011-22.
163. Flood A, Velie EM, Sinha R, et al. Meat, fat, and their subtypes as risk factors for colorectal cancer in a prospective cohort of women. Am J Epidemiol 2003; 158: 59-68.
164. Pietinen P, Malila N, Virtanen M, et al. Diet and risk of colorectal cancer in a cohort of Finnish men. Cancer Causes Control 1999; 10: 387-96.
165. Santarelli RL, Pierre F, Corpet DE. Processed meat and colorectal cancer: a review of epidemiologic and experimental evidence. Nutr Cancer 2008; 60: 131-44.
166. Henney JT, CL. Boon, CS. Institute of Medicine (US) Committee on Strategies to Reduce Sodium Intake in the United States. 2010, Washington, DC: National Academies Press, 2010.
167. World Health Organisation (WHO). Guideline: Sodium Intake for Adults and Children. 2012.
168. World Cancer Research Fund/American Institute for Cancer Research. Continuous Update Project Expert Report 2018. Diet, nutrition, physical activity and oesophageal cancer.
169. World Cancer Research Fund/American Institute for Cancer Research. Continuous Update Project Expert Report 2018. Diet, nutrition, physical activity and lung cancer.
170. Takachi R, Inoue M, Shimazu T, et al. Consumption of sodium and salted foods in relation to cancer and cardiovascular disease: the Japan Public Health Center-based Prospective Study. Am J Clin Nutr 2010; 91: 456-64.
171. Iso H, Kubota Y. Nutrition and disease in the Japan Collaborative Cohort Study for Evaluation of Cancer (JACC). Asian Pac J Cancer Prev 2007; 8 Suppl: 35-80.
172. Sauvaget C, Lagarde F, Nagano J, et al. Lifestyle factors, radiation and gastric cancer in atomic-bomb survivors (Japan). Cancer Causes Control 2005; 16: 773-80.
173. Ngoan LT, Mizoue T, Fujino Y, et al. Dietary factors and stomach cancer mortality. Br J Cancer 2002; 87: 37-42.
174. Botterweck AA, van den Brandt PA, Goldbohm RA. A prospective cohort study on vegetable and fruit consumption and stomach cancer risk in The Netherlands. Am J Epidemiol 1998; 148: 842-53.
175. Galanis DJ, Kolonel LN, Lee J, et al. Intakes of selected foods and beverages and the incidence of gastric cancer among the Japanese residents of Hawaii: a prospective study. Int J Epidemiol 1998; 27: 173-80.
176. Kato I, Tominaga S, Matsumoto K. A prospective study of stomach cancer among a rural Japanese population: a 6-year survey. Jpn J Cancer Res 1992; 83: 568-75.
177. Kato I, Tominaga S, Ito Y, et al. A prospective study of atrophic gastritis and stomach cancer risk. Jpn J Cancer Res 1992; 83: 1137-42.
178. Nomura A, Grove JS, Stemmermann GN, et al. A prospective study of stomach cancer and its relation to diet, cigarettes, and alcohol consumption. Cancer Research 1990; 50: 627-31.
179. Tatematsu M, Takahashi M, Fukushima S, et al. Effects in rats of sodium chloride on experimental gastric cancers induced by N-methyl-N-nitro-N-nitrosoguanidine or 4-nitroquinoline-1-oxide. J Natl Cancer Inst 1975; 55: 101-6.
180. Fox JG, Dangler CA, Taylor NS, et al. High-salt diet induces gastric epithelial hyperplasia and parietal cell loss, and enhances Helicobacter pylori colonization in C57BL/6 mice. Cancer Research 1999; 59: 4823-8.
181. Furihata C, Ohta H, Katsuyama T. Cause and effect between concentration-dependent tissue damage and temporary cell proliferation in rat stomach mucosa by NaCl, a stomach tumor promoter. Carcinogenesis 1996; 17: 401-6.
182. World Cancer Research Fund/American Institute for Cancer Research. Continuous Update Project Expert Report 2018. Meat, fish and dairy products and the risk of cancer. Available at dietandcancerreport.org
183. Loomis D, Guyton KZ, Grosse Y, et al. Carcinogenicity of drinking coffee, mate, and very hot beverages. Lancet Oncol 2016; 17: 877-8.
184. International Agency for Research on Cancer (IARC). IARC Monographs on the Evaluation of Carcinogenic Risks to Humans. Volume 51: Coffee, tea, mate, methylxanthines and methylglyoxal. 1991.
185. Szymanska K, Matos E, Hung RJ, et al. Drinking of mate and the risk of cancers of the upper aerodigestive tract in Latin America: a case-control study. Cancer Causes Control 2010; 21: 1799-806.
186. Vassallo A, Correa P, De Stefani E, et al. Esophageal cancer in Uruguay: a case-control study. J Natl Cancer Inst 1985; 75: 1005-9.
187. De Stefani E, Munoz N, Esteve J, et al. Mate drinking, alcohol, tobacco, diet, and esophageal cancer in Uruguay. Cancer Research 1990; 50: 426-31.
188. Rolon PA, Castellsague X, Benz M, et al. Hot and cold mate drinking and esophageal cancer in Paraguay. Cancer Epidemiol Biomarkers Prev 1995; 4: 595-605.
189. Sewram V, De Stefani E, Brennan P, et al. Mate consumption and the risk of squamous cell esophageal cancer in Uruguay. Cancer Epidemiol Biomarkers Prev 2003; 12: 508-13.
190. De Stefani E, Deneo-Pellegrini H, Ronco AL, et al. Food groups and risk of squamous cell carcinoma of the oesophagus: a case-control study in Uruguay. Br J Cancer 2003; 89: 1209-14.
191. Lubin JH, De SE, Abnet CC, et al. Mate drinking and esophageal squamous cell carcinoma in South America: pooled

results from two large multicenter case-control studies. Cancer Epidemiol Biomarkers Prev 2014;23: 107-16.
192. Andrici J, Eslick GD. Mate consumption and the risk of esophageal squamous cell carcinoma: a meta-analysis. Dis Esophagus 2013; 26: 807-16.
193. Rapozo DC, Blanco TC, Reis BB, et al. Recurrent acute thermal lesion induces esophageal hyperproliferative premalignant lesions in mice esophagus. Exp Mol Pathol 2016; 100: 325-31.
194. Johnson S, Koh WP, Wang R, et al. Coffee consumption and reduced risk of hepatocellular carcinoma: findings from the Singapore Chinese Health Study. Cancer Causes Control 2011; 22: 503-10.
195. Hu G, Tuomilehto J, Pukkala E, et al. Joint effects of coffee consumption and serum gamma-glutamyltransferase on the risk of liver cancer. Hepatology 2008; 48: 129-36.
196. Inoue M, Yoshimi I, Sobue T, et al. Influence of coffee drinking on subsequent risk of hepatocellular carcinoma: a prospective study in Japan. J Natl Cancer Inst 2005; 97: 293-300.
197. Shimazu T, Tsubono Y, Kuriyama S, et al. Coffee consumption and the risk of primary liver cancer: pooled analysis of two prospective studies in Japan. Int J Cancer 2005; 116: 150-4.
198. Bravi F, Bosetti C, Tavani A, et al. Coffee reduces risk for hepatocellular carcinoma: an updated meta-analysis. Clin Gastroenterol Hepatol 2013; 11: 1413-21.
199. Sang LX, Chang B, Li XH, et al. Consumption of coffee associated with reduced risk of liver cancer: a meta-analysis. BMC Gastroenterol 2013; 13: 34.
200. Salomone F, Galvano F, Li Volti G. Molecular bases underlying the hepatoprotective effects of coffee. Nutrients 2017; 9: 85.
201. Otake T, Fukumoto J, Abe M, et al. Linking lifestyle factors and insulin resistance, based on fasting plasma insulin and HOMA-IR in middle-aged Japanese men: a cross-sectional study. Scand J Clin Lab Invest 2014; 74: 536-45.
202. Shang F, Li X and Jiang X. Coffee consumption and risk of the metabolic syndrome: a meta-analysis. Diabetes Metab 2016; 42: 80-7.
203. Dickson JC, Liese AD, Lorenzo C, et al. Associations of coffee consumption with markers of liver injury in the insulin resistance atherosclerosis study. BMC Gastroenterol 2015; 15: 88.
204. Shimazu T, Inoue M, Sasazuki S, et al. Coffee consumption and risk of endometrial cancer: a prospective study in Japan. Int J Cancer 2008; 123: 2406-10.
205. Giri A, Sturgeon SR, Luisi N, et al. Caffeinated coffee, decaffeinated coffee and endometrial cancer risk: a prospective cohort study among US postmenopausal women. Nutrients 2011; 3: 937-50.
206. Gunter MJ, Schaub JA, Xue X, et al. A prospective investigation of coffee drinking and endometrial cancer incidence. Int J Cancer 2011; 131: E530-6.
207. Je Y, Hankinson SE, Tworoger SS, et al. A prospective cohort study of coffee consumption and risk of endometrial cancer over a 26-year follow-up. Cancer Epidemiol Biomarkers Prev 2011; 20: 2487-95.
208. Nilsson LM, Johansson I, Lenner P, et al. Consumption of filtered and boiled coffee and the risk of incident cancer: a prospective cohort study. Cancer Causes Control 2010; 21: 1533-44.
209. Friberg E, Orsini N, Mantzoros CS, et al. Coffee drinking and risk of endometrial cancer – a population-based cohort study. Int J Cancer 2009; 125: 2413-7.
210. Stensvold I and Jacobsen BK. Coffee and cancer: A prospective study of 43,000 Norwegian men and women. Cancer Causes Control 1994; 5: 401-8.
211. Ferrini RL, Barrett-Connor E. Caffeine intake and endogenous sex steroid levels in postmenopausal women. The Rancho Bernardo Study. Am J Epidemiol 1996; 144: 642-4.
212. Nagata C, Kabuto M, Shimizu H. Association of coffee, green tea, and caffeine intakes with serum concentrations of estradiol and sex hormone-binding globulin in premenopausal Japanese women. Nutr Cancer 1998; 30: 21-4.
213. London S, Willett W, Longcope C, et al. Alcohol and other dietary factors in relation to serum hormone concentrations in women at climacteric. Am J Clin Nutr 1991; 53: 166-71.
214. Wu T, Willett WC, Hankinson SE, et al. Caffeinated coffee, decaffeinated coffee, and caffeine in relation to plasma C-peptide levels, a marker of insulin secretion, in U.S. women. Diabetes Care 2005; 28: 1390-6.
215. Kotsopoulos J, Eliassen AH, Missmer SA, et al. Relationship between caffeine intake and plasma sex hormone concentrations in premenopausal and postmenopausal women. Cancer 2009; 115: 2765-74.
216. Williams CJ, Fargnoli JL, Hwang JJ, et al. Coffee consumption is associated with higher plasma adiponectin concentrations in women with or without type 2 diabetes: a prospective cohort study. Diabetes Care 2008; 31: 504-7.
217. Yamashita K, Yatsuya H, Muramatsu T, et al. Association of coffee consumption with serum adiponectin, leptin, inflammation and metabolic markers in Japanese workers: a cross-sectional study. Nutr Diabetes 2012; 2.
218. Cust AE, Kaaks R, Friedenreich C, et al. Metabolic syndrome, plasma lipid, lipoprotein and glucose levels, and endometrial cancer risk in the European Prospective Investigation into Cancer and Nutrition (EPIC). Endocr Relat Cancer 2007; 14: 755-67.
219. Luhn P, Dallal CM, Weiss JM, et al. Circulating adipokine levels and endometrial cancer risk in the prostate, lung, colorectal and ovarian cancer screening trial. Cancer Epidemiol Biomarkers Prev 2013; 22: 1304-12.
220. Lee WJ and Zhu BT. Inhibition of DNA methylation by caffeic acid and chlorogenic acid, two common catechol-containing coffee polyphenols. Carcinogenesis 2006; 27: 269-77.
221. Olthof MR, Hollman PCH, Katan MB. Chlorogenic acid and caffeic acid are absorbed in humans. J Nut 2001; 131: 66-71.
222. Lee K-A, Chae J-I, Shim J-H. Natural diterpenes from coffee, cafestol and kahweol induce apoptosis through regulation of specificity protein 1 expression in human malignant pleural mesothelioma. J Biomed Sci 2012; 19: 60.
223. Cavin C, Holzhaeuser D, Scharf G, et al. Cafestol and kahweol, two coffee-specific diterpenes with anticarcinogenic activity. Food and Chemical Toxicology 2002; 40: 1155-63.
224. International Agency for Research on Cancer (IARC). IARC Monographs on the Evaluation of Carcinogenic Risks to Humans. Volume 100, Part C: Arsenic, metals, fibres and dusts. 2012.
225. Chung CJ, Huang YL, Huang YK, et al. Urinary arsenic profiles and the risks of cancer mortality: A population-based 20-year follow-up study in arseniasis-endemic areas in Taiwan. Environ Res 2013; 122: 25-30.
226. Tsuda T, Babazono A, Yamamoto E, et al. Ingested arsenic and internal cancer: a historical cohort study followed for

33 years. Am J Epidemiol 1995; 141: 198-209.
227. Chen CL, Chiou HY, Hsu LI, et al. Ingested arsenic, characteristics of well water consumption and risk of different histological types of lung cancer in northeastern Taiwan. Environ Res 2010; 110: 455-62.
228. Baastrup R, Sorensen M, Balstrom T, et al. Arsenic in drinking-water and risk for cancer in Denmark. Environ Health Perspect 2008; 116: 231-7.
229. Singh AP, Goel RK and Kaur T. Mechanisms pertaining to arsenic toxicity. Toxicol Int 2011; 18: 87-93.
230. Yang C, Frenkel K. Arsenic-mediated cellular signal transduction, transcription factor activation, and aberrant gene expression: implications in carcinogenesis. J Environ Pathol Toxicol Oncol 2002; 21: 331-42.
231. Chen CL, Chiou HY, Hsu LI, et al. Arsenic in drinking water and risk of urinary tract cancer: a follow-up study from northeastern Taiwan. Cancer Epidemiol Biomarkers Prev 2010; 19: 101-10.
232. Michaud DS, Wright ME, Cantor KP, et al. Arsenic concentrations in prediagnostic toenails and the risk of bladder cancer in a cohort study of male smokers. Am J Epidemiol 2004; 160: 853-9.
233. Kurttio P, Pukkala E, Kahelin H, et al. Arsenic concentrations in well water and risk of bladder and kidney cancer in Finland. Environ Health Perspect 1999; 107: 705-10.
234. Lewis DR, Southwick JW, Ouellet-Hellstrom R, et al. Drinking water arsenic in Utah: a cohort mortality study. Environ Health Perspect 1999; 107: 359-65.
235. Hsueh YM, Chiou HY, Huang YL, et al. Serum beta-carotene level, arsenic methylation capability, and incidence of skin cancer. Cancer Epidemiol Biomarkers Prev 1997; 6: 589-96.

30 Gender and nutrition

Sabina Saccomanno, Anna di Tullio and Carlo De Collibus

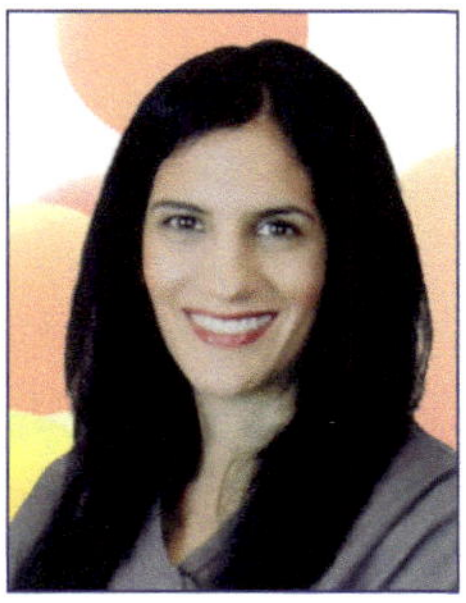

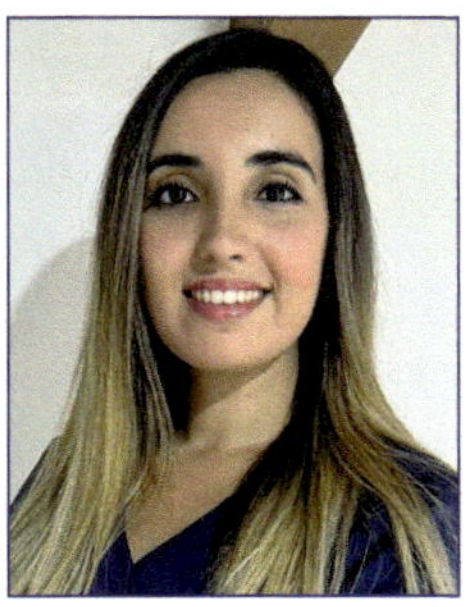

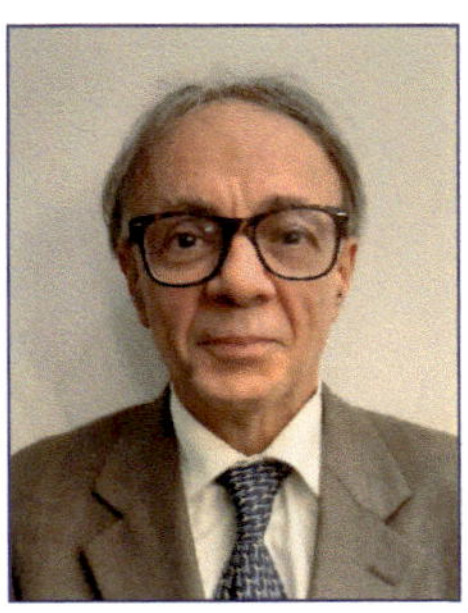

Gender medicine aims to understand the mechanisms by which gender-related differences affect the state of health and the onset and course of many diseases, as well as prevention and outcome of therapies. In fact, although men and women are subject to the same pathologies, they present very different symptoms, disease progression and response to treatments. Hence the need to pay particular attention to the study of gender, inserting this "new" dimension of medicine in all medical areas.

30.1 Nutrition in general, diseases and their prevalence in females

There are many gender differences in chronicity, more evident in advanced ages. An example concerns the calculation of cardiovascular risk using the risk card of the Italian Heart Project. It was found that non-diabetic and non-smoking women never reach a high level of risk, while for smokers this risk level is not reached until age 60-69, with significantly high cholesterol and systolic blood pressure values. Diabetic women have a significantly higher risk of coronary heart disease and tend to develop more cardiovascular events than diabetic men. The impact of diabetes on the risk of coronary death not only nullifies the "female advantage" but is significantly higher in women than men. As for obesity, its consequences are worse than men because diabetic complication is much more pronounced among obese women.

Pathologies of the psyche are also unfortunately more frequent in women, and they are increasing. In particular, depression is the main cause of disability for women aged 15-44. As for neurological diseases, the prevalence of Alzheimer's dementia is significantly higher in women. Among the medical disciplines, endocrinology is probably the one that is mostly involved with issues related to gender medicine. Hormones, in fact, determine male or female gender, but their role is much more complex, as they also are responsible for men and women presenting important differences in health. In fact, the most common endocrinological diseases, namely thyropathies and diabetes, have marked gender differences. For example, thyroid disorders are present in women 5-8 times more than in men.

Bronchial asthma is a widespread chronic inflammatory respiratory pathology, the prevalence of which is greater in boys during childhood (male/female ratio of

Sabina Saccomanno, DDS
Department of Life, Health and Environmental Sciences, University of L'Aquila, L'Aquila, Italy

Email: sabinasaccomanno@hotmail.it

Anna di Tullio, SLT
Speech Therapist in Private Practice

Carlo De Collibus,
Coordiantor of "External Health Management", INPS General Medical Legal Coordination, Rome, Italy

2:1), while in puberty there is an inversion of this ratio. It is probable that the hormonal changes present in women between 11 and 14 years of age, and in the subsequent variations of the menstrual cycle, are responsible for this reversal of prevalence between the two sexes. In fact, the activity exerted by female sex hormones on the release of inflammatory cytokines involved in the pathogenesis of the asthmatic reaction has been demonstrated [1].

A high percentage of women with asthmatic pathology (about 40-50%) show significant worsening of symptoms during the preovulatory phase, associated with a preponderant secretion of estrogen and low levels of progesterone [2].

Research on gender differences in the immune response focused on two main aspects: the endocrinological aspect, i.e., the effects of sex hormones, and the genetic aspect, i.e., the effect of sex chromosomes, which are involved in the immune response.

Even in the field of oncology, epidemiological studies have highlighted significant gender differences also in the incidence, aggression, progression, prognosis and response to therapy in many types of tumors common to the two genders. Excluding skin cancer, the five most frequently diagnosed cancers among men are prostate cancer (18.1%), colorectal cancer (14.8%), lung cancer (14.3%), bladder cancer (11%) and kidney cancer (4.6%). Among women, the most frequently diagnosed tumors are breast cancer (29.3%), colorectal cancer (12.6%), lung cancer (11.1%), thyroid cancer (5.8%) [3, 4]. A 2009 study on 23,800 women in Germany reported that they were diagnosed with one of these three gynecological cancers: cervical cancer (20.3%), endometrial cancer (48.5%) or ovarian cancer (31.2%) [5].

Gender differences exist in obesity: understanding how and why metabolic processes differ in the two genders will allow doctors to target and customize gender-based therapies. The two genders differ in the distribution of adipose tissue: males tend to accumulate more visceral fat, which leads to the classic "apple" body shape, which has been strongly correlated to an increased cardiovascular risk, while females accumulate more subcutaneous and interstitial fat before menopause, a feature that offers protection against the negative consequences associated with obesity and metabolic syndrome. After menopause, the deposition of fat is similar to that in the male and is also accompanied by a parallel increase in metabolic risk.

Obstructive sleep apnea (OSA) occurs with a prevalence of 9% in women and 24% in men (male/female ratio of 3:1). The higher prevalence in men seems to be related to endocrine factors; moreover, there is evidence of an increased level of androgens in women suffering from this pathology. In postmenopause the difference in prevalence between the two sexes is no longer evident and in females a 3-fold increase in the risk of OSAs has been described. Obesity is frequently related to OSAs and constitutes its main risk factor.

Osteoporosis is a disease that affects the female gender most but has an impact that is far from negligible even in men, for whom it can have more serious consequences. It is estimated that around one in five men over 50 years of age, worldwide, will sooner or later suffer a fracture due to osteoporosis. In most cases, in men, even after a fracturing event, the disease is not diagnosed and treated. For a man, a life-long risk of suffering a fracture (up to 27% in those over 50 years of age) is higher than the risk of developing prostate cancer (11.3%), but few are aware of it. As with women, the mortality rate after a femur fracture increases with age and is higher in the 12 months after the event. However, in the first 6 months, mortality is approximately double in men compared to women of the same age. In general, although fragility fractures are more prevalent among women, mortality rates following a fracture are higher in men and men are more likely to report serious consequences after the event. Men, therefore, should be aware of the risks they run and seek to prevent the disease also through nutrition, reduce modifiable risk factors and pay attention to those that cannot be modified. The risk factors for osteoporosis for men are largely superimposable to those of women, but two more factors can be added: the lack of testosterone (primary or secondary hypogonadism) and the possible use of androgen deprivation therapy (ADT), a treatment used in some cases to fight prostate cancer. In the presence of these risk factors, any man between 50 and 69 years of age should undergo a computerized bone mineralometry to assess whether he has osteoporosis. The examination to evaluate bone density should be performed in any case once a man reaches age 70, and if the man has already suffered a fracture following a fall after age 50, if he is being treated with steroids or ADT and if he has low testosterone levels.

The study of gender in relation to bone metabolism is particularly interesting since men have a greater bone mass than women, which makes osteoporosis less frequent in them by a 1:4 ratio for women and 1:10 for men. This figure has completely shifted the focus on female osteoporosis both with regards to diagnosis: out of 1,000 MOCs 55 are conducted on men and 945 in women; prevention: many women take calcium and vitamin D supplements during menopause; therapeutic strategies: for many women, hormone replacement therapy is available to correct estrogen deficiency in menopause. About 20% of all femur fractures occur in the males while the incidence of vertebral fractures is about half that of those in females. However, mortality and morbidity from vertebral and femoral fractures are higher in males than in females because osteoporosis in males is often not diagnosed.

30.2 Nutrition and body weight

Scientific research has revealed differences in food consumption and eating behavior in the two genders [6]. Studies conducted in modern Western societies report associations between gender and specific foods, in which meat (especially red), alcohol and abundant portion sizes are associated with the male gender, while vegetables, fruit, fish and acidic dairy products (such as yogurt or soft cheeses) are associated with females. Among the most relevant differences in the two genders are the relationship between eating habits and awareness of health and the relationship between eating behavior and weight control. Women generally show a tendency to give preference to healthier foods and are much more interested in the importance of food choices and eating behavior to stay in good physical shape. This attitude is reflected in the nutritional pattern. The higher intake of fruit and vegetables represents one of the elements that characterize the dietary profile of the female gender. Excess weight represents an important risk factor for many chronic diseases, such as cardiovascular diseases, diabetes and some types of neoplasms. Worldwide, since 1980 there has been an increase in the prevalence of overweight and obesity, with a greater increase between 1992 and 2002 followed by a slowdown, then a plateau or slower growth in the last decade, especially in developed countries. As an example, according to data from the Organization for Economic Co-operation and Development (OECD) based on self-reported weight and height, in Italy obesity would affect 10.4% of the population over 15 years of age or more, one of the lowest values recorded in Europe. In more rigorous studies that measured weight and height, the prevalence of obesity in Italy in adults over 20 years of age would be 18.6% in males and 17.7% in females, but still lower than the average of Western European countries (20.5% in males and 21% in females). If the data for adults places Italy among those with a lower prevalence, the same cannot be said for children: the comparison of children age 6-9 among 12 European nations showed that, unfortunately, obesity for Italian children is among the highest [7].

30.3 Gender-related differences

To understand how biological differences can influence or be related to nutrition, it is important to know the different physiological stages of life in different genders.

30.3.1 Girls

A study found that high consumption of fruit and vegetables appears to be protective against cervical intraepithelial neoplasia (CIN). A diet rich in antioxidants, minerals and vitamins would also prevent the progression of transient and persistent human papilloma virus (HPV) infections to high-grade CIN 2 and 3 (including *in situ* cervical cancer). The protective effect of diet is not significant for high-risk HPV persistent infections and invasive cervical cancer [8]. However, since the evidence is not available from controlled studies, it is important to monitor vaccination for HPV and rubella especially in girls.

30.3.2 Women

A woman has certain and specific nutritional needs during the various periods of her life, from puberty to menopause. Gender nutrition can support these needs through the integration of fundamental nutrients such as iron, which is necessary for the formation of red blood cells and to contribute to energy metabolism. Regular intake of iron in women is required to cope with blood losses due to the menstrual cycle, while vitamin C is useful to increase iron absorption. Calcium intake is of paramount importance, especially leading up to adolescence, for the formation of bones and the maintenance of normal bone density throughout life, having women a greater risk of developing osteoporosis with menopause. Folic acid is useful for its role in the formation of red blood cells and the consequent contribution to the reduction of tiredness and fatigue; it is also an important substance for women of childbearing age, as a prevention of embryonic malformations such as spina bifida. Folic acid is found in leafy vegetables, spinach, citrus, cereals and beans.

30.3.3 Female puberty

During puberty, young women often have a concern about their body image and weight. In some cases, this concern can lead girls to undertake, without medical or parental supervision, low-calorie and often unbalanced diets, as they are self-designed and self-managed. During puberty, two types of eating disorders can occur, which have now become "a social epidemic", as a result of the globalization of social models and stereotypes and the cultural transformations of family eating habits [9].

Anorexia nervosa

Anorexia causes the reduction or interruption of the usual diet, with an 85% reduction in normal weight for one's age, sex and height. It is a consequence of the refusal to eat food, determined by an intense fear of gaining weight or becoming fat. Often, an anorexic person begins by avoiding all foods deemed fatty and concentrating on "healthy" and low-calorie foods, with an obsessive attention to the caloric content and composition of the foods and the weighing scale. Meals are frequently avoided or consumed with extreme slowness, mulling over each swallowed bite. According to the Italian Institute of Health (ISS), in anorexic persons, the body is perceived and experienced in an altered way, with an excess of attention to the form and with the frequent refusal to admit the seriousness of the current underweight condition [10]. All eating disorders are more frequent in females than in males: in studies conducted on clinical populations, men represent 5-10% of all cases of anorexia nervosa, and 10-15% of cases of bulimia nervosa.

Bulimia nervosa

People with bulimia tend to ingest an excessive amount of food, followed by a deep sense of guilt, for which they tend to punish themselves by vomiting, ingesting diuretic pills and laxatives with the intention of losing weight. In the long run, bulimic subjects enter a phase of depression and self-loathing and try to hide this behavior from others. Eventually physical form and appearance end up becoming a permanent obsession and having strong repercussions on one's self-esteem. A study by Wilson and Shafran [11] indicated that bulimia is more responsive than anorexia to cognitive behavioral therapy rather than other psychological or drug treatments.

30.4 Food and puberal development

Nutrient requirements during puberal development increase rapidly, until then gradually reaching adult levels, to support body growth (for example, iron needs doubles in females). In particular, the need for protein, iron, calcium and vitamins A, C and D increases. It is important to maintain a balanced body weight. Leptins, substances produced by fat cells, are produced in greater quantities in overweight girls and this can accelerate puberal development. Even endocrine disruptors, molecules that interact with normal hormonal function found in various substances including plant protection products, can cause alterations such as early puberty, infertility and polycystic ovary syndrome. Therefore, it becomes essential to keep an eye on the quality of the food, especially meat, fish and dairy products, but also vegetables, fruit and cereals, and it is always better to bring untreated or organic food to the table.

Juvenile acne is very common in puberal females, due to the increase in sex hormones, which occurs markedly during this age. In particular, the presence of androgens induces an enlargement of the sebaceous glands present in the hair follicle that increase the production of sebum that promotes bacterial proliferation. Individual factors also contribute to the genesis of juvenile acne, such as a genetic predisposition, the intake of certain medications, stress and incorrect nutrition.

30.5 Pregnancy

During pregnancy, it is essential to follow a balanced diet, introducing the calories and nutrients necessary to stay healthy and to ensure the formation of new tissues and energy reserves that will be used during breastfeeding. The availability of polyunsaturated fatty acids in the mother affects the intake of nutrients by the fetus. During pregnancy, a strong transfer of lipids occurs, which are mobilized from maternal deposits to the fetus through the placenta. Essential fatty acids are very important for neonatal growth, especially in regard to omega-3. It is important to include fish in the diet at least once a week from the thirtieth week of gestation until the end of breastfeeding. This inclusion of fish or omega-3 in the diet is useful both for fetal development (greater birth weight) and for the mother since it improves pregnancy (the healthy presence of essential fatty acids decreases the risk of premature births) and reduces the incidence of postpartum depression. The intake of omega-3, in fact, is needed by the child for the correct development of the central nervous system and the cardiovascular system. Long-chain polyunsaturated fatty acids usually found in fish such as salmon, tuna and mackerel, in fruit such as avocado, in seeds, eggs, legumes, walnuts and hazelnuts, are fundamental in fetal and neonatal development for the formation of new tissues and, in particular, cell membranes [12]. Supplemental nutrients such as iodine, vitamins and other deficient elements are needed if the diet is unbalanced. Iodine is a constituent of thyroid hormones and is therefore implicated in a correct morphogenesis of organs and systems, as well as in the thermogenesis and metabolism of carbohydrates, proteins and fats. A deficiency of iodine causes cretinism, hypothyroidism and smaller infants compared to gestational age. It is also important to monitor the use of drugs and certain medications in fertile women to avoid the use of potentially embryotoxic drugs, improve overall lifestyle and limit the use of sugars to prevent pregnancy diabetes [13].

30.6 Menopause

With menopause, the usual balance between estrogen, progesterone and testosterone breaks apart. Specifically, a woman undergoes a drop in estrogen secondary to the shutdown of ovarian function while these hormones continue to be produced, albeit at lower concentrations, by the adrenal glands, by the cells of the adipose tissue and skin, and by the liver and kidneys. It is important for a woman to compensate through nutrition this relative prevalence of androgens, typical of the arrival of menopause. This is a delicate phase in which, wanting to modulate body changes and prevent the onset of pathologies, certain foods should be reduced, for example aged cheeses, hard-boiled eggs and red meat. The consumption of these foods should be reduced due to their specific amino acid profile which activates the production of androgenic hormones at the adrenal level, precisely those which are in excess in women once the ovarian activity has ceased. Through gender-based nutrition it is important to stimulate the intake of cholesterol as much as possible into the synthesis pathway of estrogen, so as to compensate for the estrogen drop in menopause. It is not only important to reduce animal proteins, but it is also important to pay attention to the glycemic index of foods to eliminate or reduce refined sugars and flours and increase or introduce whole grains and legumes as well as good fats such as extra virgin olive oil, avocado, walnuts and oil seeds. Moreover, it is essential to activate liver functions with consumption of olive oil. The liver, in fact, has a very important role in the production and metabolism of estrogen after menopause.

30.7 Boys

Ankyloglossia, or significant shortening of the free lingual portion (lingual frenulum or frenum), is an anatomical condition characterized by the limitation of the movement of the tongue, which can have a strong impact on its function, including interfering in the formation of the dental arches and their subsequent occlusion. This condition affects males more than females, with a ratio of 3:1 and with an incidence of 5% reported at birth [14]. A study by Walsh et al. [15] indicated that a diagnosis of ankyloglossia was more likely to be found in boys, with private insurance, and from a higher than median income level suggesting that socioeconomics, cultural aspects and local practices play a role in the diagnosis and treatment of a restricted lingual frenum. In early childhood, the clinical presentation of symptomatic ankyloglossia involves breastfeeding difficulties [16] with evidence of irritability due to poor nutrition, inability to breastfeed by the mother and poor weight gain of the baby [17]. The mother of a baby with ankyloglossia may experience pain during breastfeeding, resulting in ulceration, bleeding, infections or mastitis of the nipple, poor milk release due to inadequate sucking or incomplete emptying. Breastfeeding difficulty can lead to maternal and child frustration, maternal anxiety, feelings of failure or inadequacy and premature abandonment of breastfeeding [18]. An early diagnosis at birth is important to prevent feeding problems in the child [19]. Teething also appears later in boys than in girls.

30.8 Male puberty

Adolescence is characterized by an uncontrolled explosion of physical, social, psychological and sexual changes, the acceptance of which may require a period of adjustment. In males, this process starts later than in females. In such a delicate and complex phase, nutrition plays a fundamental role, and it is precisely at this age, in fact, that the foundations are laid for proper nutrition. Proper nutrition will allow the completion of an adequate psychophysical development and will contribute to the prevention of certain diseases such as: osteoporosis (a consequence of poor bone mineralization in adolescence); the appearance and/or persistence of obesity (and related complications); eating disorders (anorexia and bulimia) which show their peak in adolescence. In men, during puberty, it is appropriate to include nutrients such as calcium and phosphorus in the diet, to support the rapid accumulation of skeletal mass. In particular, different quantities of nutrients intake are necessary, based on the different needs of the two genders. In this period, great discomforts and fears appear, which are reflected in a possible conflictual relationship with food and with one's body image. In this phase, the adolescent affirms his autonomy and often shuns all kinds of regulations and controls, even in the diet: meal irregularities are frequent (food is often eaten outside the home in the form of numerous snacks) with the consumption of snacks, carbonated drinks or alcoholic drinks, fashionable foods and impromptu meals. Being overweight is always a wake-up call. Abdominal fat must be kept under control because it indicates a slowed metabolism, a diet too rich in sugars and an imbalance between ingested and burned calories. High-loaded foods/glycemic index in fact lead to an increase in abdominal and visceral fat.

Acne is a chronic disease of the sebaceous hair follicle that most often develops during puberty. In its most typical form, so-called common acne affects about 80% of teenagers between 12 and 20 years old, with a prevalence in the male gender. Various studies have shown an association between acne and milk consumption and dairy derivatives. The cause would be the presence in the milk of hormones (estrogen, progesterone, androgenic precursors, etc.) some of which would be implicated in the development of pimples (comedogenesis). In addition, milk contains bioactive substances that act on the pilosebaceous unit (glucocorticoids, IGF1, TGF-beta, etc.). According to some researchers, the hormonal influence is mainly linked to the consumption of cheese, in fact, its fermentation would determine a greater production of testosterone in milk starting from its precursors. An important role seems to be the BMI (Body Mass Index). Some studies show not gaining weight, and therefore not taking foods that promote weight gain is a factor that protects against acne. Foods that seem to have a protective effect against acne are fish, fruit and vegetables.

Onychophagy is an oral habit that consists in biting fingernails or cuticles that begins at the age of 3-4 years and is common in both children and adults. While its prevalence increases during adolescence, it decreases in the following years and is higher in male adolescents than in females [20]. This disorder, if left untreated, tends to affect the correct development of dental occlusion and oral functions.

30.9 Men

Men, like women, have certain nutritional needs. Gender nutrition is useful to ensure a good amount of vitamins and minerals that provide multiple benefits during the various stages of development. In particular, magnesium helps normal muscle function, including the heart muscle. By means of a balanced diet, it is appropriate to maintain optimal levels of B vitamins, which contribute to the normal male energy metabolism, which has a greater energy requirement than women.

30.10 Andropause

In men, andropause is a process that occurs more gradually than female menopause and is not easily identifiable. Over time, a progressive drop in testosterone occurs. Body weight control is essential, as fat converts testosterone into estrogen, accelerating the process of loss of this male hormone. Considering that hypertrophy of the prostate is created in andropause, it is recommended to increase the consumption of beta-carotene and alpha-carotene, such as lycopene, contained in tomatoes, strawberries and berries. It is important to introduce nutrients in the diet that can inhibit the enzyme responsible for the breakdown of testosterone, but also foods with a high content of vitamin E, zinc and fatty acids, useful in counteracting urinary inflammation and incontinence, improving functionality of the bladder muscles. During the andropause state, a balanced gender diet is aimed at compensating for male nutritional deficiencies, and it represents the first form of prevention that starts at the table.

30.11 Elders

With aging, physiological changes of the organism occur, which tend to change daily behaviors, ranging from physical activity to nutrition. In the elderly, one of the main health objectives is to avoid malnutrition and dehydration. For the elderly, malnutrition doesn't just mean a lack of food. There are factors that lead older people to eat less due to a lack of appetite, the physical difficulty in preparing meals or difficulty in swallowing. At other times the problem is, for reason of convenience, the elderly prefer ready-made foods, which are too rich in salt, fat and calories but poor in vitamins and minerals. There are thus two opposite conditions, both very dangerous for health: on the one hand excessive weight loss and, on the other, being overweight or obese, with a lack of certain nutrients. The elderly generally tend to drink little because, with age, the sense of thirst decreases and, therefore, they must be encouraged to a greater consumption of liquids in order not to dehydrate. Many elderly (especially women) who have an active social life, or must go shopping or be out of the house for a while, don't want to drink to avoid needing to go to the bathroom while not home. Also, achieving the goal of proper nutrition in the elderly is not at all easy because of comorbidities that may be present, such as heart problems, hypertension, neurological diseases (Alzheimer, Parkinson, etc.). All of these conditions often force older people to take medications that can affect the assimilation of nutrients and appetite. Sarcopenia, i.e., the reduction of muscle mass, is physiological and is progressive and is related to an increase in the risk of falls, an increase in physical disability and a reduction of basal metabolism, bone density and insulin sensitivity. The absence of adequate physical activity and the excessive supply of energy through food are the main reasons why a particularly high rate of being overweight and obesity occurs in the elderly.

Eating is not only a physiological necessity. Many psychological aspects in the elderly can also influence diet and sometimes make the relationship with food really complicated. For example, some of the physical changes typical of aging can transform the pleasure of a lunch with friends into an embarrassing moment. Chewing poorly, due to dental problems or the presence of unstable prostheses, pushes many elderly people to avoid "difficult" food and sometimes even to avoid an invitation to lunch or dinner for fear of showing such a discomfort to others. Taste and smell decrease over time with the risk that all prepared foods have the same flavor so being at the table becomes only a habit, sometimes even a burden. Elders often have an insufficient intake of vitamins from the diet, especially of group B, specifically B12, B6 and B9, or folic acid which is unfortunate as there are studies that correlate this deficiency with memory deficits and related diseases, starting with senile dementia. There is also a risk of vitamin D deficiency, which is activated in the body by exposure to sunlight. In this case the deficiency is related to an increased risk of osteoporosis, already present in the elderly due to poor physical activity. Furthermore, research has shown that there is a strong correlation between the deficiency of vitamin D and a lower response of the immune system, that is, the defense of the body. Even in this case therefore it may be appropriate to reintegrate, after consulting with the attending physician, supplements based on vitamin D, also in association with vitamin A (essential for the health of the eyes and skin). Vitamin C is a powerful antioxidant, and as such in old age it helps counteracting the effects of aging [21-23].

As we can see men and women have different nutritional deficiencies and needs. It is therefore very important, both as a preventive aspect, and when general health conditions are complicated by different diseases, to contact an expert who will be able to advise the best foods for a healthy and correct gender focused nutrition.

REFERENCES

1. Shilovskiy IP, Dyneva ME, Kurbacheva OM, Kudlay DA, Khaitov MR. The Role of Interleukin-37 in the Pathogenesis of Allergic Diseases. Acta Naturae 2019; 11(4): 54-64.
2. Tan KS, McFarlane LC, Lipworth BJ. Paradoxical downregulation and desensitization of beta2-adrenoceptors by exogenous progesterone in female asthmatics. Chest 1997; 111(4): 947-51.
3. https://www.airc.it/cancro/prevenzione-tumore/alimentazione/guida-menu/lalimentazione-negli-over-65
4. https://www.airc.it/cancro/informazioni-tumori/cose-il-cancro/numeri-del-cancro
5. Waldmann A, Eisemann N, Katalinic A. Epidemiology of Malignant Cervical, Corpus Uteri and Ovarian Tumours - Current Data and Epidemiological Trends. Geburtshilfe Frauenheilkd 2013; 73(2): 123-9.
6. Arganini C, Turrini A, Saba A, Virgili F, Comitato R. Gender differences in food choice and dietary intake in modern western societies. In: Public Health - Social and Behavioral Health, ed. Maddock J. (Rijeka: InTech Open Access Publisher), 2012; pp. 83-102.
7. Organisation for Economic Co-operation and Development (OECD). Overweight and obesity. In OECD Factbook 2013: Economic, Environmental and Social Statistics.
8. Chih HJ, Lee AH, Colville L, Binns CW, Xu D. A review of dietary prevention of human papillomavirus-related infection of the cervix and cervical intraepithelial neoplasia. Nutr Cancer 2013: 65(3): 317-28.
9. http://www.salute.gov.it/portale/donna/dettaglioContenutiDonna.jsp?lingua=italiano&id=4470&area=Salute%20donna&menu=patologie
10. https://www.epicentro.iss.it/anoressia/
11. Wilson GT, Shafran R. Eating disorders guidelines from NICE. Lancet 2005; 365(9453): 79-81.
12. Duttaroy AK, Basak S. Maternal dietary fatty acids and their roles in human placental development. Prostaglandins Leukot Essent Fatty Acids 2020; 155:102080.
13. Mack LR, Tomich PG. Gestational Diabetes: Diagnosis, Classification, and Clinical Care. Obstet Gynecol Clin North Am 2017; 44(2): 207-17.
14. Ballard JL, Auer CE, Khoury JC. Ankyloglossia: assessment, incidence, and effect of frenuloplasty on the breastfeeding dyad. Pediatrics 2002; 110(5): e63.
15. Walsh J, Links A, Boss E, Tunkel D. Ankyloglossia and Lingual Frenotomy: National Trends in Inpatient Diagnosis and Management in the United States, 1997-2012. Otolaryngol Head Neck Surg 2017; 156(4): 735-40.
16. Campanha SMA, Martinelli RLC, Palhares DB. Association between ankyloglossia and breastfeeding. Codas 2019; 31(1): e20170264.
17. Martinelli RL, Marchesan IQ, Berretin-Felix G. Lingual

frenulum protocol with scores for infants. Int J Orofacial Myology 2012; 38: 104-12.
18. Walsh J, Tunkel D. Diagnosis and Treatment of Ankyloglossia in Newborns and Infants: A Review. JAMA Otolaryngol Head Neck Surg 2017; 143(10): 1032-9.
19. Kotlow L. Diagnosis and treatment of ankyloglossia and tied maxillary fraenum in infants using Er:YAG and 1064 diode lasers. Eur Arch Paediatr Dent 2011; 12(2): 106-12. Review.
20. Tanaka OM, Vitral RW, Tanaka GY, Guerrero AP, Camargo ES. Nailbiting, or onychophagia: a special habit. Am J Orthod Dentofacial Orthop 2008; 134(2): 305-8.
21. de Oliveira DL, Hirotsu C, Tufik S, Andersen ML. The interfaces between vitamin D, sleep and pain. J Endocrinol 2017; 234(1): R23-R36.
22. Gominak SC. Vitamin D deficiency changes the intestinal microbiome reducing B vitamin production in the gut. The resulting lack of pantothenic acid adversely affects the immune system, producing a "pro-inflammatory" state associated with atherosclerosis and autoimmunity. Med Hypotheses 2016; 94: 103-7.
23. Gominak SC, Stumpf WE. The world epidemic of sleep disorders is linked to vitamin D deficiency. Med Hypotheses 2012; 79(2): 132-5.

31

Relationships between chewing and obesity in bariatric elderly

Marlei Braude Canterji and Simone Augusta Finard

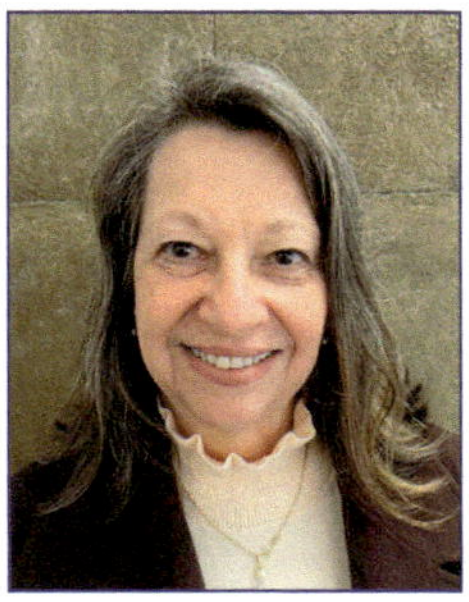

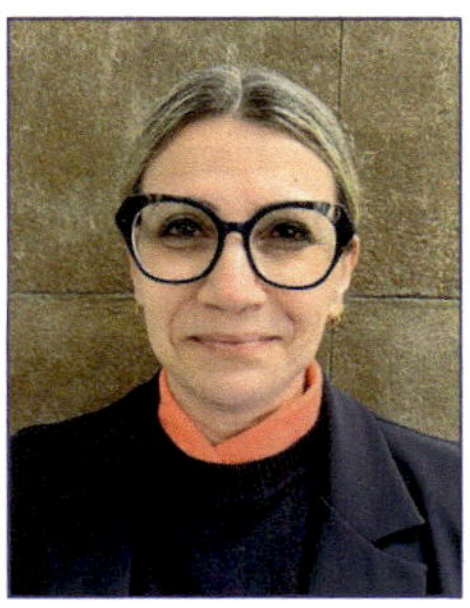

31.1 Introduction

Chewing (also called mastication) is a physiological act that occurs gradually, depending on the patterns of growth, development and maturation of the craniofacial complex, the nervous system and the dental occlusion guides [1]. The masticatory function, as well as speech and swallowing, includes movements of contraction and relaxation of the muscles responsible for the preparation of the food bolus, whose activity is initiated voluntarily [2]. In humans, the orofacial structures, including the temporomandibular joint (TMJ), perform movements of cutting, dividing and crushing solid foods, called *comminution* of food, inside the oral cavity. The movement of the mandible, performed by the coordination between the various chewing muscles, plays an important role in the fragmentation of the food [3].

Obesity is a chronic disease characterized by an excessive accumulation of adipose tissue in the organism [4-6] which causes individuals to have important consequences for their health, such as a reduction in life expectancy and quality [5]. Social, cultural, genetic, environmental and lifestyle changes are considered as causes of obesity [7].

Aging, a natural and physiological process of the organism, implies morphophysiological changes in the oral cavity that directly influence the health and quality of life of the elderly [8]. It has been confirmed that compromised oral structures and functions, along with aging itself, besides affecting the quality of life, can interfere with feeding, with socializing, and with emotional and psychological functions. These results were found in a sample of elderly with mean age of 77.5 years from São Paulo, Brazil [9].

In this chapter, the possible relationships between mastication and obesity present in elderly individuals who qualify for Bariatric Surgery (BS) will be discussed, considering the close connection between these aspects, their importance and their interference in the individuals' post-surgery quality of life. Due to the interface with the functional aspects related to chewing and obesity, mainly, to orofacial motricity, traditional speech therapy has been occupying an increas-

Marlei Braude Canterji
Speech Therapist at the Study Group on Obesity and Metabolic Surgery.
Porto Alegre, Brazil

Email: marleib@hotmail.com

Simone Augusta Finard
Speech Therapist at the Physiatrics and Rehabilitation Service of Hospital de Clínicas de Porto Alegre, Brazil

Email: simone.finard@yahoo.com.br

ingly important role within the bariatric surgery teams. The historical term "speech therapy" currently includes treatment of most orofacial dysfunctions affecting sucking, chewing, swallowing, speech, breathing and the proper rest position of lips and tongue.

31.2 Obesity

The prevalence of being overweight and obese since childhood has increased significantly. In a study on the risk indicators for oral health and obesity, it was found that this prevalence increased dramatically among children between six and twelve years of age. One-third of the 12-year-old children in the sample already had excessive abdominal adiposity, of this third 27.3% had oral diseases, 19.7% were obese and 16.5% had both conditions [10].

The degree of obesity is measured by the Body Mass Index (BMI), elaborated by Quetelet and published in *Physique Sociale* in 1869 [11]. This index is used as an international measure that characterizes the ideal weight and indicates if it is below or above the recommended index. It also indicates its relationship with possible associated diseases since obesity increases the risks for these occurrences. The main comorbidities associated with obesity are diabetes, hypertension, hyperlipidemia, obstructive sleep apnea [12], dyslipidemia [13], orthopedic problems, respiratory problems, heart disease, type 2 diabetes and a prevalence of Metabolic Syndrome (MS) [14] that may be above 50% [15].

Because of the prevalence of overweight and obese patients, the number of BS has been increasing, since it is considered the most effective treatment for obesity of any of the techniques currently used. This type of intervention, which began in the 1950s in the USA, became an affordable option in the late 1990s to a greater number of individuals diagnosed with these disorders [16].

International guidelines suggest that the patient's criteria for BS should include, first of all, control of eating behavior to eat less and more slowly, and secondly, a functional dental status that provides good masticatory function, in order to avoid physiological complications such as vomiting, diarrhea, pain and dumping syndrome [17, 18].

Considering the theme discussed in this chapter, it is important to emphasize that obesity has been associated with oral disorders such as periodontal disease, disturbances that affect the formation of the bolus of food and can favor the swallowing of food faster and with greater voracity [19], caries [20], dental wear [21, 22], and xerostomia [23].

31.3 Chewing

The stomatognathic system (SGS), comprising teeth, jaws and associated soft tissues, presents a specific biological and functional structure well integrated in the organism, that is, changes that may occur in other structures of the body can trigger immediate negative effects in the SGS. Similarly, disorders in some of the SGS, especially those affecting dental occlusion and the TMJ, may be reflected in distant organs and systems, for example the gastrointestinal system, due to inefficient chewing. Changes in ear structures, following pathological temporomandibular dysfunction, may affect the function of the ears and neck pain (cervicalgia), may be induced by a dysfunctional SGS [24].

The importance of the tongue is emphasized here because the tongue is involved in chewing, swallowing, sucking, breathing and speaking. In sucking, the tongue is responsible for performing rhythmic and repetitive movements, when it is adequately positioned to create the necessary pressure for suction. During chewing, the tongue facilitates the mixing of the food together with the saliva after being crushed by the teeth. In swallowing, the tongue is responsible for the propulsion of food toward the esophagus [25] making it a fundamental structure of the ingestion process [26]. Thus, many disorders can affect the musculature of the upper esophageal sphincter (UES), in the periodontium and the TMJ, causing speech and chewing alterations [25, 27, 28].

Chewing is considered the first stage of digestion and, related to the integrity of the gastrointestinal system, is a fundamental function for the good digestion of hard and/or fibrous foods [29]. Chewing is a complex function that involves digestive activities [30, 31] and is not limited to mandibular mouth opening and closing movements [4, 29]. Chewing is considered as a facilitator of the initial stages of digestion, stimulating the production of saliva and activating the cephalic controls that begin the assimilation of food [32].

Modification of food into absorbable nutrients is the main attribute of the digestive system [33], and the food enters through the oral cavity where it is disintegrated with the aid of teeth and muscles during chewing, followed by swallowing [34].

The masticatory function involves the following muscles: the temporalis, the lateral and medial pterygoids, the masseters, the anterior and posterior bellies of the digastric, the sternocleidomastoids and the trapeziuses [24]. All these muscles coordinate their contraction with other muscle groups, such as: the 17 muscles of the tongue, the facial muscles, especially the buccinator and the orbicularis oris of the lips. As for the functional aspects of chewing, food intake, the crushing and comminuting of food are considered the most important stomatognathic functions [35].

It is important to reiterate that effective mastication requires the use of specific features of the orofacial region, including the chewing muscles and tongue, as well as the teeth, the periodontium, saliva, a healthy oral mucosa and a coordination of an intact neuromuscular system [36-38].

The TMJ plays a decisive role in this process since its biomechanics allow the mandibular movements to occur. The movements performed by the mandible during mastication should be rotation and lateralization [39], regular and effortless [40]. The muscles involved in the masticatory process are responsible for part of the energy required to move the mandible [41]. Many of them, which are found around the oral cavity and in the anterior region of the neck, are involved in masticatory movements, controlled and harmonized in a surprisingly skillful manner [42].

Masticatory muscles can be divided into: mandibular closing group (necessary to bite) such as the masseters, the temporalis and the medial pterygoid muscles; and the mandibular opening group (to open the mouth and capture food) such as the lateral pterygoids, the supra- and the infrahyoid muscles [41].

The muscles of the tongue collect the food and direct it toward the occlusal surface, in coordination with the facial muscles and with the rhythmical mouth opening and closing. During the lowering of the mandible, the fibers of the buccinator muscle compress the cheeks against the maxilla [43]. The buccinator is an accessory muscle to the mastication and by extending between the orbicularis oris and the superior constrictor muscles it exerts a synergistic force called the Buccinator Mechanism. By contracting, these muscles are also responsible for the containment of the food while it's cut by the incisor teeth and during the grinding of the food under the direct pressure of the molar teeth, preventing the food from being pocketed into the vestibule [44]. Moreover, the way in which the teeth occlude during mastication is important for the health and comfort of the whole system [41, 45].

The opening of the mandible is performed by the suprahyoid and infrahyoid muscles. The group of suprahyoid muscles comprises the mylohyoid, the digastric, the stylohyoid and the geniohyoid. There are authors who do not consider the digastric muscle as a participant in mastication although it does exert an important function in the mandibular movement. The group of the infrahyoid muscles comprises the omohyoid, the sternohyoid and the thyrohyoid [41].

Ideal chewing in individuals with natural teeth, dentofacial balance and normal TMJ occurs when the food is retained and bit with the incisor teeth, when the formation of the food bolus occurs while maintaining a lip seal, without the presence of chewing noise, without exaggerated recruitment of the perioral musculature, with symmetric mandibular lateralization and muscular strength and performed bilaterally and alternately [1, 46, 47]. However, food can also be introduced in the mouth after being partitioned or torn with the fingers or by biting the food with lateral teeth, or chewing can be performed bilaterally and simultaneously, or unilaterally, with vertical mandibular movements, and without lip seal [46].

The alternated bilateral mastication pattern is considered most efficient because it stimulates the periodontal membrane, the chewing muscles and the TMJ on both sides, thus strengthening the proprioceptive neuromuscular circuits and favoring greater occlusal stability [24]. It has been suggested that the balance of interdental contact during the performance of the masticatory function is essential for the health and comfort of the SGS [4, 48, 49]. Thus, mastication is considered most appropriate when it involves and stimulates the teeth and supporting structures alternately, allowing for the balanced transfers of forces, and when the muscles function with alternating periods of work and rest [24], favoring synchronicity and a functional muscle balance [49, 50].

A unilateral chewing pattern can occur without significant signs and symptoms as it can be considered an adaptive mechanism to ensure minimal trauma to the periodontium, teeth and joints. This pattern of mastication is often found in individuals with temporomandibular disorders (TMD) and occlusal interference on the balance side [24].

The speed of masticatory movements varies according to each masticatory cycle, the type of food and the individual who chews. The speed, duration and shape of mastication varies according to the type of occlusion, the type of food and the presence of dysfunction [4]. Considering these chewing parameters, in a study that proposed a protocol for clinical evaluation of masticatory functions, it was observed that the slower the mastication, the better the grinding of the food, that is, a good food bolus was formed. However, when chewing is fast, it does not promote good food grinding, that is, the formation of the bolus is incomplete or inadequate, and food residues remain scattered in the oral cavity, making food difficult to swallow and compromising its digestion [51].

Chewing also stands out in its impact on the abil-

Table 31.1 Classification of Body Mass Index (BMI)

Classification	*BMI (kg/m²)*
Under weight	< 18.5
Normal	18.5-24.9
Overweight	25.0-29.9
Grade I Obesity	30.0-34.9
Grade II Obesity	35.0-39.9
Grade III Obesity	> 40.0

ity of an individual to pay attention. In a systematic review article, we identified 22 references on the effect of chewing on cognition, based on criteria established by the authors. Among the publications, 14 (64%) presented on the positive effects of chewing on attention. It was also found significant improvement in mood and stress reduction due to the influence of chewing [52].

31.4 Obesity and bariatric surgery

Table 31.1 presents the BMI calculation, which is done by dividing the mass of the individuals in kilograms by the square of their height in meters (kg/m^2), and the resulting classification, or the degree of obesity, according to this index.

According to the classification, individuals with Grade I Obesity present a moderate risk for the onset of diseases, cases with Grade II Obesity present a serious risk for the onset of these diseases, and the results classified as Grade III Obesity are considered at very serious risk for associated diseases [12-15].

In addition to leading to compromised health and risk of death, obesity can lead to metabolic syndrome [16]. In this syndrome, there is insulin resistance, which diminishes in the tissues, forcing the pancreas to produce it, thus raising insulin levels in the blood. This set of metabolic risk factors also increases the chances of developing a stroke [53].

The USA has the highest number of bariatric surgeries performed, and with Brazil, the second country with the highest number of procedures, the total is more than 500,000 surgeries per year. In Brazil the number of bariatric surgeries increased by 7.5% in 2016 compared to the previous year, in addition, women represent 76% of the patients [54, 55]. It is currently the most frequently performed procedure for obesity not only in the USA but also in Canada and the Asia-Pacific regions, as well as in the regions of Europe and Latin America and South America [56].

31.4.1 Risks and benefits of bariatric surgery

The anatomical changes undergone in the gastrointestinal tract, after BS, imply the occurrence of nutritional and metabolic deficiencies [57]. These deficiencies can trigger severe protein-calorie malnutrition and poor fat absorption, as well as deficiencies of Vitamins B12 and D, iron and calcium. Knowing this, for the prevention of these complications, it is necessary to maintain the follow-up and monitoring of the patient in the postoperative period [58].

Despite the risk inherent to the procedure, it was identified that the change in physical appearance and weight loss would imply higher life value, improved social relations, increased self-esteem and, consequently, better health care [59]. In addition to these benefits, it was also verified that the patients submitted to BS reported changes in lifestyle and quality improvement regarding physical, psychological and social relationships [60]. A greater willingness to work toward the health goals was identified, due to weight reduction and the metabolic modifications of most of the comorbidities evaluated. Improvement of the physical conditions, satisfaction during physical activities and increased libido was also reported, once the main comorbidity was resolved and others improved [60, 61].

31.4.2 Surgical procedures

Regarding surgical procedures specifically, there are several approaches indicated and, among them, there are two main methods: Vertical Gastrectomy and Roux-en-Y gastric bypass (gold standard) [62, 63].

31.4.3 Vertical gastrectomy

Vertical gastrectomy (Fig. 31.1) is a surgical technique that shows good results; therefore, it encounters great acceptance in many centers in different countries. Also called a gastric sleeve, it is a restrictive procedure that consists of removing the greater curvature of the stomach, starting from 4-6 cm from the pylorus to the esophagogastric angle, leaving the new reservoir with a tubular and elongated shape [62, 64].

Some of the advantages described with vertical gastrectomy are the absence of problems of malabsorption, as this procedure does not alter the contact of food with the intestinal walls and, consequently, with their respective digestive enzymes. Besides these advantages, it does not imply digestive anasto-

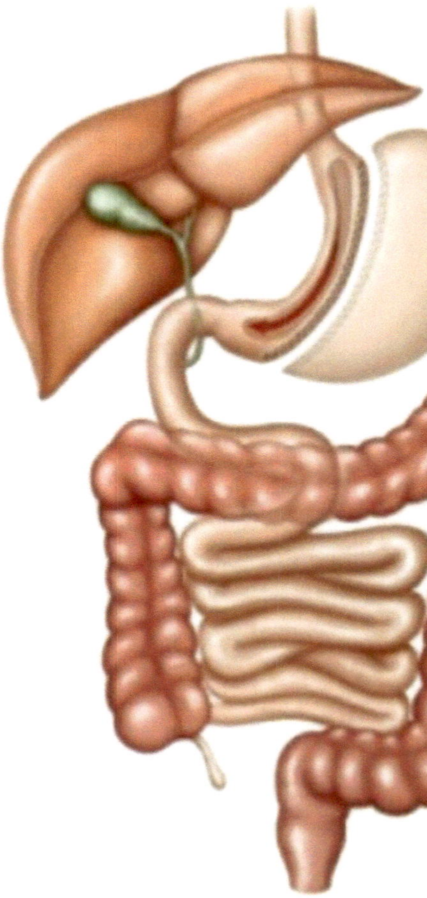

Fig. 31.1 Vertical gastrectomy.
[https://www.sbcbm.org.br/tecnicas-cirurgicas-bariatrica/]

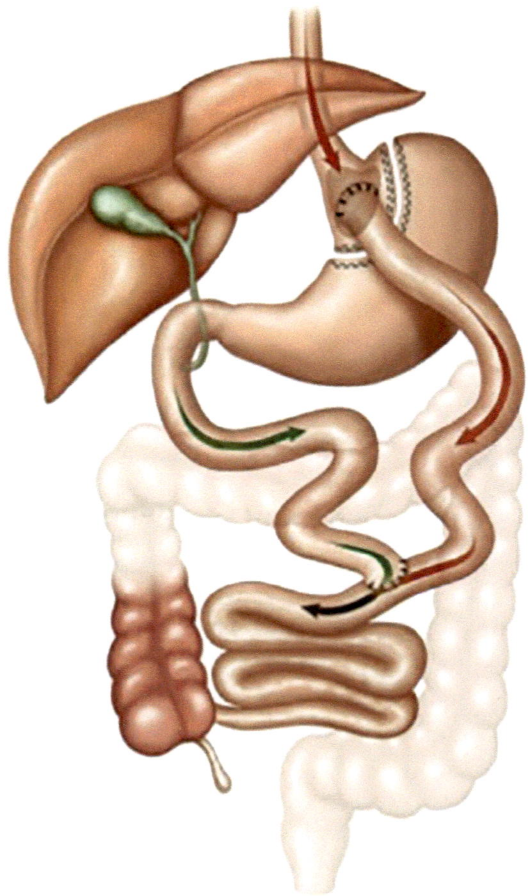

Fig. 31.2 Roux-en-Y gastric bypass.
[https://www.sbcbm.org.br/tecnicas-cirurgicas-bariatrica/]

moses and offers a lower risk of postoperative complications when compared to other BS [64, 65].

31.4.4 Roux-en-Y gastric bypass

The procedure called Roux-en-Y Gastric Bypass or Fobi-Capella Surgery is considered a gold standard in BS [65] and is known as one of the three most common surgeries used for severe obesity [66]. As a mixed intervention, it combines the modification of nutrient uptake by the intestine with decreased stomach capacity as mechanisms for weight loss (Fig. 31.2). It is also characterized by a greater restrictive component, since it implies a gastric bypass with reconstitution of Roux-en-Y intestinal transit, which makes food intake limited and modifies the production of hormones that modulate hunger and satiety [65-69].

31.5 Chewing and bariatric surgery

Chewing is an oral function of fundamental importance when considering morbid obesity. It has been confirmed that the quality of life in this population was negatively influenced by socioeconomic factors and oral diseases when compared with subjects with normal weight. Oral diseases are also considered as part of the individual's metabolic condition, compromising the general health of the senior obese patient. Thus, oral health care programs for obese elderly people, implemented by a multidisciplinary team, would imply a positive impact on the general health of the obese [70].

A study that explored the relationship between chewing and body weight of toothed individuals, evaluated 64 subjects with both normal weight and complete dentition as well as subjects overweight and obese. The individuals were evaluated based on food consumption and number of masticatory cycles, measuring the duration of mastication before swallowing. In adults, there was a significant negative relationship between BMI, number of masticatory cycles and chewing duration. The results suggested that mastication was associated with body weight of healthy toothed adults [54]. These results corroborated a previous study that showed that subjects with normal weight ate more slowly than individuals with overweight and obesity [71].

In relation to the pharyngoesophageal structures, it is known that the oral cavity has the function of controlling hunger, appetite and satiety, besides being responsible for accepting the food, determining chewing and swallowing of food or its rejection, and generating protective mechanisms such as spitting or vomiting [34]. Appetite is related to the desire for food ingestion, satiety refers to the self-limiting aspect of eating [34], and the control of these sensations is performed by the hypothalamus [72].

Considering the sensory aspects related to food consumption, tactile receptors play a decisive role in oral physiology, besides stimulating the sensation of touch, as they are responsible for the recognition of important motor reactions, such as the chewing reflex [73].

The act of chewing food, thus properly forming a bolus, and interacting with different textures, consistencies and types of food in a meal, would assist in the activation of the gustative sensation (taste). The grounding or comminution of the food during chewing allows a larger number of molecules to interact with the taste receptors, therefore changing the type of food during a meal contributes to the impairment or neutralization of the sensory adaptation effect, thus keeping the oral sensory system alert [74].

As for the masticatory process, it is also reported that if there is a muscular imbalance, then inadequate chewing patterns and, possibly, inadequate swallowing patterns may occur [43]. Therefore, the knowledge of how the masticatory function is performed supports the need for (re)habilitation of the bariatric patient, leading to a more adequate dietary behavior, in both the short and the long term. Inefficient chewing can cause myofunctional orofacial disorders, gastrointestinal disorders and even nutritional deficiencies [75-77].

As previously mentioned, the main purpose of mastication is to grind the food into smaller and smaller particles, preparing them for swallowing and digestion [24, 41, 46]. Chewing is considered a pleasant action that takes advantage of the sensations coming from smell, taste, touch and vision thus forming a contextualized environment for the reception of the food. It is part of a speech therapist's practice to inform the bariatric patients that, at the moment they feel hungry, chewing becomes pleasurable; on the other hand, when the stomach is sated, there is a stimulus that ceases this sensory information [4, 41, 78].

Chewing is the essential function in the prevention of myofunctional disorders and the maintenance of an acquired muscle tone [30, 79]. Regarding swallowing, even though the function is not emphasized in this process, it is known that it may be affected by poor respiration [80] and chewing [77]. Thus, masticatory training facilitates the stimulation of the lip seal, which is important for nasal breathing and facilitates the preparation of food boluses, which promotes an adequate swallowing pattern [46].

Educating the patient regarding the relation between all these functions would be relevant so that one of the main therapeutic goals can be achieved: the restoration of muscular functional balance [79, 81]. As a result of the incoordination of respiration with chewing, there is a possibility that the food bolus may not be well crushed and may lead to gagging [77].

Regarding the feeding of patients with mixed techniques, there is the possibility of presenting episodes of vomiting that may be justified by inadequate chewing, food intake greater than its new capacity or by velocity higher than its flow rate [4, 82, 83]. Moreover, working on masticatory force would facilitate the strengthening of the jaw lifting muscles, favoring the postural balance of the mandible when resting [46, 84].

The acquisition of a new muscular pattern can only be acquired and preserved (automated) through functional training, that is, chewing is necessary before a new chewing pattern can be acquired [46].

Regarding the rehabilitation process, in particular for the ingestion and intraoral manipulation of solid foods, several aspects are analyzed, such as the presence of the following [48]:

- Bilateral or unilateral chewing
- Ability to form a bolus of pasty or liquid consistency
- Lip seal
- Exaggerated periorbicular movements
- Predominantly rotational or vertical movements in chewing
- Lower lip interposition
- Exaggerated movements of the tongue, noises or clicks.

Following BS, during the rehabilitation period, attention should be paid to the selection of foods, as reaching a level of a new food processing or pattern of eating will depend on relearning to chew and even swallowing. The amount ingested will initially be minimal and only liquid, and, for some time, it will remain in small amounts in order to maintain a target weight [85].

31.5.1 Chewing and the obese elderly

Regarding the modifications that occur throughout life with regards to the stomatognathic system and the digestive process, we have identified the following impacting features [86]:

- Absence or loss of dentition
- Use of dental prostheses
- Decreased salivary production
- Atrophy of the taste buds
- Changes in esophageal peristalsis
- Atrophy of the gastric mucosa
- Decrease in number of gastrointestinal wall cells
- Decreased production of gastric secretions
- Increased pH and slower gastric emptying
- Decreased metabolism of dose-dependent drugs
- Decreased protein synthesis with risk of hepatotoxicity
- Decreased lean body mass
- Higher prevalence of biliary lithiasis
- Decreased absorption of calcium
- Increased number of diverticula
- Atrophy of the intestinal mucosa
- Hypotonia of the abdominal wall
- Decreased motor function of the colon.

Based on these modifications which occur over time, it is agreed that a balanced and more appropriate diet is necessary, considering the consistencies and textures which allow the elderly to chew effectively so that the absorption of the nutrients occurs effectively [87, 88]. It is emphasized here that the orofacial function alteration most often reported by the elderly is chewing difficulty, since even in the presence of dentures, they do not process the food in their mouths with the same efficiency of young adults. There is an increased oral transit time of the food bolus, which slows down the overall eating time [89].

Although the effects of aging on mastication have not been defined, previous studies, including experimental studies with animal models, suggest that with increasing age more bites are needed for optimal oral processing and bolus formation, possibly and specifically due to changes in muscle morphology and physiology [90].

A study on the performance of the masticatory function concluded that mastication strongly depends on a stable occlusion, either with natural dentition or dental prosthesis. Thus, it would be fundamental to analyze the interface of chewing with the insidious dental losses associated with aging, since tooth loss would affect the masticatory performance due to a diminished occlusal support [91].

The findings reported in a recent study are even more striking, as they characterized chewing as an indispensable oral function related to physical, mental and social health throughout life. The study, which investigated the influence of changes in chewing on cognition, more specifically in relation to memory loss, reports that the elderly tend to have masticatory dysfunction due to tooth loss and weakness of the masticatory muscles and such changes or modifications would potentially result in impaired cognitive function [92].

Considering the functional losses, it was reported that the elderly present a high prevalence of TMD identified through TMJ palpation, although of a mild degree, mainly in females, and weakness of the masticatory and cervical muscles, detected in the course of the examination [93].

In elderly patients with a diagnosis of obesity, typical metabolic changes associated with aging are added to obesity, such as glucose intolerance as well as a 20% decrease in the basal metabolic rate between 30 and 90 years of age. Apart from metabolic disorders, and among other aspects, the presence of locomotion difficulties – associated or not with systemic diseases – can lead to a sedentary lifestyle [94].

There are three relevant implications that directly affect chewing in the elderly and impact their diet choices: (1) the relationship between age, dentition and masticatory efficiency; (2) the connection between objectively measured chewing functions; (3) age implications and impact of dentition on nutrition, morbidity and mortality [4, 95, 96]. The inability to chew adequately with normal rotational movements may lead the patient to ingest very limited textures and diets, as mastication changes may be characterized by an over 50% decrease in muscular bite force compared to young individuals, thus causing health problems and a reduction in their eating pleasure [36, 97]. This decrease in bite force can be evidenced by the atrophy of the muscles responsible for this orofacial function, or by the decrease of biochemical efficiency due to alterations of the muscular ligaments [4, 98].

Adequate chewing, not only for its alimentary and nutritional aspects, and oral health as a whole, besides contributing to the proper functioning of the organism, assist with the maintenance of social interactions which are fundamental for a healthy aging [29].

As previously described, considering the structural losses that occur over the years, besides the effects associated with the lack of oral health care, maintaining an efficient masticatory function would bring benefits, not only to food processing, but also to the cognitive and behavioral aspects, such as attention, mood and stress relief [99, 100].

31.5.2 Food consumption and quality of life of the bariatric elderly

The reduction of masticatory performance as a result of tooth loss has an adverse effect on dietary intake

[101, 102] which may impact general health, affecting activities of daily living and quality of life [103, 104]. There are many factors that interfere with chewing, in addition to the number of functional teeth or maximum bite force [105]. Periodontal status is one of those aspects that impacts masticatory performance, which may also vary according to the different areas of occlusal support. These factors may serve as evidence to establish new standards for properly assessing masticatory performance in elderly people and they confirmed the importance of providing dietary guidelines to those elderly affected by tooth loss or periodontal disease [91].

It should be emphasized here that elderly should be made aware of orofacial myofunctional changes [87] that may occur over the years, which would then require a voluntary change in what has become an automatic but inadequate behavioral pattern. Post-surgery patients should be aware of a new eating mechanism with the purpose of facilitating the reintroduction of food after BS. Specifically in cases of obesity in the elderly, it is necessary for BS to have well-defined indications, thus careful evaluation is essential to identify the risks and what would be the real benefits of the procedure [48, 106, 107]. Speech therapists are the professionals who best can treat the elderly candidates for BS, by contributing to the maintenance of their quality of life through providing and highlighting information about the masticatory process and the changes that occur in it. This is an extremely important approach in the prevention of further disorders or to prevent their progression [108, 109]. Moreover, successful aging includes enjoying the pleasure of eating, which contributes to the maintenance of socio-communicative interactions [94, 106].

One of the essential guidelines given to the patient in relation to the BS postoperative period is the need for follow-ups by the multidisciplinary team. Important aspects, which would require an interdisciplinary approach, would be to recognize, favor and facilitate the promotion of a significant change in the patients, while retaining the best of their original essence, so that they can recognize themselves after surgery [110].

After bariatric surgery, all obese patients, considering the state of their dentition, presented a modification in the kinematics of chewing. The effects of masticatory behavior on the granulometry or texture of the food bolus formed would depend on the dental state and the type of food. Even so, further studies are needed to better understand the impact of dental status on eating and nutritional behavior in obese individuals [17].

From a speech therapy point-of-view, patients are recommended to organize their meals and to be able to anticipate them and/or always carry snacks to avoid being hungry. Called *masticatory shortage* in a previous study [111], the recommendation is to also increase the number of masticatory cycles. Following these recommendations makes the treatment successful, as there is a decreased likelihood of compulsive eating. In some studies, oral exposure time (time in which the food is in the mouth) was also associated with a lower bite force pattern [112] and an increase in the number of chews [113], which would imply a sensation of satiety [114, 115] and a decrease in voracity [116].

It is of fundamental importance for the bariatric patient to be tended by a team of specialized professionals who demonstrate sensitivity and respect, since obesity is a chronic disease with a multifactorial etiology. The multidisciplinary team may comprise a surgeon with specific training, a gastroenterologist, a nutritionist, a psychiatrist and/or psychologist, a physiotherapist, an anesthesiologist, a speech pathologist, nurses and nursing assistants familiar with the management of these patients [66].

The success criterion for speech therapists treating bariatric patients, is that they must be able to eat any kind of food, with varied textures and consistencies in both their daily routine and social events [108], in the short term and especially in the long term, thus preventing health risks and improving their quality of life [106].

REFERENCES

1. Junqueira P. Avaliação miofuncional. In: Marchesan IQ, Organizadora. Fundamentos em fonoaudiologia: aspectos clínicos de motricidade oral. 2ª ed. Rio de Janeiro: Guanabara Koogan; 2005, pp.19-27.
2. Marchesan IQ. Deglutição. Diagnóstico e possibilidade terapêuticas. In: Marchesan IQ (Org). Fundamentos em fonoaudiologia: aspectos clínicos de motricidade oral. 2ª ed. Rio de Janeiro: Guanabara Koogan; 2005, pp. 51-8.
3. Van der Bilt A. Assessment of mastication with implications for oral rehabilitation: a review. J Oral Rehabil 2011; 38: 754-80.
4. Canterji MB, Corrêa SPM. Fonoaudiologia e nutrição trabalhando a qualidade de vida alimentar. In: Franques ARM, Loli MAS. Novos corpos, novas realidades: reflexões sobre o pós-operatório da cirurgia da obesidade. SAo Paulo: Vetor; 2011, pp. 327-37.
5. Fandiño J, Benchimol AK, Coutinho WF, Appolinário JC. Cirurgia bariátrica: aspectos clínico-cirúrgicos e psiquiátricos. Rev Psiquiatr RS 2004; 26: 47-51.
6. National Institute of Health, National Heart, Lung and Blood Institute. Clinical guidelines on the identification, evaluation, and treatment of overweight and obesity in

adults. Obes Res 1998; 6(Suppl 2): 51s-209s.
7. Sichieri R, Moura EC. Análise multinível das variações no índice de massa corporal entre adultos, Brasil, 2006. Rev Saúde Pública 2009; 43(Suppl 2): 90-7.
8. Malheiros VS, Miranda AF. Alterações bucais no idoso: Breves orientações. R Odontol Planal Cent. Jan-Jun 2016; 6(1): 1-7.
9. Rihs LH, Costa AM, Torres LHN, Neri AL, Guariento ME, Cintra FA, Delboux MJ, Sousa MLR. Oral health of elderly with different frailty levels from the city of Campinas, São Paulo, Brazil. Rev Ciênc Méd 2013; 22(3): 157-65.
10. Tubert-Jeannin S, Pichot H, Rouchon B, Pereira B, Hennequin M. Common risk indicators for oral diseases and obesity in 12-year-olds: a South Pacific cross sectional study. BMC Public Health 2018; 18: 112.
11. Deurenberg P, Weststrate JA, Seidell JC. Body mass index as a measure of body fatness: age- and sex-specific prediction formulas. Br J Nutr 1991; 65: 105-14.
12. Buchwald H, Avidor Y, Braunwald E, Jensen MD, Pories W, Fahrbach K, Schoelles K. Bariatric Surgery: A Systematic Review and Meta-analysis. J Am Medical Assoc 2004; 292(14): 1724-37.
13. Silva EM, Sanches MD. Perfil Lipídico de Obesos Antes e Após a Derivação Gástrica a Fobi-Capella. Rev Col Bras Cirurg 2006; 33(2): 91-5.
14. Pedrosa IV, Burgos, MGPA, Souza NC, Morais CN. Aspectos Nutricionais em Obesos Antes e Após a Cirurgia Bariátrica. Rev Col Bras Cirurg 2009; 36(4): 316-22.
15. Vigitel Brasil 2015. Vigilância de fatores de risco e proteção para doenças crônicas por inquérito telefônico: estimativas sobre frequência e distribuição sociodemográfica de fatores de risco e proteção para doenças crônicas nas capitais dos 26 estados brasileiros e no Distrito Federal em 2015 [recurso eletrônico]/Ministério da Saúde, Secretaria de Vigilância em Saúde, Departamento de Vigilância de Doenças e Agravos não Transmissíveis e Promoção da Saúde. Brasília: Ministério da Saúde, 2016. 160p.
16. Sociedade Brasileira de Cirurgia Bariátrica e Metabólica. http://www.sbcbm.org.br/wordpress/numero-de-cirurgias-bariatricas-no-brasil-cresce-75-em-2016/ (Accessed on 18/04/2018).
17. Godlewski AE, Veyrune JL, Nicolas E, Ciangura CA, Chaussain CC, et al. Effect of Dental Status on Changes in Mastication in Patients with Obesity following Bariatric Surgery. PLoS ONE 2011; 6(7): e22324.
18. Bastos A, Falcão C, Pereira A, Pereira A, Alves C. Obesity and periodontal disease. Brazilian Research in Pediatric Dentistry and Integrated Clinic 2005; 5(3): 57-61.
19. Pataro AL, Costa FO, Cortelli SC, Cortelli JR, Abreu MH, Costa JE. Association between severity of body mass index and periodontal condition in women. Clin Oral Investig 2012; 16(3): 727-34.
20. Levine R. Obesity and oral disease -a challenge for dentistry. Br Dent J 2012; 213(9): 453-6.
21. Barron RP, Carmichael RP, Marcon MA, Sandor GK. Dental erosion in gastroesophageal reflux disease. J Can Dent Assoc 2003; 69(2): 84-9.
22. Biccas BN, Lemme EM, Abrahao LJ Jr, Aguero GC, Alvariz A, Schechter RB. Higher prevalence of obesity in erosive gastroesophageal reflux disease. Arch Gastroenterol 2009; 46(1): 15-9.
23. Modeer T, Blomberg CC, Wondimu B, Julihn A, Marcus C. Association between obesity, flow rate of whole saliva, and dental caries in adolescents. Obesity (Silver Spring) 2010; 18(12): 2367-73.
24. Molina OF. Fisiopatologia craniomandibular: oclusão e ATM. São Paulo: Pancast; 1989.
25. Furlan RMMM. Avaliação quantitativa da força axial da língua em indivíduos com grave diminuição da força lingual. [Trabalho de conclusão de curso]. Belo Horizonte, MG: UFMG; 2008.
26. Silva Netto CR. Deglutição no feto, no infante, no adulto, no idoso. 2ª ed. São Paulo: Funpec-Editora; 2012.
27. Junqueira PS. A investigação da mastigação em indivíduos portadores de classe III de Angle. Pró-Fono. 1992; 4: 29-31.
28. Felício CM. Desenvolvimento normal das funções estomatognáticas. In: Ferreira LP, Befi- Lopes DM, Limongi SCO, Organizadores. Tratado de fonoaudiologia. São Paulo: Roca; 2004, pp. 195-211.
29. Canterji MB, Nisa-Castro SAF. O envelhecimento da motricidade oral: aspectos da mastigação. In: Terra NL, Dornelles B, Organizadores. Envelhecimento bem sucedido. Porto Alegre: EDIPUCRS; 2002, pp. 355-60.
30. Tanigute CC. Desenvolvimento das funções estomatognáticas. In: Marchesan IQ, Organizadora. Fundamentos em fonoaudiologia: aspectos clínicos de motricidade oral. 2ª ed. Rio de Janeiro: Guanabara Koogan; 2005, pp. 1-6.
31. Allied Health Sciences Section Ad Hoc Nutrition Committee, Aills L, Blankenship J, Buffington C, Furtado M, Parrott J. ASMBS Allied Health Nutritional Guidelines for the Surgical Weight Loss Patient. Surg Obes Relat Dis 2008; 4(5 Suppl): S73-S108.
32. Power ML, Schulkin J. Anticipatory physiological regulation in feeding biology: cephalic phase responses. Appetite 2008; 50: 194-206.
33. Arasaki CH, Del Grande JC. Fundamentos da fisiologia gastrointestinal. In: Garrido Júnior AB, Ferraz EM, Barroso LF, Marchesini JB, Szegö T. Cirurgia da obesidade. São Paulo: Atheneu; 2006, pp. 23-8.
34. Douglas CR. Funções gerais desenvolvidas pela boca. In: Douglas CR. Tratado de fisiologia aplicada à fonoaudiologia. São Paulo: Robe; 2002, pp. 285-8.
35. Marchesan IQ. Motricidade oral. São Paulo: Pancast; 1993.
36. Lamy M, Mojon P, Kalykakis G, Legrand R, Butz-Jorgensen E. Oral status and nutrition in the institutionalized elderly. J Dentistry 1999; 27: 443-8.
37. Baum BJ, Ship JA. The oral cavity. In: Hazzard WR, Bierman EL, Blass JP, Ettinger WHJ, Halter JB. Principles of geriatric medicine and gerontology. 3rd ed. New York: McGraw-Hill; 1994, pp. 431-9.
38. Rahal A, Goffi-Gomez MVS. Electromyographic study of the masseter muscle during maximal voluntary clenchung and habitual chewing in adults with normal occlusion. Rev Soc Bras Fonoaudiol 2009; 14: 160-4.
39. Ide Y, Nakazawa K. Anatomical atlas of the temporomandibular joint. Tokyo: Quintessence; 1991.
40. Marchesan IQ. Atuação fonoaudiológica nas funções orofaciais: desenvolvimento, avaliação e tratamento. In: Andrade CRF, Marcondes E. Fonoaudiologia em pediatria. São Paulo: Sarvier; 2003, pp. 3-22.
41. Okeson JP. Fundamentos de oclusão e desordens temporo-mandibulares. 2ª ed. Porto Alegre: Artes Médicas; 1992.
42. Bray GA, Popkin BM. Dietary fat intake does affect obesity! Am J Clin Nutr 1998; 68: 1157-73.
43. Felício CM. Desordens temporomandibulares: diagnóstico fonoaudiológico e terapia. In: Felício CM, Organizador.

Fonoaudiologia aplicada a casos odontológicos: motricidade oral e audiologia. São Paulo: Pancast; 1998, pp. 91-125.
44. Castillo Morales R. Terapia da regulação orofacial. São Paulo: Memnon; 1999.
45. Ash MM, Ramfjord SP. Introdução à oclusão funcional. São Paulo: Panamed; 1987.
46. Motta AR, Perilo TVC. Terapia fonoaudiológica em mastigação (como eu trato). In: Marchesan IQ, Silva HJ, Berretin-Felix G, Organizadoras. Terapia fonoaudiológica em motricidade orofacial. São Paulo: Pulso; 2012, pp. 139-46.
47. Gomes LM, Bianchini EMG. Caracterização da função mastigatória em crianças com dentição decídua e dentição. Rev Cefac 2009; 11: 324-33.
48. Canterji MB. Evaluación miofuncional orofacial en cirugía bariátrica. In: Susanibar F, Marchesan I, Parra D, Dioses A. Tratado de Evaluación de Motricidad Orofacial y áreas afines. Madrid: Editorial EOS; 2014, pp. 253-62.
49. Bianchini EMG. Mastigação e ATM: avaliação e terapia. In: Marchesan IQ, Organizador. Fundamentos em fonoaudiologia: aspectos clínicos da motricidade oral. 2ª.ed. Rio de Janeiro: Guanabara Koogan; 2005, pp. 45-58.
50. Trawitzki LVV, Grechi TH, Giglio LD. Terapia fonaoudiológica em mastigação (como eu trato). In: Marchesan IQ, Silva HJ, Berretin-Felix G, Organizadoras. Terapia fonoaudiológica em motricidade orofacial. São Paulo: Pulso Editorial; 2012, pp. 23-38.
51. Whitaker ME, Trindade Jr AS, Genaro KF. Proposta de protocolo de avaliação clínica da função mastigatória. Rev Cefac 2009; 11(supl 3): 311-23.
52. Hirano Y, Onozuka M. Chewing and attention. A positive effect on sustained attention. BioMed Res Int May 2015. In: http://dx.doi.org/10.1155/2015/367026 (Accessed on 19/03/2019).
53. Rosenbaum P, Ferreira SRG. An update on the cardiovascular risk of metabolic syndrome. Arq Bras End & Metab 2003; 47 (3): 220-7.
54. Zhu B, Haruyama Y, Muto T, Yamazaki T. Association between eating speed and metabolic syndrome in a three-year population-based cohort study. J Epidemiol 2015; 25: 332-6.
55. Branco-Filho AJ, Nassif LS, Menacho AM, Aurichio RAE, Siqueira DED, Fernandez RM. Treatment of morbid obesity with vertical gastrectomy. ABCD Arq Bras Cir Dig 2011; 24 (1): 52-4.
56. Angrisani L, Santonicola A, Lovino P, Formisano G, Buchwald H, Scopinaro N. Bariatric Surgery Worldwide 2013. Obes Surg 2015; 25: 1822-32.
57. Bordalo LA, Mourão DM, Bressan J. Nutritional deficiencies after bariatric surgery: why they happen? Acta Med Port 2011; 24: 1021-8.
58. Malinowski SS. Nutritional and metabolic complications of bariatric surgery. Am J Med Sci 2006; 331 (4): 219-25.
59. Shiri S, Gurevich T, Feintuch U, Beglaibter N. Positive psychological impact of bariatric surgery. Obes Surg 2007; 17 (5): 663-8.
60. Lemos MCM. Quality of life of patients undergoing bariatric surgery in the municipality of cascavel. Arq Ciên Saúde 2006; 10: 155-63.
61. Faria O, Pereira VA, Gangoni CMC, Lins RD, Leite S, Rassi V, et al. Morbid obese patients treated with gastric bypass at Roux-en-Y gastric bypass: analysis of 160 patients. Brasília Med 2002; 39: 26-34.
62. Nassif LS, Menacho AM, Aurichio RAE, Siqueira DED, Fernandez RM. Treatment of morbid obesity with vertical gastrectomy. ABCD Arq Bras Cir Dig 2011; 24 (1): 52-4.
63. Bennett JM, Mehta S, Rhodes M. Surgery for morbid obesity. Postgrad Med J 2007; 83: 8-15.
64. Brethauer SA, Hammel JP, Schauer PR. Systematic review of sleeve gastrectomy staging and primary bariatric procedure. Surg Obes Relat Dis 2009; 5: 469-75.
65. Hallowell PT, Stellato TA. Avoidance of complications in older patients and Medicare recipients undergoing gastric bypass. Arch Surg 2007; 142: 506-12.
66. Brazil. Federal Council of Medicine. Safe standards for the surgical treatment of morbid obesity, defining indications, procedures and staff. CFM Resolution N° 1.942/2010. Available at: http://www.portalmedico.org.br/resolucoes/cfm/2010/1942_2010.htm (Accessed on 10/07/2011).
67. Monteforte M, Turkelson C. Bariatric surgery for morbid obesity. Obes Surg 2000; 10: 391-40.
68. Leite MAM, Rodrigues MPF. Surgical procedures. Historical introduction. In: Garrido Júnior AB, Ferraz EM, Barroso LF, Marchesini JB, Szegö T. Obesity surgery. São Paulo: Atheneu; 2006, pp. 141-8.
69. Andrew B, Alley JB, Aguilar CE, Fanelli RD. Barrett's esophagus before and after Roux-en-Y gastric bypass for severe obesity Surg Endosc. Aug 2017. https://link.springer.com/article/10.1007%2Fs00464-017-5768-6.
70. Yamashita JM, Moura-Grec PG, Freitas AR, Sales-Peres A, Groppo FC, Ceneviva R, Sales-Peres SHC. Assessment of Oral Conditions and Quality of Life in Morbid Obese and Normal Weight Individuals: A Cross-Sectional Study. PLoS ONE 2015; 10 (7): e0129687.
71. Laessle RG, Lehrke S, Duckers S. Laboratory eating behavior in obesity. Appetite 2007, 49: 399-404.
72. Guyton AC, Hall JE. Regulação neural da circulação e o controle rápido da pressão arterial. In: Guyton AC, Hall JE. Tratado de fisiologia médica. Rio de Janeiro: Guanabara Koogan; 1997, pp. 191-201.
73. Douglas CR. Fisiologia da função sensorial. In: Douglas CR. Tratado de fisiologia aplicada à fonoaudiologia. São Paulo: Robe; 2002, pp. 97-105.
74. Silva Netto CR. Paladar: gosto, olfato, tato e temperatura: fisiologia e fisiopatologia. São Paulo: Funpec; 2007.
75. Almeida PIA. Fonoaudiologia estética facial. Rio de Janeiro: Revinter; 2008.
76. Marchesini JB, Marchesini JCD, Marchesine SD, Cambi MPC, Frare RC, Strobel R. Derivações biliopancreáticas com gastrectomia distal (operação de Scopinaro) e gastrectomia vertical com preservação do piloro (duodenal switch de Hess e Marceau). In: Garrido Júnior AB, Barroso FL, Marchesini JB, Szegö T. Cirurgia da obesidade. São Paulo: Atheneu; 2006, pp. 163-71.
77. Marchesan IQ, Krakauer LH. A importância do trabalho respiratório na terapia miofuncional. In: Marchesan IQ, Bolaffi, Gomes ICD, Zorzi JL, Organizadores. Tópicos em fonoaudiologia. São Paulo: Lovise; 1995, pp. 155-60.
78. Orthlieb JD, Brocard D, Schittly J, Maniera-Ezvan A. Descrição da oclusão. In: Orthlieb JD, Laplenche O. Oclusão: princípios práticos. Porto Alegre: Artmed; 2002, pp. 28-36.
79. Tessitore A. Abordagem mioterápica com estimulação de pontos motores da face. In: Marchesan IQ, Bolaffi, Gomes ICD, Zorzi JL, Organizadoras. Tópicos em fonoaudiologia. São Paulo: Lovise; 1995, pp. 75-82.
80. Krakauer LH. Alterações de funções orais nos diversos tipos faciais. In: Marchesan IQ, Bolaffi, Gomes ICD, Zorzi JL, Organizadoras. Tópicos em fonoaudiologia. São Paulo: Lovise; 1995, pp. 147-54.

81. Bianchini EMG. A cefalometria nas alterações miofuncionais orais: diagnóstico e tratamento fonoaudiológico. São Paulo: Pró-Fono; 1993.
82. Quadros MRR, Savaris AL, Ferreira MV, Branco-Filho AJ. Intolerância alimentar no pós-operatório de pacientes submetidos à cirurgia bariátrica. Rev Bras Nutr Clin 2007; 22: 15-9.
83. Mottin CC. Bypass gástrico com anel por laparotomia. In: Silva RS, Kawahara NT, Organizadores. Cuidados pré e pós-operatórios na cirurgia da obesidade. Porto Alegre: AGE; 2005, pp. 180-94.
84. Cunha DA, Silva HJ. Terapia fonaudiológica em respiração oral (como eu trato). In: Marchesan IQ, Silva HJ, Berretin-Felix G. Organizadores. Terapia fonoaudiológica em motricidade orofacial. São Paulo: Pulso; 2012, pp. 87-109.
85. Cambi MPC, Marchesini JB. Acompanhamento clínico, dieta e medicação. In: Garrido Júnior. AB, Barroso FL, Marchesini JB, Szegö T. Cirurgia da obesidade. São Paulo: Atheneu; 2006, pp. 255-72.
86. Cuppari L. Nutrition guide: adult clinical nutrition. Barueri: Manole, 2014.
87. Amaral AKFJ, Regis RMFL. Stomatognathic system in the elderly. In: Hilton JS, Cunha DA, Organizers. The stomatognathic system: anatomophysiology and development. São Paulo: Pulse; 2011, pp. 129-44.
88. Silva SM, Chemin S, Martinez S. Menu: practical guide for elaboration. São Paulo: Roca, 2014.
89. Logemann JA, Pauloski BR, Rademaker AW, Colangelo LA, Kahrilas PJ, Smith CH. Temporal and biomechanical characteristics of oropharyngeal swallow in younger and older men. J Speech Lang Hear Res 2000; 43: 1264-74.
90. Krekeler BN, Connor NP. Age-Related Changes in Mastication Are Not Improved by Tongue Exercise in a Rat Model. Laryngoscope Jan 2017; 127(1): E29- E34.
91. Kosaka T, Ono T, Kida M, Kikui M, Yamamoto M, Yasui S, Nokubi T, Maeda Y, Kokubo Y, Watanabe M, Miyamoto Y. A multifactorial model of masticatory performance: the Suita study. J Oral Rehabil 2016; 43: 340-7.
92. Fukushima-Nakayama Y, Takehito O, Hayashi M, Inoue M, Wake H, Takashi O, Nakashima T. Reduced Mastication Impairs Memory Function. J Dent Res 2017; 96(9): 1058-66.
93. Camacho JGDD, Oltramari-Navarro PVP, Navarro RL, Conti ACCF, Conti MRA, Marchiori LLM, Fernandes KBP. Signs and symptoms of Temporomandibular Disorders in the Elderly. CoDAS 2014; 26(1): 76-80.
94. Pajecki D, Santo MA, Kanagi AL, Riccioppo D, Cleva R, Cecconello I. Functional assessment of older obese patients candidates for bariatric surgery. Arq Gastroenterol 2014; 51(1): 25-8.
95. Ministério da Saúde. Epidemiologia: relevância do problema e conceito e classificação. Brasília: O Ministério; 2006, pp. 16-26. [Cadernos de Atenção Básica n.12. Serie A. Normas e Manuais Técnicos] http://189.28.128.100/nutricao/docs/geral/doc_obesidade.pdf (Accessed on 3/11/2011).
96. Ship JA, Duffy V, Jones JA, Langmore S. Geriatric oral health and its impact on eating. J Am Geriatr Soc 1996; 44: 456-64.
97. Davies PM. Recomeçando outra vez. São Paulo: Manole; 1997.
98. Plant RL. Anatomy and physiology of swallowing in adults and geriatrics. Otolaryngol Clin North Am 1998; 31: 477-88.
99. Onyper RSV, Carr TL, Farrar JS, Floyd BR. Cognitive advantages of chewing gum. Now you see them, now you don't. Appetite 2011; 57(2): 321-8.
100. Tucha L, Simpson W. The role of time on task performance in modifying the effects of gum chewing on attention. Appetite 2011; 56(2): 299-301.
101. Sheiham A, Steele JG, Marcenes W, Lowe C, Finch S, Bates CJ et al. The relationship between dental status, nutrient intake, and nutritional status in older people. J Dent Res 2001; 80: 408-13.
102. Nowjack-Raymer RE, Sheiham A. Association of edentulism and diet and nutrition in US adults. J Dent Res 2003; 82: 123-6.
103. Takata Y, Ansai T, Awano S, Sonoki K, Fukuhara M, Wakisaka M et al. Activities of daily living and chewing ability in an 80-year-old population. Oral Dis 2004; 10: 365-8.
104. Takata Y, Ansai T, Awano S, Fukuhara M, Sonoki K, Wakisaka M et al. Chewing ability and quality of life in an 80-year-old population. J Oral Rehabil 2006; 33: 330-4.
105. Lepley CR, Throckmorton GS, Ceen RF, Buschang PH. Relative contributions of occlusion, maximum bite force, and chewing cycle kinematics to masticatory performance. Am J Orthod Dentofacial Orthop 2011; 139: 606-13.
106. Canterji MB, Corrêa SBM, Vargas GS, Pereira JLR, Finard SA. Speech, hearing and language sciences therapy in bariatric surgery of the elderly: case report. ABCD Arq Bras Cir Dig 2015; 28(Supl.1): 86-7.
107. Silva ASG, Tanigute CC, Tessitore A. A necessidade da avaliação fonoaudiológica no protocolo de pacientes candidatos à cirurgia bariátrica. Rev CEFAC 2014; 16(5): 1655-68.
108. Canterji MB. Fonoaudiologia e cirurgia bariátrica. São José dos Campos, SP: Pulso; 2012.
109. Canterji MB, Corrêa SPM. Terapia miofuncional orofacial em casos submetidos à cirurgia bariátrica. In: Silva HJ, Marchesan IQ, Tomé MC (Eds.). Tratado das Especialidades em Fonoaudiologia. São Paulo: Roca; 2014, pp. 386-93.
110. Franques ARM, Pacheco ESC. Acompanhamento psicológico no pós-operatório da cirurgia bariátrica. In: Segal A, Franques ARM. Atuação multidisciplinar na cirurgia bariátrica. A visão da COESAS-SBCBM. São Paulo: Miró Editorial; 2012, pp. 149-157.
111. Gonçalves RFM, Cheter EZ. Perfil mastigatório de obesos mórbidos submetidos à gastroplastia. Rev CEFAC Mai-Jun 2012; 14(3): 489-97.
112. Santos AC, Silva CAB. Força de mordida em pacientes candidatos à gastroplastia. Arq Bras Cir Dig 2013; 26(4): 315-8.
113. Zhu Y, Hollis JH. Increasing the Number of Chews before Swallowing Reduces Meal Size in Normal-Weight, Overweight, and Obese Adults. J Acad Nut Diet 2014; 114(6): 926-31.
114. Forde CG, van Kuijk N, Thaler T, Graaf C, Martin N. Oral processing characteristics of solid savoury meal components, and relationship with food composition, sensory attributes and expected satiation. Appetite 2013; 60: 208-19.
115. Godoy CMA, Caetano AL, Viana KRS, Godoy EP, Barbosa ALC, Ferraz EM. Food tolerance in patients submitted to gastric bypass: The importance of using an integrate and interdisciplinary approach. Obes Surg 2012; 22: 124-30.
116. Canterji MB, Finard SA. Intervenção fonoaudiológica em pacientes submetidos à cirurgia bariátrica. In: Silva HJ, Tessitore A, Motta AR, Cunha DA, Berretin-Felix G, Marchesan IQ. Tratado de Motricidade Orofacial. Pulso Editorial: São José dos Campos; 2019, pp. 763-76.

32 Anorexia nervosa and bulimia: psychological factors and oral implications

Mauro Bernabei and Marina Angela Visco

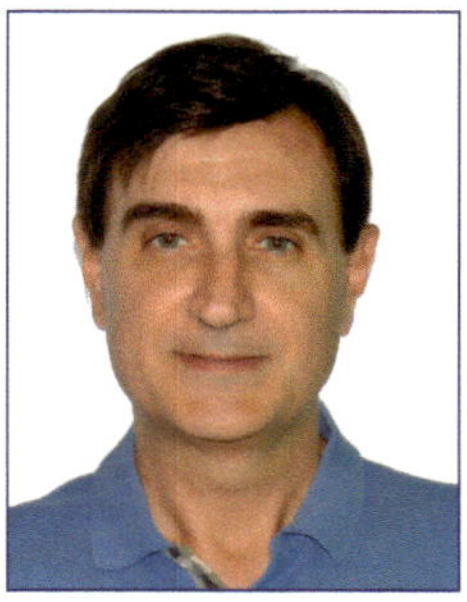

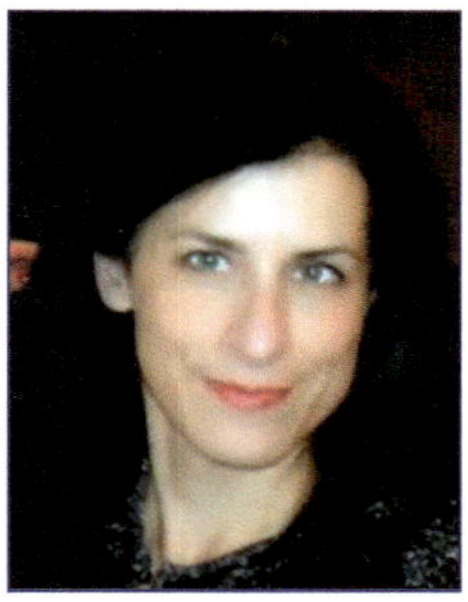

32.1 Introduction

Eating disorders are a wide group of psychopathological disorders characterized by the refusal or the excessive consumption of food (e.g., anorexia, bulimia, binge-eating disorder). The difficulties in the alimentary sphere represent the manifest expression, which takes shape "in the body", of a profound suffering of the subject. Around the food and its consumption revolve a quantity of meanings, of affective and relational experiences manifested through distorted or chaotic eating behaviors [1].

Although the diagnosis and the treatment of eating disorders pertain to mental health clinicians, the oral health practitioners can play an important role. They may be the first to detect an eating disorder [2-3] and they may have a role in informing the patient and the family for the first time.

Furthermore, the choices made by the specialist during treatment should also take into consideration the psychological characteristics of the patients and the consequent implications in dental therapies.

In this chapter we will focalize on the two main eating disorders affecting patients, *anorexia* and *bulimia*, which create complex and important connections between mental health clinicians and dental healthcare providers.

32.2 Definition and diagnostic criteria of anorexia nervosa and bulimia

The most used definitions of eating disorders are provided by the American Psychiatric Association's *Diagnostic and Statistical Manual of Mental Disorders DSM-V* [4].

The principal characteristic of anorexic patients is the obsessive need to decrease their body weight, so they tend to achieve weight control mainly by food abstention, which can be sometimes associated with intensive physical activity and/or other compensative behaviors.

According to the DSM-V, anorexia nervosa is characterized by:

- Restriction of energy intake relative to requirements, leading to a significant-

Mauro Bernabei, MD
Università Cattolica del Sacro Cuore, Rome, Italy

Email: maurobernabei@outlook.it

Marina Angela Visco, PhD
eCampus University, Novedrate, Como, Italy

ly low body weight in the context of age, sex, developmental trajectory and physical health. Significantly low weight is defined as a weight that is less than minimally normal or, for children and adolescents, less than minimally expected.
- Intense fear of gaining weight or of becoming fat, or persistent behavior that interferes with weight gain, even though at a significantly low weight.
- Disturbance in the way in which one's body weight or shape is experienced, undue influence of body weight or shape on self-evaluation, or persistent lack of recognition of the seriousness of the current low body weight.

The DSM-V includes the two subtypes of anorexia nervosa: *restrictive type,* where weight loss is accomplished primarily through dieting, fasting and/or excessive exercise, and *binge eating/purging type,* with recurrent episodes of binge eating or purging behavior in the last three months, i.e., self-induced vomiting, or the misuse of laxatives, diuretics or enemas.

Notably, in the DSM-V amenorrhea was eliminated as a diagnostic criterion for anorexia nervosa. Unlike the previous DSM-IV, the DSM-V also introduced severity specifiers for anorexia nervosa. Severity is determined by weight status: mild (Body Mass Index or BMI more than 17), moderate (BMI: 16-16.99), severe (BMI: 15-15.99) and extreme (BMI less than 15).

On the other hand, the essential features for specific diagnosis of bulimia are a persistent preoccupation with eating, binge eating, a strong fear of weight gain and inappropriate compensatory methods to prevent weight gain.

According to the DSM-V definition, the diagnostic criteria for bulimia are:
- Recurrent episodes of binge eating. An episode of binge eating is characterized by both:
  - Eating in a discrete period of time (e.g., within any 2-hour period), an amount of food that is definitely larger than what most individuals would eat in a similar period of time under similar circumstances;
  - A sense of lack of control over eating during the episodes (e.g., a feeling that one cannot stop eating or control what or how much one is eating).
- Recurrent inappropriate compensatory behaviors to prevent weight gain, such as self-induced vomiting; misuse of laxatives, diuretics or other medications; fasting; or excessive exercise.
- The binge eating and inappropriate compensatory behaviors both occur, on average, at least once a week for 3 months.
- Self-evaluation is unduly influenced by body shape and weight.
- The disturbance does not occur exclusively during episodes of anorexia nervosa.

As for anorexia nervosa, the DSM-V introduced severity specifiers for bulimia. In this disorder, severity is based on the average frequency of inappropriate compensatory behaviors (i.e., self-induced vomiting, laxative use, diuretic use, excessive exercise): mild (an average of 1-3 episodes per week), moderate (an average of 4-7 episodes per week), severe (an average of 8-13 episodes per week) and extreme (14 or more episodes per week).

So, in the DSM-V the diagnosis of bulimia has a frequency requirement of once weekly for binge-eating and weight-compensatory behaviors, a lower frequency than the twice weekly requirement of the DSM-IV.

Eating disorders rank as the third most common chronic illness in female adolescents, with an incidence of up to 5% [5-6]. In the DSM-V, the diagnostic criteria necessary for eating disorders became less restrictive. However, only limited research has assessed the impact of the newly introduced DSM-V criteria and severity specifiers across incidence of eating disorders diagnoses [7-9].

32.3 Psychological factors

The importance of psychological factors and interpersonal dynamics in the pathogenesis of eating disorders is widely recognized in literature. Eating disorders occur primarily in females, and adolescence is a major risk period for the development of these disorders [10].

Some authors underline temperamental and personality traits (e.g., dependency on others' approval) [11], traumatic factors (e.g., physical and sexual abuse, serious negligence suffered during childhood) [12], and family situations (e.g., enmeshment) in the etiology of eating disorders.

From a psychological point of view, it can be observed that eating is the first communication channel between children and their caregivers. It is one of the first ways to establish an affective relationship, through which the parent can respond to the child's vital needs and convey love and attention.

From nursing to weaning, feeding is a fundamental moment in which the quality of the relationship between the child and the parents is built. Within this fundamental affective function, it is essential for the caregiver to recognize the personal rhythms of the child and to decode his or her signals, helping the child to progressively discriminate her feelings, distinguishing hunger from other needs that she may be perceiving.

During growth, eating thus acquires an emotional value and became a way of expressing affection, primarily in the relationship between parents and child. In this way, the child may establish an equivalence between feeding and parental care and attention, and can create dysfunctional relational patterns within the family, which lead to the child's stimulation of excessive and/or unregulated eating.

As previously stressed, research has shown that anorexia nervosa and bulimia nervosa typically occur during adolescence and that onset thereafter is uncommon [13-17].

Adolescence can be defined as a period of "crisis" – Laufer defines it as a "developmental breakdown" [18] – during which the difficulties related to the transition process and the physical and psychological changes can affect many areas.

Adolescence is a process rather than a specific age or a developmental step that begins at puberty with a transformation and ends with the maturation of a quietly defined identity [19]. If these processes, for various reasons (for vulnerability, for a deficit of basic experiences or for any external circumstances) exceed the capacity of thought processing, manifestations of distress and even specific diseases could appear. So, a problem can express itself with conflicts with both the body and nutrition. In this scenario, diet becomes the instrument through which the attempt to control and manipulate one's body image may repair the weakness and the conflict in one's personal identity.

32.4 Oral manifestation of eating disorders

The medical complications of eating disorders are multiple and mainly attributable to nutritional deficiencies and erroneous weight control practices (Table 32.1).

Patients with eating disorders (EDs) are more likely to develop dental complications compared to other dental patients [20]. Besides the psychiatric symptoms, the effects of chronic self-induced starvation and vomiting can cause significant changes of the oral cavity health.

Most of the effects of EDs on oral health are reflected on the dental surface, periodontal tissues, oral mucosa and salivary glands. Because of the dental and oral exposure to stomach acids from frequent vomiting, these patients often have dental complica-

Table 32.1 Medical problems of eating disorders

System	*Starvation*	*Purging/vomiting*
Blood	Anemia Thrombocytopenia Leucopenia	
Cardiovascular	Bradycardia Hypotension	Arrhythmias and sudden death Cardiac failure, ECG abnormalities
CNS	Cerebral changes Cognitive damage	Epileptic fits Tetany
Endocrine	Ovarian changes Amenorrhea Reduced estrogen and progesterone Increased cortisol and growth hormone Diabetes insipidus	
Gastrointestinal	Delayed gastric emptying and poor motility Malabsorption	Esophageal ulcers Constipation and/or diarrhea
Liver	Raised enzymes Fatty infiltration	
Musculoskeletal	Osteoporosis Pathological fractures	Myopathy
Renal	Reduced glomerular filtration	Electrolyte abnormalities: reduced Na and K, increased P and Mg
Skin/hair	Loss of head hair Fur-like hair	

tions such as cavities, dental erosion, loss of restorations, abscesses, crumbling teeth, salivary gland swelling and pain.

With the changes in nutrition over the last 20 years, multiple studies have reported dental erosion due to overconsumption of carbonated beverages especially among teenagers.

However, because these types of dental erosion usually progress gradually, patients usually do not experience symptoms such as pain induced by cold fluids, and even when symptoms do occur, the pain is minimal [21]. Instead in patients with EDs, dental erosion may progress quickly often associated with severe cold induced pain [22].

The severity of dental erosion varies among patients with EDs and is not associated with the eating disorder's duration but only frequency of vomiting and consequent exposure of the teeth and soft tissues of the oral cavity to the stomach acids.

The most common dental symptoms presented by patients with bulimia, with or without anorexia, are pain caused by the tooth erosion with exposure of the dentin resulting in thermal sensitivity up to developing pulpitis. It takes about two years of frequent vomiting to cause this damage.

Since 1990, numerous articles linking EDs and oral health have been published because a dental emergency may be the patient's first contact with a health professional. In general, anorexic patients are more than 15% below ideal body weight whereas bulimic patients are within 10% of ideal weight or can even be overweight.

Because of all this, people with anorexia will look thin while people with bulimia are less readily identifiable from their outward appearance. Patients with bulimia usually do not present signs and symptoms of the disease and most of these patients show normal body weight.

This is the main reason why dentists may be the first healthcare professional to recognize the early symptoms of a previously undiagnosed case of eating disorder. The effects of self-induced starvation and chronic vomiting can cause significant and often irreversible changes in the dentition and in the oral cavity, besides the complex medical and psychiatric symptoms.

32.5 Dental erosion

Several epidemiological studies [23] have investigated the prevalence of dental erosion, defined as the chemical dissolution of dental hard tissues, as the most common oral manifestation in patients with EDs, who practice self-induced vomiting. This causes regurgitation of acidic gastric contents into the oral cavity, thereby making teeth more susceptible to enamel demineralization and erosion as vomitus passes through the oral cavity. Such erosion is characterized by a chemical rather than a bacterial dissolution and leads to uniform and glossy surfaces, in contrast to abrasion, which is caused by mechanical wear with the dental erosion appearing flat.

In 1939, Holst and Lange [24], inspired by a 1929 publication by Fleury, coined the term "perimylolysis" to describe decalcification of the dentition due to chronic regurgitation. The authors noted that "gastric dysfunction" with vomiting produced a destruction of coronal tooth tissue. The tooth erosion was caused by both the acidic composition of the vomitus and the acid retention.

The impact of eating disorders on oral health was initially reported by Hellstrom [25] describing perimyolysis as "a loss of enamel and dentin on lingual surfaces as a result of chemical and mechanical effects, mainly caused by gastric regurgitation contained and exacerbated by movements of the tongue".

Erosion can take place on all surfaces of the teeth. But the most frequent sites in patients with bulimia nervosa and anorexia nervosa are the lingual/palatal and occlusal surfaces of the posterior teeth [26]. The teeth appear smooth and glossy with rounded margins [27].

Factors that may influence the severity of dental erosion in patients with EDs include duration and frequency of vomiting incidents per day; the degree of acid dilution by means of water rinsing or drinking neutralizing liquids, such as milk; and timing of tooth cleansing particularly after a vomiting incident.

Studies suggest that a significant pre-vomiting water consumption can effectively protect the teeth from acid [28]. Recent studies also showed that cleaning the teeth with a toothbrush immediately after each vomiting episode is harmful because the softened, demineralized tooth surface, due to etching acid onto the teeth, is more susceptible to toothbrush abrasion compared with subjects who only rinsed their mouth or did nothing [29]. Therefore, to avoid worsening of dental erosion, oral hygiene after vomiting should always include a thorough oral rinse with water, bicarbonate or other liquids, such as milk, to neutralize the acid in the oral cavity and to allow remineralization of dental surfaces before careful tooth brushing [30].

Patients with anorexia nervosa and bulimia nervosa tend to consume an excessive amount of acidic drinks and foods, such as acidic sports drinks during physical activity [31]. They may also make abnormal use of some caffeinated and carbonated drinks, either to boost energy levels or to decrease the hunger stimulus by increasing dilation of the stomach [32]. Some patients also use lemon (juice or slices) and vinegar to diminish mechanism regulating hunger [33]. Patients with anorexia and bulimia nervosa also tend to consume excessive sugary drinks, sweets and sugary chewing gum not only have energy, but also to allay the constant feeling of hunger.

The critical pH for chemical erosion of the surface enamel is approximately 5.5 and about 6.7 in the exposed dentin. In general, carbonated drinks and citrus juice have a pH of about 3.0, higher than the pH able to dissolve the tooth. Therefore, regular consumption of these acidic products can cause chronic oral acidity, which can increase the severity of the initial dental erosion caused by vomiting [34].

The risk of caries is high because of the frequency and quantity of refined sugars ingested. The bacteria present in the oral cavity, such as *Streptococcus mutans*, which are attached to the dental structures, metabolize the sugars consumed thus producing acids such as lactic acid. These oral acids lower the oral pH, induce the demineralization of the enamel and further promotes the growth of aciduric microorganisms such as *S. sobrinus*, *Lactobacillus spp.* and *Candida spp.*

However, even in the presence of oral acidity induced by the consumption of acidic or sugary foods, the teeth will physiologically repair after a certain period. Salivary pH depends on the concentration of bicarbonate dissolved in saliva and an increase in bicarbonate concentration causes an increase in oral pH. Salivary bicarbonate content depends on salivary flow [35]. The bicarbonate concentration ranges from 1 mmol/L in unstimulated saliva to almost 60 mmol/L at high flow rates.

Bicarbonate is the most important buffer system in saliva but only at high flow rates. When saliva is not stimulated, the bicarbonate ion level is too low to be effective with the consequence that unstimulated saliva is poorly buffered [35]. For the remineralization process it is therefore essential to neutralize the acid pH of the oral cavity.

Quantitative and qualitative changes in saliva reduce its buffering and remineralizing capacity [36]. It is however accepted that quantita tive rather than qualitative variations influence the buffering effect of saliva in patients with EDs [37]. Saliva, which pH normally ranges between 5.5 and 8.0, loses its buffer capacity when it's below pH 5.0 and can no longer neutralize the acids present in the oral cavity [38].

It is generally accepted that this can be attributed to the side effects of commonly used psychoactive drugs, including antidepressants and antipsychotic drugs [39]. Psychiatrists should also be aware that antidepressants will decrease the amount of saliva, thus increasing the risk of caries and erosion. The abuse of laxatives and diuretics [40], binges and starvation, which lead to electrolyte imbalances, have serious dental implications, influencing saliva may further aggravate the problem.

For patients suffering from EDs, the consumption of sugars is often the most important source of calories and prohibiting these patients from consuming sugary foods is likely to be fatal [41]. As such, the progression of dental erosion should be slowed by changing the way patients consume sugary foods or by changing their oral hygiene behavior after consumption, for example by rinsing the mouth with water or with substances that can act as a buffer such as bicarbonate.

32.6 Dental caries

Dental caries becomes a problem in individuals whose diet is rich in cariogenic food, who have poor oral hygiene and manifest salivary disturbances [42].

Several of studies have investigated the association between dental caries and EDs [43]. It has been demonstrated that the frequency distribution of aciduric microbes (including *S. mutans*, *Lactobacilli* and yeasts) was significantly higher in bulimics when compared to medically healthy individuals with dental caries [43]. It has been reported that most patients with EDs consume high-sugar snacks several times daily which may in turn provide a source of nourishment to the cariogenic microbes residing in the oral cavity [44].

Simultaneously, the use of anti-depressants by several psychiatric patients may induce xerostomia in these individuals. It is noteworthy that a dry oral environment (coupled with poor oral health maintenance) may allow dental plaque to stagnate on teeth surfaces thereby facilitating the activity and multiplication of cariogenic microbes on fermentable carbohydrates. Many patients suck citrus flavored candies to help managing xerostomia but unwittingly they increase the potential for caries.

With patients with EDs, a collaborative treatment approach that requires both dental and psychological skills is indicated. It is essential that dentists understand that the patients have no voluntary control over their behavior.

It is important to make these patients feel reassured that the dental treatment will continue while the patient is in psychotherapy, so that they do not feel rejected or abandoned. However, the usual dental procedures to restore form and function must wait. In patients with EDs it is essential to neutralize the acids present in the oral cavity with adequate oral hygiene instructions, rinse with fluoride (using a 0.05% sodium fluoride concentration twice a day) and rinse with sodium bicarbonate. Using a device during vomiting, such as a bite, may limit dental erosion.

Any dental emergencies can be treated using temporary procedures such as preformed crowns, calcium hydroxide and acid-resistant composite resin. Artificial saliva for bulimics with reduced salivary production may be useful, as well as vitamin C supplements for gingival bleeding. Any permanent restoration is contraindicated as long as the eating disorder is not under control.

32.7 Periodontal disease

Periodontal disease is characterized by inflammation of the supporting structures of teeth including gingiva, periodontal ligament, root cementum and alveolar bone with poor oral hygiene maintenance being the most common risk factor. The etiology of periodontal disease is complex and multifactorial. Any factors that influence the composition of the microbiota may have an influence on both the establishment and progression of periodontal conditions.

It is well documented in the literature how periodontal disease is directly associated with the patient's age. Therefore it is a rather rare disease in patients suffering from EDs, which are relatively young individuals. Severe vitamin C deficiency has been reported to be associated with the development of a periodontal syndrome called "scorbutic gingivitis". It has been suggested that avitaminosis C in patients with EDs may play a role in periodontal disease in these individuals [45].

32.8 Oral mucosa

It is well accepted that saliva is important as a lubricant of the oral mucous membranes. Any change in quality, quantity and buffering capacity of saliva on the mucous membranes is related to chronic irritation due to direct contact of acidic contents on the mucosa.

Reduced intake of vitamins and other nutrients, as well as general metabolic alterations and iron deficiency anemia, can significantly influence the physiological trophism of the oral mucosa up to mucosal atrophy. A vitamin deficiency of the B group, in particular B1, B6 and B12, is classically associated with a decrease in epithelial cell turnover. Mucosal atrophy can also cause a diffuse oral burning sensation, which may be more intense on the tongue (glossodynia). This is particularly evident on the tongue where the association with erythema may result in atrophic glossitis. Trauma to the mucosa, particularly to that of the pharynx and soft palate, is believed to arise as a result of inserting foreign objects into the oral cavity to induce vomiting.

Mucosal lesions such as those induced by trauma are frequently secondarily infected by candida organisms. Angular cheilitis, a form of chronic oral candidiasis, has been reported in patients with EDs. Oral candidiasis is associated with both nutritional deficiencies and salivary dysfunction. Many oral mucosal lesions are due to acid during vomiting (epithelial erosion) which may impair repair and the regenerative potential of the oral mucosa and may induce neoplastic tissue changes.

32.9 Salivary glands

Dry and cracked lips, burning sensation in the mouth (especially on the tongue) and parotid gland swellings have been reported to be common in patients with EDs. This reflects a negative impact on the salivary glands caused by frequent vomiting, starvation and use of antidepressant drugs that result in hyposalivation.

It has been reported that most patients with EDs often have enlarged parotid glands. The onset and extension of the parotid swelling is proportional to the duration and severity of the purging behavior. In the early stages of eating disorder, the enlarged gland may appear only sometimes, but when the eating disorder will progress, the swelling becomes more persistent. The etiology of the enlargement of the salivary glands is uncertain but some authors have associated parotid enlargement with the recurrent vomiting episodes, because of the chronic stimulation of the glands during vomiting.

32.10 Conclusion

Eating disorders, such as anorexia and bulimia nervosa, are a serious concern for the oral health of patients presenting unique psychological, medical, nutritional and dental models.

Treatment of eating disorders needs to take a multi-disciplinary approach, and would ideally include not only mental health clinician and medical teams, but also dental healthcare providers [46].

Dentist may be the first to identify sign and symptoms of eating disorders, and early detection and intervention play a key role in the recovery of this pathology. Furthermore, knowledge of the patient's psychological characteristics is important for the correct management of dental treatment. The dentist must be aware of the important dynamics going around the issues of control. With the right approach, the dentist can help the patient feel in control of his or her mouth and body. Some individuals are resistant to acknowledging their eating disorder and are reluctant to accept treatment. The prognosis depends on the nature and extent of the personality disorder, which can range from mild to severe. Any extensive dental treatment undertaken without psychological treatment of the underlying problem is obviously doomed to failure. Therefore, any dental procedures to restore form and function must consider the psychological condition of the patient [47].

REFERENCES

1. Lo Russo L, Campisi G, Di Fede O, Di Liberto C, Panzarella V, Lo Muzio L. Oral manifestations of eating disorders: a critical review. Oral Dis 2008; 14(6): 479-84.
2. Walsh JM, Wheat ME, Freund K. Detection, evaluation, and treatment of eating disorders the role of the primary care physician. J Gen Intern Med 2000; 15(8): 577-90.
3. DeBate RD, Tedesco LA, Kerschbaum WE. Knowledge of oral and physical manifestations of anorexia and bulimia nervosa among dentists and dental hygienists. J Dent Educ 2005; 69(3): 346-54.
4. American Psychiatric Association. Diagnostic and statistical manual of mental disorders (DSM-5®). American Psychiatric Pub, 2013.
5. Fisher M, Golden NH, Katzman DK, et al. Eating disorders in adolescents: A background paper. J Adolesc Health 1995; 16: 420-37.
6. Croll J, Neumark-Sztainer D, Story M, Ireland M. Prevalence and risk and protective factors related to disordered eating behaviors among adolescents: Relationship to gender and ethnicity. J Adolesc Health 2002; 31: 166-75.
7. Smith KE, Ellison JM, Crosby RD, Engel SG, Mitchell JE, Crow SJ, Peterson CB, Le Grange D, Wonderlich SA. The validity of DSM-5 severity specifiers for anorexia nervosa, bulimia nervosa, and binge-eating disorder. Int J Eat Disord 2017; 50(9): 1109-13.
8. Serrano-Troncoso E, Cañas L, Carbonell X, Carulla M, Palma C, Matalí J, Dolz M. Diagnostic Distribution of eating disorders: Comparison between DSMIV-IV TR and DSM-5. Actas Esp Psiquiatr 2017; 45(1): 32-8.
9. Vo M, Accurso EC, Goldschmidt AB, Le Grange D. The Impact of DSM-5 on Eating Disorder Diagnoses. Int J Eat Disord 2017; 50(5): 578-81.
10. Leon GR, Fulkerson JA, Perry CL, Cudeck R. Personality and behavioral vulnerabilities associated with risk status for eating disorders in adolescent girls. J Abnorm Psychol 1993; 102(3): 438-44.
11. Matsunaga H, Kaye WH, McConaha C, Plotnicov K, Pollice C, Rao R. Personality disorders among subjects recovered from eating disorders. Int J Eat Disord 2000; 27(3): 353-7.
12. Carter JC, Bewell C, Blackmore E, Woodside DB. The impact of childhood sexual abuse in anorexia nervosa. Child Abuse Negl 2006; 30(3): 257-69.
13. Garfinkel PE, Lin E, Goering P, Spegg C, Goldbloom DS, Kennedy S, Kaplan AS, Woodside DB. Bulimia nervosa in a Canadian community sample: prevalence and comparison of subgroups. Am J Psychiatry 1995; 152(7): 1052-8.
14. Hudson JI, Pope HG Jr, Jonas JM, Yurgelun-Todd D, Frankenburg FR. A controlled family history study of bulimia. Psychol Med 1987; 17(4): 883-90.
15. Kendler KS, MacLean C, Neale M, Kessler R, Heath A, Eaves L. The genetic epidemiology of bulimia nervosa. Am J Psychiatry 1991; 148(12): 1627-37.
16. Striegel-Moore RH, Franko DL, Thompson D, Barton B, Schreiber GB, Daniels SR. An empirical study of the typology of bulimia nervosa and its spectrum variants. Psychol Med 2005; 35(11): 1563-72.
17. Woodside DB, Garfinkel PE, Lin E, Goering P, Kaplan AS, Goldbloom DS, Kennedy SH. Comparisons of men with full or partial eating disorders, men without eating disorders, and women with eating disorders in the community. Am J Psychiatry 2001; 158(4): 570-4.
18. Laufer ME and Laufer M. Adolescence and Developmental Breakdown: A Psychoanalytic View. Karnac Books, 1995.
19. Pavan L. Adolescence between temporary crisis and breakdown evolution. Interdisciplinary Journal of Family Studies, XIX, 2/2014.
20. Hermont AP, Pordeus IA, Paiva SM, Abreu MH, Auad SM. Eating disorder risk behavior and dental implications among adolescents. Int J Eat Disord 2013, 46: 677-83.
21. Cronin RJ Jr, Cagna DR. Causes of severe tooth wear. Jpn Dental Outlook 2003, 101: 254-65.
22. Otsu M, Suzuki A, Hasegawa I, Miyauchi M, Karibe H, Okada T, Ishii T, Yamaoka M, Ichijyo T, Sato T. Dental problems in patients with eating disorder accompanied by self-induced vomiting – Oral environment. Jpn J Psychosom Med 2006, 46: 960-96.
23. Hamilton J. Eating disorders: the untold story. CDS Review 1996; 89: 10-8.
24. Holst JJ, Lange F. Perimylolysis. A contribution towards the genesis of tooth wasting from non-mechanical causes. Acta Odontol Scand 1939; 1: 36-47.
25. Hellstrom I. Oral complications in anorexia nervosa. Scand J Dent Res 1977; 85: 71-86.
26. Parry J, Shaw L, Arnaud MJ, Smith AJ. Investigation of mineral waters and soft drinks in relation to dental erosion. J Oral Rehabil 2001; 28(8): 766-72.
27. Frydrych AM, Davies GR, McDermott BM. Eating disorders and oral health: a review of the literature. Aust Dent J 2005; 50(1): 6-15; quiz 56.
28. Otsu M, Hamura A, Ishikawa Y, Karibe H, Ichijyo T, Yoshinaga Y. Factors affecting the dental erosion severity of patients with eating disorders. Biopsychosoc Med 2014; 8: 25.
29. Meurman JH, ten Cate JM: Pathogenesis and modifying factors of dental erosion. Eur J Oral Sci 1996; 104: 199-206.
30. Hamasha AA, Zawaideh FI, Al-Hadithy RT: Risk indicators associated with dental erosion among Jordanian school children aged 12-14 years of age. Int J Paediatr Dent 2014; 24: 56-68.

31. Messias DC, Turssi CP, Hara AT, Serra MC: Sodium bicarbonate solution as an anti-erosive agent against simulated endogenous erosion. Eur J Oral Sci 2010; 118: 385-88.
32. Jarvinen VK, Rytomaa II, Heinonen OP. Risk factors in dental erosion. J Dent Res 1991; 70: 942-7.
33. Del Signore A, Campisi B, Di Giacomo F. Characterization of balsamic vinegar by multivariate statistical analysis of trace element content. J AOAC Int 1998; 81(5): 1087-95.
34. Lussi A, Jaeggi T, Zero D: The role of diet in the aetiology of dental erosion. Caries Res 2004, 38: 34-44.
35. Levine JM, Walton BE, Franko DL, Jimerson DC. Serum amylase in bulimia nervosa: clinical status and pathology. Int J Eat Disord 1992; 12: 431-9.
36. Hurst PS, Lacey JH, Crisp AH. Teeth, vomiting and diet: a study of the dental characteristics of 17 anorexia nervosa patients. Postgrad Med J 1977; 53: 298-305.
37. House RC, Bliziotes MM, Licht JH. Perimolysis: unveiling the surreptitious vomiter. Oral Surg 1981; 51: 152-5.
38. Valentine AD, Anderson RJ, Bradnock G. SalivarypH and dental caries. Brit Dent J 1978; 144: 105-7.
39. Kleier JK, Aragon SB, Averbach RE. Dental management of the chronic vomiting patient. J Am Dent Assoc 1984; 108: 618-21.
40. Harrison JL, George LA, Cheatham JL, Zinn J. Dental effects and management of bulimia nervosa. Gen Dent 1985; 33: 65-8.
41. Crow SJ, Peterson CB, Swanson SA, Raymond NC, Specker S, Eckert ED, Mitchell JE. Increased mortality in bulimia nervosa and other eating disorders. Am J Psychiatry 2009; 166: 1342-6.
42. Touyz S, Liew V, Tseng P, Frisken K, Williams H, Beumont P. Oral and dental complications in dieting disorders. Int J Eat Disord 1993; 14: 341-7.
43. Bretz WA, Krahn DD, Drewnowski A, Loesche WJ. Salivary levels of putative cariogenic organisms in patients with eating disorders. Oral Microbiol Immunol 1989; 4(4): 230-2.
44. Studen-Pavlovich D, Elliott MA. Eating disorders in women's oral health. Dent Clin North Am 2001; 45(3): 491-511.
45. Hamilton J. Eating disorders, the untold story. CDS Rev 1996; 89(4): 10-8.
46. Johansson AK, Johansson A, Unell L, Norring C, Carlsson GE. Eating disorders and signs and symptoms of temporomandibular disorders: a matched case-control study. Swed Dent J 2010; 34(3): 139-47.
47. Levinson NA. Oral manifestations of eating disorders: Indications for a collaborative treatment approach. The Eating Disorders. Blinder BJ, Chaitin BF and Goldstein RS (Eds), PMA Publishing Corp. New York, 405-411, 1998.

Section 5 Foods' new frontiers

33 Imaging evaluation of foods and subjects under dietary regimen: new frontiers

Davide Bellini, Nicola Panvini, Daniela Prosperi, Damiano Caruso and Andrea Laghi

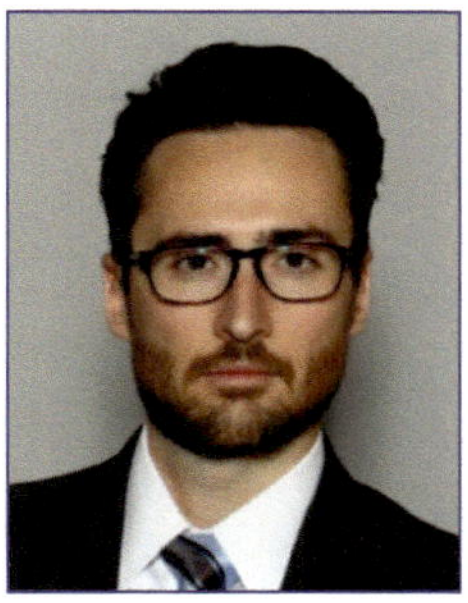

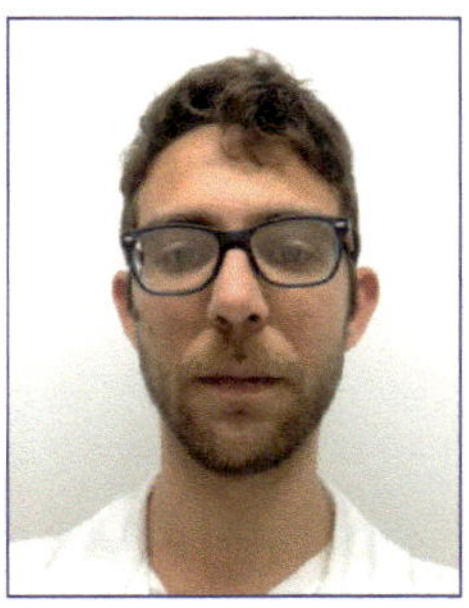

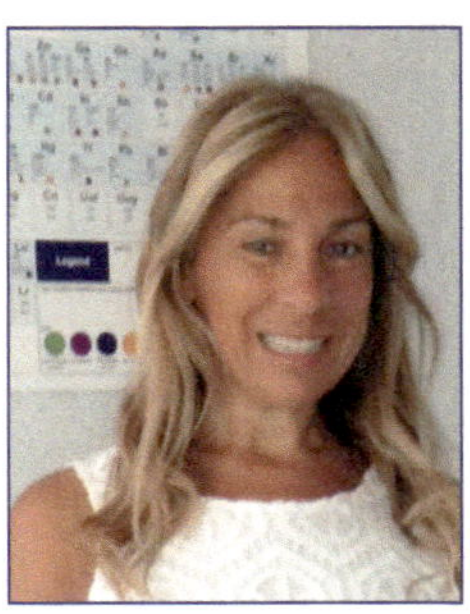

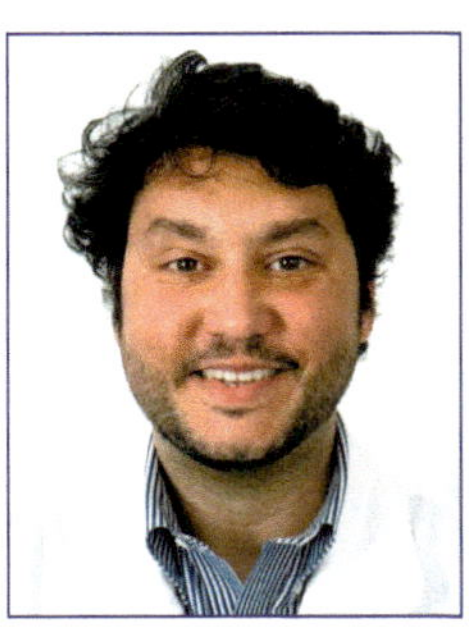

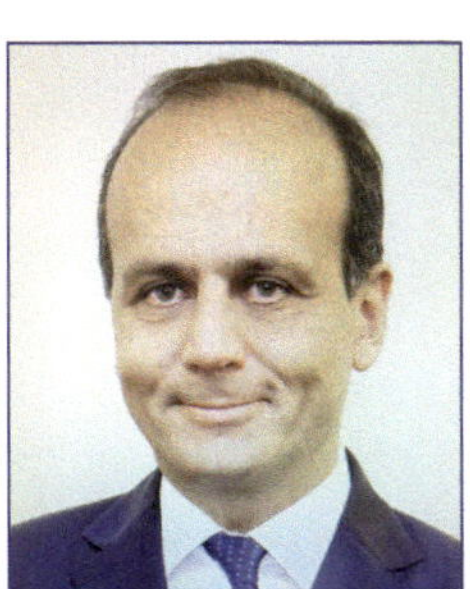

33.1 Introduction

Non-invasive, objective methods to evaluate subjects under dietary regimen are of upmost importance. Diagnostic imaging techniques such as dual energy x-ray absorptiometry (DXA), computed tomography (CT), magnetic resonance imaging (MRI) and ultrasonography (US) are emerging as accurate tools to assess human body anatomy, composition and consequently nutrition status. Moreover, emerging evidence documented their role in the evaluation of foods' texture and for monitoring foods' quality during processing.

In this chapter we'll explore the methodologies and the value of imaging techniques used to assess human body composition in research and clinical settings, while also focusing our attention on the most common pathologies that can affect the entire gastrointestinal tract and that can negatively influence patients under dietary regimen.

33.2 Imaging and food quality control

Modern challenges in food science require a new understanding of the determinants of food quality and safety. Traditional assessment procedures such as mechanical or chemical methods are destructive and time-consuming that can-

Davide Bellini, MD
Department of Radiological Sciences, Oncology and Pathology, Sapienza University of Rome; I.C.O.T. Hospital, Latina, Italy

Email: bellinidavide29@gmail.com

Nicola Panvini MD
Department of Radiological Sciences, Oncology and Pathology, Sapienza University of Rome; I.C.O.T. Hospital, Latina, Italy

Daniela Prosperi MD
Nuclear Medicine Unit; Sant'Andrea University Hospital, Rome, Italy

Damiano Caruso MD, PhD
Department of Medical Surgical Sciences and Translational Medicine, Sapienza University of Rome; Sant'Andrea University Hospital, Rome, Italy

Andrea Laghi, MD
Department of Medical Surgical Sciences and Translational Medicine, Sapienza University of Rome; Sant'Andrea University Hospital, Rome, Italy

Email: andrea.laghi@uniroma1.it

not respond to the contemporary food industry demands. Application of advanced imaging modalities such as MRI has seen impressive successes and fast growth over the past decade.

The MRI has been proven to be an effective non-invasive technique for quality assessment in a wide variety of food products. MRI is a non-ionizing, non-invasive technology that is widely used in diagnostic radiology. Using radio waves and a powerful magnet linked to a computer, the MRI can create detailed pictures of the human body but also of objects and foods. With the advancement of technologies, new techniques for MRI are shifting the paradigm of imaging evaluation from a qualitative to a quantitative point of view. The most interesting quantitative MRI methods in food evaluation, currently considered are diffusion weighted imaging (DWI), which is able to evaluate movements of water molecules; diffusion tensor imaging (DTI), which is a kind of diffusion weighted MRI that measures diffusion coefficients in several directions; and MRI spectroscopy, which is able to detect small molecular markers.

Specific MR sequences can easily identify and quantify molecular composition of foods, computing for example the distribution of muscle and fat, which are very important elements in the tastiness, texture and smell of meat and fish products.

Magnetic resonance imaging is helpful in determining the distribution, size, volume and shape of the adipose tissues in live fish [1] and different meat types [2, 3]. DWI can be used to determine the amount of oil uptake in the meat during frying [4, 5]. DTI can delineate muscle fibers orientation and distribution, evaluating complex structural information such as fiber type and diameter, and allowing correlation with muscle metabolic characteristics.

Evaluation of salt and water distribution using DWI sequences is well reported in literature. The diffusion pattern of restriction is significantly different in various meat tissues. During curing, for example, the meat microstructure greatly changes, and the diffusion coefficient increases. MRI is also applied in monitoring and optimizing brining of fish products.

Magnetic resonance can be used to monitor the structural events occurring during cooking, final rising of dough and baking in order to enhance these processes [6]. The strength of this method and its large applicability are confirmed by the fact that MRI has also been regarded as a useful method for the evaluation of texture and structure of foods such as lasagna, pasta, potato and noodles during and after cooking [7].

Last but not least, there is a plethora of studies reporting the use of MRI in the evaluation of agricultural products and post-harvest sorting and processing [8], in soil, root, stem and leaf water content as well as produce transport [9]. Some of the most common applications are: performing internal quality assessment and monitoring for ripening of almost all vegetables and fruits; evaluating the effects of chitosan (a natural biocontrol active ingredient) on the maturity and conservation of citruses; distinguishing mealy (soft and over ripened) from fresh fruits; studying the infestation of apples by the peach moth; and investigating water content in kiwis.

33.3 Liver imaging

Nonalcoholic fatty liver disease (NAFLD) is an emerging cause of hepatocellular carcinoma, liver transplantation and liver-related mortality affecting approximately 30% of Western populations. The NAFLD encompasses a wide spectrum of pathological conditions ranging from hepatic steatosis to nonalcoholic steatohepatitis (NASH) and cirrhosis, and is frequently associated with comorbidities such as obesity, diabetes mellitus, hypertension and dyslipidemia [10]. Dietary intervention consisting of hypocaloric diet alone or combined with physical exercise plays a pivotal role in the therapeutical management of NAFLD and has been shown to effectively improve the histopathological features of NASH and overall morbidity and mortality rates in these patients [11]. Liver biopsy is the gold standard for diagnosis of NAFLD, nevertheless, biopsy is invasive, costly, and it is subject to sampling variability and potential complications. Therefore, MRI, which is a non-invasive tool for accurate grading and quantification of liver steatosis, is currently recognized as the reference standard technique to monitor patients with NAFLD who underwent dietary restriction and need to assess response to treatment. Moreover, MRI can be used to accurately estimate the degree of hepatic fibrosis, which has been demonstrated to be an independent predictor of liver-related mortality in NAFLD [12].

Magnetic Resonance spectroscopy is the most sensitive MRI-based technique for hepatic fat quantification, being able to measure the hepatic proton density fat fraction (PDFF), which represents the proportion of protons bound to the fat among the total number of protons in the liver. However, MR spectroscopy has considerable limitations as it is a time-consuming technique and not widely available on all MRI scanners. In addition, it can lead to unrepresentative results because, similarly to liver biopsy, it typically measures data from just a single region of the liver parenchyma [13].

Multi-echo chemical shift MRI is a valuable alternative to MR spectroscopy, which allows to estimate whole liver PDFF with high sensitivity and excellent correlation with histopathologic analyses. Multi-echo chemical shift may be used during the follow-up of patients with NAFLD to monitor the effects of dietary regimen and has been shown to be able to detect small changes in liver fat content following dietary intervention, with an accuracy even superior to liver biopsy [14].

33.4 Upper gastrointestinal tract imaging

The introduction of multidetector row systems has renewed interest in imaging of the upper gastrointestinal (GI) tract by means of CT. Optimal upper GI CT studies require adequate luminal distension and the administration of intravenous contrast material to accurate detect walls' abnormalities and enhancement occurring in inflammatory and neoplastic processes. Gastric distension is usually obtained by ingestion of 500-1000 mL of water just before starting the examination. Positive oral contrasts should not routinely used as they can mask the walls' enhancement after intravenous contrast administration and are generally reserved for selected cases when the presence of fistulas or perforation is suspected. Additionally, administration of antiperistaltic agents, such as scopolamine N-butylbromide, can be useful to prevent contractures that may mimic pathological wall thickening or strictures. CT gastrography is a recent imaging technique that takes advantage of several reconstruction methods, such as multiplanar reformation, transparent imaging, and 3D volume rendering virtual gastroscopy to provide comprehensive evaluation of various gastric diseases (Fig. 33.1). Gastric distension for CT gastrography is usually achieved by oral ingestion of negative contrast agents mixed with effervescent granules. After that, intramuscular injection of an antispasmolytic agent is performed to reduce bowel peristalsis and the patient is then scanned in both prone and supine position [15].

Over the last decade, MRI has progressively become an important imaging method for the detection and characterization of diseases of the upper GI tract. Magnetic resonance protocols for upper GI evaluation usually entail the acquisition of T2-weighted single-shot and breath-hold 2D or 3D T1-weighted gradient echo (GRE) before and after the administration of gadolinium-based contrast agents. To obtain optimal distension and reduce motion artifacts, approximately 1000 mL of water are administered orally before the examination, followed by intramuscular injection of a bowel paralytic drug such as scopolamine or glucagon [16]. Cine-MR imaging with fast

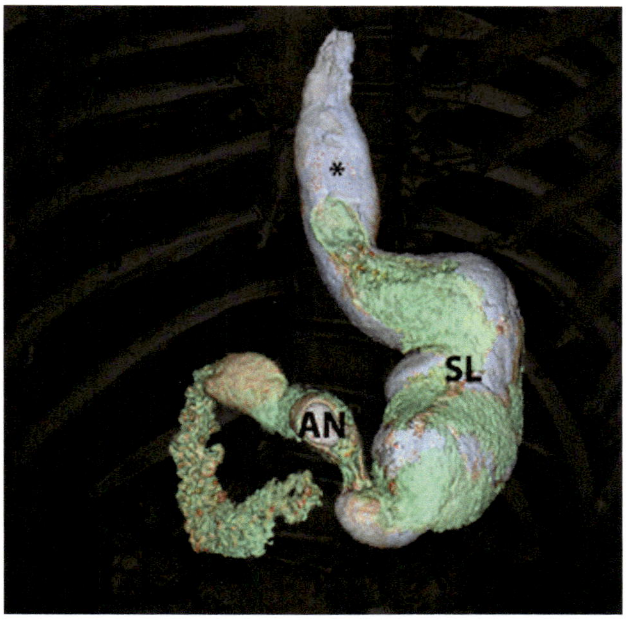

Fig. 33.1 3D volume rendering reconstruction of a CT exam. The image shows gastric morphology and volume of a patient after "Sleeve Gastrectomy", a surgical procedure that restricts the volume of the stomach consequently reducing the amount of food that can be ingested. The gastric sleeve volume was segmented to show the dilatation of the sleeve (SL), hiatal hernia (*) and the antrum (AN).

T2-weigthed pulse sequences is an accurate technique for non-invasive evaluation of gastrointestinal motility, playing an important role in the assessment of several functional esophageal and gastric disorders, without the burden of employing ionizing radiations or endoluminal catheters. In addition, MR may be useful to evaluate gastric emptying, by using a test meal mixed with paramagnetic agents and plotting the changes in gastric volume over time [17].

33.5 Small bowel imaging

The small bowel is habitually known to be a challenging anatomical district to evaluate by imaging. However, the significant technical improvement which occurred in the last decades have led to a progressive increase in the use of cross-sectional imaging techniques, such as ultrasounds (US), multidetector computed tomography (MDCT) and MRI, that now are widely recognized as fundamental tools for the diagnosis and management of a large variety of disorders that may affect the small intestine. Unlikely traditional barium studies and endoscopy, cross-sectional imaging yields the opportunity to evaluate not only luminal, but also transmural and extra-enteric disease, and has replaced barium examinations as first-line imaging technique for the assessment of patient with known or suspected small bowel diseases.

Small bowel imaging requires the bowel loops to be adequately distended before image acquisition to ensure high diagnostic accuracy. Bowel distension can be achieved with two different techniques: enteroclysis or enterography. Enteroclysis dictates the administration of 1500-2000 mL of enteral contrast media through a nasojejunal tube inserted by fluoroscopic guidance. To avoid impairment of mucosal enhancement (uptake of contrast medium by the inner layer of the intestinal wall) when using intravenous contrast agents, neutral contrast agents such as water or polyethylene glycol (PEG) solutions are usually employed, rather than using diluted barium or iodinated positive contrasts. For enterography instead, bowel distension is obtained by oral administration of contrast media approximately 30-40 minutes before starting the examination. Although enteroclysis provides generally better bowel distension, especially for the duodenum and jejunum, than enterography, the latter is usually preferred in the clinical practice due to its easiness and the higher patient tolerability [18].

Small bowel US is a cheap and widely available technique that can be used to successfully evaluate small bowel disease processes. It is well tolerated, does not entail radiation exposure, and allows dynamic evaluation of bowel loops and repeated examination. However, diagnostic accuracy is significantly influenced by the individual operator's skill and experience. Small bowel US require pre-procedural fasting, to limit intraluminal gas, and the use of high-frequency (5-17 MHz) linear probes. Additional information regarding bowel and mesenteric vascularity can be obtained using color or power Doppler imaging. Small intestine contrast ultrasounds (SICUS), also known as hydrosonography, is performed after obtaining bowel distension with oral administration of echo-poor liquid contrasts, most commonly PEG solutions. The SICUS allows better proximal bowel evaluation and has been shown to improve diagnostic accuracy and to reduce inter-observer variability [18]. In the last years, moreover, Contrast-enhanced US (CEUS) with intravenous microbubble contrast agents has been increasingly adopted for small bowel imaging, especially in patients with Crohn's disease (CD) [19].

Multidetector CT enterography/enteroclysis showed high diagnostic accuracy for a variety of pathological conditions arising from the small bowel. Given its widespread availability and rapid scanning time, MDCT is the imaging modality of choice to evaluate the small bowel in acute setting, with high reliability in detecting life-threatening pathologies such as acute gastrointestinal bleeding, small bowel ischemia or obstruction [20]. Radiation exposure is the major concern regarding the use of MDCT enterography/enteroclysis, especially for younger patients and for those affected by chronic conditions such as irritable bowel disease (IBD) as they require repeated imaging over their lifetime. Nonetheless, it should be noted that many effective strategies for radiation dose reduction have been recently developed, such as lowering the tube voltage, automatic exposure control, and the use of iterative reconstruction, which can allow reduction up to 50% of the delivered radiation dose [21].

Magnetic resonance enterography/enteroclysis (MRE) is a relatively recent imaging technique that is progressively taking on a role as the imaging modality of choice for the evaluation of several inflammatory and non-inflammatory small bowel diseases. The main strengths of MRE are: the lack of exposure to ionizing radiations and iodinated contrast media; the ability to provide functional dynamic evaluation of the small bowel motility and distension; and its excellent soft tissue contrast, superior to that obtained with CTE. Major limitations include: restricted availability, higher cost, and variability in image quality (depending on patient's compliance and breath-holding capacity). However, due to the absence of radiation exposure, MRE is the best-suited imaging modality to asses chronic small bowel diseases that develop early in the life, such as CD and celiac disease, which may require multiple serial examinations to evaluate disease progression and monitor the response to treatment [22].

Many different enteric contrast agents are available to achieve bowel distension before MRE, and these can be divided into three classes, depending on the signal intensity that they produce on T1- and T2-weighted images: positive contrast agents (high signal intensity on both T1- and T2-weighted images, such as dilute gadolinium solutions, or manganese containing fluids, like blueberry juice); negative contrast agents (low signal intensity on both T1- and T2-weighted images, such as superparamagnetic iron oxide solution in air); and biphasic contrast agents (high signal intensity on T1-weighted images and low signal intensity on T2-weighted imaging, such as water or PEG solutions) (Fig. 33.2). Biphasic agents are the most commonly adopted, leading to optimal contrast between bowel lumen and enhancing walls or endoluminal masses on T1-weighted images obtained after intravenous contrast media administration [23].

The lack of radiation exposure during MRE allows for repeated acquisitions at various points in time to obtain dynamic cine-MRI images. Cine-MRI provides functional information for non-invasive as-

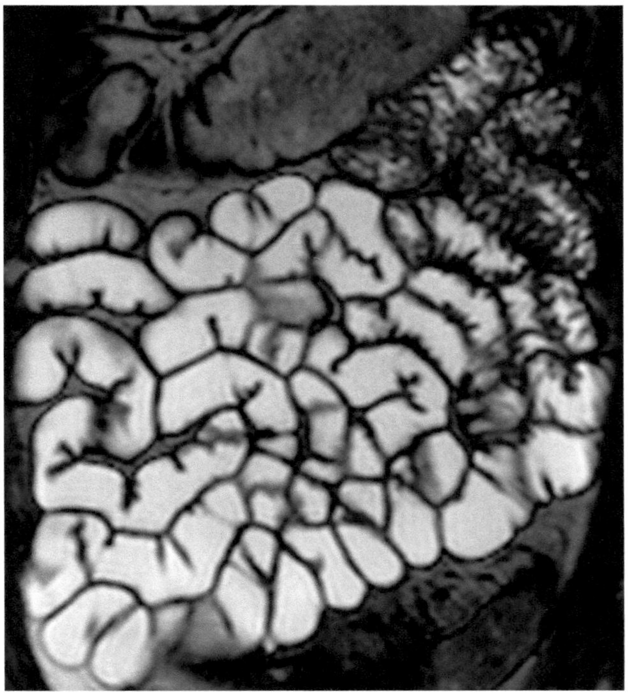

Fig. 33.2 MR enterography. Coronal balanced SSFP image clearly depicts well distended ileal loops after ingestion of biphasic oral contrast. Endoluminal oral contrast appears hyperintense on T2-weighted images and is easily distinguished from the bowel wall, which appears hypointense.

sessment of bowel motility and has been recently investigated with promising results for the evaluation of both organic diseases, such as IBD, and functional disorders such as irritable bowel syndrome (IBS) [24].

33.6 Large bowel imaging

In the last decades, cross-sectional imaging has become a fundamental technique for the assessment of large bowel, progressively replacing conventional double-contrast barium enema and fluoroscopic studies in a wide range of clinical scenarios. Due to recent advances in both patient preparation and image acquisition, and to the ability to provide valuable transmural evaluation, cross-sectional imaging is currently regarded as the modality of choice for non-invasive large bowel evaluation, allowing optical colonoscopy to be reserved for tissue sampling and therapeutic intervention in a variety of clinical indications [25].

Computed tomography colonography (CTC), also known as virtual colonoscopy, is a minimally invasive, patient-friendly, safe and accurate imaging modality for colon evaluation (Fig. 33.3). The CTC consists in three consecutive phases: bowel preparation, colonic distension and image acquisition. Bowel preparation has the objective to clean the colonic lumen of bulky contents that may mimic or hide pathological endoluminal findings and to tag any solid or fluid residual [26]. Both these targets can be optimally achieved with a reduced bowel-cleansing regimen consisting of oral administration of a colon-cleansing agents (1000 mL of PEG solutions) the evening before the examination followed by a fecal tagging agent (60 mL of sodium diatrizoate and meglumine diatrizoate solution) to be orally administered the day of the examination, without the need for any dietary restriction [27]. Adequate colonic distension can be obtained with manual room air administration through a rectal catheter or, preferably, by using an automated low-pressure CO_2 insufflator, that allows for improved reproducibility of colonic distension and reduces patient's discomfort. Image acquisition involves two consecutive scanning, the first with the patient in prone position and the second supine, to allow for redistribution of tagged stools and residual fluid and for visualization of the entire colonic wall. Additional decubitus scans can be obtained as a problem-solving series when colonic segments are collapsed on standard acquisition images. Several dose reduction strategies, such as reducing tube current and voltage, and using automatic exposure control and iterative reconstruction, can be incorporated in CTC acquisition protocol to perform very low-dose CTC (lower than 3-5 mSv) without affecting diagnostic accuracy [28]. The CTC is a safe examination, with few contraindications, namely acute abdominal conditions such as diverticulitis or acute phase of IBD or recent colonic surgery, and a very low complication rate (i.e., perforation).

The CTC has been proven to accurately detect colorectal cancers and large adenomas (≥ 10 mm), with diagnostic performance and detection rates comparable to those observed for colonoscopy. The role of CTC in different clinical scenarios has been defined by the consensus guidelines on indications of CTC developed by a team of gastrointestinal radiologists and endoscopists and jointly published by the European Society of Gastrointestinal and Abdominal Radiology (ESGAR) and the European Society of Gastrointestinal Endoscopy (ESGE) [29]. Major indications for CTC include incomplete, failed, or unfeasible colonoscopy, evaluation of non-mucosal lesion detected at colonoscopy, and opportunistic colorectal cancer screening of average-risk individuals. In addition, CTC plays a pivotal role in the evaluation of diverticular disease, both when the diagnosis is still unknown as well as for the assessment of patients with symptomatic chronic diverticular disease. Based on its ability to provide comprehensive endoluminal and extraluminal evaluation, CTC can confirm the

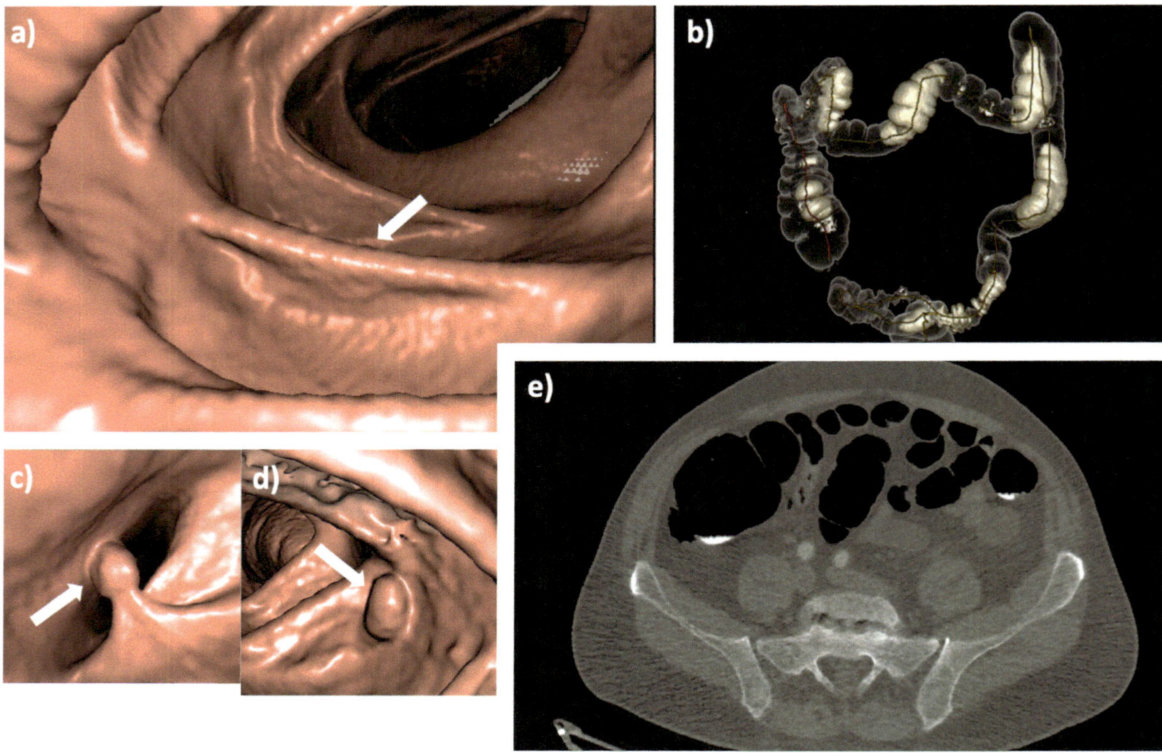

Fig. 33.3 Computed tomography (CT) colonography, also known as Virtual colonoscopy. Classic 2D image of abdomen is reported in **e**). From that image, multiplanar reconstruction and 3D endoluminal view (**a**, **c**, **d**) can be easily obtained, resembling endoscopic view. **b**) CT 3D reconstruction with iconographic effect similar to double contrast barium enema, where the entire colon can be displayed in one single image, obtaining a comprehensive evaluation of the colon. In **c**) and **d**) are reported two different polypoid lesions, a pedunculate polyp with a thin peduncle arising from the fold in **c**); a sessile polyp with large base of implant in **d**).

diagnosis of diverticular disease and detect underlying malignancies or unknown complications, such as peridiverticular abscesses or fistulas. Determination of the severity of a disease by the means of CTC-based scores can be used as a tool for therapeutic management decisions, providing relevant information to guide conservative or surgical treatment [30].

Two different strategies for bowel distension for MR colonography have been described: bright-lumen and dark-lumen strategies, depending on distension agents' appearance on T1-weighted images. Bright-lumen techniques consist of water mixed with dilute gadolinium chelate administration either rectally, orally or both. Dark-lumen colonography involves either rectal gas insufflation (room air or CO_2) or rectal water administration and require intravenous administration of a gadolinium-based contrast agent for optimal visualization of colonic walls. Bowel preparation prior MR colonography can be achieved either by colon cleansing or by fecal tagging. Bowel cleansing generally entails a full cathartic preparation combined with a liquid diet the day before the examination. Fecal tagging requires the oral ingestion of tagging agents (barium-based or paramagnetic agents for dark- and bright-lumen strategies, respectively) in association with a low-fiber diet. Eventually, image acquisition is performed with three-dimensional T1-weighted and two-dimensional T2-weighted pulse sequences acquired in both supine and prone position. MR colonography can also be performed concurrently with MR enterography providing comprehensive evaluation of both small and large bowel to asses disease activity, severity, and the presence of complications in patients with IBD [31]. Although MR colonography yields high diagnostic accuracy for the detection of colorectal cancers and adenomas greater then 6 mm, approaching that of CTC and colonoscopy, it's widespread adoption in clinical practice has yet to be realized, mainly due to its limited availability and the necessity of fluid enema and intravenous contrast administration, with increased costs, patient discomfort, and overall technique complexity [32].

33.7 Biometric imaging techniques to assess body composition in dieting patients

Body composition refers to the amount of fat and lean tissues in human body. Although body weight and body mass index (BMI) are well known indexes of health status, most researchers agree that they are rather inaccurate measures, especially for elderly individuals and for those patients with specific clinical conditions. For instance, individuals may present with weight stability while gaining fat and losing lean mass.

Imaging techniques such as dual energy x-ray absorptiometry (DXA), CT and MRI, routinely used in the clinical setting, are gaining importance in the assessment of body composition, focusing on the value of lean soft tissue (LST) to predict nutrition status.

The DXA is the most used imaging tool in the clinical practice. During a DXA scan, low-radiation x-rays of 2 different photon energy go through the body and are identified by a detector that measures their attenuation by soft tissue and bone at each pixel. Bone mineral mass and density, as well as fat and fat-free soft tissues, can be quantified at the whole-body and regional levels as DXA is precise, accurate, safe, fast and non-invasive. Regional measurements of body composition can also be obtained. Drawbacks are related to radiation exposure.

CT is considered the gold-standard imaging method for body composition analysis at the tissue organ level. Tissue attenuations, measured using Hounsfield unit, are reported on 2D images using a gray scale. Bone, skeletal muscle and adipose tissue, as well as visceral organs, have specific Hounsfield unit ranges, allowing for their identification in the cross-sectional images [33-35]. Advantages are related to high image resolution, quantitative body composition at the tissue-organ level and reproducibility. However, radiation exposure cannot be ignored, costs are significant, and dedicated specialized medical radiologists are required for image evaluation.

MRI is a very useful imaging method, commonly used in clinical radiology. The MRI scanners use very strong magnetic fields and radio waves, which interact with the protons in tissues to create a signal that is then processed to form detailed images from any part of the body. It allows a multiparametric approach and it has high spatial resolution and high contrast resolution. One of its most common applications is the quantification of lipid content within skeletal muscle using "chemical shift" imaging techniques. The fat content of the liver and changes during a dietary regimen can also be assessed (Fig. 33.4). Due to the lack of radiations, it is considered the safest imaging method. Therefore, it can be used in children and for monitoring patients during longitudinal studies. However, the high cost, the required high technical expertise, and the time related to the procedure, especially for the whole-body assessment, hinder the routinely implementation of this method.

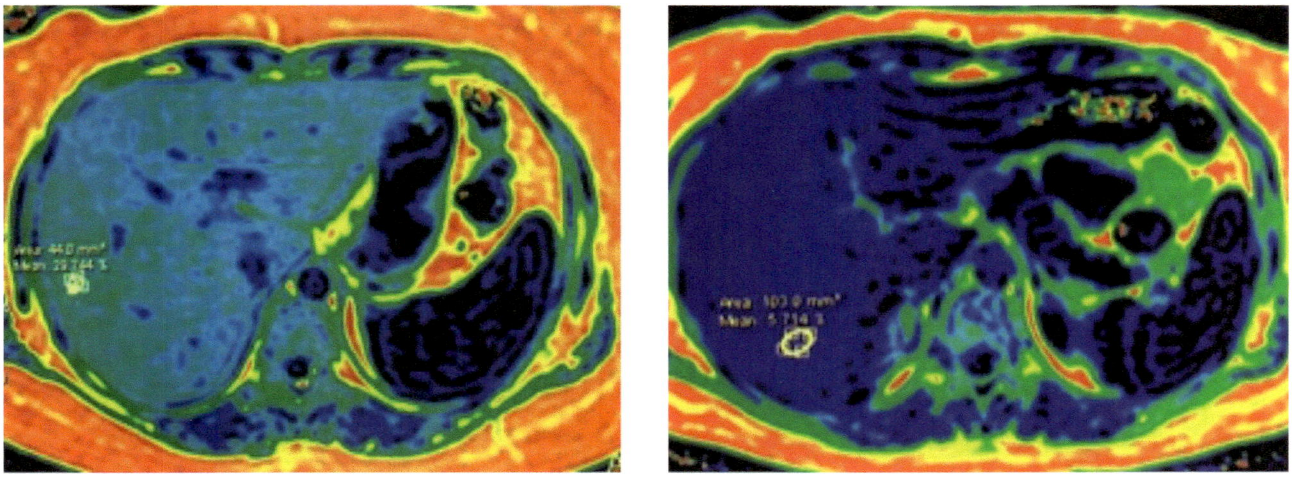

Before diet: Fat Fraction, 29% **After diet: Fat Fraction, 5%**

Fig. 33.4 Fat-fraction maps displayed in color. Serial liver MRI exams can be used to demonstrate changes in liver fat during therapy. Serial proton density fat-fraction (PDFF) maps obtained with complex-based MRI were acquired in a 52 year-old man with hypertriglyceridemia undergoing multidrug therapy and dietary regimen to lower serum triglycerides. Follow-up MRI demonstrates reduction in hepatic PDFF (from 29% to 5%).

REFERENCES

1. Wu J-L, Zhang J-L, Du X-X, et al. Evaluation of the distribution of adipose tissues in fish using magnetic resonance imaging (MRI). Aquaculture 2015; 448: 112-22.
2. Toussaint C, Fauconneau B, Médale F, et al. Description of the heterogeneity of lipid distribution in the flesh of brown trout (Salmo trutta) by MR imaging. Aquaculture 2005; 243: 255-67.
3. Ballerini L, Hogberg A, Borgefors G, et al. A segmentation technique to determine fat content in NMR images of beef meat. IEEE Transactions on Nuclear Science 2002; 49: 195-9.
4. Clerjon S, Kondjoyan A, Bonny JM, et al. Oil uptake by beef during pan frying: impact on fatty acid composition. Meat Sci 2012; 91: 79-87.
5. Horigane AK, Motoi H, Irie K, Yoshida M. Observation of the Structure, Moisture Distribution, and Oil Distribution in the Coating of Tempura by NMR Micro Imaging. Journal of Food Science 2003; 68: 2034-9.
6. Shaarani SM, Nott KP, Hall LD. Combination of NMR and MRI quantitation of moisture and structure changes for convection cooking of fresh chicken meat. Meat Sci 2006; 72: 398-403.
7. Gonzalez JJ, McCarthy KL, McCarthy MJ. Textural and structural changes in lasagna after cooking. Journal of Texture Studies 2000; 31: 93-108.
8. Jha SN, Matsuoka T. Non-Destructive Techniques for Quality Evaluation of Intact Fruits and Vegetables. Food Science and Technology Research 2000; 6: 248-51.
9. Van As H. Intact plant MRI for the study of cell water relations, membrane permeability, cell-to-cell and long distance water transport. J Exp Bot 2007; 58: 743-56.
10. Friedman SL, Neuschwander-Tetri BA, Rinella M, Sanyal AJ. Mechanisms of NAFLD development and therapeutic strategies. Nat Med 2018; 24: 908-22.
11. Chalasani N, Younossi Z, Lavine JE, et al. The diagnosis and management of nonalcoholic fatty liver disease: Practice guidance from the American Association for the Study of Liver Diseases. Hepatology 2018; 67: 328-57.
12. Patel V, Sanyal AJ, Sterling R. Clinical Presentation and Patient Evaluation in Nonalcoholic Fatty Liver Disease. Clin Liver Dis 2016; 20: 277-92.
13. Esterson YB, Grimaldi GM. Radiologic Imaging in Nonalcoholic Fatty Liver Disease and Nonalcoholic Steatohepatitis. Clin Liver Dis 2018; 22: 93-108.
14. Noureddin M, Lam J, Peterson MR, et al. Utility of magnetic resonance imaging versus histology for quantifying changes in liver fat in nonalcoholic fatty liver disease trials. Hepatology 2013; 58: 1930-40.
15. Kondo H, Kanematsu M, Goshima S, et al. Abdominal multidetector CT in patients with varying body fat percentages: estimation of optimal contrast material dose. Radiology 2008; 249: 872-7.
16. Martin DR, Danrad R, Herrmann K, Semelka RC, Hussain SM. Magnetic resonance imaging of the gastrointestinal tract. Top Magn Reson Imaging 2005; 16: 77-98.
17. de Jonge CS, Smout A, Nederveen AJ, Stoker J. Evaluation of gastrointestinal motility with MRI: Advances, challenges and opportunities. Neurogastroenterol Motil 2018; 30(1).
18. Masselli G, Gualdi G. MR imaging of the small bowel. Radiology 2012; 264: 333-48.
19. Serafin Z, Bialecki M, Bialecka A, Sconfienza LM, Klopocka M. Contrast-enhanced Ultrasound for Detection of Crohn's Disease Activity: Systematic Review and Meta-analysis. J Crohns Colitis 2016; 10: 354-62.
20. Sheedy SP, Kolbe AB, Fletcher JG, Fidler JL. Computed Tomography Enterography. Radiol Clin North Am 2018; 56: 649-70.
21. Del Gaizo AJ, Fletcher JG, Yu L, et al. Reducing radiation dose in CT enterography. Radiographics 2013; 33: 1109-24.
22. Laghi A, Paolantonio P, Hassan C. Small bowel imaging. Semin Roentgenol 2009; 44: 99-110.
23. Santillan CS. MR imaging techniques of the bowel. Magn Reson Imaging Clin N Am 2014; 22: 1-11.
24. Hoad C, Clarke C, Marciani L, Graves MJ, Corsetti M. Will MRI of gastrointestinal function parallel the clinical success of cine cardiac MRI? Br J Radiol 2019; 92(1093): 20180433.
25. Pickhardt PJ. Noninvasive radiologic imaging of the large intestine: a valuable complement to optical colonoscopy. Curr Opin Gastroenterol 2010; 26: 61-8.
26. Laghi A. CT Colonography: an update on current and future indications. Expert Rev Gastroenterol Hepatol 2016; 10: 785-94.
27. Bellini D, De Santis D, Caruso D, et al. Bowel preparation in CT colonography: Is diet restriction necessary? A randomised trial (DIETSAN). Eur Radiol 2018; 28: 382-9.
28. Chang KJ, Yee J. Low-Dose Computed Tomography Colonography Technique. Radiol Clin North Am 2018; 56: 709-17.
29. Spada C, Stoker J, Alarcon O, et al. Clinical indications for computed tomographic colonography: European Society of Gastrointestinal Endoscopy (ESGE) and European Society of Gastrointestinal and Abdominal Radiology (ESGAR) Guideline. Eur Radiol 2015; 25: 331-45.
30. Flor N, Maconi G, Cornalba G, Pickhardt PJ. The Current Role of Radiologic and Endoscopic Imaging in the Diagnosis and Follow-Up of Colonic Diverticular Disease. AJR Am J Roentgenol 2016; 207: 15-24.
31. Rimola J, Ordas I. MR colonography in inflammatory bowel disease. Magn Reson Imaging Clin N Am 2014; 22: 23-33.
32. van der Paardt MP, Stoker J. Current Status of Magnetic Resonance Colonography for Screening and Diagnosis of Colorectal Cancer. Radiol Clin North Am 2018; 56: 737-49.
33. Andreoli A, Garaci F, Cafarelli FP, Guglielmi G. Body composition in clinical practice. Eur J Radiol 2016; 85: 1461-8.
34. Goodpaster BH, Thaete FL, Kelley DE. Composition of skeletal muscle evaluated with computed tomography. Ann N Y Acad Sci 2000; 904: 18-24.
35. Mattsson S, Thomas BJ. Development of methods for body composition studies. Phys Med Biol 2006; 51: R203-228.

34 Eating in space

Luca Revelli, Maria Cristina Fabbri and Antonio Valassina

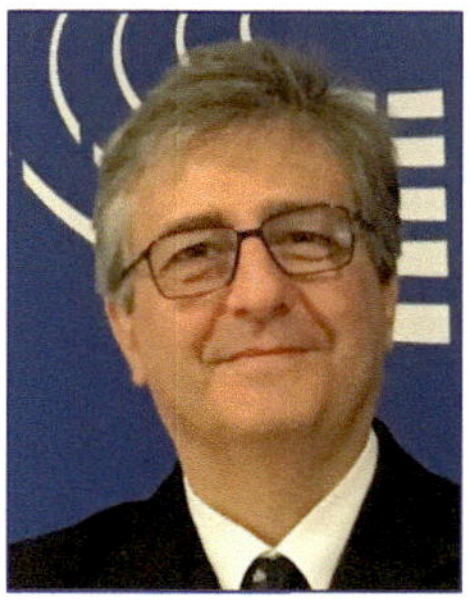

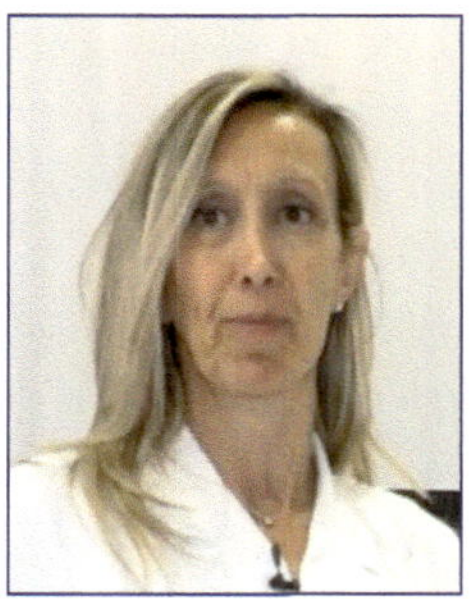

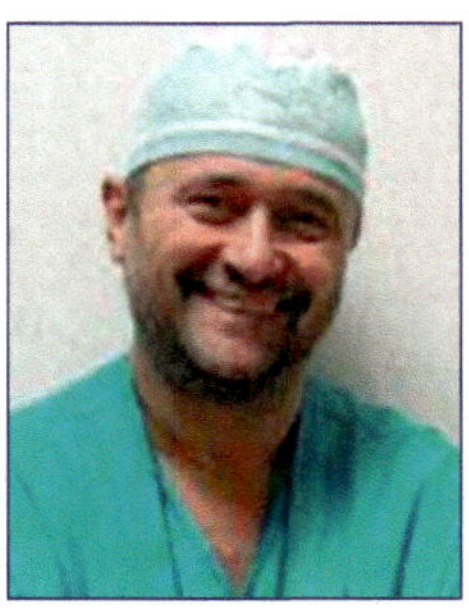

34.1 Food for Travel

The decisive factor in the Napoleonic wars was the supply, transportation and – above all – the preservation of food for the soldiers.

On the plain of Austerlitz (South Moravia, Czech Republic) the masterpiece of the French general was developed (1805): comparable to that of Hannibal in Canne (216 BC, Canne della Battaglia, BAT, Puglia, Italy).

On the Slovak plain (as well as in the Tavoliere delle Puglie) there were no refrigerators or canned food. **Napoleon** had to feed 70,000 soldiers adequately and satisfactorily. The secret weapon was **salt**.

Explorers and **travelers** throughout history have had to develop methods for **preserving food** and **carrying** enough food for their journeys. This problem was especially difficult during the time when people made **long sea voyages** on sailing ships. Great explorers like **Christopher Columbus**, **Ferdinand Magellan** and **Thomas Cook** carried **dried foods** and **foods preserved** in salt and brine.

More recently, **refrigeration** and **canning** have provided solutions to the problem of **food preservation**. However, space travel required that new methods be devised for keeping foods edible [1].

Foods taken into space must be **light-weight**, **compact**, **tasty** and **nutritious**. They must also keep for long periods without refrigeration. A variety of "space menus" must provide each astronaut with about **2,500 or more calories** per day.

Luca Revelli, MD
Professor, Fondazione Policlinico Universitario A. Gemelli IRCCS,
Università Cattolica del Sacro Cuore, Rome, Italy

Email: luca.revelli@unicatt.it

Maria Cristina Fabbri, MD
Fondazione Policlinico Universitario A. Gemelli IRCCS,
Università Cattolica del Sacro Cuore, Rome, Italy

Email: fabbrimariacristina@gmail.com

Antonio Valassina, MD
Fondazione Policlinico Universitario A. Gemelli IRCCS,
Università Cattolica del Sacro Cuore, Rome, Italy

Email: antonio_valassina@yahoo.it

34.2 The Sixties

Soviet cosmonaut **Yuri Gagarin** was the first man to travel in space (April 12, 1961). On board the **Vostok 1** spaceship, food was stored in 160 grams aluminum tubes, similar to those for toothpaste. For lunch: two portions of meat and puree and one of chocolate cream.

On February 20, 1962, **John Glenn** was the first American to eat in space. The astronaut wanted to call his spacecraft **Friendship 7** in honor of the first seven astronauts of the **US Mercury-Atlas 6** space program.

At that time, it was not known if **ingestion** and **absorption** of nutrients were possible in a state of zero gravity. Glenn's consumption of applesauce, packed in a tube, and xylose sugar tablets with water, demonstrated that people could eat, swallow, and digest food in a weightless environment.

Mercury Program (1961-1963) space food included food packaged in bite-sized cubes, freeze-dried powders, and semiliquid foods (such as ham salad) stuffed into aluminum tubes.

While Glenn and the other Mercury astronauts experienced no problems in chewing, drinking, swallowing, or digesting, the food was not considered very delicious.

Project Gemini (1961-1966), conducted between **project Mercury** and **Apollo**, was NASA's second human spaceflight program. The Gemini spacecraft carried a two-astronaut crew. For this mission, **NASA** developed more elaborate foods. The tubes were abandoned, and the **freeze-dried products** were packaged in special plastic containers. The menu included shrimp cocktails, chicken, vegetables, pudding and apple juice.

Dehydrated, freeze-dried, and bite-sized foods, coated with gelatin or oil to prevent crumbling, were introduced during Gemini. On-board hydrogen-oxygen fuel cells provided a source of water that could be used to moisten dehydrated or freeze-dried foods.

A freeze-dried meal would be rehydrated using a water gun to inject cold water into the package. After cutting the package open with scissors, the meal was then ready to eat.

34.3 One giant leap for mankind

The **Apollo program** (1968-1972) was the first to have hot water. This made rehydrating foods easier, and improved taste and quality. Apollo astronauts were the first crew members to use the *spoonbowl*, a utensil that eliminated having to consume food into the mouth directly from the package.

Apollo 11 launched from Cape Kennedy on July 16, 1969, carrying Commander Neil Armstrong, Command Module Pilot Michael Collins and Lunar Module Pilot Edwin "Buzz" Aldrin. An estimated 650 million people watched Armstrong's televised image and heard his voice describe the event as he took ***"...one small step for a man, one giant leap for mankind"*** on July 20, 1969.

Before leaving – in the euphoria of the moment – in front of cameras and journalists, Neil Amstrong asked himself: *"Will I find a good Chef on my trip?"*.

34.4 The seventies

The next major advancement in the quality and variety of space food occurred in 1973 during the **Skylab Program**. Skylab was a space mission after Apollo, in which the third stage of a **Saturn V rocket** was converted into a space station. The space station had a full galley in which the astronauts could cook and eat meals of their own choosing. Skylab relied on solar cells for power, instead of water-producing fuel cells. Dehydrated foods were limited in order to conserve the water supply. Skylab was equipped with a refrigerator so that frozen foods could be carried. This included what became the astronauts favorite dish: ice cream.

34.5 Food in space

Space food in popular culture ranges from liquid meals of various viscosities – think Stanley Kubrick's *"2001: A Space Odyssey"* – to a miracle pill containing a day's worth of nutrition.

But the reality is very different [2].

There's a **psychological experience** that comes with eating. People don't want to take all their meals through a straw. They don't want to swallow a pill for all their nutrition, and the pill wouldn't be as bioavailable as the food itself.

It's necessary, in terms of the human experience: that **people eat**.

In the crew, the absence of gravity reduces the sense of smell and of a large part of the **sense of taste**: all foods must therefore be seasoned with special sauces that enhance their flavors.

Food packaging must be particularly careful to withstand the extreme conditions of space. Everything must be strictly under **vacuum**; just a minimal amount of oxygen inside the package can definitively compromise the content and make it inedible.

The dehydration process of the food and the cold sterilization to which they are subjected, deprives the food of most of the vitamins and proteins: for this reason the crew must however supplement their diet with complementary micronutrients.

34.6 The present

Astronauts live aboard the **International Space Station** (ISS) for as long as six months at a time.

Periodically, an automated spacecraft such as the **ESA Automated Transfer Vehicle**, or the Russian **Progress**, reaches the Station, loaded with fresh fruit, water and ready meals.

According to NASA, astronauts are given more than 200 food and beverage choices to select from. About 8 to 9 months before launch, astronauts join a food evaluation session where they sample foods and pick breakfast, lunch, dinner and snacks, from scrambled eggs to macaroni and cheese.

Some of the food astronauts eat are dehydrated, to save on space and weight. These foods typically come in snippable packages, so water generated by shuttle fuel cells can be added. Other foods, like fruits, fish and meat, are thermostabilized or irradiated to kill microorganisms and enzymes.

Salt and **pepper** come in liquid form. **Coffee** and **juices** come as powder.

For ISS crew members, their menu repeats every eight days. On holidays, they can request special items that remind them of home. They also get "**psychological support kits**" from friends and family that can contain special treats

34.7 The way to Mars

With missions lasting years, the issue of menu fatigue escalates to a serious problem. One of the solutions is to **allow the crew to cook**.

Astronauts can make endless variations. And there's a bonus: it improves social cohesion. It's possible to hare food and to talk about it: a basic human thing.

Someday, **hydroponic growth** labs could allow astronauts to grow vegetables, soybeans and rice.

Space agencies haven't yet explored this avenue in practice for a few key reasons: cooking requires **water** and **energy** (two things that are extremely precious in space). It also requires time, and astronauts lead very busy lives completing their orders. Finally, humans in space are currently in microgravity, where cooking isn't possible.

Weightlessness requires more energy; the body is never truly at rest at zero gravity, so astronauts must eat accordingly, consuming 3,000 calories a day.

34.8 Astronaut food

An optimal diet, paired with constant exercise, is essential to counteract the effects of spaceflight on the human body. Bone loss, muscle atrophy and depleted nutrient stores such as protein, fat and vitamin D are among the negatives of space travel.

Research shows that **energy intake** in orbit is usually lower than on Earth [3] – some even call it "***spaceflight anorexia***". From tubes to cans and rehydratable packages, space food has evolved to meet nutritional requirements and boost crew morale.

Food in space tastes different: it is like eating with a cold and a reduced appetite follows.

Alongside such healthy dishes as Indian fish curry and crab cakes, the NASA menu includes chocolate pudding, lemon curd cake and apricot cobbler.

NASA has even been known to send **birthday cakes** to astronauts.

34.9 App

EveryWear is an iPad-based application that collects physiology and medical data from astronauts on the ISS. It is connected to wearable biomedical sensors that record exercise, heart rate and sleep quality.

Its main use is as a **food diary**. The astronaut simply scans the barcode of the food with the built-in tablet camera, classify it as breakfast, lunch, dinner or snack, and add how much water was consumed.

The crew can also add food by tapping on a specific product. The app comes loaded with a database containing all the food on the Space Station, both in English and in Russian. If something is not listed yet, there is an option to take a picture.

An added value of the tool is that it connects the astronaut with nutrition experts on Earth, some 400 km below. Ground teams receive the information and can suggest the best combination of meals for a healthy stay in orbit.

34.10 Space travel and nutrition

Nutrition has played a critical role throughout the history of exploration, and space exploration is no exception. While a one-to-two-week flight aboard the Space Shuttle might be analogous to a camping trip, adequate nutrition is absolutely critical when spending several months aboard the ISS or several years on a mission to another planet [4]. To ensure adequate nutrition, space-nutrition specialists must know how much of various individual **nutrients** astronauts need, and these nutrients must be available in the spaceflight food system. To complicate matters, spaceflight **nutritional requirements** are influenced by many of the **physiological** changes that occur during spaceflight.

34.11 Space physiology

Spacecraft, the space environment, and weightlessness itself impact human physiology. Clean air, drinkable water, and effective waste collection systems are required for maintaining a habitable environment. Without the Earth's atmosphere to protect them, astronauts are exposed to a much higher level of radiation than individuals on the Earth.

Weightlessness impacts almost every system in the body, including those of the **bones**, **muscles**, **heart**, **blood vessels** and **nerves** [5].

Bone loss, especially in the legs, is significant during spaceflight. This is most important on flights longer than 30 days, because the amount of bone lost increases as the length of time in space increases. Weightlessness also increases excretion of calcium in the urine and the risk of forming **kidney stones**.

Many nutrients are important for healthy bones, particularly **calcium** and **vitamin D**. When a food containing calcium is eaten, the calcium is absorbed by the intestines and goes into the bloodstream. Absorption of calcium from the intestines decreases during spaceflight. Even when astronauts take extra calcium as a supplement, they still lose bone mass.

On Earth, the body can produce **vitamin D** after the skin is exposed to the sun's ultraviolet light. In space, astronauts could receive too much ultraviolet light, so spacecraft are shielded to prevent this exposure. Because of this, all the astronauts' vitamin D has to be provided by their **diet**. However, it is very common for vitamin D levels to decrease during spaceflight.

Sodium intake is also a concern during spaceflight because space diets tend to have relatively high amounts of sodium. Increased dietary sodium is associated with increased amounts of **calcium** in the urine and may relate to the increased risk of **kidney stones**.

Bone is a living tissue and is constantly being remodeled. This remodeling is achieved through the breakdown of existing bone tissue (resorption) and the formation of new bone tissue (affixing of new bone on the trabeculae of the marrow and in the cortex). During spaceflight, bone resorption increases significantly, and formation either remains unchanged or decreases slightly. The net effect of this imbalance is an important loss of bone mass.

It is not clear whether bone mass lost in space is fully replaced after returning to Earth. It is also unclear whether the quality (or strength) of the replaced bone is the same as the bone that was there before a spaceflight. Preliminary data seem to show that some crew members do indeed regain their preflight bone mass, but this process takes about two or three times as long as their flight. Another no less important aspect of the loss of total bone quantity is the loss of bone quality. In fact, in the absence of gravity, there is also a loss of the mineralization capacity of the bone matrix with consequent aspects similar to osteomalacia. The final picture of the damage suffered by the bone is therefore that of an **osteoporomalacia**.

The changes in bone during spaceflight are very similar to those seen in certain situations on the ground. There are similarities to **osteoporosis** in the elderly, and even in the bones of the skeleton affected by **motor paralysis**. While osteoporosis has many causes, the result seems to be similar to spaceflight bone loss. Paralyzed individuals have biomechanical and biochemical changes very similar to those of astronauts. This is because in both cases the bones are not being used for support. In fact, one of the ways spaceflight bone loss is studied is to have people lie in bed for several weeks. Using this approach, scientists attempt to understand the mechanisms of bone loss and to test ways to counteract it. If they can find ways to successfully counteract spaceflight bone loss, doctors may be able to use similar methods to treat people with osteoporosis or paralysis, while taking into account metabolic differences in the elderly and biomechanical differences due to the absence of active movement in paralyzed patients.

Muscle. Loss of body weight (mass) is a consistent finding throughout the history of spaceflight. Typically, these losses are small (1 to 5% of body mass), but they can reach 10 to 15% of preflight body mass. Although a 1% body-weight loss can be explained by the loss of body water, most of the observed loss of body weight is accounted for by the loss of muscle and adipose (**fat**) tissue. Weightlessness leads to the loss of muscle mass and muscle volume, weakening muscle performance, especially in the legs. The loss is believed to be related to a **metabolic stress** associated with spaceflight. These findings are similar to those found in patients with serious diseases or trauma, such as burn patients.

In any case, in astronauts, these rapid mass losses of adipose tissue, muscle tissue and especially bone tissue are not associated with evident movements or enzymatic alterations such as to be able to demonstrate the phenomena of myolysis or lipolysis linked to serious metabolic disorders. Also, for this reason, it is very difficult to identify the exact mechanisms that govern the trophism of the tissues subjected to earth gravity and their rapid dystrophy in the absence of gravity.

Exercise routines have not succeeded in maintaining muscle mass or strength of astronauts during spaceflight. Most of the exercises performed have been **aerobic** (e.g., treadmill, stationary bicycle). Use of resistance exercise, in which a weight (or another person) provides resistance to exercise against, has been proposed to aid in the maintenance of both muscle and bone during flight. Ground-based studies (not done in space) of resistance exercise show that it may be helpful, not only for muscles but also for bones. Studies being conducted on the ISS are testing the effectiveness of this type of exercise for astronauts.

Blood. A decrease in the mass of red blood cells is also a consistent finding after short- and long-term spaceflight. The actual composition of the blood changes little because the amount of fluid (blood **plasma**) decreases as well. The net result is that the total volume of blood in the circulatory system decreases. While this loss is significant (about 10 to 15% below preflight levels), it seems to be simply an adaptation to spaceflight, with no reported effect on body function during flight.

The initial loss of red blood cells seems to happen because newly synthesized cells (which are not needed in a smaller blood volume) are destroyed until a new steady state is reached. One consequence of the increased destruction of red blood cells is that the **iron** released when they are destroyed is processed for storage in the body. Too much iron may be harmful and is thus a concern for long space missions.

34.12 Living in space

The ISS represents the beginning of an era of **humans living and working in space**, with the potential for a permanent human presence in space.

Nutrition will play a vital role in ensuring the health and safety of spacefaring individuals, whether they are in low Earth orbit or on journeys to the moon, Mars, or beyond. Finally, the creation of conditions of artificial gravity appears to be the key to optimizing the nutritional intake, guaranteeing a fundamental metabolic balance in long sidereal journeys.

A more complete understanding of the effects of weightlessness in space flight will not only help humans explore the universe, but will provide the information necessary to maintain human health and improve disease treatment here on Earth.

REFERENCES

1. Bourland CT. Advances in Food Systems for Space Flight. Life Support Biosph Sci 1998; 5(1): 71-7.
2. Lane HW, Smith SM. Nutrition in Space. In: Modern Nutrition in Health and Disease, 9th edition, eds. M. E. Shils, J. A. Olson, M. Shike, and A. C. Ross. Baltimore: Williams & Wilkins, 1998.
3. Smith SM, Davis-Street JE, Rice BL, Nillen JL, Gillman PL, Block G. Nutritional status assessment in semiclosed environments: ground-based and space flight studies in humans. J Nutr 2001; 131(7): 2053-61.
4. Smith SM, Lane HW. Gravity and space flight: effects on nutritional status. Curr Opin Clin Nutr Metab Care 1999; 2(4): 335-8.
5. Smith SM, Lane HW. Nutritional Support. In: Principles of Clinical Medicine for Space Flight, ed. Michael R. Barratt and Sam L. Pool. New York: Springer-Verlag, 2002.

35 Food and diving

Luca Revelli, Ersilia Biondi and Emanuela Traini

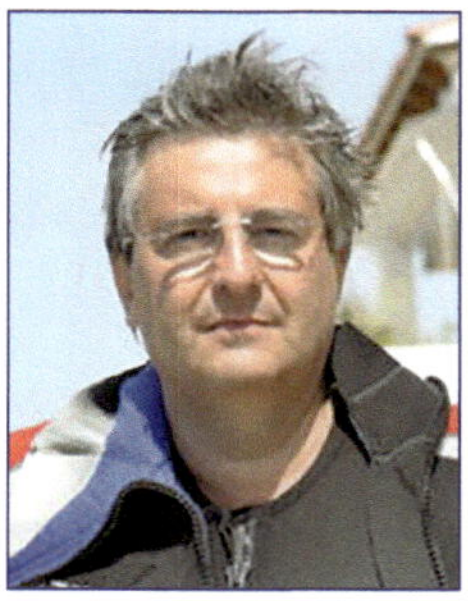

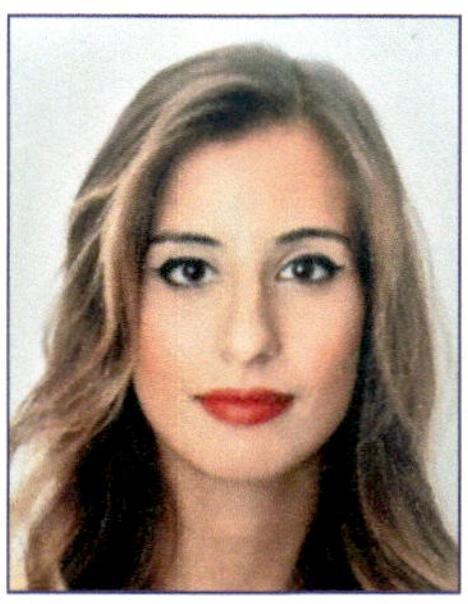

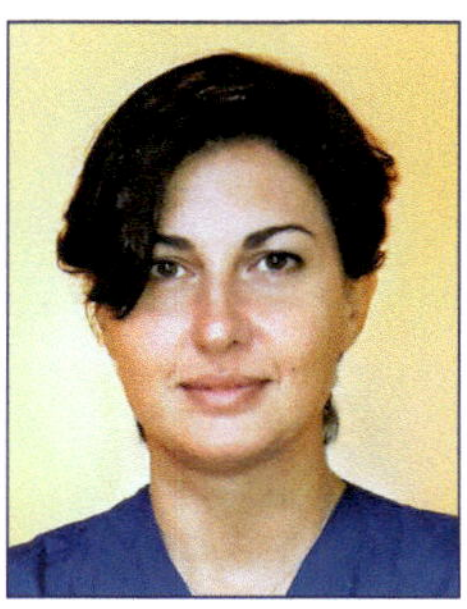

35.1 The unknown blue planet

The underwater world is basically unknown.

The topography of the ocean floor is much less detailed than the maps of the Moon, Mars or Venus.

Seas and oceans cover about 361 million km^2 of the earth's surface, that is to say that: **over 70% of the globe is covered by water**. For this reason, the Earth is called "the blue planet": looking at it from space it appears, in fact, like a huge blue-turquoise mass.

Only 5% of the seabed has been topographically mapped, which means that 65% of our entire planet remains relatively unknown.

Unlike moons and planets, **undersea soil cannot be mapped with radars**, because sea water hinders the penetration of satellite radio waves. To be able to obtain high-resolution images of the seabed, scientists need a series of sophisticated and expensive sonar techniques. But the sea and oceans are part of our life: just think of **anthropic activities** (fishing, navigation, international trading, renewable energy production, oil drilling, etc.), sports and recreational activities, food and medicinal sources and the role of water masses in environmental homeostasis. Their study is a potential source of discoveries that could prove useful in understanding many current problems, from **climate change** to the treatment of certain **diseases**.

35.2 Man and the sea

The sea attracts men.

Looking at the Earth at night you can see that the coastal areas are the most illuminated. The peripheries of the continents are more populated than the heart of the continents: over a third of humanity lives in the coastal areas. The attraction of the sea is due to fishing resources, but even more to the tempering action on the climate and the opening to maritime traffic.

Luca Revelli, MD
Professor, Fondazione Policlinico Universitario A. Gemelli IRCCS,
Università Cattolica del Sacro Cuore, Rome, Italy

Email: luca.revelli@unicatt.it

Ersilia Biondi, MD
Fondazione Policlinico Universitario A. Gemelli IRCCS,
Università Cattolica del Sacro Cuore, Rome, Italy

Emanuela Traini, MD
Fondazione Policlinico Universitario A. Gemelli IRCCS,
Università Cattolica del Sacro Cuore, Rome, Italy

The sea hosts 3/4 of the life of the planet. The food obtained from the sea is the main source of proteins for about half of the world's population.

However, direct knowledge of the sea is modest. The Mariana Trench, the deepest ocean depression (–11 thousand meters) in the northwest Pacific (between the Philippines, Japan and New Guinea) was explored in 1960 by Don Walsh and Jacques Piccard with the Trieste bathyscaphe. In 2012 James Cameron, a Canadian director and oceanographer, reached the bottom of the Trench with a single-seater submarine, the *Deepsea Challenger*. But this was a "spot" experience. After all, very little is known. Only a few species of abyssal fish, never seen by humans, are being discovered.

On the other hand, the depths that divers can reach are very limited.

Man's first approach to the sea was apnea (free-diving, breath-holding). In Ancient Greece and in Roman times people used to dive to find food, collect sponges, repair ships (or sink them). But until we found a way to breathe underwater, the dives were short and convulsive.

In the 16th century a diving bell was used; in the 19th century the first divers appeared, breathing the air pumped from the surfaces through a tube. It was only in 1943 that the first Self-Contained Underwater Breathing Apparatus (SCUBA) was created by Jacques Yves Cousteau and Emile Gagnan. With the Scuba air system, it is possible to descend to 45 meters (**recreational**, **sport** or **tourist** dive). For greater depths (**technical immersion**), different gas mixtures (helium, hydrogen, oxygen, etc.) or closed systems (**rebreather**) are used in which the exhaled air, rich in CO_2, is regenerated with oxygen. **Professional dives**, practiced for work, require a fee and are generally at high depths (up to three hundred meters, **saturation dives**).

In apnea or with scuba tanks the depths that are reached are always very modest. Today there are many free divers who exceed 100 meters, but these are always record attempts and not exploratory dives. The same with scuba: the record with mixtures (technical immersion) is over 330 meters.

In 1992 Comex, a French diving company, conducted a series of **experimental dives** to 2,133 feet (650 meters) of seawater in a hyperbaric research chamber in France. For two hours one diver went to 2,300 feet (701 meters), which is the deepest a human has gone under pressure (71.1 atmospheres) to date.

35.3 Underwater environment

Exposure to an underwater (UW) environment for **recreational** or **professional** purposes is increasing across the globe. Worldwide, the number of annual diving licenses has tripled during the last 25 years. There are about 6 millions of **active scuba divers** worldwide, performing at least 5 dives in a year [1].

Divers Alert Network (DAN) 2014 data shows there are 3.174 million recreational scuba divers in America, of which 2.351 million dive 1 to 7 times per year (**causal recreational divers**) and 823,000 dive 8 or more times per year **(core recreational divers)** [2].

Males make up 61% of casual and 72% of core participants.

As a recreational activity, scuba diving challenges individuals with some **uncommon environmental stresses** including increased ambient pressure, raised partial pressure of inhaled gasses, enhanced resistance to breathing, cold water immersion, and increased resistance to movement by dragging diving equipment [3]. All these factors result in a range of **physiological effects**, **metabolic stresses** and potentially **pathophysiological consequences**, including the risk of drowning. Consequently, these stresses elicit a physiological adaptive response affecting multiple systems (**diving reflex**: bradycardia, peripheral vasoconstriction, average increase in blood pressure, diverting blood flow to the brain, heart, and lungs: serves to conserve oxygen until breathing resumes and to delay potential brain damage) [4].

Multiple factors may affect hemodynamic such as: changes in pressure and ventilation of a high-density gas mixture which increases afterload [5]; hyperoxia that slows heart rate; the increase in hydrostatic pressure that can modify the excitability and conduction speed [6]. Moreover, immersion increases the preload while prolonged exposure to cold and hyperbaric pressure also plays a role increasing afterload and slowing the heart rate [4, 7].

35.4 One K calories per dive

Scuba dive is one of the **most calories-consuming** sports activities.

The metabolic adaptations and, in particular, the consumption of calories in immersion do not depend only on **movement** (it is a truly "complete" activity, more than swimming) as on **thermal dispersion**.

A single leisure **boat dive** in warm, tropical waters, **burns** an average **300 calories** per hour, equivalent to hiking or a brisk walk.

An average **shore dive** in temperate water can burns as much as **600 calories** per hour (about the same as jogging).

There is also the energy consumption linked to the **preparation** of the dive (assembly of the equipment and reaching the dive site) and the disassembly and

35.1 Immersion calorie consumption calculator

(modified from: Hyperbaric Center of Ravenna, Italy)

Calorie consumption	*1001*	*Kcal*
Body weight	89	Kg
Dive time	50	minutes
Water temperature	24	°C
Wetsuit thickness	5	mm
Thermal conductivity of the suit	0.00002	Kcal/ms °C
Wetsuit surface	2	square meters

washing of the equipment. All these elements (preparation, movement, heat dispersion, disassembly) would lead to a consumption of up to almost **a thousand calories per immersion** (also in relation to a whole series of variables ranging from water temperature, the presence of drift, the type of equipment, the type of gas breathed, the time and depth of the dive).

There are very refined programs for the evaluation of calorie consumption during dive which also consider: the weight of the diver; the thickness, the thermal conductivity and the size of the suit (Box 35.1).

35.5 BMI, hydration and alcohol

Some diet-dependent factors increase the risk of **Decompression Pathology** (DP), an almost exclusive disease of scuba divers. Among them: a **high BMI** (excess of adipose tissue), **dehydration** and **alcohol abuse**.

It has been shown that the higher the rate of **adipose tissue**, the greater the risk of DP. Fat is considered a "slow tissue", that is, one of those tissues that lets inert gas (nitrogen) enter more slowly than the others: in the same way, however, it gets rid of it less quickly.

Nutritional status is of fundamental importance for those who face UW activities.

A **thin diver** is more easily victim of the cold: in the water the dispersion of the heat is 25 times greater than in the air. In addition, breathing air (or other compressed mixtures) removes more heat than normobaric breathing (at 1 atm = 760 mmHg). This phenomenon is accentuated if helium-containing mixtures are breathed (*heliox, heliair, trimix*). Being cold can facilitate the early onset of muscle fatigue, due to the depletion of energy reserves used for thermoregulation and can decrease the nitrogen elimination rate.

The **excess of adipose tissue** instead predisposes to poor physical shape, less resistance to stress and sudden efforts, increased predisposition to nitrogen narcosis and increased risk of DP.

During the dive, there is a **redistribution of liquids** from the tissues to the bloodstream, which leads to an increase in diuresis and a consequent loss of fluids. In fact, the stimulus to urination under water and – above all – to re-emergence is known.

In the thirty minutes after emergence, the reverse process takes place, i.e., the liquids return from the circulation to the tissues (**relative dehydration**). It is therefore very important to drink a lot in the hour following the dive. Water is essential to thin the lymph and counteract the overload of the lymphatic vessels responsible for the drainage of the connective tissue (prevention of DP).

Water is considered a real "drug" in DP treatment.

It is very important to drink 2-3 liters of **water** within the 24 hours preceding the dive and it is necessary to remember the rule of **hydration**, particularly in case of occasional dives.

Water losses are significant even during short dives, due to gas exchange, ventilation and metabolic modification.

Not all types of drinks and liquid supplements are appropriate. For example: the **orange juice** usually has strong acidity and can cause problems for those with a particular tendency to GastroEsophageal Reflux Disease (GERD); **milk** that has a very long digestion process especially when taken with solid foods; the so-called "**energy drinks**" for athletes should be avoided too because they often contain sugars, extra calories and superfluous salts. **Mineral salts** and supplements should never be taken before diving because they can cause cramps and gastrointestinal disorders. It is useful to remember to ban also **coffee** and alcoholic beverages that act as diuretics and can contribute to dehydration.

Alcohol frighteningly dehydrates even in small percentages, just think of the typical diuretic effect of beer, and not only: underwater the psychotropic substances really do have a bad effect. It seems that the surrounding pressure increases alcohol concentration, and therefore the neurological toxicity of each psychotropic substance. If it is never a good idea to dive in conditions of **psychic alteration**, the worst of all is to dive after having taken alcohol: the multiplication of the effects of psychic slowing adds dehydration and changes in the circulatory phase.

In addition to mental clarity, alcohol can also have negative consequences on cold tolerance, muscle endurance and its effect combined with environmental pressure which would favor the onset of **nitrogen narcosis**.

Alcohol should account for about 4% of the daily calorie amount (a glass of wine). Obviously far from diving.

35.6 Digestibility of food

Another important consideration must be made regarding the digestion time of the various foods: it is necessary not to weigh down the stomach which, otherwise, would take precious energy away from the body to digest food.

The fatter the foods, the longer their residence time in the stomach; the same is true for lightly chewed or ingested whole foods.

On the contrary, liquid foods, soups and drinks (avoiding alcohol and carbonated drinks) are by far the most digestible foods that leave the stomach in the shortest time compared to all the others.

35.7 Recreational diving

Recreational divers don't need special foods or supplements. It is sufficient to make **balanced meals** (carbohydrates 60%, fat 30-35%, vegetable or animal proteins 10-15%).

An important rule is to take in moderation foods that contain **simple carbohydrates** such as sweets or biscuits and have many calories but a low nutritional value. It would be better to privilege complex carbohydrates (potatoes, rice, legumes) that stimulate a lower insulin response than simple sugars.

Fats are not well considered in main diets, yet they can be valid allies for diving and are in any case essential elements for nutrition. Fats significantly reduce the sense of hunger and represents an important source of energy, but they must be taken in moderation. A particular attention should be paid on foods containing oleic acid such as olive oil and animal fats should be avoided before immersion.

Some people have the bad habit of skip **breakfast** in the morning, especially before an immersion, in order to feel lighter and snappy. However, this is a fallacy and an enormous mistake since several calories are burned during the dive in order to keep the body warm. Although, breakfast should be light, preferably based on tea, yogurt, cereals, a small portion of fruit or albumen. These are highly energetic foods which give the right contribution of calories that are transformed into energy, but it is necessary not to exceed with **proteins** otherwise the risk of dehydration can occur. The ideal daily dose is 0.8 g of protein per kilogram of body weight and both athletes and common people should not go further or have an over-abundant breakfast (it could cause **seasickness** especially for those who are not used to sea sports).

It is possible to have some **snacks between dives**: bananas, dried fruit, cereals, yogurt and fruit are recommended. Make sure to eat at least 2 hours before going underwater to give the body time to digest.

Diving immediately after eating can cause a slight state of discomfort.

35.8 The day of the dive

We recommend a light breakfast without fat, sugar and heavy oils. A breakfast of **cereals**, **fruit**, **yogurt**, **toast** and even **eggs** and a piece of **dark chocolate** will give enough energy to deal with a dive. Ingestion of 30 g of dark chocolate 90 minutes before scu-

35.2 PLANNING A DIVE

Before diving the consumption of foods with a very high glycemic index increase the lactic acid that may affect performances.
Planning a dive, it is necessary to balance the diet from the night before, preferring a **dinner** with a **medium-high glycemic index**.

Day before the dive
Dinner: pasta with olive oil, salad with fresh tomatoes, avocado and spinach, salmon steak or fish.
Drink 2/3 L of water (or soft drinks) during the day before immersion.

Day of the dive
Breakfast: tea and a toast with jam, half a banana, a piece of dark chocolate.
Drink three glasses of water.
Snack (2 h before dive): cereals, a portion of almonds.
One glass of water.

After the dive
Fresh fruit or bread, in order to reintegrate with easily digestible sugars that quickly enter the bloodstream.
Only after a few hours make a complete (but not too heavy) meal with a small amount of pasta and fresh fish.
Dinner: boiled vegetables or mixed salad, chicken or turkey.
The rule of drinking a lot is always valid.

ba diving prevents post-dive endothelial dysfunction, as the antioxidants contained in dark chocolate probably scavenge free radicals [8] (Box 35.2).

Another important recommendation is to make an adequate water load. **Infusions** (tea, herbal teas), **fruit juices** (not citrus) and **water** are essential to prevent dehydration during diving.

Before a dive, the consumption of (too much) **coffee** is not recommended: caffeine acts as a diuretic and can contribute to dehydration [9].

It is good to wait a couple of hours from breakfast before diving into the water and/or getting on the boat with diving equipment.

Those suffering from **seasickness** should avoid heavy breakfasts and prefer a "**dry diet**" based on dry biscuits, toasts, cheeses and crackers, which usually help to absorb gastric acids.

35.9 Repetitive dives

In case of repetitive dives, during surface intervals, it is advisable to have a snack with carbohydrate-rich foods, such as: bananas, fruit, cereal bars, energy bars, yogurt and biscuits. This will provide instant energy for the next dive.

On "full day dive" in the Mediterranean (especially in Italy) the so-called "**spaghetti**" with tomatoes is often organized: an excellent opportunity to socialize (and to eat a good dish) but to be postponed after the last dive. The other usual dish that should be preferred – possibly – is "**bruschetta**" (slice of "homemade" toasted bread) with olive oil and salt or "**panzanella**" with the addition of pieces of fresh tomato.

Bananas are perhaps the most popular snack of the surface range: but not all boat owners allow their consumption on board. An **old superstition** claims that **bananas bring bad luck to sailors**. But it is also said that: "*You could stay ashore (with a banana in your hand) while your buddies will leave for the most beautiful dive in life!*"

Foods rich in starches should be avoided during the surface interval: the goal is to replenish the energies and fluids for the next dive. For this reason, it is always recommended – as usual – to ensure proper rehydration by drinking mainly non-carbonated water.

35.10 Competitive and professional dives

Athletes often and wrongly focus on maximizing the strength-to-weight ratio, which requires a food strategy that enables a maintenance or **increase in muscle mass** and a decrease in **fat mass**.

Divers who follow restrained dietary patterns with the goal of maintaining or losing weight may develop multiple risk factors that could compromise their state of nutrition and health. In fact, **competitive diving** involves strength, power, balance and flexibility, all of which require a satisfying daily need of energy and nutrients. There is a wrong tendency for some divers to focus on **protein intakes**, while overlook the importance of **carbohydrate** and **fat**. This restrictive dietary practice leading to low energy availability also results in: premature fatigue, frequent injuries and poor athletic performance.

The powerful and anaerobic nature of diving, requiring adequate muscle glycogen and stored phosphocreatin, suggests that divers should consume diets that are absolutely **well balanced in all macronutrients**. This consumption should be well integrated with **micronutrients** (vitamins, macroelements such as calcium and magnesium, microelements such as iron) to avoid an increase in hunger-related cortisol that could compromise bone and muscle mass.

35.11 Saturation diving

Commercial (professional) diving is an occupation that involves prolonged exposure to an **"extreme" environment** (for depth, temperature, visibility, movement difficulties, etc.) which is thought to cause disruptions of physiological and metabolic homeostasis. These physiological concerns may be alleviated and supported by **appropriate nutritional intake**, whilst enhancing performance in saturation divers.

Saturation diving is when the inert gas-breathed by a diver dissolves in the body's tissues and reaches equilibrium with the ambient pressure at the diver's depth (no more gas can be absorbed by the tissues, they're fully saturated). This is **Henry's law** (1803), named for British chemist William Henry. Tissues saturate at various speeds, but most are saturated in 24 hours.

It is a diving technique that allows divers to reduce the risk of **decompression sickness** when they work at great depths for long periods of time. Once saturated, decompression time does not increase with further exposure. Saturation divers typically breathe a helium-oxygen mixture to prevent **nitrogen narcosis** (at shallow depths saturation diving has done on nitrox mixtures).

It is a very specialized form of diving; of the 3,420 commercial divers employed in the United States in 2019, (commercial diving) only 10 percent were saturation divers.

35.12 Energy intake

Saturation divers required approximately 53 kcal/kg Body Mass (BM) a day. According to this an 80 kg expert diver would require 4,240 kcal daily (value obviously variable).

Increased energy expenditure is attributed to thermal stress caused by the helium-oxygen environment and water temperature. In addition, breathing for divers is much more exhausting than other athletes, due to the high density of the gases [10].

35.13 Antioxidants and oxidative stress

Saturation dives involve **long-term stays** (several days to weeks) in a closed environment with an increased partial pressure of oxygen. Saturation diving and exposure to oxygen-rich environments in general lead to oxidative damage. The hyperoxic and hyperbaric environment is enormously different from what is physiologically programmed for humans, and may impact on both human health and performance [5].

Underwater divers are exposed to increased gas density, increased partial pressures and increased physiological dead space. **Hyperoxia** could lead to the production of **Reactive Oxygen Species** (ROS) that cause damage to cell structures and interacting proteins, lipids and nucleic acid [11]. Exposure to **oxygen-rich environments** can lead to oxidative damage too, increased lipid peroxidation and DNA damage, increased body iron stores and changes in status of some vitamins, especially folate [11].

The imbalance between **ROS** and **antioxidant** is implicated with diabetes, cardiovascular/neurodegenerative disorders and several types of cancer.

The full effect of saturation diving on **redox physiology** is yet to be ascertained, in particular other factors such as the chronic high-pressure exposure and the effect of inert gas mixtures (combination of oxygen and helium and/or nitrogen), which may improve the oxidative stress. However, it is certain that while the adaptative response during intermittent exposure to oxidized particles may be possible, the prolonged and chronic exposure to hyperoxia within the saturation chamber causes greater magnitude of **oxidative stress** [12].

The **antioxidant status** of the diver become a very important mechanism in the protection against injuries and diet has an important role. **Antioxidants** – such as **vitamin C** and **E** – are absolutely recommended to be beneficial in reinforcing endogenous antioxidant reserves.

A varied diet, rich in **fruit** and **vegetables,** is highly recommended to provide sufficient micronutrients to support physiological processes, such as **vitamin B12**, and **folate** intake that facilitate red blood cell production. Some studies showed that the correct dose and supplementation of **vitamin C** should be at least 600 mg, and 150 mg for **vitamin E** per day. This amount of vitamins diminishes oxidative damage in the liver.

Another consideration of **redox homeostasis** is the reduced endogenous antioxidant enzyme activity; therefore, a dietary intake to elevate both **SOD** and **Glutathione Peroxidase** (GPX) may be prudent. Dietary intakes can support these enzymes such as **selenium** intake to increase GPX activity and **zinc** intake, which may elevate SOD.

35.14 Macronutrients

35.14.1 Carbohydrates

Diving-specific training and competition are primarily **anaerobic** with a high reliance on **phosphocreatine** and **glycogen**.

Current carbohydrate recommendations, if we consider general population, are between 45 and 65% of total calorie intake [13]. To allow sufficient intake of all three macronutrients, divers should consume a diet that provides 3-8 g/kg/day of carbohydrate. However, divers should avoid carbohydrate-loading strategies that maximize glycogen stores because they could compromise flexibility.

Before training or a competition, a meal or snack scheduled 1-4 hours before exercise should provide adequate fluid, be relatively low in fat and fiber to facilitate gastric emptying and minimize gastrointestinal distress, contain carbohydrate, be moderate in protein, be composed of familiar foods, and be well tolerated by the athlete because blood sugar fluxes in 3-hour units.

35.14.2 Proteins

Divers may find themselves in a catabolic state. In this case a higher protein intake is required to reduce skeletal muscle loss.

Total daily protein intake to optimize the adaptation from daily training and promote recovery after exercise is approximately 1.2-1.7 g/kg body mass [14]. It may be conceivable that higher protein intakes are required in divers: it appears appropriate to propose that under the extreme condition and physiological challenges, the ideal intake for saturation divers should be kept at a moderately increased level, which is 1.3 g/kg BM a day of high-quality protein. This quote is above the recommended daily allowance for the general population (which is currently 0.8 g/kg BM a day) in order to prevent muscle loss while in an energy-deficient state and to satisfy creatine synthesis.

On the other hand, protein oxidation requires lots of **fluids** (almost twice as much as the utilization of carbohydrates and fats) and this is particularly critical in divers, because this can lead to dehydration. Since the protein surplus elimination systems are normally efficient, a consumption not exceeding our recommendations is not to be considered at risk.

35.14.3 Fats

High-fat diets are not ideals for athletes. But it is demonstrated that exercise under acute **hyperoxic conditions** lowers the Respiratory Exchange Ratio (RER) of exercise (compared to normoxia). That means increased fat oxidation.

Fat is an important source of **energy**, **fat-soluble vitamins** and **essential fatty acids**.

That is why divers should consume fats at the recommended level of **20-25% of total calories** intake to help ensure that total energy requirements are met.

35.15 Micronutrients

35.15.1 Vitamin B12 and folate

A **reduction in hemoglobin** concentration is consistently reported after deep saturation dives. This may be due to a downregulation of erythropoietin (EPO) concentration or to a toxic effect of the hyperoxia associated with the dives resulting in an increased destruction rate of erythrocytes [15].

During diving, blood hemoglobin reduces immediately after decompression from professional saturation diving, compatible with acclimatization to the **hyperbaric hyperoxia**. The primary cause of reduced hemoglobin concentration is the attenuation of the rate of red blood cell production. For this reason, it is appropriate that saturation divers should consume sufficient levels of **vitamin B12** and **folate**, which are involved in the production red blood cells and are linked to EPO activity.

For saturation divers recommendations for vitamin B12 are 2.4 µg/day.

After a saturation dive, consistent decrease in RBC folate is significant, and therefore it is suggested that folate intake corresponding to the Recommended Daily Allowance (RDA) of 400 µg/day is appropriate. However, it is advised that the intake does not exceed the recommended upper tolerable limit of 1000 µg/day. **Folic acid** is found in vegetables, mainly in green leafy ones (spinach, chard, endive), in broccoli, but also in red turnips, asparagus, artichokes, rocket, legumes (beans, chickpea peas), and in citrus fruits. Hazelnuts, walnuts and pistachios are also good sources of folic acid.

Iron also has an important role in hematological processes. The decline in red blood cell content causes iron accumulation during saturation. For this reason, a dietary intake of iron should be monitored in divers. Current RDA for iron is 18 mg/day [16].

There are two forms of dietary iron: heme and non-heme. Most **non-heme** iron is from plant sources, while **heme** iron is derived from hemoglobin. It is found in animal foods that originally contained hemoglobin, such as red meats, fish, and poultry (meat, poultry, and seafood contain both heme and non-heme iron). The body absorbs the most iron from heme sources.

35.15.2 Vitamin D

Vitamin D is known to promote the **mineralization of bones** by enhancing calcium and phosphorus absorption. This micronutrient has a pivotal role in helping enhancing muscle protein anabolism, improving immune function, regulating calcium homeostasis and therefore overall bone health. In fact, bone is a nutritionally modulated tissue, meaning dietary intake can have a significant impact on it and **bone health** has been shown to be one of the few documented long-term diseases associated with saturation diving.

Expert and professional divers may be deprived of exposure to UBV radiation from sunlight, and this condition can cause inadequate or deficient levels of **serum 25[OH]VitD**.

It has been proposed that supplementation with 2000 IU daily is sufficient to maintain serum 25[OH] VitD levels in divers [17].

35.16 Hydration

Renal function undergoes significant variations during mixed-gas saturation diving.

The daily urine flow **increases rapidly** on compression to a value of 700-1000 mL/day above the predictive level, then **slightly drops** to a steady level of approximately 500 mL/day above the predictive level. During decompression, the diuresis **slowly disappears**, and the urine flow returns to the control level towards the end of the decompression [18].

These changes in renal function generally occur with no significant changes in plasma osmolality and glomerular filtration rate, indicating that the **renal tubular transport**, not the filtered load, of salt and water is altered in hyperbaric environment.

Nevertheless, the **hypohydration** that results from this condition is thought to cause a range of adverse health and performance consequences.

Hot humid environments can lead to marked dehydration in the pre-dive period if adequate amounts of fluid are not consumed. Standby divers are also at risk of dehydration and thermal stress injury under these conditions. It is enormously important for divers to maintain euhydration, a goal that is also hindered by the sweat produced during what is considered a very high-consumption sport [19]. Adequate amounts of non-alcoholic fluid should be consumed for 24 hours prior to the start of a dive. Five mL of fluid per kg of body weight (about 400 mL, or 12 fl. oz. in an 80 kg diver) should be consumed within 1 hour before diving.

35.17 Endorphins and microgravity

Under water it is possible to "fly": to move in all directions.

Playing with microgravity. Stop at any depth, enjoying a completely different dimension.

Scuba tanks and regulators – then – allow an incredible experience: breathing in the water. Experiencing this sensation can be a great joy that is renewed with every dive.

Good visibility, absence of current, tepid water, richness of the seabed can transform this experience into a large **production of endorphins**, endogenous opioids, which contribute so much to well-being.

35.3 Foods not recommended in compensation problems

- **Alcohol** (causes vasodilation with secondary swelling of the mucous membranes)
- **Excess of proteins** (causes water retention with secondary increase in the thickness of the mucous membranes)
- **Milk and derivatives** (lactose can cause water retention and consequent swelling of the mucous membranes)
- **Citrus fruits** (contain histamine and cause swelling of the mucous membranes)

35.4 Food rules on the days of diving

- For **breakfast**, prefer milk tea as the latter is less digestible.
- **Lunch** with pasta, rice or cereals, vegetables and fruit. If an afternoon diving is planned, do not exceed with fatty foods and avoid alcohol.
- Always **drink** abundantly before and after diving (at least 2 liters of water).
- Have a **snack** with fruit and liquids.
- For **dinner** eat proteins (meat, fish, legumes), with vegetables and fruit.
- Eat plenty of **fruit** and **vegetables**. These foods perform important functions in the fight against free radicals and make potentially harmful substances that insinuate themselves through food or breathing, harmless.
- Eat **carbohydrate-rich foods** regularly (pasta, rice, cereals)
- On the **day of diving** consume light and digestible food.
- If you do more than one dive a day, eat something just before bedtime.
- If you do two or more dives a day, do not overdo it with foods that contain or release **histamine** especially between one dive and another (chocolate, strawberries, tomatoes, shellfish, cold cuts, fermented cheeses, dried fruit)
- Mineral salts, trace elements and vitamins are important. A **balanced diet** is sufficient to cover its needs.

REFERENCES

1. Revelli L, Addolorato G, D'Amore A, Carrozza C, Giubileo G, Puiu A, Lombardi CP, Bellantone R, Gasbarrini G; Progetto Abissi 2005 Dive Medical Group. Neuroendocrine and psychological assessment in a guinness 10 days scuba dive. Int J Sports Med 2007; 28(10): 848-52.
2. Professional Association of Diving Instructors. Worldwide certification history. http://www.padi.com/padi/en/footerlinks/certhis to rynum.aspx (Accessed May 2020).
3. Boussuges A, Lafay V. Modifications de la fonction cardiaque en plongée sportive [Changes in cardiac function during recreational diving]. Arch Mal Coeur Vaiss. 1997 Feb;90(2):263-8. [Article in French].
4. Puiu A, Giubileo G, Addolorato G, Revelli L, Gasbarrini G, Bellantone R, D'amore A, Lombardi CP, Carrozza C. Stress monitoring in a Guinness 10-days scuba dive. Laser Physics 2007; 17: 448-52.
5. Doolette DJ, Mitchell SJ. Hyperbaric conditions. Compr Physiol 2011; 1(1): 163-201.
6. Deb SK, Swinton PA, Dolan E. Nutritional considerations during prolonged exposure to a confined, hyperbaric, hyperoxic environment: recommendations for saturation divers. Extrem Physiol Med 2016; 5: 1.
7. Doubt TJ: Cardiovascular and thermal responses to SCUBA diving. Med Sci Sports Exerc 1996; 28: 581-6.
8. Theunissen S, Balestra C, Boutros A, De Bels D, Guerrero F, Germonpré P. The effect of pre-dive ingestion of dark chocolate on endothelial function after a scuba dive. Diving Hyperb Med 2015; 45(1): 4-9.
9. Benardot D, Zimmermann W, Cox GR, Marks S. Nutritional recommendations for divers. Int J Sport Nutr Exerc Metab. 2014 Aug;24(4): 392-403.
10. Paciorek JA: Nutrition for a 350 MSW working dive. Undersea Biomed Res 1985; 12.
11. Hong SK, Bennett PB, Shiraki K, Lin Y, Claybaugh JR. Mixed-gas saturation diving. Compr Physiol 2011 [https://doi.org/10.1002/cphy.cp040244].
12. Brubakk AO, Ross JA, Thom SR. Saturation diving; physiology and pathophysiology. Compr Physiol 2014; 4(3): 1229-72.
13. IOM. Dietary reference intakes for Energy, carbohydrate, fibre, fat, fatty acids, cholesterol, protein and amino acids. Washington DC: National Academic Press; 2005.
14. Phillips SM, Van Loon LJ. Dietary protein for athletes: from requirements to optimum adaptation. J Sports Sci 2011; 29 Suppl 1: S29-38.
15. Revelli L, Vagnoni S, D'Amore A, Di Stasio E, Lombardi CP, Storti G, Proietti R, Balestra C, Ricerca BM. EPO modulation in a 14-days undersea scuba dive. Int J Sports Med 2013; 34(10): 856-60.
16. Hofsø D, Ulvik RJ, Segadal K, Hope A, Thorsen E. Changes in erythropoietin and haemoglobin concentrations in response to saturation diving. Eur J Appl Physiol 2005; 95(2-3): 191-6.
17. Smith SM, Davis-street JE, Fesperman JV, Smith MD, Rice BL, Zwart SR. Nutritional status changes in humans during a 14-day saturation dive: the NASA extreme environment mission. J Nutr 2004; 134: 1765-71.
18. Sagawa S, Claybaugh JR, Shiraki K, Park YS, Mohri M, Hong SK. Characteristics of increased urine flow during a dry saturation dive at 31 ATA. Undersea Biomed Res 1990; 17: 13-22.
19. Shiraki K, Konda N, Sagawa S, Nakayama H, Matsua M. Body heat balance and urine excretion during 4day saturation dive at 4 ATA. Undersea Biomed Res 1982; 9: 321-33.
20. Revelli L, D'Alatri L, Scorpecci A, D'Amore A, De Corso E, Lombardi CP, Fetoni AR. ENT function in a 14-days guinness scuba dive. Int J Sports Med 2012; 33(1): 31-5.

SECTION 6 Social and cultural aspects of food

36 The encounter between religion and food

Sabina Saccomanno, Daniele Laganà and Licia Coceani Paskay

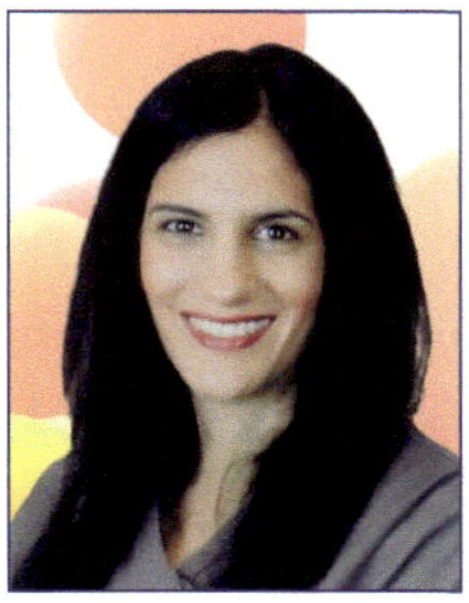

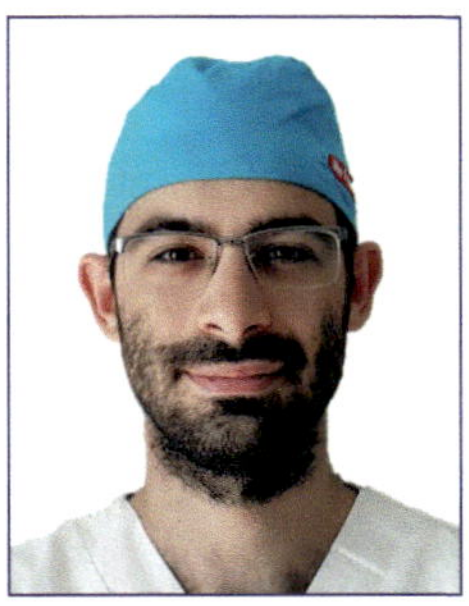

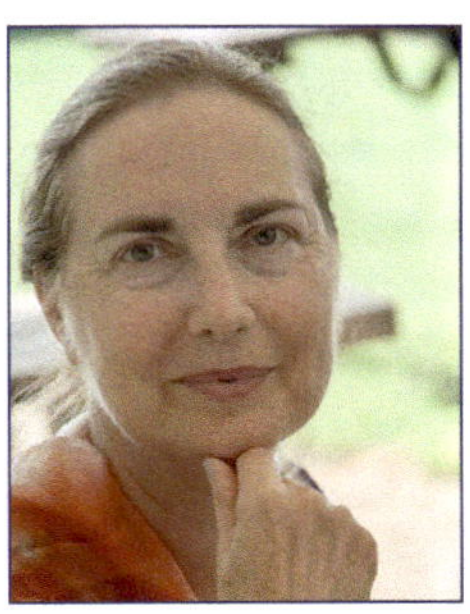

In the context of the cultural differences of different peoples, food plays a decisive role not only for anthropological, climatic, territorial and geographical reasons, customs and traditions, but above all for the link with the religious dimension.

Common traits in the various religions are the recognition of food as a gift from God. In fact, in the Bible, Deuteronomy, 8:10 states: "*When you eat and are satisfied, you are to bless the LORD, your God for the good land that He has given you.*" Hence the importance of prayer as thanksgiving and blessing for the food received, while abstinence and fasting as well as community and celebration, become forms of encounters with God and generally includes a particular menu with which the faithful praises God in joy.

Please note that various geographical areas may use slightly different spelling for the same concepts.

36.1 Foods and nutrition in Christianity

Christianity is almost devoid of food bans, thanks to the New Covenant which canceled the Jewish restrictions in terms of food: for this purpose, the episode of the trance of St. Peter, as recounted in the Acts of the Apostles (Acts 10. 10-16) is particularly indicative [1]. In this episode, Peter was praying and became hungry. While his meal was being prepared, he had a trance in which he saw animals, reptiles and birds and a voice told him to get up, kill and eat those animals. He replied that he has never "eaten anything impure or unclean" to which the voice answered: "*Do not call anything impure that God has made clean*". Likewise, in the Gospel (New Testament) there is an explicit reference to the overcoming of dietary limitations in which Jesus tells the crowd: "*What goes into someone's mouth does not defile them, but what comes out of their mouth, that is what defiles them.*" (Mt 15:11).

Sabina Saccomanno, DDS
Department of Life, Health and Environmental Sciences, University of L'Aquila, L'Aquila, Italy

Email: sabinasaccomanno@hotmail.it

Daniele Laganà, DDS
Full Professor, Dental School, University of L'Aquila, Italy

Email: daniele.lagana@outlook.it

Licia Coceani Paskay, MS, CCC-SLP
Speech-Language Pathologist, Private Practice
Los Angeles, USA

Email: lcpaskay@gmail.com

36.1.1 Fasting and abstinence in the Catholic Church

The only nutritional precepts observed by Catholics are fasting during the days of Ash Wednesday, the beginning of the Lenten (Lent) period, and fasting on Good Friday, the day of the Passion of Jesus. Abstinence (but not fasting) is recommended on all Fridays of the year, unless they coincide with a solemnity. In accordance with the Apostolic Constitution Paenitemini of Paul VI and the Code of Canon Law [2, 3], *fasting* consists in the consumption of a single meal a day, possibly accompanied by two light lunches during the morning and in the evening, extremely modest in quantity and quality, while *abstinence* means the exclusion from meals or dishes containing meat, even though it is still possible to eat eggs, dairy products and condiments including animal fat such as butter or lard. All the faithful from age 14 are required to abstain, while only the faithful of age 14 to 60 are required to be fasting. In addition, canon law contemplates the possibility that the Episcopal Conferences may grant the replacement of the observance of fasting or abstinence with other forms of penance, such as works of charity or exercises of piety.

36.1.2 Fasting in the Orthodox Church

Unlike Catholicism, the practice of fasting in orthodoxy assumes a much tighter frequency and a divergent formulation, in which there is an edict for abstinence from animal proteins, alcohol and oil, with a diet essentially based on bread, pasta, rice, fruit, vegetables, olives, crustaceans and mollusks; this fast is observed every Wednesday and Friday of the year, as well as in four specific periods: the Great Lent (seven weeks before Easter), the Fast of the Apostles (eight days after Pentecost until June 28th), the Fast of Ascension (from August 1st to 14th) and the Christmas fast (from November 15th to December 24th) [4].

36.1.3 Fasting in other Christian denominations

Fasting is practiced by Anglicans, as it is foreseen by the Book of Common Prayer, and by Methodists, in which John Wesley himself recommended it every Friday except Christmas and every day from awakening until early afternoon [5, 6]. Currently this type of fasting is considered as a work of piety and is prescribed on some holidays for the faithful and on Wednesdays and Fridays for the clergy. In the other Protestant denominations fasting is considered a spiritual exercise therefore carried out freely by the faithful.

36.2 Foods and nutrition in Judaism

Judaism provides a set of dietary rules, defined as *kashrut*, which distinguishes what is *kosher*, or allowed, and what is *taref* or *trief*, which is prohibited [7]. The source of these rules is the Torah, which provides for a subdivision of food according to the criterion of purity, regarding the species of animals consumed. The oral tradition, as explained by the Talmudic Rabbis, explains their method of preparation. Some explain that there are hygienic-sanitary reasons in these provisions while others give a symbolic value to food bans, as in the case of birds of prey, due to their aggressiveness. The food classification distinguishes the environment in which the animals live, that is, land, water and air, and establishes permitted or prohibited edible species for each of them.

36.2.1 Land animals

The essential requirements for terrestrial quadrupeds are the possession of a bipartite claw, that is, a hoof completely divided in two, and being a ruminant.

From the scientific point-of-view, ruminants constitute a suborder having the Latin name of Ruminantia and was classified in 1777 by the Italian Dr. Giovanni Antonio Scopoli. Ruminants are characterized by the presence of a *concamerated* stomach, which is divided into rumen, reticulum, omasum and abomasum, and by the behavior of rumination, a characteristic digestive process which involves a double oral chewing with an intermediate passage inside the gastric compartments of the rumen and the reticulum to then flow into the gastric compartments of the omasum and the abomasum. To the suborder belong the families of the Tragulidae (such as mouse deer and chevrotain), of the Moschidae (musk deer), of the Cervidae (including deer in general, reindeer or caribou, and moose or elk), of the Giraffidae (giraffes and okapi), of the Antilocapridae (pronghorns) and of the Bovidae (including cattle, sheep, goats, gazelles and antelopes).

The forbidden edible quadrupeds belong to the Camelidae family (including camels, dromedaries and llamas), the Leporiadae family (hares and rabbits), the Equidae family (horses, donkeys and zebras) and the Suidae family (pigs and wild boars) (Table 36.1).

Furthermore, the consumption of Invertebrata

(sub-kingdom classified by Lamarck, but no longer in use today), of the class of Reptilia and the order of Carnivora (including dogs, cats, wolves and bears) is strictly prohibited; the only exception is a type of locust, which is allowed as food.

Table 36.1 Mainland edible animals

Tarèf/Trief	*Kosher*
Hare/rabbit	Cattle
Camel	Goat
Donkey/horse	Deer
Pig/Wild boar	Sheep

36.2.2 Water animals

The rules regarding aquatic species is the contextual presence of fins and scales (such as carp or trout), however there are exceptions to this criterion with regard to the Clupidae family (including herring and sardines) which develops scales after birth and the Scombridae family (including tuna and mackerel) that loses them when coming out of the water.

Instead, the entire phylum of Mollusca (including mussels, oysters, clams, octopuses, squid and cuttlefish), the subphylum of Crustacea (including lobsters, shrimps and scampi), the superfamily of Pinnipedia (seals, walruses and sea lions) and the infraorder of the Cetacea (including whales, dolphins, killer whales and sperm whales are prohibited (Table 36.2).

Fish, in contrast to permitted animals and fowl, are not "ritually slaughtered".

Table 36.2 Main water edible animals

Tarèf	*Kosher*
Clams	Mackerel
Mussels	Sardines/Herrings
Calamari/Squid	Tuna
Octopus	Carp/Trout
Shrimps	Salmon

36.2.3 Air animals

The main requirement for Kosher birds is the absence of rapacity, to which are added the presence of two legs in the front position and two legs in the rear position and the fact that they do not catch food on the fly. Among the clearly permitted aerial species are the Anatidae family (including geese and swans) due to the rounded beak or the Phasianidae family (including roosters, hens, ducks, pheasants, and turkey) due to the fingers joined by membrane, while the ostrich, owls and the vultures are explicitly prohibited along with, for peculiar historical reasons, Canadian geese (Table 36.3).

Table 36.3 Main flying edible animals

Tarèf	*Kosher*
Ostrich	Chicken/Pheasant
Owl	Turkey
Vulture	Domestic Goose/Ducks
Canadian geese	Quail/Doves

36.2.4 The Ritual Slaughter

Shechitah involves cutting the trachea and esophagus, causing rapid and consistent bleeding which reduces the suffering of the animal at the hands of the *shochèt*, a professional figure who makes a blessing before performing this task. This rite emphasizes that eating animal meat is not a human right, but a generous concession from God. Furthermore, a careful inspection of the animal is necessary to ensure that it does not suffer from diseases or malformations such as to make it tarèf, that is, impure.

Any time shechitah is performed, kissùyi hadam is also performed, which is the rite of covering the blood. In this rite, the leaked blood is hidden with dirt and soil to cover it from the sight of man. Within seventy-two hours of slaughtering, the meat must be subjected to salting, a process consisting of immersing the animal in salty water for a certain amount of time, to leach out the remaining blood through subsequent washing of the meat under running water.

36.2.5 Further religious dietary rules

The Bible forbids the consumption of one specific part of the animal body: the sciatic nerve because it commemorates the wounding of Jacob's thigh during his wrestling bout as stated in Genesis 32:25. In this regard, Ashkenazi Jews of Germanic origin do not eat a particular cut of beef meat (commonly known as *filet mignon)* which surrounds the sciatic nerve while Sephardic Jews of Spanish origin have the custom of removing the sciatic nerve in order to eat the meat around it.

Furthermore, there are three mentions in the Bible which prohibit the cooking a baby goat in its mother's milk, which is interpreted by the Rabbis to not cook and eat a mixture of meat and milk products together.

36.3 Foods and nutrition in Islam

Islam also considers food bans based on the commands of its own sacred text, the Quran, which prohibits the consumption of alcoholic beverages and haram (illicit) meats, while nutrition with halal (lawful) is permitted. The Second Sura explicitly refers to this distinction: "O men, eat what is lawful and pure of what is on earth, and do not follow in the footsteps of Satan. Indeed, he is your declared enemy" (II, 168).

The number of haram foods seems to overlap with the tarèf ones, in all probability due to the continuity that Mohammed claimed with respect to the patriarch Abraham. The differences do not exist so much in the animals considered lawful, which almost coincide with rare exceptions (such as rabbits), that are contextually halal and tarèf, but rather in the Jewish prohibition of mixing meat and milk and in the Islamic prohibition of the consumption of alcohol (Table 36.4).

Table 36.4 Food differences between Hebraism and Islam

Food	*Hebraism*	*Islam*
Rabbit	Tarèf	Halal
Mixing meat and milk	Tarèf	Halal
Alcohol	Kosher	Haram

36.3.1 Slaughter and prayer

Even Islamic slaughter, the *dhabiha*, is somewhat similar to the Jewish *shechitah*, essentially differing in the absence of a specific figure for this procedure, but being possible to implement it by any adult male Abrahamite who is aware of all Islamic precepts on ritual slaughter.

A characteristic of Islamism that differs from the Jewish rite is the *basmala*, the prayer that must be pronounced before eating a meal and whose translated text is: "In the name of the gracious and merciful God".

36.3.2 Ramadan

One of the five pillars of Islam is fasting during the month of Ramadan, which each year falls in a different season because the Islamic calendar is based on the 28 days lunar month. The Second Sura also defines it as "the month in which the Quran was sent down as a guide for men and clear proof of right direction and salvation" (II, 185).

Fasting constitutes a complete abstention from any food, including drinking water, from dawn to sunset, with a few exceptions such as young children, people who are sick or pregnant women. The fasting ends with the *maghrib*, that is the sunset prayer, followed by the *iftar*, the dinner that traditionally begins with one or three dates, emulating the similar behavior of Muhammad in this circumstance.

Traditionally, *iftar* is a family dinner often consumed in parks during the warm months. The end of Ramadan is celebrated with the *Eid-el-fitr* feast, in which multiple families get together to consume traditional foods that vary in different geographical regions, but that most often include large serving plates of lentils, fish, chicken, lamb or other halal meats, potatoes, and various vegetables. Plenty of spices and herbs, also reflecting the geographical influences on Islamic food, are used to enhance flavor, such as chili pepper, cardamom, garlic, cloves, parsley or curry. Both the *iftar* and any major Islamic feast feature plenty of sweets, often made with honey (the only food that never decays), almonds, pistachios, dry coconut or dried figs. Because of the abundance of food prepared for Eid, a tenet of Islam is to share the Eid feast with the poor.

36.4 Foods and nutrition in Hinduism

Hinduism, also called Sanatana Dharma (Eternal Order), has been applying specific food guidelines since they were written in the Vedas, the ancient sacred texts of Hinduism and subsequently in the Upanishads text [8]. In the Vedas it is written that: "*One becomes worthy of salvation when no living being is killed*", so much so that observant Hindus are strictly vegetarians although they can eat eggs (Table 36.5). Moreover, the cow is considered a sacred animal and blessed for providing milk, butter and other dairy products. Furthermore, apart from the prohibition of

Table 36.5 Hindu Diet

Prohibited	*Allowed*
Cow Meat	Fruits, veggies, grains, pulses
Alcohol (for Brahmins only)	Eggs, milk and dairy

eating animals, members of the Brahmin priestly caste are prohibited from drinking alcohol.

Over time, some of the strict rules about not eating meat and fish were reconsidered and codified. Hinduism considers the body a temple and therefore only "pure" foods should be allowed inside as food becomes energy. Therefore, regardless of the type of food consumed, it is imperative the blessing of the food, as a show of gratitude, and whenever possible fresh fruits and vegetables are eaten.

Currently, food in Sanatana Dharma is divided in three broad categories: Sattvic, Rajasic and Tamasic [9].

Sattvic foods are supposed to be easy to digest, they help people being compassionate, loving, forgiving, perceptive, content and moderate. The Sattvic food includes fruits such as mango, apples, bananas, fresh fruit juices, coconut and peaches; vegetables such as lettuce, parsley and sweet potato; dairy products such as organic milk and yogurt; grains and beans such as rice, yellow lentils and kidney beans.

Rajasic foods are characterized by being salty, sour, acidic, hot (as in chili pepper hot) and loaded with spices. They are foods considered tempting or stimulant and consequently they favor strong emotions such as anger or hate. Rajasic foods include sour apples, chilies, garlic, onions, hot peppers, eggplants, pickled veggies and dairy products such as sour milk and sour cream. Rajasic foods also include chicken meat, shrimps and fish in general.

Tamasic foods are heavy foods and do include meat. Because of their nature, Tamasic foods make people feel tired, sleepy and depressed, but can be consumed in small amounts. Tamasic foods include onions and garlic, mushrooms, pumpkin, white flour, aged cheese and even food leftovers.

Because of its geographical and climatic origin, foods consumed by Hindus reflect the agricultural availability as well as medical necessity. Rice features prominently and accompanies every meal. Due to lack of refrigeration and to prevent food spoiling, curry sauce (made with turmeric or curcumin) and other spices (ginger, chili pepper, cardamom, garlic among others) are heavily used and occupy a large part of the traditional Hindu food preparation. These spices are well known in pharmacopeia to have various health benefits, in keeping with the tradition that food is also a medicine. Moreover, most foods are thoroughly cooked and even tea is rigorously prepared with boiling water.

In this brief and general review of food and nutrition in the four main religions, it's possible to see how where the specific religion originated dictated most of the rules and regulations that then crossed time and boundaries often unchanged [10].

The sacred sphere has been enveloping philosophy, social mores, hygiene, medicine, pharmacopeia and traditional culture for thousands of years and survives even in the current tendency to globalism.

REFERENCES

1. La Bibbia di Gerusalemme, a cura della Conferenza Episcopale Italiana, Dehoniane, 2009.
2. Costituzione apostolica Paenitemini, Paolo VI, Libreria Editrice Vaticana, 1966.
3. Codice di Diritto Canonico e leggi complementari commentato, a cura di Juan Ignacio Arrieta, Coletti a San Pietro, 2018.
4. Catechismo ortodosso, San Nikolaj Velimirovic, Le vie della Cristianità, 2019.
5. The Book of Common Prayer 1559: The Elizabethan Prayer Book, a cura di John E. Booty, University of Virginia Press, 2005.
6. An Introduction to World Methodism, Kenneth Cracknell, Cambridge University Press, 2005.
7. Kosher, halal, bio. Regole e mercati, Elena Toselli, FrancoAngeli, 2018.
8. Veda: introduzione ai testi sacri indiani, Alessandra Consolaro, Xenia, 2000.
9. Sattvic, Rajasic and Tamasic Food. https://www.nithyananda.org/Nithyananda-eNcyclopedia/Sattvic%20Rajasic%20Tamsic%20Food.html
10. Religione come cibo e cibo come religione a cura di Omar Marchisio, FrancoAngeli, 2004.

The authors wish to thank Rabbi Dr. Joseph Schames, for additional editing of the section on Jewish food and traditions; to Ms. Hena Mohiuddin. for additional editing of the section on Islamic food and traditions; and to Mahadev Parameswaran, PhD, for additional editing of the section on food and traditions in Hinduism.

37 The Mediterranean diet

Sabina Saccomanno, Vincenzo Quinzi, Rebecca Jewel Manenti,
Silvia Giancaspro, Giuseppe Marzo

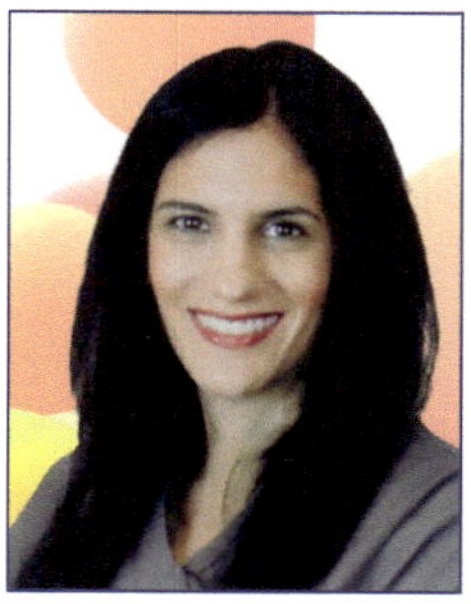

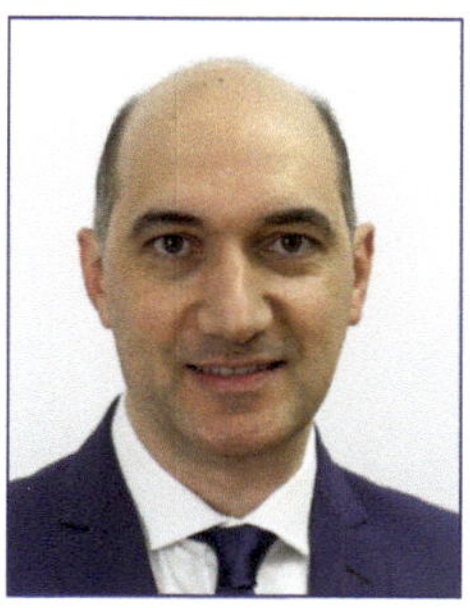

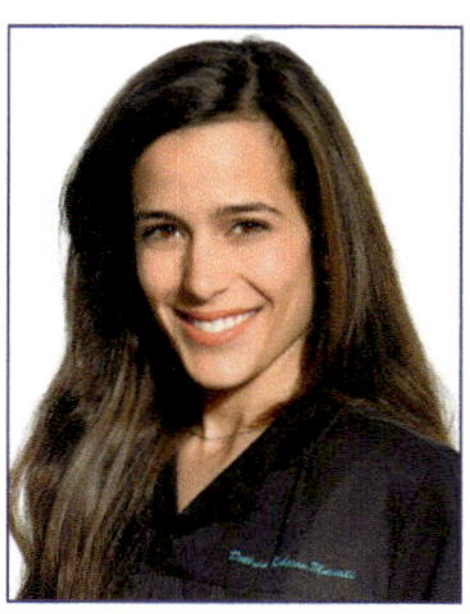

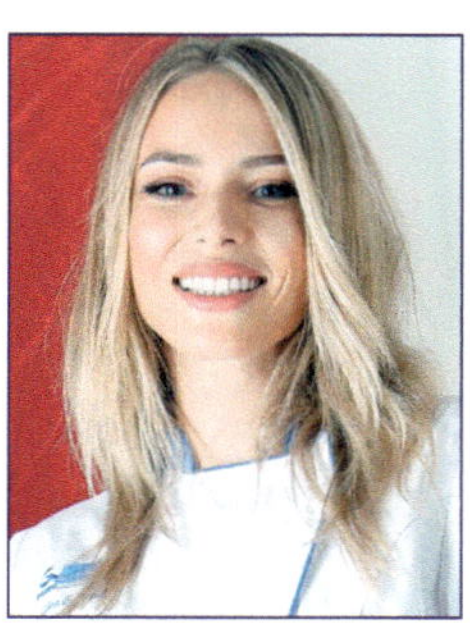

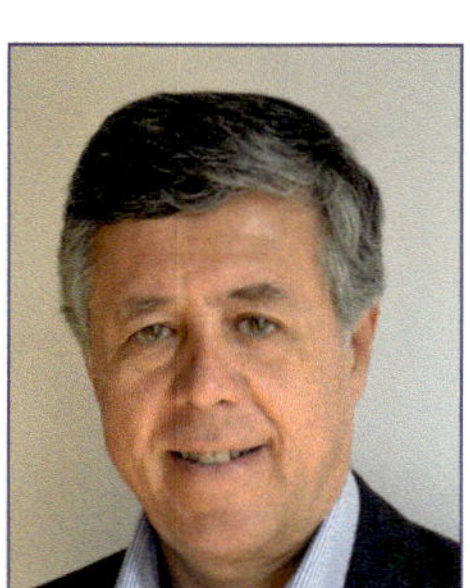

37.1 Mediterranean diet: general description and pyramids

The Mediterranean diet (MD) is a nutritional model with proven health and ethical value, so much that since 2010 UNESCO attributed it the coveted recognition of *intangible cultural heritage of humanity* [1]. The MD was first defined by Ancel Keys as being the diet low in saturated fat and high in vegetable oils, observed in the early 1960s in South Italy, Crete and other areas of Greece [2, 3]. The definitions include guidelines for high intake of extra virgin (cold pressed) olive oil, vegetables including leafy green vegetables, fruits, cereals, nuts and pulses/legumes, moderate intakes of fish and other meat, dairy products and red wine and low intakes of eggs and sweets.

The MD is characterized by an adequately balanced combination of fruit and vegetables, fish, cereals and polyunsaturated fats, with a reduced consumption of meat and dairy products and a moderate intake of alcohol, primarily red wine [4]. Most commonly, recommended numbers of servings for these food groups are represented as a diet pyramid. Diet pyramids are considered a useful way to display the general principles of a diet including approximate recommendations for quantities of food groups (i.e., those consumed in greatest quantities appear in the largest base section of the pyramid) [5]. The Mediterranean diet pyramid, as recommended by the *Fundación Dieta Mediterránea*, promotes a high consumption of cereals, fruits and vegetables, low consumption of red meats and sweets and moderate consumption of dairy, poultry and fish. Additionally, the diet also includes moderate consumption of wine and use of olive oil (replacing other forms of fats) as essential components of the diet. Both these factors can be considered reasonable recommendations, given past evidence of health benefits for cardiovascular health associated with olive oil and moderate alcohol consumption [6, 7]. Moreover, high intake of dairy products is not advised in the landmark publications on the MD and health [8, 9].

Sabina Saccomanno, DDS
Department of Life, Health and Environmental Sciences, University of L'Aquila, L'Aquila, Italy

Email: sabinasaccomanno@hotmail.it

Vincenzo Quinzi, DDS; Rebecca Jewel Manenti, DDS; Silvia Giancaspro, DDS;
Giuseppe Marzo, MD
Department of Life, Health and Environmental Science, University of L'Aquila, L'Aquila, Italy

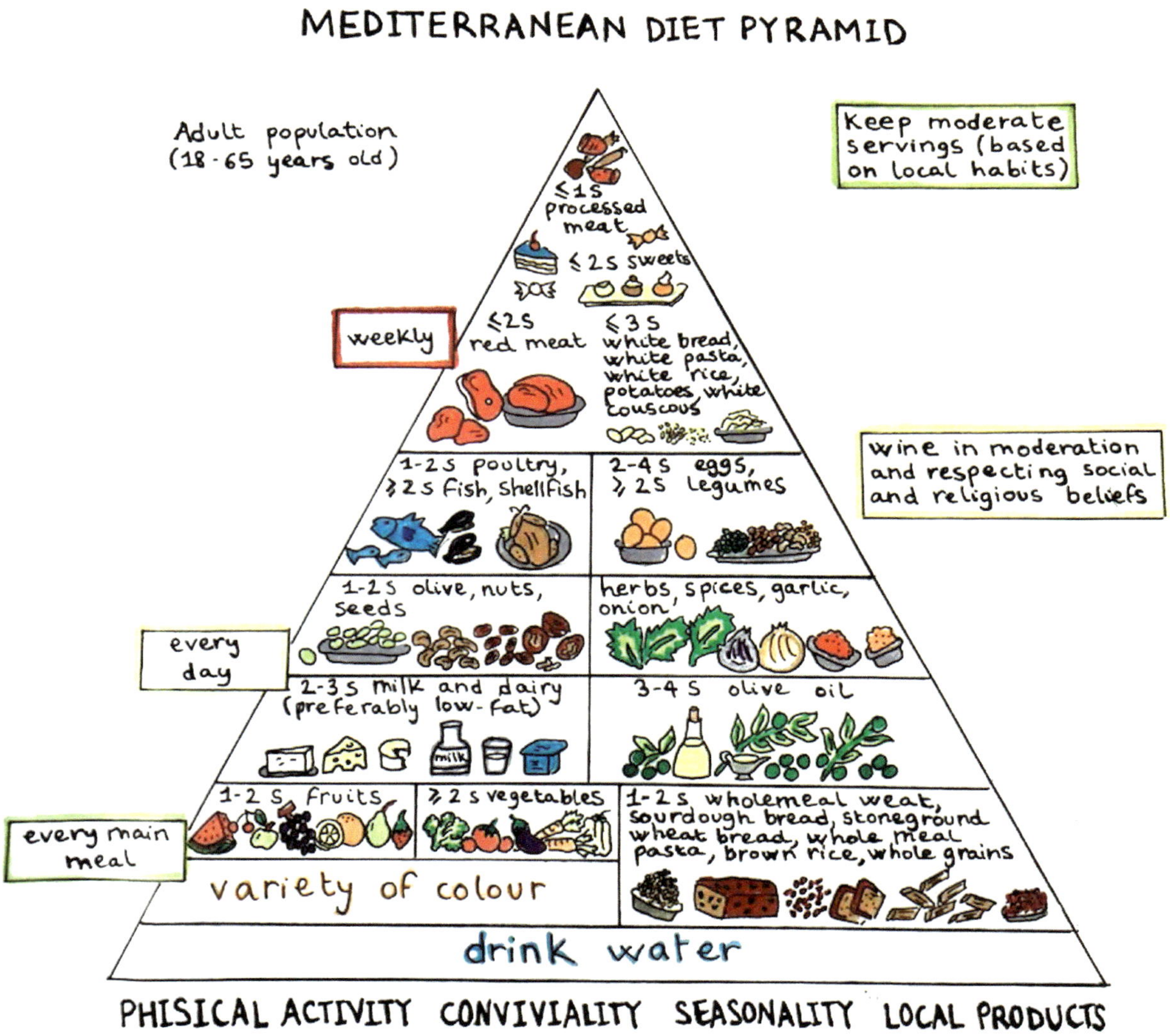

Fig. 37.1 Mediterranean diet pyramid (Image by Giulia Giancaspro, adapted from [5]).

37.2 Mediterranean diet: general health improvement

The exact mechanism by which a traditional MD exerts its beneficial effects in lowering the risk of developing cardiovascular disease, certain cancers and other metabolic conditions is not known. Many interrelated and overlapping factors have been hypothesized to play a role (Fig. 37.1).

The five most important mechanisms, which can mediate the pro-health and pro-longevity effects of the traditional MD, are as follows: (a) lipid-lowering effect; (b) protection against oxidative stress, inflammation and platelet aggregation; (c) modification of hormones and growth factors involved in the pathogenesis of cancer; (d) inhibition of nutrient sensing pathways by specific amino acid restriction; (e) gut microbiota-mediated production of metabolites influencing metabolic health [9]. Scientific evidence has shown that the adoption of the MD is a protective factor against the onset of various types of cancer, cardiovascular disease, aging and obesity. As shown by the European Prospective Investigation into Cancer and Nutrition (EPIC) study, the MD is most effective in the prevention of several chronic diseases, including cancer [4]. The Dietary Guidelines Advisory Committee included the MD among highly beneficial dietary patterns for the prevention of overweight and obesity, cardiovascular diseases (CVD), type 2 diabetes, colorectal cancer and postmenopausal breast cancer [3]. Populations living in the area of Mediterranean Sea showed a decrease incidence of cancer, compared with those living in regions of North Europe or the USA, which has been attributed to healthier dietary habits [9]. Many elements of the MD eating pattern are associated with improved health and longevity The MD exerts protective effects in elderly subjects with and without baseline of chronic diseases. The bioactive food components have a potential preventive action on cancer [10]. The nutrients that are found in abundance in the MD have anti-cancer, anti-inflammatory, anti-obesity properties and together contribute to the maintenance of a healthy status. The anti-tumor effects of the MD are mostly due to the combination of antioxidant elements, fiber and polyunsaturated fats. This dietary pattern is therefore essential as a preventive measure against the onset of cancer and other chronic diseases but also to reduce health care costs [4]. A recent meta-analysis conducted by Grosso et al. [11] has linked the association between MD adherence and CVD incidence and mortality. They found an important decrease of incidence of coronary heart disease, myocardial infarction and stroke. The most protective effects are associated to higher consumption of olive oil, fruits, vegetables, legumes, nuts and moderate intake of wine (especially red wine) [12]. A recent paper examined the effects of Italian Mediterranean Diet (IMD) and Italian Mediterranean Organic Diet (IMOD) on body composition and laboratory parameters in healthy subjects and in patients with Chronic Kidney Disease (CKD) [13]. Therefore, the impact of IMD and IMOD on decrease of cardiovascular risk factors and on the progression of renal disease was investigated. The authors demonstrated that the IMOD diet, according to "Nicotera Diet", was able to reduce the total plasma homocysteine (tHcy), phosphorus and albuminuria levels in CKD patients and to ameliorate the cardiovascular risk profile in both populations examined [14]. Di Daniele et al. [15] have shown that the IMD promotes weight loss and reduces the growing burden of cardiovascular risk factors that typifies patients with Metabolic syndrome (MetS). Specifically, a balanced hypocaloric IMD improved significantly systolic and diastolic blood pressure and fasting glucose in 80 white Italian subjects with MetS. Moreover, the authors have observed a resolution of MetS in 52% of treated patients. Regarding longevity, the MD, together with the Mediterranean Adequacy Index (MAI) and the Healthy Diet Indicator (HDI), were studied during the Healthy Ageing: a European longitudinal study (HALE) that included men and women from ten European countries. The subjects were followed over a 10 years-time observation. The study has confirmed the protective role of MD for elderly subjects with and without baseline chronic diseases [16]. Another study confirmed that higher adherence to MD in older adults in the United-States and Israel is linked to better cognitive and physical functions. In fact, in these subjects, a faster walking speed and fewer disabilities were detected [17]. In a Greek population cohort study, Trichopoulou et al. [18] demonstrated for the first time that a higher degree of adherence to MD was correlated with a reduction in total mortality. The benefits of MD are evident in the prevention and slowing of the progression of chronic degenerative diseases. A meta-analysis highlighted that both men and women with eating habits very close to MD have about 10-20% reduced risk of dying of CVD, cancer and other causes. The MD is significantly inversely associated with both systolic and diastolic blood pressure [1]. The protective effect of olive oil (OO) on aging is confirmed by a study that has evaluated the bioactivity of OO compounds on multipotential mesenchymal stem cell (MSC) progenitor differentiation. In fact, osteoblasts and adipocytes derive from the same MSC. Santiago-Mora et al. [8] have demonstrated that oleuropein, one of the most important OO compounds, enhances osteoblastogenesis and inhibits the main adipogenesis regulators, as proliferator-activated receptor gamma (PPAR-γ), lowering the incidence of osteoporosis. The extra virgin olive oil, vegetables, fresh fruits, nuts, wine and fish contain molecules with antioxidants and anti-inflammatory properties, as monounsaturated fatty acids, fatty acids omega 3, polyphenols, flavonoids, phytosterols, vitamins, antioxidants, minerals and micronutrients. These factors act on longevity and slow the development of chronic diseases associated with aging. The diet and the natural antioxidants play an important role on these metabolic pathways affecting cancer progression [4].

37.3 Mediterranean diet: a sustainable model

The MD model in many studies has been deemed to have a lower environmental impact, mainly due to its consumption of more plant-derived products and less animal products, with respect to other current dietary patterns [19]. On an economic level, the importance of investments in preventive policies and practices is highlighted. Such strategies can prevent much higher costs than not taking action. The reduction of chronic non-communicable diseases can be implemented through the consumption of healthier foods than those consumed globally today [3]. This aspect must be taken into consideration since the broader benefits in terms of reduction of current healthcare expenditure will be particularly impactful in low and middle-income countries and families. In fact, the MD is a healthy diet since it contains a large amount of cereals, fruit and vegetables with a limited consumption of red meat and derivative products [20].

37.4 Seven Countries Study (SCS): Municipality of Nicotera (Province of Vibo Valentia) - «Italian Mediterranean Reference Diet»

The municipality of Nicotera in Calabria, a region of Italy, entered the history of national and international nutritional research as it was the center of the pilot study included in the Seven Countries Study (SCS) [21, 22].

Between 1958 and 1961 the study was extended to sixteen cohorts of 40-59-year-old men residing in population centers in Finland, Japan, Greece, Italy, the former Yugoslavia, the Netherlands and the United States of America. From the analysis of Nicotera's data, the prevalence of heart attack was very low (about 0.7%) and hypertension, diabetes and overweight were uncommon. The results obtained, considering the clinical investigation and lifestyle of the adults examined, led to the definition of Nicotera's diet, at that time, as the «Italian Mediterranean Reference Diet» [21].

Regarding the SCS, conducted by some of the finest scientists from all over the world, it emerged that between the nine European rural cohorts, and the Mediterranean ones (Crevalcore and Montegiorgio in Italy, Crete and Corfu in Greece and Dalmatia in the former Yugoslavia), at the 25th year follow up, presented a mortality rate from heart and coronary heart disease of 978/10,000, while the non-Mediterranean ones (Slavonia and Velika Krsna in the former Yugoslavia and Eastern and western Finland) had a double mortality rate of 1,947/10,000 [23, 24]. The diets of the two groups were very different. Olive oil, cereals, fruit, vegetables and wine during meals were mostly present in the five Mediterranean cohorts, while meat, eggs, cheeses and animal fats were found in Finland and in former Yugoslavia, where alcoholic beverages such as beer and spirits were usually consumed between meals [24].

37.5 Mediterranean Adequacy Index (MAI)

The Mediterranean Adequacy Index (MAI) was established in the 1990s by Adalberta Alberti-Fidanza [25]. It indicates the degree of adequacy of the dish/menu compared to the Italian Mediterranean Diet of Reference and it also evaluates the changes that the food components have undergone over time. The index value is obtained by dividing the sum of the percentages of total energy coming from the foods belonging to the MD (bread, cereals, legumes, potatoes, vegetables, fruit, fish, red wine, olive oil) by the sum of the percentages of energy total provided by foods not belonging to the MD (milk, cheese, meat, animal fats, margarine, sweet drinks, biscuits, cakes and sugar). The optimum value of the MAI is between 5-10 [25].

The higher the MAI, the more likely the diet will be adapted to the Mediterranean Reference Diet. Although the results of these studies indicate that the food style to aim for in a healthy life is the MD, from the 50's to today, that is, from the first Keys study, we have witnessed throughout the Mediterranean area, including Italy, a gradual disuse of this diet in favor of less healthy eating styles.

This is unfortunate, as the abundance of antioxidants is one of the main characteristics of the Mediterranean Diet of Reference, recognized as one of the primary factors in promoting and maintaining the state of health [24].

37.6 The Italian Mediterranean Organic Diet (IMOD) as a prevention of food inadequacies

The Italian Mediterranean Organic Diet (IMOD) is a balanced diet in which there is the prevalence of some typical Mediterranean food groups from organic farming such as cereals, legumes, vegetables, fresh and dried fruit, oil, virgin olive oil, fish and red wine. The appropriate combination of these foods, by qualitative and quantitative means, allows the prevention of nutritional inadequacies by excess and defect and provides nutrients and food components that have high protective effects [14, 24].

The results obtained from the general research indicate that the consumption of organic products in a MD can guarantee an effective antioxidant action capable of opposing the effects of free radicals and decreasing the inflammatory processes, which are important mechanisms in the prevention of the onset of chronic-degenerative diseases. An appropriate, organic and balanced food plan in reference to the Italian Mediterranean Diet will spare us from nitrogen fertilizers, which determine a decrease in the biological value of proteins; from potassium fertilizers, which lower magnesium and minerals; and from phosphatic fertilizers, which reduce the quantity of vitamins. It also helps to improve some blood parameters when compared to conventional non-organic products: decreases inflammatory factors (pro-inflammatory cytokines), reduces markers of oxidative stress (lipid hydroperoxides and nitrogen oxide metabolites) and markers of cardiovascular risk (homocysteine and lipoprotein profile).

For this reason, it is possible to affirm that the IMOD plays a very important role for life quality and longevity [14].

37.7 Progressive distancing from the Italian Mediterranean Reference Diet: risk factors for chronic-degenerative diseases

The lack of recognition of the Italian Mediterranean Reference Diet as a healthy food model is a weakness for humanity. The current nutritional transition, combined with environmental pollution, is creating major public health concerns, since food patterns are the main risk factors in the onset of non-communicable diseases (NCD), especially regarding cardiovascular diseases, diabetes, certain types of cancer and chronic-degenerative diseases. At least 100 years of epidemiological studies have demonstrated the associations between diet, lifestyle and the increased incidence and severity of chronic NCD.

The lack of clarity due to generic and misleading messages regarding the MD prevents the unaware consumer from knowing that there is a Mediterranean Adequacy Index (MAI) that compares diets. This index allows consumers to be able to evaluate objectively how much of their chosen diet approaches the Mediterranean one that should be taken as a reference. That's unfortunate as nutritional transition and aging of the population contribute to an increase in the impact of chronic diseases on the general quality of health. After all, non-adherence to the MD, coupled with a smoking habit and sedentary lifestyle, reduces life expectancy by 4.8 years in twenty years and by 10.7 years in forty years [25].

REFERENCES

1. D'Alessandro A, Lampignano L, De Pergola G. Mediterranean Diet Pyramid: A Proposal for Italian People. A Systematic Review of Prospective Studies to Derive Serving Sizes. Nutrients 2019; 11(6): 1296.
2. Davis C, Bryan J, Hodgson J, Murphy K. Definition of the Mediterranean Diet; a Literature Review. Nutrients 2015; 7(11): 9139-53.
3. Saulle R, Semyonov L, La Torre G. Cost and cost-effectiveness of the Mediterranean diet: results of a systematic review. Nutrients 2013; 5(11): 4566-86.
4. Di Daniele N, Noce A, Vidiri MF, et al. Impact of Mediterranean diet on metabolic syndrome, cancer and longevity. Oncotarget 2017; 8(5): 8947-79.
5. D'Alessandro A, De Pergola G. Mediterranean diet pyramid: a proposal for Italian people. Nutrients 2014; 6(10): 4302-16.
6. Sofi F, Cesari F, Abbate R, Gensini GF, Casini A. Adherence to Mediterranean diet and health status: meta-analysis. BMJ 2008; 337: a1344.
7. Trichopoulou A, Martínez-González MA, Tong TY, et al. Definitions and potential health benefits of the Mediterranean diet: views from experts around the world. BMC Med 2014; 12: 112.
8. Santiago-Mora R, Casado-Díaz A, De Castro MD, Quesada- Gómez JM. Oleuropein enhances osteoblastogenesis and inhibits adipogenesis: the effect on differentiation in stem cells derived from bone marrow. Osteoporos Int 2011; 22(2): 675-84.
9. Romagnolo DF, Selmin OI. Mediterranean Diet and Prevention of Chronic Diseases. Nutr Today 2017; 52(5): 208-22.
10. Grosso G, Buscemi S, Galvano F, et al. Mediterranean diet and cancer: epidemiological evidence and mechanism of selected aspects. BMC Surg 2013; 13 Suppl 2(Suppl 2): S14.
11. Grosso G, Marventano S, Yang J, et al. A comprehensive meta-analysis on evidence of Mediterranean diet and cardiovascular disease: Are individual components equal? Crit Rev Food Sci Nutr 2017; 57(15): 3218-32.
12. Trichopoulou A, Costacou T, Bamia C, Trichopoulos D. Adherence to a Mediterranean diet and survival in a Greek population. N Engl J Med 2003; 348(26): 2599-608.
13. Di Daniele N, Di Renzo L, Noce A, et al. Effects of Italian Mediterranean organic diet vs. low-protein diet in nephropathic patients according to MTHFR genotypes. J Nephrol 2014; 27(5): 529-36.
14. De Lorenzo A, Noce A, Bigioni M, et al. The effects of Italian Mediterranean organic diet (IMOD) on health status. Curr Pharm Des 2010; 16(7): 814-24.
15. Di Daniele N, Petramala L, Di Renzo L, et al. Body composition changes and cardiometabolic benefits of a balanced Italian Mediterranean Diet in obese patients with metabolic syndrome. Acta Diabetol 2013; 50(3): 409-16.
16. Knoops KT, Groot de LC, Fidanza F, Alberti-Fidanza A, Kromhout D, van Staveren WA. Comparison of three different dietary scores in relation to 10-year mortality in elderly European subjects: the HALE project. Eur J Clin Nutr. 2006 Jun;60(6):746-55.
17. Zbeida M, Goldsmith R, Shimony T, Vardi H, Naggan L, Shahar DR. Mediterranean diet and functional indicators among older adults in non-Mediterranean and Mediterranean countries. J Nutr Health Aging 2014; 18(4): 411-8.
18. Trichopoulou A, Kouris-Blazos A, Wahlqvist ML, et al. Diet and overall survival in elderly people. BMJ 1995; 311(7018):1457-60.
19. Serra-Majem L, Tomaino L, Dernini S, et al. Updating the Mediterranean Diet Pyramid towards Sustainability: Focus on Environmental Concerns. Int J Environ Res Public Health 2020; 17(23): 8758.
20. Willett WC, Sacks F, Trichopoulou A, et al. Mediterranean diet pyramid: a cultural model for healthy eating. Am J Clin Nutr 1995; 61(6 Suppl): 1402S-1406S.

21. Legge Regionale VALORIZZAZIONE DIETA MEDITERRANEA ITALIANA DI RIFERIMENTO DI NICOTERA. Burc n. 109 del 8 Novembre 2017 https://burc.regione.calabria.it/ricerca.jsp?q=YW5ubz0yMDE3IyMjbnVtZXJvPTEwOQ==
22. "La Dieta Mediterranea Italiana di Riferimento di Nicotera ad Expo Milano 2015" https://www.quotidianosanita.it/allegati/allegato703200.pdf
23. The 7 Countries Project-The HALE Project. https://www.sevencountriesstudy.com/about-the-study/related-studie/hale-study/
24. Relazione Senato-La Dieta Mediterranea Italiana di Riferimento https://www.senato.it/application/xmanager/projects/leg17/attachments/documento_evento_procedura_commissione/files/000/003/461/De_Lorenzo_Relazione.pdf
25. Alberti-Fidanza A, Fidanza F. Mediterranean Adequacy Index of Italian diets. Public Health Nutr 2004; 7(7): 937-41.

38 International foods: a review of their benefits

Sabina Saccomanno, Anna di Tullio and Licia Coceani Paskay

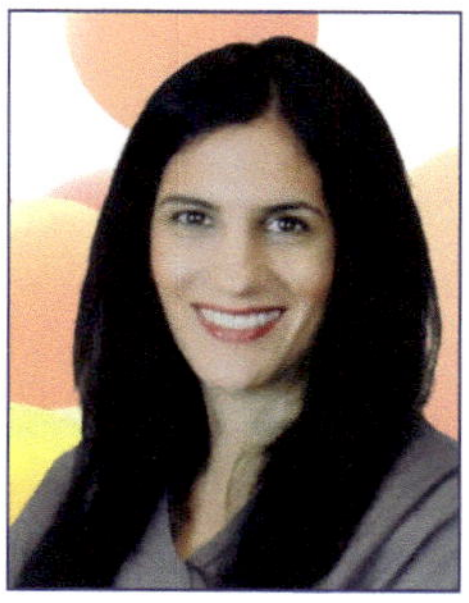
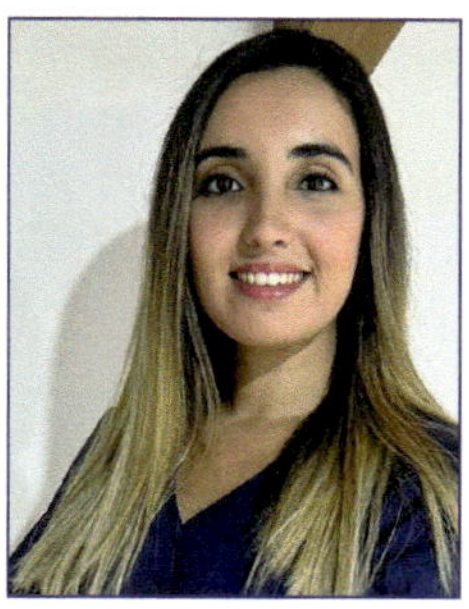
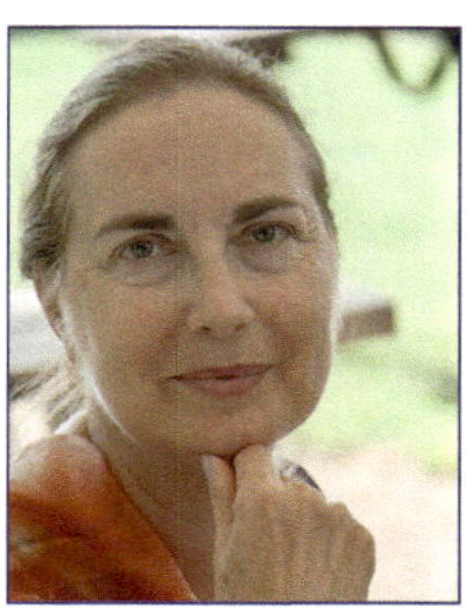

Food preparation is an integral part of a country's culture and discovering the various types of ethnic cuisines is the first step in getting to know groups of people and their traditions. Each ethnic cuisine is characterized by its own territorial distinctiveness and is the expression of a real cultural system, becoming part of a habitual local diet transmitted between and along generations. Each ethnic group adopts a different type of diet, which offers different nutrients, different degrees and cooking methods and different textures of food, but also a different approach to food intake, such as utensils used for example. In addition to its role as a sustenance, food has a huge cultural significance, so much so that it becomes part of the history and identity of a population. Many ethnic foods are made from raw materials typical of a specific area, so depending on the geographical regions, we find different diets rich in beneficial properties for health, together with local culinary traditions. Thanks to the ever-increasing number of scientific studies, today there is an increased awareness of the link that exists between health and cooking. Numerous studies report that Mediterranean cuisine, for example, has beneficial effects on health, as it helps prevent cardiovascular diseases [1], type 2 diabetes [2], neoplasms [3], stroke, depression, cognitive impairment and Parkinson's disease [4] and Alzheimer's [5]. The role of nutrition in disease prevention has promoted further research into the benefits and safety of food: balanced and healthy nutrition can become the first form of prevention that starts at the table, but also the first medicine, precisely because what we eat affects our health. In this chapter, in very generic terms, we'll explore the gastronomic cultures of the various ethnic groups, the health benefits, the culinary excellence and the traditions at the table.

38.1 European Cuisine

Northern European cuisine is characterized by the use of local ingredients: wild herbs, cloudberries, whey, Limfjord oysters, pine and juniper, but also mushrooms, nuts, game such as elk, deer and bears, with all meats provided by local hunters.

Sabina Saccomanno, DDS
Department of Life, Health and Environmental Sciences, University of L'Aquila, L'Aquila, Italy

Email: sabinasaccomanno@hotmail.it

Anna di Tullio, SLT
Speech Therapist in Private Practice

Licia Coceani Paskay, MS, CCC-SLP
Speech-Language Pathologist, Private Practice
Los Angeles, USA

Email: lcpaskay@gmail.com

The birth of the "New Nordic" culinary movement was the claim of a creative space for Nordic chefs, who proposed a traditional cuisine, in which freshness, purity, simplicity, ethics come together to embellish each dish. From the use of shells, hay and branches as kitchen utensils to the recovery of traditional methods such as drying, smoking, seasoning and pickling, the New Nordic movement looks to the past rather than the future, proposing an authentic kitchen which aims to produce food in the most natural way possible. This was, after all, the New Nordic revolution, which allowed Northern Europe to enter the empyrean of haute cuisine with such typical products as fresh, smoked and marinated salmon, whose recipe is very ancient and was born as a method of preserving fish.

In Germany the most used ingredients are meat and potatoes. Very common are the *brotsuppe*, soups made from bread with vegetables, potatoes and egg yolk; the *kartoffelsalat*, a potato salad; the *sauerkraut*, made with German cabbage, finely chopped and subjected to lactic fermentation; the *knödel,* potato balls and bread with small pieces of speck or lard and Würstel and various types of sausages, are also very popular in Germany as well as in most of Central and East Europe. A typical dessert is the apple *strudel.* Beer is the most popular and most used alcoholic drink to accompany almost all types of meal from sandwiches to sausage-based main courses, with the local Augustiner, Beck's and Bitburger being very popular.

The main dishes of French cuisine are *omelettes*, *boeuf bourgignon*, a stew of beef covered in red wine, with aromatic herbs and bacon; the *escargot*, are boiled snails and some recipes require their stuffing; *quiche Lorraine* is a shortcrust pastry shell containing a mixture of eggs, bacon and sour cream; *soupe gratinée à l'oignon* is a soup made with white onions and butter, blended with Port wine and chicken broth. The most popular traditional cheeses are the soft Brie, Camembert and Roquefort. Croissants are classic pastries for breakfast, made with yeast dough and plenty of butter. France is famous for its high quality DOP (certified origin) wines, such as Bordeaux Bergerac, Burgundy, Champagne, Sauternes-Barsac, Alsace and Beaujolais. In the late 1970s, researchers noted that residents in parts of France who were avid red wine drinkers had less heart disease than other Western populations, even though they consumed more fat and cheese in their diets. This observation has triggered numerous investigations into this so-called "French paradox". Subsequent research confirmed the presence of high concentrations of antioxidant polyphenols in the skins of red grapes. However, it should be noted that moderate consumption of any alcoholic beverages, such as beer, wine or spirits, reduces the risk of heart disease in the populations studied [6], although this issue is not completely settled yet.

At the base of Spanish cuisine we find fresh, local and seasonal products. *Gazpacho,* a cold soup made with tomato, onions, olive oil and wine vinegar, is an all-times favorite along with *tapas,* small appetizers based on meat, cheese and vegetables, and potato *tortillas,* made with fried eggs and potatoes. The best known Spanish dish is the *paella Valenciana*, a rich dish, the key ingredients of which are chicken or rabbit and vegetables, with the fish-based versions considered a traditional option in the more coastal areas. Among the typical desserts we find *churros,* sweetened pancakes, and Catalan cream, based on caramelized sugar, custard flavored with citrus peel and cinnamon.

In Greece, the most characteristic products are yogurt, salads and olives. The dishes that distinguish traditional cuisine are *horiatiki*, the rustic Greek salad made with vegetables, typically tomatoes, cucumbers and onions, and feta, the traditional Greek cheese made from sheep and goat milk, to which olives are added. Kalamata olives and capers are added to any salad and other dishes often served with *Tzatziki*, a cream that is prepared by adding small pieces of fresh cucumber to the yogurt, olive oil and intense aromatic herbes such as mint, dill and garlic. Other local favorites are *souvlaki*, skewers of pork cooked on the grill and the *moussaka*, a sort of lasagna with layers of potatoes and eggplant. Among the well known desserts is the *baklava*, pastries made with sheets of phyllo dough alternated with layers of honey and dried fruit.

38.2 Russian Cuisine

Russia covers a very large and diverse area from the point-of-view of food production and consumption and variations of some dishes have been adopted by other Eastern countries. In northern Russia and Siberia, common dishes are *pelmeni* and *vareniki,* which are dumplings filled with meat, fish, cheese, mushrooms and/or veggies. In the area closest to Europe, typical foods are based on potatoes and cabbage or turnips (along other ingredients), such as *borsht soup,* along with *piroshki* (small baked pies filed for veggies, meat or fish), *blini* (crepes), *okroshka* (cold soup made of fermented bread), salted herrings and *kasha* (buckwheat). River fish, meat and lots of rye bread are also part of the tradition, with reindeer meat in the area close to the Baltic. In areas close to Mongolia or in the south-east of Russia, lamb meat, goat's milk and mutton's meat (salted, smoked or dried) are traditional and nomadic food and prepared accordingly.

38.3 Chinese Cuisine

It is mainly based on the use of simple and traditional foods based on rice, soy, pickled vegetables, fish, eggs, fermented sauces, ginger and pork. Studies have shown the benefits of soy, from which tofu is derived, thanks to its richness in isoflavones. Soy also has been shown to help prevent the onset of cardiovascular disease and some types of cancer, such as breast and prostate cancer. These products may also have antioxidant effects that relieve hot flashes during menopause and bone loss [7]. According to some studies, ginger has a potential preventive property against some chronic diseases, in particular hypertension and coronary heart disease [8] and is effective in improving hyperlipidemia, hyperglycemia, stress oxidative and inflammation [9]. Green tea also has numerous health benefits and is widely used in China. The correlation between tea consumption and the health-related quality of life (HRQOL) among elderly Chinese was examined: habitual consumption of tea was associated with a lower incidence of disease and a consequent improvement in the quality of life [10]. A very common cooking method in Chinese cuisine is based on the use of a large hemispherical pan, the *wok*. This typical utensil allows you to prepare food through various cooking techniques, such as sautéed, steamed, fried and smoked. Cooking over high heat allows for cooking food quickly, preserving its nutritional properties, while steaming has the benefit of limiting the addition of fats, such as oil, preserving the flavor and nutritional value of food.

Traditional foods include a wide range of products, such as pickled vegetables, fish (which is a widely used protein source in the diet), salted jellyfish, fermented sauces, poultry, eggs and products derived from tofu and rice, which is the most important staple food in China and from which people obtain a caloric intake of about 80-90% of the daily intake. Ethnic foods are generally low-fat foods, with a relatively low-calorie value and require longer preparation times to achieve the desired sensory characteristics. The ingredients are cut into small pieces in order to cook quickly so as to maintain distinct flavors and a good texture, as unlike Western food, creaminess is not a favored texture. According to Chinese food culture, the consumption of food is practiced with the use of a pair of chopsticks of equal length and with a pointed end. The foods, being already cut into small pieces, are eaten quickly without the need to use a knife, which is used in food preparation, but which does not appear on the table. Chopsticks originated in ancient China, under the Shāng dynasty and are widely used in various countries of Asia, as well as in restaurants offering typical dishes from these cuisines.

Among the most typical dishes of Chinese cuisine are the dumplings, balls of pasta stuffed with meat, fish or vegetables steamed or grilled, which contain the typical flavor of Asian cuisine, where soy, ginger, cabbage are just some of the basic ingredients; the spring rolls, a thin and crunchy pastry, stuffed with a mix of vegetables and fried, often accompanied by a sweet and sour sauce or in soy sauce; rice noodles mixed with seafood, grilled fish, soy sauce and ginger; Cantonese rice, boiled and flavored with peas, pieces of cooked ham and eggs. Traditional Chinese foods have attracted attention from food scientists and technologists, from the food industry and health-promoting institutions around the world due to the values they offer. Further development of traditional techniques for preparing these foods is expected to produce economic, social and health benefits. Ethnic Chinese foods will continue to find a special niche in history, preserving Chinese culture in the modern diet, even for generations to come [11].

38.4 Indian Cuisine

It is known throughout the world for the scents of its spices, which are frequently used to flavor dishes. Some religious precepts forbid eating pork, others consider cattle sacred animals, for this reason in this kitchen we find numerous vegetarian dishes.

Several biomedical studies have focused on the beneficial properties of Indian spices, to provide scientific evidence supporting the traditional uses of these spices in cooking. Among the best known are curry, turmeric, cinnamon, cardamom, chili, cumin, coriander, mustard, garam masala and ginger. Turmeric, for example, is used for wound healing, in the treatment of rheumatic disorders, gastrointestinal symptoms and rhinitis. Studies conducted in India have explored its anti-inflammatory and antioxidant potentials, investigations have shown its anti-cancer preventive effect, which prevents the formation of cancer cells by preventing DNA damage, and anti-atherosclerotic, which helps to keep the blood cholesterol levels [12]. Furthermore, curcumin is also recognized for its strong antioxidant properties as it helps fight free radicals, prevent and delay the degenerative processes of Alzheimer's and promote health in general [13]. Spices such as turmeric, fenugreek, mustard, ginger, onion and garlic have a great variety of organic functions, and their additive or synergistic actions are a valid natural aid for the prevention and treatment of various diseases. For this reason, including spices in the diet appears to have holistic effects on human health. Some of the most common foods of India are rice, legumes, bread, yogurt and vegetables. The mango is a typical fruit of tropical and subtropical climates and widespread in India. According to studies, it has a rich source of bioactive compounds including phenols and carotenoids [14] and its main bioactive compound is mangiferin, protective against radiation-induced diseases, as well as being associated with an anti-diabetic, anti-atherogenic, anti-hyperlipidemic activity in rats and has antibacterial and antifungal effects [15].

The cooking methods of Indian cuisine are characteristic, the different tools used give particular flavors to the dishes and different textures. In India the meal is usually eaten sitting on the floor on a mat, with the plate resting on the lap. You eat with your hands to have a tactile relationship with the food and to feel its temperature and degree of cooking.

Indian cuisine is especially loved for its vegetarian dishes, not making much use of eggs and meat. Among the typical dishes we have *dosa*, a rice batter stuffed with *masala dosa*, the spicy filling of potatoes, onion, curry, turmeric, coriander, rice and lentils; chicken with curry, served on a bed of white rice; *tandoori* chicken consists of chicken marinated in a yogurt sauce, spices called *tandoori masala* and then traditionally cooked in tandoori clay ovens; *samosa*, a crunchy appetizer, the flour dough wraps a filling of chopped, spiced and pan-cooked ingredients, such as potatoes, onions, lentils, meat; *biryani* is a dish of boiled basmati rice to which many spices and various ingredients cooked separately are added: meat, fish, vegetables.

38.5 Japanese Cuisine

The Japanese diet is varied and rich in white rice and traditional food such as fish, vegetables, seaweed, legumes such as soy, meat, milk, oils, fruit and fermented condiments, such as the popular *wasabi* (obtained from Japanese radish), ginger and sesame. The lipid and protein contents differ from those of Western diets due to the high consumption of fresh fish, in particular tuna and salmon stand out. Among the most popular Japanese recipes are *sushi*, white rice balls wrapped in a layer of seaweed with a fish filling. Another famous dish is *nigiri*, rice balls with fish or shellfish on top; *maki*, which are rice with fish or vegetables in a sheet of *nori* seaweed. *Sashimi*, on the other hand, is a dish based on raw fish, without rice. *Tempura* is fried shrimp and vegetables battered with rice flour and then fried; *Soba* is spaghetti made with flour and water seasoned with broth; *Udons*, on the other hand, is noodles prepared with whole wheat flour. Then there is *ramen*, a soup based on spaghetti or noodles accompanied by fish or meat. Ramen is a popular and inexpensive food choice with students and workers on both sides of the Pacific Ocean, due to its ease of preparation when using a freeze dry mix that only requires water and being microwaved; popular restaurants also offer *kaiten*, where sushi plates flow in front of customers.

Japanese cuisine is low-calorie and complete with a source of fatty acids such as omega-3 and isoflavones, contained in soy. Seaweed is a typical plant food rich in fiber and each variety has its own specific properties. They are excellent antioxidants and anti-inflammatories plus they contain a good percentage of vitamins, proteins and mineral salts. Seaweed is a source of iodine and chlorophyll that purifies the body and promotes oxygenation of the blood, stimulating thyroid function. Some algae (such as spirulina) have high iron concentrations, suitable for nutrition by those suffering from anemia [16]. Japanese cuisine leans toward cold dishes and a typical dish is sushi, made with rice, fish and seaweed. According to a study conducted in 2017, people with a higher adherence to Japanese dietary guidelines have a lower risk of death especially from cardiovascular and cerebrovascular diseases. The results of this study suggest that a balanced consumption of grains, vegetables, fruits, meat, fish, eggs, soy products, dairy products, confectionery and alcoholic beverages can contribute to longevity by decreasing the risk of death, mainly from cardiovascular disease [17].

38.6 African Cuisine

Africa is a vast continent with many different climates and cultural influences on food [18]. The coastal swath of North Africa was dominated by the Ottoman Empire for about 400 years and currently almost all the coastal and the Sub-Saharan countries are predominantly or exclusively Muslim, therefore their food production and consumption follows specific, general and local religious rules. The food from the tropical band of the continent is reflected in the richness of flavors from the eastern portion of Africa, such as Ethiopia or Eritrea and, and from the western countries such as Ivory Coast and Ghana. The southern region of Africa, having a more tempered climate, allows production of many foods (and even wine) that reflects both the ancestral richness and simplicity of ingredients as well as the colonial influence exerted there for centuries.

The basic food of African cuisine is fresh vegetables and cereals, with which different types of soups and stews are prepared, with proteins and some type of starch, rice or possibly yams. Dietary fiber, very common in the African diet, has beneficial effects on food-related diseases. Dietary fiber is known to relieve constipation, useful in reducing the incidence of colon cancer, and help reduce cardiovascular disease and diabetes. Cereals in an African diet provide a significant amount of vitamin E and selenium, which is important for their antioxidant and anticancer properties. Phytochemicals play a protective role against some chronic diseases and the phytoestrogens present in grains are believed to have protective properties and reduce the risk of cancer. The main dishes of many African cuisines are made of cereals (corn, millet, sorghum, teff), roots and tubers (cassava, cocoyam, sweet potatoes), green bananas or plantain. Treculia africana is a fruit that is eaten as a main dish and can be considered a valid alternative to rice and potatoes. Unlike fish, meats are not very common in this cuisine, as are dairy products; a small amount of food of animal origin can be added to the meal to improve the taste and protein value, providing iron and vitamins, especially vitamin A and folate. Many traditional African foods contain large amounts of oils, including palm or canola oil. Fried foods are common, such as fried plantains, chickpeas and yams [19] as they may reflect the difficulty to refrigerate food and the need to fry, boil or bake most foods. In most African communities, people rely on one or two staple crops that provide most of the energy supply to family members. The most common are corn, teff, cassava, sweet potato, sweet potato, plantain and enset. To balance their diet, consumers supplement staple foods with legumes or foods from animal sources that are rich in protein and oil.

Traditionally, *Aspalathus linearis* (Rooibos) is a plant used in South Africa to obtain red tea, which has antioxidant, chemopreventive and phenolic compound properties, and has an immune modulating effect and an anti-allergenic action. Free radicals can damage DNA in cells and increase the risk of chronic disease. Antioxidants, such as polyphenols, are able to bind free radicals before they become harmful to the body. A traditional African fruit is the Java plum, widespread in Uganda and introduced by the Indians in 1900. It is traditionally consumed for the treatment of asthma; the fruits are eaten especially by young children. Studies conducted on this fruit have revealed that Java plum seeds have a high antioxidant content [15]. Food distribution within the traditional family is often related to the hierarchical position, with the head of the family receiving priority in eating from the common bowl, while women and children can only serve themselves after the elders and men are satisfied, receiving therefore a smaller share of food. This custom results in undernourishment for the most vulnerable groups, which is common to other communities in Asia and the Middle East. A general rule of thumb is to give each a different amount of food, but the same share of taste. Among the typical dishes we find cous cous, a base of coarsely ground wheat, boiled and combined with the most diverse ingredients such as vegetables, meat, fish, dried fruit; The tajine, named for the pan where it is cooked. Tajine is a main course dish mainly made of meat; Harissa sauce which is a very spicy sauce made with red chillies and aromatic herbs; Sauce d'avocat: a typical appetizer from the Democratic Republic of the Congo (formerly, Zaire) is based on avocado, anchovies, onions, garlic, seasoned with mayonnaise. In African cuisine neither sausages nor dairy products are widespread.

38.7 North American Cuisine

North America includes Canada, the USA and Mexico. Nowadays traditional foods can be found everywhere but still every country retains something in particular. Since the 1990s, American cuisine typically features a single dish of meat with a side dish of potatoes, or vegetables, with sauces for dressing and desserts as a culinary specialty: apple pie, glazed donuts, cookies and cheesecakes. Among the classic meaty dishes of North America one can find barbecue ribs, beef or pork ribs, in barbecue sauce; Buffalo Wings, a spicy dish strictly eaten with your hands, forks and knives are banned from the table and Chili Cheese Dog, a variation of the classic hot dog, with chili and cheese. The meat sold in fast food restaurants, such as hot dogs and hamburgers, has a soft consistency, which does not require vigorous chewing. The number one ordered food in the United States is pizza, of all varieties, but uppermost in the pizza group is one with pepperoni and cheese topping. California is the land of wine, especially as regards the more classic reds such as Cabernet Sauvignon and Chardonnays. In the northernmost regions of the upper Midwest, fish and dairy dishes are common, thanks to fishing and farms In New England, you'll find dishes famous for seafood. Vermont is known for cheddar-type cheese. The standard American diet (SAD) [20] includes an excessive consumption of calories from refined carbohydrates, animal fats and added sugars and lacks many nutrients, such as those found in whole grains, fruits and vegetables. This dietary pattern, which also includes excessive sodium intake, contributes to elevating current levels of overweight and obesity, as well as diet-related illnesses and conditions such as type 2 diabetes mellitus, hypertension and heart disease. The 2005 American Diet Guidelines (DGAs) recommend that Americans eat more nutritious foods, including fruits and vegetables (particularly dark green – and orange – colored vegetables, starchy, legumes, beans and peas), grains (especially whole grains) and to choose low-fat dairy products. Lean meats (including beef and poultry), fish, eggs, nuts, seeds, as well as foods low in fat and added sugar are also recommended [6, 20].

Canada and Alaska (a state that is part of the USA) share the characteristics of foods available at high latitude and the social reality of having a large swath of the population sparsely scattered on the territory and living of a subsistence, seasonal diet. The First Nation people, including the Inuit, still survive mostly by hunting and some gathering [21]. Prominent feature of local diets (except for large cities, where any food is available) is meat such as that of caribou (moose), seals, whales, game and migratory birds which are usually smoked and/or salted. The most famous fish is the Alaskan salmon, valued for its peach-colored meat and versatility of preservation, being consumed grilled in season, or smoked and salted for the winter months. Shellfish is also harvested in Alaska and along both coasts of Canada. Roots and berries, especially blueberries are the traditional and seasonal fresh vegetables and fruit. The lack of vitamins derived from vegetables is often mitigated by eating other items. For instance, strips of whale skin and blubber, usually consumed raw, called *muktuk* is rich in vitamin C, which is also found in kelp and in berries. Vitamins A and B are found in fish oil, especially salmon, along with plenty of omega-3 fatty acids, while fish heads are a good source of calcium. In the past, hard labor at sub-freezing temperatures easily counterbalanced a diet that would not be healthy for city dwellers nowadays, but the healthy lifestyle of the First Nation people is a testimony to the importance of culture and tradition in food gathering and consumption.

38.8 Mexican Cuisine

Mexican cuisine is characterized by very strong and spicy flavors, thanks to the extensive use of multiple varieties of chillies. Mexican dishes contain many ingredients with beneficial properties, being rich in proteins, minerals and vitamins. Moreover, they vary according to the region, given the strong climatic difference and the different Spanish influence typical of certain areas. However, there are typical dishes present in any place in Mexico such as: tacos, served with guacamole sauce, based on avocado, onion, lime and in some cases Tabasco; burritos, made up of tortillas rolled and stuffed with chicken meat cooked with onion, spices and hot sauces, often served with rice and beans; chili, a spicy stew made from chilli, meat, tomatoes and beans. Tex-Mex cuisine, a variant of Mexican cuisine that has undergone the influence of Texan cuisine, is widespread in the border area that separates the United States from Mexico. Once the Mexican migrants arrived in the United States, they struggled to find some of the main ingredients to prepare the typical dishes, making up for these shortcomings by creating a more "American" version of the tradition. The most famous Mexican bread is the tortilla, a type of flat bread, crunchy and soft, made of corn flour and stuffed in various ways, with which the enchiladas are prepared, which have a filling of beans, beef or chicken, covered with tomato sauce and baked in the oven. Fajitas, cooked on a cast iron plate and served with cheese, guacamole and lettuce sauce and the nachos, in which the corn tortilla is cut into deep-fried triangles and then garnished with various sauces and ingredients such as cheese, beans, chili, peppers, olives, onions.

Also prominent in Mexico is cocoa. The first uses of cocoa date back to the Mayans who were the first to create a cocoa plantation. Cocoa's uses were the most varied: its seeds were used to buy goods and slaves, but above all they were ground with stones to make drinks to which spices and honey were added.

38.9 Cuisine from Central America

The ingredients that stand out in Central American cuisine are rice, legumes, plantains and potatoes that accompany almost all dishes, often fortified with spices such as garlic, cumin, oregano, paprika, chilli and vegetables, especially pumpkin and avocado. The most famous ingredient in all of Central America is corn: this cereal is the basis of various typical dishes such as tortillas, nacatamales and tamales. The typical dishes par excellence are tacos, burritos which are tortillas with a filling based on meat, onions and spices. The most substantial dishes revolve around the use of meat, especially pork, while the use of fish is not frequent.

Caribbean cuisine is very rich and varied, with dishes that are the results of a fusion of different cuisines including: African, French, Spanish and Indian. The main ingredients of Jamaican cuisine are local fruits such as mango, papaya, coconuts and meats such as chicken, pork, goat and fish, shellfish, all accompanied by spices. Usually before the meal it is customary to bring rice and beans to the table.

Cuban cuisine leans towards grilled or fried fish, seafood, prawns and pork as the protagonists at the table. With the fat parts of the pig, the Cubans prepare the famous chicharrones, salty snacks. A typical Cuban dish is Ajiaco which is a typical soup, with meat, especially beef or veal, corn, garlic, onions, avocado, at least two varieties of potatoes (criolla and pastuza), guasca, eggs, cream. Among the spices, cumin, pepper, sweet paprika, oregano.

38.10 Cuisine from South America

Argentine cuisine is characterized by the use of meat and wheat flour, originating from Spanish and Italian cuisine, especially due to the great migration by these nationalities to Argentina. It is known for its quality meat and many meals are based on meat, such as Asado, the roast; the Parilla, a grilled meat, with different types of cuts used; Empanadas, cornmeal pastry dumplings filled with meat, onions, olives, hard-boiled eggs and spices, with a crescent shape, can be fried or baked.

Brazilian cuisine has rice and beans as its basic products, while cassava is used as flour. Dried meat, fish, long and rich skewers of grilled meat are widespread. The traditional dish is Feijoada, made with rice, black beans, pork and beef. Among the typical fish dishes we find the Caranguejo, or crab and shrimp. Rice is also widely used, often flavored with garlic, black olives or tomatoes. Among the most famous dishes made with exotic fruits we find the fried plantain, which is often crushed and fried twice, usually served as an appetizer, and coconut sweets which is another of the main ingredients of Brazilian cuisine. Brazil is the largest coffee producer in the world and has held this record for over 150 years.

Chilean cuisine has fish at the base of many dishes. La Cazuela is one of the most popular traditional dishes: it consists of a soup made from vegetables (such as corn, potatoes and squash) and meat, usually chicken The cultivation of various protein-rich vegetables, such as potatoes, tomatoes and cassava are among the foods most common in the Andean regions of Peru, Chile and Ecuador. Among the typical sweets, the Dulce de Leche stands out, a dessert made with milk and sugar that is obtained by cooking these two ingredients until they are caramelized.

38.11 Australian Cuisine

In Australian cuisine, both meat and fish dishes are characteristic, often cooked on the grill. The most common Australian fish is the *barramundi*, found only in parts of the Pacific, along with the Tasmanian salmon. Other fish specialties are the *balmain bug*, a crustacean found only in Oceania, mussels and oysters. The most popular way to eat fish in Australia is the traditional English-derived Fish and Chips. Among the meat dishes on the barbecue, kangaroo, lamb and duck stand out. A meat dish for a quick meal is the steak sandwich of beef grilled between two slices of bread, with butter, fresh vegetables, beetroot and sauces. One of the most popular products is *vegemite*, a sticky and dark salty paste, produced with yeasts to which vegetable extracts are added and used to spread it on toast with butter. Another universal dish is the meat pie, a savory pie filled with meat and various sauces, very tasty and used as a snack.

Very interesting also the food groups, dietary practices, and nutrition guideline, from birth to old age, available in New Zeland, a country where the Maori traditions and values are deeply engraimed in the local society and mirror other pacific islands [22].

38.12 Conclusion

This chapter meant to highlight the diversity of foods available, the derived eating habits and the nutritional characteristics of those foods coming from selected geographical area, with the understanding that reducing continents in a few text line does not do any justice to the incredible variety of options spread on the territory. In the following pages, Tables 38.1, 38.2 and 38.3 will illustrate a variety of a still limited list of foods, both natural and manmade and their area of origin. Centuries ago, every community had available a type of food that often was really exclusive only of that area, as it was dependent on indigenous plants and animals. Now with the advent of globalization the same foodstuff can be found basically in every continent, especially in large cities. With the recent movement of reclaiming the origin of a food or eating practice, there is more attention to the nutritional value, and the historical and geographical characteristics defining and distinguishing various foods, which can only enrich and enhance the experience and the enjoyment of food, something that we cannot and do not want to be without.

Table 38.1 Types of fruits from all over the world

Fruit	*Origin*	*Characteristics, properties and chewability*
Citruses	**Italy and around the Mediterranean Sea**	A wrinkled and resistant peel covers a white and compact rind that contains the juicy pulp divided into segments, with a typical sour and sugary or bitter taste. Citrus fruits such as lemon, orange, mandarin, bergamot, cedar, grapefruit are rich in vitamin C, have astringent, antioxidant, disinfectant properties, and have the benefit of counteracting gingivitis and stomatitis, for the supply of vitamin C. The taste is sour, and the acid taste stimulates salivation, therefore citrus fruits are contraindicated in the presence of salivary stones.
Olives	**Greece and around the Mediterranean Sea**	Kalamata olives, the fruit of the olive tree, are traditionally consumed in Mediterranean countries. Black olives are more mature and consistent, as they contain more monounsaturated fats, while green ones are richer in water and mineral salts. Extra virgin olive oil is obtained from olives, a specialty appreciated all over the world, for its aromatic taste and numerous health benefits, as it protects against coronary heart disease and some types of cancer. Olives have a firm texture and are flavorful and slippery.
Wine Grapes and Table Grapes	**France, Italy, Australia, Chile, Argentina and California**	Grapes contain mineral salts, potassium, manganese, copper, phosphorus, magnesium, silicon, chlorine and iron. Its berries can be black, pink or white. The flavor, always sweet, is enhanced by subtle aromas linked to the varieties and the soil where the vine grows. Contains vitamins A, B1, B2, C, PP and triterpenes [23]. These nutritional principles, combined with polyphenols, ensure that grapes have an antioxidant, antitumor and antiviral effect, in particular thanks to revestratol, and can be useful in problems related to blood circulation. During ripening the berry gradually accumulates a mixture of glucose and fructose in the pulp cells and loses acidity. In unripe fruits the peel is astringent due to the presence of reactive tannins with salivary proteins. During the ripening there is a decrease in this reactivity which progressively leads to a lower sensation of tannin in the grapes. The consistency of the grape influences its pleasantness also based on the tactile sensations caused by chewing the pulp, which can be more or less crunchy and juicy.
Berries	**North Europe**	Blueberries, raspberries, currants, blackberries, wild strawberries, gooseberries, elderberries: these are fruits that develop in particular humidity conditions typical of the undergrowth. Their flavor is sweet and fragrant, combined with a slight acidic aftertaste, the consistency of fresh fruits is compact and crunchy, if they are dried instead, they have a softer consistency. Arctic berries are rich in vitamins B, C, E and K, mineral salts, polyphenols and have numerous benefits for the intestine, antioxidant, purifying, bactericidal, diuretic and laxative properties, they also help prevent chronic diseases and improve cognitive abilities. A study conducted on the Norwegian population shows that a diet rich in vegetables and berries reduces mortality from stroke and cancer [24].
Bananas, dates and watermelon	**Africa**	Among the fruits from this continent we find many varieties of bananas, rich in potassium and vitamin C. The flavor and texture depend on the temperature at which they ripen, and on the degree of ripeness: the fruits ripened for longer and at higher temperatures will have a soft consistency and they will be sweeter than the more unripe ones and grown in a more rigid or ventilated environment, which will therefore be more turgid and less tasty. Dates are oblong-shaped fruits, with brown color and are rich in vitamins, potassium, magnesium and phosphorus. The consistency is fleshy and homogeneous, the taste is sweet and sugary. Watermelon is a hydrating and thirst-quenching fruit because it is rich in water. The ripe fruit has a bright red pulp, fragrant and rich in seeds; the peel is smooth and hard, green in color. Watermelon improves lipid metabolism, reduces chronic inflammation [25], has anti-inflammatory, diuretic, purifying properties and produces benefits on vascular function, reducing blood pressure [26]. The pulp of the watermelon also contains vitamins A and C, potassium, phosphorus and magnesium. The texture of the watermelon is crunchy and watery, with a fresh and delicate flavor.

Table 38.1 Types of fruits from all over the world

Fruit	*Origin*	*Characteristics, properties and chewability*
Litchee and Goji Berries	**China**	Litchee has a rough red shell, while the pulp is white, with remarkable aromatic properties. The taste is sweet, the texture crunchy; it is rich in vitamin C, potassium, calcium, phosphorus. Goji berries, which have a high content of flavonoids, which makes them effective antioxidants. They can be eaten fresh, or in the dried version, which is sweeter and softer.
Japanese Medlar	**Japan**	They are more or less sweet fruits depending on the degree of ripeness, characterized by a sour note. Perfect to be eaten raw, with or without peel, they contain large seeds that lend themselves to the preparation of liqueurs such as medlar, while honey is obtained from the Japanese medlar flowers. Medlar is rich in potassium and, in smaller quantities, phosphorus and magnesium, but above all it is abundant in vitamin A, for the benefit of the skin and eyes. Unripe medlars have astringent properties, while when ripen they have good bowel regulatory capabilities. The consistency of the freshly picked medlar is very hard, the taste is sour, and the rind is very clear; once ripe, its texture is mushy, the color darkens and the sour taste becomes particularly sweet.
Avocado	**Australia, Mexico**	Among the most popular exotic fruits in Australia we have the avocado, consumed simply, with salt and lemon, as an accompaniment to various foods. In Mexico it's called aguacate and it's the main ingredient of guacamole, a smooth sauce served with crunchy corn tortilla chips. The avocado has multiple beneficial properties, as it is rich in vitamins, minerals, fibers and antioxidants, fatty acids, its consumption reduces cardiovascular risk, increases the sense of satiety and reduces cholesterol. The texture is soft and buttery, the taste is delicate.
Mango	**South America**	Mango is rich in vitamins A, B and C, water, fructose, dietary fiber and minerals, especially potassium, calcium, phosphorus and magnesium; it has antioxidant, antitumor and anti-inflammatory properties, thanks to Lupeol (Saalem, 2009). Fresh, ripe mangoes have a sweet, slightly sour taste and a soft texture. Dried mango, on the other hand, requires a more energetic incision and chewing.
Pitaya (Dragon Fruit)	**Cuba**	The Pitaya, known as Dragon Fruit, has a white and foamy pulp, woven with very thick black seeds, also very widespread in the countries of Southeast Asia. It is a fruit rich in water, vitamins B1, C, E, iron, phosphorus and mineral salts as well as antioxidants. The flavor is light, delicate and refreshing, the texture is soft and watery.
Carambola	**India**	Carambola is an exotic bittersweet fruit, with a particular star-shaped section and a bright yellow color, rich in fiber and vitamin C; is native to India and Sri Lanka has spread throughout Southeast Asia. The texture is crunchy, and the flavor is sour, tart and slightly spicy.
Acai and Maracuja (Passion Fruit)	**Brazil**	Acai, originally from Brazil, is now grown throughout Latin America; the fruits are berries with shades of color ranging from purple to dark blue, they are an effective antioxidant, thanks to the rich presence of anthocyanins; they are also endowed with fiber, vitamins A and C, calcium. Widely used in herbal medicine, a concentrated oil is extracted, considered an anti-aging remedy for the skin. Maracuja, known as passion fruit, is another exotic fruit native to Brazil, has an oval shape, a consistent purple skin and a soft and sweet pulp, studded with edible black seeds. The consistency of the pulp is gelatinous, fragrant and with a characteristic sweet-sour taste.
Papaya	**Mexico**	Papaya has excellent nutritional properties: it contains antioxidant vitamins (A, C, E) which stimulate the immune defenses; many fibers, and low fat, it has an orange pulp with a delicate and soft texture and a sweet taste, with edible black seeds.

Table 38.1 Types of fruits from all over the world

Fruit	*Origin*	*Characteristics, properties and chewability*
Coconut	**Caribbean Islands and Thailand**	Coconut is a fruit wrapped in a fibrous, woody and very hard shell. The internal part consists of a white pulp with a pleasant, sweet and delicate flavor, containing coconut milk. Coconut is an important source of potassium but also contains other minerals such as magnesium, copper, phosphorus, zinc and iron. Contains natural sugars, vegetable fibers and amino acids. It is also a source of some vitamins, with particular reference to vitamins B, C, E and K. Coconut oil supports the development of bones and teeth, preventing tooth decay [27]. According to studies, coconut has a positive effect on bone metabolism, may be useful in preventing osteoporosis, and represents a possible intervention to slow down the bone loss observed after menopause [28]. The consistency of coconut is firm and watery, requiring vigorous and prolonged chewing.
Cherries	**Turkey**	This fruit has a round or heart-shaped shape, with a red color. Contains vitamins of group B, C and K and minerals such as potassium, manganese, copper and magnesium. The red color of the skin and pulp indicates a very high content of anthocyanins and other phenolic compounds with antioxidant action. These compounds are accumulated during ripening, especially in the skin, and contribute to the flavor of the fruit with their characteristic astringency. Ripe cherries have a firm and crunchy texture, a fleshy, firm flesh and a glossy, bright skin. Sour cherries contain a lower sugar content, while the deep red cherry variety is more tender to chew. Cherries have anti-inflammatory, antioxidant, anticarcinogenic effects for breast cancer [29]. Some studies suggest that the consumption of cherry, or fruit juice, can improve memory and cognitive processes in elderly people with mild forms of dementia and can have a relaxing effect and promote sleep in individuals with insomnia problems.
Pineapple	**Paraguay**	The pineapple has a firm and juicy texture, the scent is sweet and intense, and the color is bright yellow. The central part of the pineapple is the richest in bromelain: it has a fibrous consistency, which requires a more vigorous chewing. This fruit has a high content of water, fiber, mineral salts and vitamins of groups C and B. It contains an enzyme, bromelain, which helps digestion, has an anti-inflammatory, anti-edematous action and has antiproliferative and proapoptotic effects against cancer in the colon [30].
Cantaloupe (melon) and Honeydew	**Central and Eastern Asia**	Fruit with an oval shape, slightly wrinkled skin and a light color, depending on the variety it can have white or orange pulp, it is consistent and fragrant. Contains vitamins A, B and C, is rich in iron and is excellent for replenishing the losses of mineral salts. It has refreshing, laxative, purifying and moisturizing properties. The texture of the melon is firm and juicy, the taste is sweet.
Nuts: hazelnuts, pistachios, almonds, walnuts, pecans, macadamia	**Italy, Iran, Brazil, Hawaii**	Nuts are highly energetic, rich in proteins, fibers, minerals and monounsaturated fats, capable of lowering cholesterol. Hazelnuts, along with almonds, are rich in vitamin E and are a source of phytosterols, an important substance for the prevention of cardiovascular disease. Pistachios are rich in phosphorus, a mineral that contributes to increasing glucose tolerance. For this reason, their intake has been evaluated as a possible ally in the prevention of type 2 diabetes. Almonds, considered a typical Italian food product, are rich in vitamin E, magnesium and calcium. Walnuts are rich in B vitamins, in particular B1 and B6, but also vitamin E, folic acid and calcium. Brazil nuts and macadamia nuts are rich in selenium which has antioxidant, detoxifying and anticancer properties. Nuts are typically crunchy and flavorful, requiring vigorous chewing.

Table 38.2 Bread types worldwide

Type	*Origin*	*Characteristics and chewability*
Lefse	**Norway**	It is a flat-shaped focaccia, mixed with potatoes, which make the consistency of this bread softer to chew. It is typical of parties and is used as a stuffed roll, sweet or savory. In this bread the flour is replaced with potatoes, as the soil of the cold regions of Northern Europe is ideal for the cultivation of tubers.
Dark Rye Bread	**Finland**	It is a bread made with 100% Finnish rye flour and this gives it a crunchy texture, a dark color and a slightly acidic flavor. Other varieties are also popular in Finland, containing oats, barley and wheat
Pretzel and Pumpernickel	**Germany**	This bread was designed by a monk and has a characteristic ring shape with the two ends knotted, which is inspired by the position of the praying Christians, with the arms folded over the chest and each hand touching the opposite shoulder. It is made with soft wheat flour, malt, brewer's yeast and water, in addition to baking soda. In some regions, lard is also added or wholemeal, spelled or other grain flour is used. On the glaze created by the alkaline solution before cooking it is sprinkled with coarse salt or sesame seeds. It is said that an apprentice baker fell asleep while cooking the pretzel: once awake and convinced that the bread was not yet ready, since the fire had gone out, he gave it a second baking, hardening them. At first the owner of the oven went on a rampage but then, tasting the result, he discovered that the texture and flavor were excellent and lasted longer than the soft ones. Another famous bread is the Pumpernickel, with a compact consistency and dark color, it has an intense and decisive flavor; it is prepared with rye flour and then cooked very slowly in the oven in special metal boxes. After being baked and cooled, this bread is served in very thin slices.
Baguette	**France**	It is the typical French bread, with an elongated shape, famous for the contrast between the crunchy crust and the delicate crumb, it is savored both with sweet and salty, as an accompaniment to main meals.
Pan de Hogaza	**Spain**	It is a round and large Spanish loaf, a typical food consumed by shepherds and farmers. It is mentioned several times in literary works, such as Don Quixote, and constitutes a sort of gastronomic and cultural heritage of Spain. Rye flour was originally used for the dough, today wheat flour with a small percentage of bran. The rind is dry and thick and the crumb dense, requires vigorous chewing.
Pita	**Greece**	It is the typical bread of Greek cuisine, with a round shape, it is a type of leavened bread made from wheat flour, usually open and stuffed inside with pieces of roasted meat and vegetables. Its preparation involves cooking in the oven at a very high temperature (370 °C), so as to allow the bread to swell, giving it a soft consistency.
Mantou and Baozi	**China**	Mantou is a typical Chinese buns whose dough involves the use of wheat, water and yeast, to be arranged in loaves of about 4 centimeters; originally considered a luxury food (due to the presence of wheat flour), it is currently a very popular snack. Steaming makes the consistency soft and delicate. Another popular bread is Baozi, which has a dough similar to Mantou, but is filled with meat, vegetables, lotus seeds or cream of beans. The seasoned filling stimulates salivation and facilitates the swallowing of this bread.
Naan	**India**	It is the typical Indian bread that accompanies traditional meals. Made from wheat, it is cooked in a tandoori oven and served hot; it is often spread with ghee, clarified butter, which gives a more slippery consistency making it easier to prepare this bread for eating.
Curry Bread and Nikuman	**Japan**	Curry Bread is characterized by the curry filling: a piece of dough with a circular shape fried or baked in the oven, then wrapped with flaky breadcrumbs. The crust is crunchy, while the filling is tender. Another very popular bread is Nikuman, whose dough is made with water, salt and flour, while the traditional filling is based on pork; the taste is strengthened with sesame oil and lard or with mixtures of spices such as curry. Small round shaped buns are steamed and kept warm in special containers. The tender consistency is determined by steaming.
Himbasha	**Eritrea**	In Eritrea, Himbasha is famous, as a holiday bread, slightly sweet, although made in many different versions. Cardamom seeds give it a distinctly aromatic flavor.

Table 38.2 Bread types worldwide

Type	*Origin*	*Characteristics and chewability*
Injera	**Ethiopia**	Injera is widespread in Ethiopia, it is a bread made with teff, a very simple cereal, and then seasoned with various spices. It has a slightly acidic taste, is fermented and cooked on stone plates and is also used as a container to accommodate stews or to pick up food morsels.
Pancake	**Canada**	It is a type of bread prepared with milk, sugar, yeast, butter, flour and eggs, whose soft dough is then baked on hot plates. It is eaten for breakfast, usually accompanied by eggs, Canadian bacon, ham or sausage or served as a dessert in combination with berries or the typical Canadian maple syrup.
Oat bread	**United States of America**	Oat bread is the oldest produced in the United States of America, since oats were the easiest cereal to grow by the first populations; originally a bread with a thick crust and very compact and tasty crumb, it has, over time, given the low quantity of gluten, partially replaced oat flour with wheat flour. The consistency is solid and compact, requiring modest chewing.
Tortilla	**Mexico**	It is the typical Mexican bread, with a flat, crunchy and soft shape, made of corn flour and stuffed in various ways. It has a basically neutral flavor to contain rich fillings. The piadina goes well with pure ingredients, rarely with cooked dishes, unlike the tortilla that goes with real dishes. The most classic piadina is prepared with local cold cuts and cheeses.
Casabe	**Cuba**	Cuban bread has a long and thin shape and there is the particular addition of lard to the dough. Another typical bread is Casabe, the bread of the Indians. Of ancient tradition, it derives from a dough based on cassava flour and salt, therefore completely gluten-free. This amalgam must be molded into thin discs to be cooked until golden brown on cast iron pans.
Bammy	**Jamaica**	Bammy is the typical Jamaican bread, made by mixing cassava, a popular South American tuber, into the dough, a Jamaican flat bread traditionally baked on a hot plate and served for breakfast to accompany fish.
Pão de queijo	**Brazil**	It is the typical Brazilian bread: these are small round sandwiches filled with cheese. The dough is made from tapioca or cassava flour, eggs, milk and typical local cheese made with cow's milk. The consistency is made very soft by the presence of milk.
Hallulla and Corn Bread	**Chile**	Hallullas are small soft rolls particularly popular in Chile and consumed on holidays, to be garnished as desired. Hallullas are made by adding powdered milk and melted lard to the basic dough made of flour, water, salt and yeast. Another characteristic bread of South Chile is the corn bread, prepared with corn flour of which there are regional versions, differently adapted for different types of cooking.
Damper	**Australia**	The typical bread, made with flour, milk, salt and butter and traditionally cooked over campfires; the dough is softened with butter and milk, made into a medium-sized round loaf and cooked on cast iron pans soaked in oil. The presence of oil and butter makes the consistency of the dough soft when chewed.

Table 38.3 Types of fish and their characteristics

Type of fish	*Local usage*	*Characteristics and chewability*
Salmon	**Norway**	Among the most popular typical products are fresh, smoked and marinated salmon, whose recipe is very ancient and was born as a method of preserving fish. Norwegian Salmon is a fjord specialty famous around the world for its high standards of excellence and quality in the seafood sector. The nutritional supply of Norwegian salmon is extraordinary as it is low in saturated fat but rich in omega-3 polyunsaturated fatty acids. It also contains significant amounts of vitamins A, D and B12. Its role is especially important in the prevention of many diseases, and in particular cardiovascular and degenerative diseases such as Alzheimer's. In addition, in an *in vitro* model, Hemli H et al demonstrated in 2002 that EPA present in fatty fish (especially salmon, tuna and mackerel) would be able to neutralize some types of cancer cells, favoring their apoptosis and thus covering a potentially interesting role in the prevention of some forms of cancer, such as lymphomas. Other popular fish dishes are Skrei, a Nordic cod, cod, stockfish, salted and smoked herring. Caviar is mainly used for parties and anniversaries, from a nutritional point of view it contains many vitamins and proteins, it is rich in sodium and cholesterol. The consistency of the salmon is firm and elastic, it stimulates salivation due to the salting process it undergoes.
Bacalhau	**Portugal**	It is a low-fat protein fish whose origin is linked to the period of exploration voyages. In the 16th century, in fact, the Portuguese had the custom of fishing for cod in the waters of the North Atlantic and preserving it in salt. The long preservation of the fish allowed sailors and fellow citizens on the mainland to have large quantities of food at a very low cost. According to tradition, there are 365 cod-based recipes, one for each day of the year; among those most popular are the Bacalhau à Gomes de sà, cooked in a casserole with potatoes, onions and hard-boiled eggs; à Bràs, scrambled eggs with cod, onions and potatoes; com Natas, cod flan with onions, potatoes, béchamel and cream. The consistency of the cod is soft, because, before being cooked, it is soaked to desalt it and to soften the meat.
Barramundi	**Australia**	With its aboriginal name, this fish is one of the dishes that best represent Australia. It is both a fresh and saltwater fish, with a delicate flavor, which does not support breading or frying, which is why it is preferred to cook on the grill or roast, often seasoned with basil and lime, or melted butter. Shellfish is also widespread and has been a major source of protein for the original inhabitants of Australia for thousands of years.
Shrimps and Prawns	**China**	Seafood is used in various recipes in Chinese cuisine, especially shrimp such as shrimp rolls, crunchy on the outside and with a soft filling inside and crispy dragon clouds. Fish and prawns are consumed in large quantities usually boiled, to maintain the delicacy of fish, such as carp and sea bass, and represent the greatest source of vitamins.
Sushi and Sashimi	**Japan**	Most of the dishes of Japanese cuisine are based on fish, eaten fresh; given its geographic conformation made up of islands, it has developed an economic culture almost exclusively based on fishing from the beginning. Among the most common varieties we find tuna, eel, Fugu, a puffer fish, which must be treated properly before being served, because it is poisonous. Raw fish is consumed, such as in sushi and sashimi, but also fried, a typical dish is *tempura*, and grilled *robatayaki*, with which flavored fish skewers are prepared. The texture of raw fish suggests its freshness: a sashimi prepared with fresh fish must appear compact, cold, non-sticky and bright in color. On the other hand, when the consistency is so soft that the fish splits easily, it is rubbery, slimy, a sticky substance is noted to the touch and the color is opaque, the fish is not fresh.
Lobster	**Maine (USA)**	The preferred cooking method for lobsters is boiling and the most popular condiment for its pulp is melted butter. The consistency of the pulp of lobster fished in Canada is firm, compact and with a strong flavor, while the Maine lobster has less pulp, but is more tender and has a more delicate flavor. Also very popular is the lobster bisque, a rather thick and salty soup with chewy bits of lobster.
Dungeness Crab	**San Francisco (USA)**	The famous red crabs are the emblem of this Californian city. Their meat is considered a real delicacy, constitutes 25% of the animal's weight and is characterized by a sweet and delicate flavor that makes it particularly pleasant on the palate. Fishing for these large crustaceans represents a tradition deeply rooted in the local culture. The most traditional method of preparation is boiling, while the most particular recipe that best blends the concept of "fast" cuisine with traditional cuisine based on seafood is a *bread bowl,* a round loaf of bread filled, as if it were a bowl, of a thick soup made from crab, seafood, especially clams, and vegetables.

Table 38.3 Types of fish and their characteristics

Type of fish	*Local usage*	*Characteristics and chewability*
"Blue Fish"	**Mediterranean Sea**	The popular sardines, herrings, anchovies mackerels, and bonitos are fish of medium-small size and with blue, tiny and soft scales, hence the collective name of *blue fish*. They are rich in omega-3 and unsaturated fats, which are good for a child's development; their meats are fatty and full of easily digestible oils. Among the precious substances for our body these fish provide vitamin A, vitamin B and vitamin D, calcium, selenium, iodine, zinc, phosphorus, fluorine and potassium, in addition to the abundance of proteins with a high biological value. In recipes they are best accompanied by citrus fruits, and can be prepared marinated or grilled, perfect for draining the fat, which is a typical feature of blue fish. Sometimes blue fish is flavored with raisins, to sweeten its flavor

Table 38.4 Types of meat

Type of meat	*Local usage*	*Characteristics and chewability*
Jamón Ibérico	**Spain**	Jamón Ibérico is a very famous Spanish ham, obtained from the Alentejano pig breed (or similar), also known as "black ibérico"; this breed, mainly bred in the western part of the peninsula and in Portugal, is typically dark in color, which is why abroad it is better known as Pata Negra (Spanish for "black hoof"), it has an intense and juicy flavor and a consistency wrinkled and oily, thanks to the quality of the intramuscular fat.
Beef Steaks and Roast Beef	**United States of America**	In steak houses across the country, it is possible to taste various meat specialties: the American Black Angus beef steak stands out, known for its marbling, or for the uniform distribution of fat in the cut of meat, a characteristic that makes the meat more tender, juicy and tasty. The quality and degree of cooking determine the texture of the meat. The "rare" cooking is rare, it is the softest and easily chewable consistency; "medium" cooking requires more intense chewing; "well done" cooking has a lower quantity of liquid component, and therefore requires vigorous and prolonged chewing. Roast beef, and its variance *brisket*, is a slow cooked slab of marinated beef, usually cooked to a rare consistency, sliced thin and served hot or cold. Because of its cooking and slicing methods, the meat requires less chewing than a regular steak.
Beef	**Argentina**	Argentine meat is recognized as a culinary excellence around the world. Delicious, succulent, rich in B vitamins, an excellent source of iron and with a high content of essential amino acids, it expresses its best qualities when cooked on the grill, seasoned with the right amount of salt, a lively fire and turning it only once. The consistency depends on the cut, the part under the ribs is the most tender and elastic. Asado, the classic roast beef, is cooked on a grill placed next to the flame almost vertically. It is a particularly slow cooking, which serves to enhance the flavor and texture of the meat.
Würstel	**Austria and Germany**	It is a typical product of street food, which was born in Vienna: a sausage made of pork meat finely minced. Its refined flavor lends itself to different types of cooking, as it can be grilled, barbecued, boiled, fried or smoked. They are flavored and often served with curry, cheese and spicy sauces. In Germany there are many varieties of frankfurters, among which two basic types stand out: *rohwürste*, which is a raw würst, therefore a salami to be sliced, and *kochwürste*, the würst to be boiled, sauteed, grilled or fried, depending on the variety. They are made with pork, beef or veal and can look whitish, dark red or brown. The inside texture is full-bodied, firm and juicy, while the outside is crunchy.
Kebab	**Iran**	It is a dish based on roasted meat and its name derives from the particular method of cooking the meat that takes place on a vertical spit: the "doner kebab". The meat used can be mutton, lamb, veal, but also chicken, turkey or pork. The meat is first cut into pieces and then marinated with a mixture of herbs and spices, before being placed on the spit for cooking. It has a juicy and spicy texture.
Peking Duck	**China**	Named after old Beijing, the duck is cooked slowly in the oven after undergoing a very long preparation process, which includes boiling, lacquering with honey syrup and drying. It is cut into very thin crepes folded into a triangle and served with a vegetable and leek broth. The skin is thin and crunchy, while the meats are tender and delicate in flavor.
Foie Gras	**France and Hungary**	Foie Gras is one of the most famous products of French haute cuisine, traditionally consumed during the holidays. It is a duck or goose liver pate, marinated in Port wine and Cognac. The texture is buttery and velvety, sweet and greasy, eaten spread on bread.

REFERENCES

1. Mattioli AV, Palmiero P, Manfrini O, Puddu PE, Nodari S, Dei Cas A, Mercuro G, Scrutinio D, Palermo P, Sciomer S, Di Francesco S, Novo G, Novo S, Pedretti RFE, Zito A, Parati G, Pedrinelli R, Farinetti A, Maiello M, Moscucci F, Tenaglia RL, Sucato V, Triggiani M, Cugusi L, Scicchitano P, Saba PS, Ciccone MM. Mediterranean diet impact on cardiovascular diseases: a narrative review. J Cardiovasc Med (Hagerstown) 2017; 18(12): 925-35.
2. Esposito K, Giugliano D. Mediterranean diet and type 2 diabetes. Diabetes Metab Res Rev 2014; 30 Suppl 1: 34-40.
3. Schwingshackl L, Schwedhelm C, Galbete C, Hoffmann G. Adherence to Mediterranean Diet and Risk of Cancer: An Updated Systematic Review and Meta-Analysis. Nutrients 2017;9(10).
4. Psaltopoulou T, Sergentanis TN, Panagiotakos DB, Sergentanis IN, Kosti R, Scarmeas N. Mediterranean diet, stroke, cognitive impairment, and depression: A meta-analysis. Ann Neurol 2013; 74(4): 580-91.
5. Miranda A, Gómez-Gaete C, Mennickent S. Role of Mediterranean diet on the prevention of Alzheimer disease. Rev Med Chil 2017; 145(4): 501-7.
6. Hasler CM. Functional foods: benefits, concerns and challenges - a position paper from the american council on science and health. J Nutr 2002; 132(12): 3772-81.
7. Xiao Y, Zhang S, Tong H, Shi S. Comprehensive evaluation of the role of soy and isoflavone supplementation in humans and animals over the past two decades. Phytother Res 2018; 32(3): 384-94.
8. Wang Y, Yu H, Zhang X, Feng Q, Guo X, Li S, Li R, Chu D, Ma Y. Evaluation of daily ginger consumption for the prevention of chronic diseases in adults: A cross-sectional study. Nutrition 2017; 36: 79-84.
9. Wang J, Ke W, Bao R, Hu X, Chen F. Beneficial effects of ginger Zingiber officinale Roscoe on obesity and metabolic syndrome: a review. Ann N Y Acad Sci 2017; 1398(1): 83-98.
10. Pan CW, Ma Q, Sun HP, Xu Y, Luo N, Wang P. Tea Consumption and Health-Related Quality of Life in Older Adults. J Nutr Health Aging 2017; 21(5): 480-6.
11. Li JR, Hsieh YH. Traditional Chinese food technology and cuisine. Asia Pac J Clin Nutr 2004; 13(2): 147-55.
12. Krishnaswamy K. Traditional Indian spices and their health significance. Asia Pac J Clin Nutr 2008; 17 Suppl 1: 265-8.
13. Ahmed T, Gilani AH. Therapeutic potential of turmeric in Alzheimer's disease: curcumin or curcuminoids? Phytother Res 2014; 28(4): 517-25.
14. Kim Y, Brecht JK, Talcott ST. Antioxidant phytochemical and fruit quality changes in mango (*Mangifera indica* L.) following hot water immersion and controlled atmosphere storage. Food Chemistry 2007; 105(4): 1327-34.
15. Bovell-Benjamin AC. Bioactivity, Benefits and Safety of Traditional and Ethnic Foods. Ensuring Global Food Safety: Exploring Global Harmonization. 2010, Elsevier Inc.
16. Kurotani K, Akter S, Kashino I, Goto A, Mizoue T, Noda M, Sasazuki S, Sawada N, Tsugane S. Quality of diet and mortality among Japanese men and women: Japan Public Health Center based prospective study. BMJ 2016; 352: i1209.
17. Iwagaki Y, Sakamoto Y, Sugawara S, Mizowaki Y, Yamamoto K, Sugawara T, Kimura K, Tsuduki T. Identification of Characteristic Components and Foodstuffs in Healthy Japanese Diet and the Health Effects of a Diet with Increased Use Frequency of these Foodstuffs. Mol Nutr Food Res 2017; 61(12).
18. Ruth K Oniang'o, Joseph M Mutuku, Serah J Malaba. Contemporary African food habits and their nutritional and health implications. Asia Pacific J Clin Nutr 2003; 12(3): 231-6.
19. Jakub KE, Turk MT, Fapohunda A, Zoucha R. Cultural Beliefs, Perceptions, and Practices of Young Adult Offspring of African Immigrants Regarding Healthy Eating and Activity. J Transcult Nurs 2018; 29(6): 548-54.
20. Grotto D and Zied E. The Standard American Diet and Its Relationship to the Health Status of Americans. Nutr Clin Pract. 2010 Dec;25(6):603-12.
21. Robinson, A. Country Food (Inuit Food) in Canada. The Canadian Encyclopedia. 2018. https://www.thecanadianencyclopedia.ca/en/article/country-food-inuit-food-in-canada
22. Ministry of Health. Food and Nutrition Guidelines for Healthy Infants and Toddlers (Aged 0–2): A background paper (4th Ed). 2008. Partially Revised December 2012.
23. Saleem M. Lupeol, A Novel Anti-inflammatory and Anti-cancer Dietary Triterpene. Cancer Lett 2009; 285(2): 109-15.
24. Hjartåker A, Knudsen MD, Tretli S, Weiderpass E. Consumption of berries, fruits and vegetables and mortality among 10,000 Norwegian men followed for four decades. Eur J Nutr 2015; 54(4): 599-608.
25. Becraft A, Sturm M, Pierce G, Mendez R, Shay N. Hepatic Metabolomic Analysis in Mice Fed a High Fat Diet with Watermelon and Watermelon Byproducts Shows Improved Lipid Metabolism and Reduction of Chronic Inflammation (P06-023-19). Curr Dev Nutr 2019; 3(Suppl 1): nzz031.P06-023-19.
26. Figueroa A, Wong A, Jaime SJ, Gonzales JU. Influence of L-citrulline and watermelon supplementation on vascular function and exercise performance. Curr Opin Clin Nutr Metab Care 2017; 20(1): 92-8.
27. Wallace TC. Health Effects of Coconut Oil-A Narrative Review of Current Evidence. J Am Coll Nutr 2019; 38(2): 97-107.
28. Morii Y, Matsushita H, Minami A, Kanazawa H, Suzuki T, Subhadhirasakul S, Watanabe K, Wakatsuki A. Young Coconut Juice Supplementation Results in Greater Bone Mass and Bone Formation Indices in Ovariectomized Rats: A Preliminary Study. Phytother Res 2015; 29(12): 1950-5.
29. Layosa MA, Lage N, Talcott S, Talcott S, Pedrosa M, Chew B, Noratto G. Dark Sweet Cherry phenolics as Dietary Chemopreventive/therapeutic Compounds for Aggressive Breast Cancer Cell Growth with No Toxicity to Normal Breast Cells (FS13-03-19). Curr Dev Nutr 2019; 3(Suppl 1): nzz030.FS13-03-19.
30. Romano B, Fasolino I, Pagano E, Capasso R, Pace S, De Rosa G, Milic N, Orlando P, Izzo AA, Borrelli F. The chemopreventive action of bromelain, from pineapple stem (Ananas comosus L.), on colon carcinogenesis is related to antiproliferative and proapoptotic effects. Mol Nutr Food Res 2014; 58(3): 457-65.